EMERGENCY MEDICINE REVIEW

Preparing for the Boards

EMERGENCY MEDICINE REVIEW

Preparing for the Boards

Richard A. Harrigan, MD
Professor of Emergency Medicine
Department of Emergency Medicine
Temple University School of Medicine
Philadelphia, Pennsylvania

Jacob W. Ufberg, MD
Associate Professor and Residency Director
Department of Emergency Medicine
Temple University School of Medicine
Philadelphia, Pennsylvania

Matthew L. Tripp, MD
Assistant Medical Director and Director of Service Excellence
Department of Emergency Medicine
Santa Clara Valley Medical Center/California Emergency Physicians
San Jose, California

Imaging Editor

Thomas Costantino, MD
Associate Professor of Emergency Medicine
Department of Emergency Medicine
Temple University School of Medicine
Philadelphia, Pennsylvania

Manuscript Manager

Linda Kruus, PhD
Temple University School of Medicine
Philadelphia, Pennsylvania

ELSEVIER
SAUNDERS

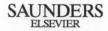

3251 Riverport Lane
St. Louis, Missouri 63043

EMERGENCY MEDICINE REVIEW: PREPARING FOR THE BOARDS   ISBN: 978-1-4160-6191-5

Notices

Knowledge and best practice in this field are constantly changing. As new research and experience broaden our understanding, changes in research methods, professional practices, or medical treatment may become necessary.

Practitioners and researchers must always rely on their own experience and knowledge in evaluating and using any information, methods, compounds, or experiments described herein. In using such information or methods they should be mindful of their own safety and the safety of others, including parties for whom they have a professional responsibility.

With respect to any drug or pharmaceutical products identified, readers are advised to check the most current information provided (i) on procedures featured or (ii) by the manufacturer of each product to be administered, to verify the recommended dose or formula, the method and duration of administration, and contraindications. It is the responsibility of practitioners, relying on their own experience and knowledge of their patients, to make diagnoses, to determine dosages and the best treatment for each individual patient, and to take all appropriate safety precautions.

To the fullest extent of the law, neither the Publisher nor the authors, contributors, or editors assume any liability for any injury and/or damage to persons or property as a matter of products liability, negligence or otherwise, or from any use or operation of any methods, products, instructions, or ideas contained in the material herein.

Library of Congress Cataloging-in-Publication Data

Emergency medicine review : preparing for the boards / [edited by] Richard Harrigan, Matthew Tripp, Jacob Ufberg.—1st ed.
  p. ; cm.
  ISBN 978-1-4160-6191-5
  1. Emergency medicine—Outlines, syllabi, etc. 2. Emergency medicine—Examinations, questions, etc. I. Harrigan, Richard. II. Tripp, Matthew. III. Ufberg, Jacob.
  [DNLM: 1. Outlines. 2. Emergency Medicine—methods. WB 18.2 E5295 2010]
  RC86.92.E44 2010
  616.02′5—dc22

                2010016623

Publishing Director: Judith Fletcher
Acquisitions Editor: Stefanie Jewell-Thomas
Associate Developmental Editor: Joanie Milnes
Publishing Services Manager: Linda Van Pelt/Anne Altepeter
Senior Project Manager: Priscilla Crater/Cheryl A. Abbott
Design Direction: Steven Stave
Illustrator: Lesley Frazier

To my daughters, Quinn and Kelly, who continue to ask the best questions and be the perfect answer.

R. A. H.

To Amy, Hayden, Robby, and Jenna, who continue to make every day my best day yet.

J. W. U.

To all Temple EM faculty who took the time to teach.

M. L. T.

Contributors

Jeffrey Barrett, MD
Assistant Professor
Emergency Medicine
Assistant Clerkship Director
Department of Emergency Medicine
Temple University School of Medicine
Philadelphia, Pennsylvania

Nathan P. Charlton, MD
Assistant Professor of Emergency Medicine
University of Virginia School of Medicine
Charlottesville, Virginia

Pierre Detiege, MD, FAAEM
Clinical Assistant Professor
Section of Emergency Medicine
Louisiana State University Health Sciences Center
New Orleans, Louisiana

Manish Garg, MD, FAAEM
Clinical Associate Professor of Emergency Medicine
Associate Residency Program Director
Temple University School of Medicine
Philadelphia, Pennsylvania

Carl A. Germann, MD, FACEP
Department of Emergency Medicine
Maine Medical Center
Portland, Maine
Assistant Professor
Tufts University School of Medicine
Boston, Massachusetts

Jeffrey Green, MD, FACEP
Assistant Program Director
New York Hospital, Queens
Flushing, New York
Department of Emergency Medicine
Clinical Instructor, Weil Cornell Medical Center
New York, New York

Michael Greenberg, MD
Professor of Emergency Medicine and Public Health
Department of Emergency Medicine
Hahnemann University Hospital
Philadelphia, Pennsylvania

Sanjey Gupta, MD
Clinical Assistant Professor
Weill Cornell College of Medicine
Attending Emergency Physician
New York Hospital, Queens
Flushing, New York

Richard A. Harrigan, MD
Professor of Emergency Medicine
Department of Emergency Medicine
Temple University School of Medicine
Philadelphia, Pennsylvania

Terence Hauver, MD
Clinical Instructor
Section of Emergency Medicine
Louisiana State University Health Sciences Center
New Orleans, Louisiana

Robert G. Hendrickson, MD, FAACT, FACEP
Associate Professor of Emergency Medicine
Associate Medical Director, Oregon Poison Center
Program Director, Fellowship in Medical Toxicology
Oregon Health and Science University
Portland, Oregon

Christopher P. Holstege, MD
Chief, Division of Medical Toxicology
Associate Professor
Department of Emergency Medicine and Pediatrics
University of Virginia School of Medicine
Medical Director, Blue Ridge Poison Center
Charlottesville, Virginia

Joel Kravitz, MD, FACEP, FRCPSC
Attending Physician
Emergency Department
Director of Medical Student Education
Community Medical Center
Barnabas Health System
Toms River, New Jersey

Kenneth T. Kwon, MD
Director of Pediatric Emergency Medicine
Associate Clinical Professor
University of California Irvine Medical Center
Director, Pediatric Emergency Services
Mission Hospital/Children's Hospital
  of Orange County
Irvine, California

Tracy Leigh LeGros, MD, PhD, UHM/ABEM, FAAEM, FACEP
Clinical Assistant Professor of Emergency Medicine
Program Director, Hyperbaric Medicine Fellowship
  Program
Medical Director of Emergency Medicine Services
Louisiana State University Health Sciences Center
New Orleans, Lousiana

Alexander T. Limkakeng, Jr, MD, FACEP
Assistant Professor
Interim Director of Acute Care Research
Division of Emergency Medicine
Department of Surgery
Duke University Medical Center
Durham, North Carolina

Bernard Lopez, MD
Professor and Vice Chair for Academic Affairs
Residency Program Director
Department of Emergency Medicine
Thomas Jefferson University
Jefferson Medical College
Philadelphia, Pennsylvania

Nathanael J. McKeown, DO
Assistant Professor
Department of Emergency Medicine
Oregon Health and Science University
Portland VA Medical Center
Medical Toxicologist
Oregon Poison Center
Portland, Oregon

Heather Murphy-Lavoie, MD
Clinical Assistant Professor
Assistant Residency Director for Emergency Medicine
Associate Director for Undersea and Hyperbaric
    Medicine Fellowship
Louisiana State University School of Medicine
New Orleans, Louisiana

Andrew Lee Nyce, MD
Assistant Professor of Emergency Medicine
University of Medicine and Dentistry of New Jersey
Robert Wood Johnson Medical School at Camden
Cooper University Hospital
Camden, New Jersey

Jennifer A. Oman, MD, FACEP, FAAEM, RDMS
Associate Clinical Professor of Emergency Medicine
Department of Emergency Medicine
School of Medicine
University of California, Irvine
Irvine, California

Leslie C. Oyama, MD
Assistant Clinical Professor
Department of Emergency Medicine
University of California, San Diego
San Diego, California

Sundip Patel, MD
Assistant Director of Undergraduate Medical
    Education
Department of Emergency Medicine
University of Medicine and Dentistry of New Jersey
Robert Wood Johnson Medical School at Camden
Cooper Hospital University
Camden, New Jersey

Andrew D. Perron, MD, FACEP, FACSM
Professor and Residency Program Director
Maine Medical Center, Portland
Portland, Maine

Robert L. Rogers, MD, FACEP, FAAEM, FACP
Associate Professor of Emergency Medicine
    and Internal Medicine
Director of Undergraduate Medical Education
Department of Emergency Medicine
University of Maryland School of Medicine
Baltimore, Maryland

Bisan Salhi, MD
Assistant Professor
Department of Emergency Medicine
Emory University School of Medicine
Atlanta, Georgia

H. Edward Seibert, MD
Attending Physician
Emergency Trauma Center
Abington Memorial Hospital
Abington, Pennsylvania

Ghazala Q. Sharieff, MD
Division Director and Clinical Professor
Rady Children's Hospital Emergency Care Center
University of California, San Diego
Director of Pediatric Emergency Medicine
Palomar-Pomerado Health System/California
    Emergency Physicians
San Diego, California

Sarah A. Stahmer, MD
Associate Professor of Surgery
Residency Program Director
Division of Emergency Medicine
DukeMedical Center
Durham, North Carolina

Edward A. Stettner, MD
Assistant Professor of Emergency Medicine
Assistant Program Director, Emergency Medicine
Department of Emergency Medicine
Emory University School of Medicine
Atlanta, Georgia

Alison E. Suarez, MD, MS
Assistant Program Director
Emergency Medicine
New York Hospital, Queens
Flushing, New York

Matthew L. Tripp, MD
Assistant Medical Director and Director of Service
  Excellence
Department of Emergency Medicine
Santa Clara Valley Medical Center/California
  Emergency Physicians
San Jose, California

Jacob W. Ufberg, MD
Associate Professor and Residency Director
Department of Emergency Medicine
Temple University School of Medicine
Philadelphia, Pennsylvania

David Vearrier, MD
Core Faculty
Department of Emergency Medicine
Division of Medical Toxicology
Albert Einstein Medical Center
Philadelphia, Pennsylvania

Gary M. Vilke, MD
Professor of Clinical Medicine
Chief of Staff
University of California San Diego Medical Center
Director, Clinical Research for Emergency Medicine
University of California San Diego Medical Center
San Diego, California

David A. Wald, DO
Medical Director
William Maul Measey Institute for Clinical Simulation
  and Patient Safety
Director of Undergraduate Education
Associate Professor of Emergency Medicine
Department of Emergency Medicine
Temple University School of Medicine
Philadelphia, Pennsylvania

Steven S. Wright, MD, FACEP, MS
Instructor of Emergency Medicine in Clinical
  Medicine—Cornell
Director of Undergraduate Education
Core Faculty
Department of Emergency Medicine
New York Hospital, Queens
Flushing, New York

Gerald C. Wydro, MD
Clinical Associate Professor of Emergency Medicine
Director, Emergency Medical Services
Department of Emergency Medicine
Temple University School of Medicine
Program Director, Temple Transport Team
Director of Emergency Preparedness, Temple
  University
Philadelphia, Pennsylvania

Ernest Yeh, MD
Assistant Professor of Emergency Medicine
Assistant Director, Emergency Medical Services
Department of Emergency Medicine
Temple University School of Medicine
ALS Service Medical Director, Temple Transport
  Team
Philadelphia, Pennsylvania

This textbook was developed with you in mind—whether you are an emergency medicine resident in training; a recent graduate of an emergency medicine residency program preparing for board certification; or a seasoned practitioner who wants a focused review of the broad field of emergency medicine, perhaps in preparation for your upcoming recertification examination. Indeed, we bring to you three perspectives, each quite different, as they reflect the varied stages in our respective careers at Temple University Hospital. Richard Harrigan has been in academic emergency medicine for nearly 20 years and has completed the process of ABEM recertification. Jacob Ufberg is a veteran emergency medicine program director who is aware of what his residents need as they progress through training and subsequently ready themselves for their first encounter with the boards. Matthew Tripp was a chief resident at Temple who has recently completed board certification for the first time. Collectively, we feel that we know the wants and needs of the emergency physician community insofar as a board review book that can also serve as a study guide. We have each sampled a number of the excellent products currently available, and it has been our goal to provide you with a new and unique publication that will meet your needs as you juggle family, career, and the other balls we all keep in the air from day-to-day.

Some of the highlights of this first edition of *Emergency Medicine Review: Preparing for the Boards* follow.

- **Format.** A *bulleted format* minimizes length and maximizes convenience. We cover the entire *Model of the Clinical Practice of Emergency Medicine* (the EM Model, or "core content"). In doing so, we offer separate chapters on **Pediatrics** and **Procedures.** Larger topic areas (**Cardiovascular, Toxicology,** and **Trauma**) have been divided into two chapters each. Those topic areas that receive more weight on the board examination are correspondingly more detailed in their scope. All

chapters begin with a tabular **outline of the chapter** so you can quickly scan the topic areas contained within. Each chapter closes with a list of summary points, **"Pearls,"** which are quick and easy take-home points you will want to recall as you move on to the next chapter.

- **Authors.** All of our authors are practicing, board-certified emergency physicians. We are lucky to have some of the best in our field as contributors to this book.
- **Pictures and images.** The book contains an abundance of radiographs, CT and ultrasound images, ECGs, and clinical pictures. We hope that having these images in close proximity to the relevant text (usually on the same page) will increase the ease with which you can move through the material. We think you'll appreciate not being referred to another section of the book, or even another textbook, in search of an image for a key topic area.
- **Questions and answers.** Each chapter concludes with at least 15 questions that are followed by answers with detailed explanations; longer chapters have 40 questions. You will find an equivalent mix of "board-style" questions with shorter, fact-style questions.

We hope you find that *Emergency Medicine Review: Preparing for the Boards* meets your needs for a study guide, a review book, and a quick reference textbook. You should continue to rely on the many wonderful emergency medicine textbooks we found to be so helpful as we put together this project. It is our hope that this new book supplements those resources. Whether you are a rookie or a veteran, we wish you the best as you approach the board certification examination—and we hope our book is helpful to you in that process.

Richard A. Harrigan, MD
Jacob W. Ufberg, MD
Matthew L. Tripp, MD

Contents

Abdominal/Gastrointestinal

Andrew Lee Nyce | Sundip Patel

Abdominal wall

HERNIAS

Termed *reducible* if contents of hernia able to return to natural cavity by external manipulation. Termed *incarcerated* if unable to reduce hernia. Termed *strangulated* when vascular compromise of incarcerated hernia. Risk factors for hernias include developmental immaturity of the anatomic structures, family history, conditions that increase intra-abdominal pressure, chronic obstructive pulmonary disease (COPD), and pregnancy.

Indirect inguinal hernia

- Secondary to a persistent patent process vaginalis
- Most common hernia, usually on right
- Commonly incarcerate/strangulate, particularly in first year of life

Direct inguinal hernia

- Protrusions directly through the external inguinal ring
- Acquired defects; not through inguinal canal
- Mostly adult men; rarely incarcerate/strangulate

Femoral hernia

- Less common than inguinal hernias
- More common in women and frequently incarcerate/strangulate

Umbilical hernia

- Congenital: common and usually spontaneously seal by 3 to 4 years of age
- Acquired: more common in women and frequently incarcerate

Incisional hernia

- Herniation through surgical incision in up to 10% to 20% of postlaparotomy cases
- Obesity and postoperative wound infections are risk factors

SIGNS AND SYMPTOMS

- Majority present as asymptomatic lump on physical examination
- Incarcerated hernias: painful, may be accompanied by nausea and vomiting
- Strangulated hernia: patient may appear toxic, in addition to nausea and vomiting
- Inguinal hernias may extend into scrotum

DIAGNOSIS

- Inguinal hernia in men palpated through the external ring
- Incarcerated hernias tender to palpation
- Imaging recommended if bowel obstruction or perforation suspected

TREATMENT

- Asymptomatic/reducible hernias generally repaired electively
- May attempt to reduce recent-onset incarcerated hernia
- Ischemic bowel should *not* be reduced into abdominal cavity
- Reduction may be aided by pain medication, an anxiolytic, and placing patient in the Trendelenburg position
- Surgical fixation required if unable to reduce

Esophagus

INFECTIOUS DISORDERS

Candida infections

Immunosuppressed patients (AIDS, cancer, diabetes, alcoholism, use of corticosteroids [oral and inhaled]) at higher risk for infectious esophagitis. Candida most common etiologic agent but also consider herpes simplex virus and cytomegalovirus.

SIGNS AND SYMPTOMS

- Primarily dysphagia and odynophagia

DIAGNOSIS

- Direct visualization by endoscopy, or presumptive based on immunocompromise, signs, and symptoms

TREATMENT

- Antifungal therapy (fluconazole 200 mg daily for 2 to 3 weeks)

INFLAMMATORY DISORDERS

Esophagitis

SIGNS AND SYMPTOMS

- Odynophagia and prolonged periods of chest pain
- NSAIDS, potassium chloride, doxycycline, tetracycline, and clindamycin can induce esophageal mucosal irritation

DIAGNOSIS

- Generally clinical but advanced esophagitis diagnosed by endoscopy

TREATMENT

- Aggressive therapy with acid-suppressive medications
- Withdrawal of offending medication

Gastroesophageal reflux (GERD)

SIGNS AND SYMPTOMS

- Heartburn is classic symptom, also odynophagia, dysphagia, and acid regurgitation
- Associated with meals (high-fat foods), nicotine, ethanol, caffeine, medicines (nitrates, anticholinergics, progesterone, estrogen, calcium-channel blockers), pregnancy
- Associated with decreased esophageal motility and prolonged gastric emptying
- May present with similar symptoms to cardiac pain, worse when supine
- May present as asthma exacerbations and multiple ear–nose–throat complaints
- Over time may cause scarring, ulcerations, strictures, and Barrett's metaplasia: a premalignant condition

DIAGNOSIS

- Generally clinical; endoscopy for definitive diagnosis

TREATMENT

- Decrease acid production in stomach, enhance upper-tract motility, and eliminate risk factors for disease and offending agents
- Histamine (H_2) blockers or proton-pump inhibitors are mainstays of therapy

Caustic agents

- **Acids:** Common acids are hydrochloric and sulfuric acid
- **Alkali:** Common alkali include bleach, sodium hydroxide, and potassium hydroxide

SIGNS AND SYMPTOMS

- Severe pain, odynophagia, dysphonia, oral and facial burns, abdominal pain, vomiting, drooling, and respiratory distress

- Strong acid ingestion causes coagulation necrosis and eschar necrosis
- Strong alkaline ingestions induce deep tissue injury from liquefaction necrosis
- Household bleach (3% to 6% sodium hypochlorite) is not corrosive to the esophagus
- Acids mainly affect the esophagus and stomach
- Alkali mainly affect the esophagus

DIAGNOSIS

- Mainly clinical
- Strong acids may cause systemic acidosis, hemolysis, and renal failure
- Alkaline ingestions may cause gastric perforation and necrosis of abdominal viscera
- Upright chest x-ray (CXR) for peritoneal/mediastinal air
- Gastroenterology consult to perform endoscopy to determine extent of injury

TREATMENT

- Supportive care
- *Avoid* blind nasotracheal intubation, charcoal, nasogastric (NG) tube, dilution, and neutralization
- No consensus on steroids and antibiotics

MOTOR ABNORMALITIES

Achalasia

- The most common motility disorder and is associated with impaired relaxation of the lower esophageal sphincter (LES) and absence of esophageal peristalsis

Diffuse esophageal spasm

- Simultaneous contractions of the esophageal body with 30% of swallows

SIGNS AND SYMPTOMS

- Achalasia: may present with esophageal spasm, chest pain, and odynophagia
- Esophageal motility disorders often present with chest pain in the 5th decade
- Stress or ingestion of liquids at extremes of temperature may trigger symptoms
- Often difficult to differentiate from anginal pain

DIAGNOSIS

- Esophageal manometry is primary diagnostic modality

TREATMENT

- Achalasia: medications to decrease LES pressure, dilation, or surgical myotomy
- Esophageal spasm: medications to control reflux, smooth muscle relaxants, and/or antidepressants

STRUCTURAL DISORDERS

Boerhaave syndrome

- Full-thickness perforation of the esophagus following a sudden rise in intraesophageal pressure
- Misdiagnosed up to 50% of the time

SIGNS AND SYMPTOMS

- About 75% of cases result from sudden forceful emesis
- Usually ill appearing, neck or chest pain, fever, respiratory distress
- Pain generally left sided, radiates to back, and often with subcutaneous neck/chest wall air
- Crunching sound synchronous with the heartbeat (Hamman crunch) may be heard
- Rupture generally on left side of distal esophagus

DIAGNOSIS

- Chest x-ray generally abnormal up to 90% of time with pleural effusion, pneumomediastinum, pneumothorax, or pneumoperitoneum
- Diagnosis made by chest x-ray with water-soluble contrast or computed tomographic (CT) scan with water-soluble contrast

TREATMENT

- Broad-spectrum antibiotics and operative repair

Diverticula

- Can be found throughout the esophagus
- Pharyngoesophageal or Zenker diverticulum is present at the pharyngeal mucosa just above the upper esophageal sphincter (UES)

SIGNS AND SYMPTOMS

- Usually after 50 years old
- Transfer dysfunction and halitosis, feeling of neck mass

DIAGNOSIS

- CT scan or endoscopy

TREATMENT

- Surgical repair

Foreign body

- Pediatric patients account for up to 80% of all cases; most pediatric obstructions are in proximal esophagus as compared with the majority of adult obstructions occurring in the distal esophagus
- Five areas of esophageal constriction in children: cricopharyngeal narrowing (most common), thoracic inlet, aortic arch, tracheal bifurcation, and hiatal narrowing

SIGNS AND SYMPTOMS

- Adults: retrosternal pain, vomiting, dysphagia, choking, coughing, gagging
- Pediatric: refusal to eat, vomiting, gagging, choking, stridor, increased salivation
- Physical examination of oropharynx for foreign body and neck for subcutaneous air

DIAGNOSIS

- Radiopaque object demonstrated on radiographs of neck, chest, and/or abdomen
- Esophagogram
  - Suspected perforation: use water soluble contrast
  - Possible aspiration: use the least amount of contrast possible
  - Perforation/aspiration possible: use non-ionic contrast agent
- CT scan may be required to visualize foreign body
- Direct visualization via endoscopy

TREATMENT

- All severely symptomatic patients require observation and esophagoscopy
- Foreign bodies warranting endoscopic consultation
  - Sharp or elongated objects, multiple foreign bodies, button batteries, evidence of perforation, airway compromise, present for more than 24 hours
- Child with a nickel or quarter at the level of the cricopharyngeus muscle
- *Food impaction*
  - Remove within 12 hours
  - Avoid proteolytic enzymes (meat tenderizer)
  - Glucagon 1 mg IV RH (may repeat dose), nifedipine, or nitroglycerin may relieve impaction, but are often unsuccessful
  - Perform esophagogram postimpaction to ensure passage and follow-up endoscopy
- *Coin ingestion*
  - Coin in esophagus visible on AP radiograph (Fig. 1-1) with flat side visible
  - Method of removal: endoscopy or with Foley catheter
- *Button battery*
  - Immediate removal necessary if lodged in the esophagus secondary to potential perforation within 6 hours
  - If in stomach, allow to pass pylorus within 48 hours in an asymptomatic patient

Mallory–Weiss syndrome

- Bleeding of distal esophagus/proximal stomach from mucosa bleeding from partial thickness tear; majority at gastroesophageal junction

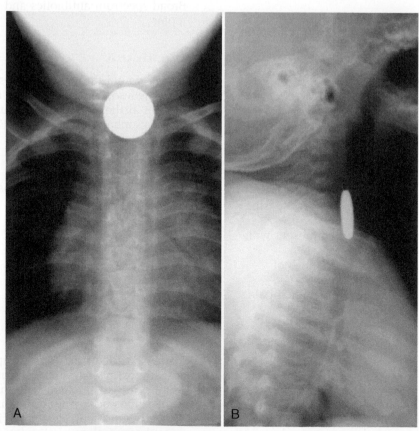

Figure 1-1. Radiographs of a coin in the esophagus. When foreign bodies lodge in the esophagus, the flat surface of the object is seen in the anteroposterior view (**A**) and the edge is seen in the lateral view. **B,** The reverse is true for objects in the trachea. (Courtesy of Beverley Newman, MD.)

SIGNS AND SYMPTOMS

- Account for 5% to 15% of upper GI hemorrhages
- Majority occur in the 4th to 6th decade of life
- Acute onset of upper GI tract bleeding following repeated retching is common presentation

DIAGNOSIS

- Based on clinical presentation and endoscopy/arteriography if required

TREATMENT

- Supportive treatment for GI tract bleeding as vast majority resolve spontaneously
- Low incidence of surgical intervention

Strictures and stenosis

- Esophageal strictures generally develop secondary to scarring from GERD at the distal esophagus

SIGNS AND SYMPTOMS

- Generally present as difficulty swallowing solids
- Schatzki ring most common cause of intermittent dysphagia with solids; common cause of "steakhouse syndrome"

DIAGNOSIS

- Thorough history and generally endoscopy

TREATMENT

- Endoscopic dilatation

Tracheoesophageal fistula

- Defect in the separation of the trachea from the esophagus; most common type: esophageal atresia with distal fistula between trachea and esophagus

SIGNS AND SYMPTOMS

- Potential for respiratory distress in first few hours in neonate for proximal fistula
- Proximal fistula can lead to massive aspiration on first feed
- Other types of fistulas present as inability to handle oral secretions, aspiration, choking, and recurrent pneumonias

DIAGNOSIS

- Inability to pass a catheter from nose/mouth to stomach
- Radiograph may show coiled tube in proximal esophagus

TREATMENT

- Respiratory support, reverse Trendelenburg position
- Operative fixation

Esophageal varices

SIGNS AND SYMPTOMS

- Develop in patients with chronic liver disease from portal hypertension (up to 60% of patients)
- About 25% bleed (higher rate in alcoholics), and 50% likelihood of recurrent bleed within 6 weeks of initial bleeding episode
- May present with hematemesis, "coffee ground" emesis, melena, or bright red blood per rectum

DIAGNOSIS

- History, physical examination, and early endoscopy
- No evidence of increased risk of iatrogenic hemorrhage from placement of NG tube

TREATMENT

- Supportive treatment for GI bleed; airway management if necessary
- Vasoactive agents and sclerotherapy have similar efficacy in establishing initial hemostasis
- Vasoactive medication such as somatostatin and octreotide cause relaxation of mesenteric vascular smooth muscle and reduce portal venous pressure without arterial vasospasm
- Empiric antibiotic therapy to cover enteric organisms
- Balloon tamponade optional if pharmacologic agents failing and endoscopy unavailable
- Main treatment for acute bleed is endoscopic ligation/sclerotherapy

TUMORS

95% of esophageal tumors are squamous cell. Men affected three times more than women. Risk factors: smoking, alcohol, and achalasia. Barrett esophagus from chronic GERD predisposes to adenocarcinoma.

SIGNS AND SYMPTOMS

- Rapid progression of dysphagia from solids to liquids
- Consider in patient more than 40 years old with new-onset dysphagia
- May present as GI bleed

DIAGNOSIS

- Early diagnosis is key through history and physical examination
- Definitive diagnosis through endoscopy and biopsy

TREATMENT

- Very poor prognosis

Liver

HEPATIC FAILURE

Diseases are divided into hepatocellular, cholestatic, and immunologic/infiltrative disorders

Cirrhosis

- Results from fibrous scarring mixed with hepatocellular regeneration in response to sustained inflammatory, toxic or metabolic insults. Common causes of liver failure include alcohol, acetaminophen, isoniazid, halothane, valproic acid, toxic mushrooms, and carbon tetrachloride.

SIGNS AND SYMPTOMS

- Historical risk factors: travel, sexual behavior, volume and duration of alcohol use, blood transfusions, needle stick exposure, intravenous drug abuse (IVDA), mushroom ingestion
- Hepatocellular necrosis (i.e., viral): anorexia, nausea/vomiting, low grade fever
- Cholestatic disease: jaundice, pruritis, clay-colored stools, dark urine
- Chronic liver disease: abdominal pain, ascites, GI tract bleeding, fever, change in mental status
- Physical findings
  - Acute liver failure: moderate liver enlargement and tenderness
  - Chronic failure: muscle atrophy, palmar erythema, cutaneous spider angiomata, parotid gland enlargement, testicular atrophy and gynecomastia

DIAGNOSIS

- **Bilirubin—marker of hepatocyte catabolic activity**
- Direct bilirubin elevates in states of biliary stasis or obstruction
- **Transaminases—markers of hepatocellular injury or death**
- Elevated levels from any hepatocyte injury: infection, ischemia, alcohol, acetaminophen
- Elevation in hundreds suggests mild injury whereas levels in thousands suggest extensive hepatic necrosis
- AST/ALT ratio >2:1 common in alcohol hepatitis (AST rarely >300 U/L)
- AST/ALT ratio <1 typical of acute/chronic viral hepatitis
- **Alkaline phosphatase—marker of cholestasis and biliary obstruction**
- Elevation associated with biliary obstruction and cholestasis
- 4 times normal suggests cholestasis
- Markedly elevated without increased bilirubin suggests lymphoma, fungal infection, sarcoidosis, tuberculosis, primary biliary cirrhosis (or bone alkaline phosphatase)
- Elevated in healthy children and pregnancy
- **Ammonia—marker of catabolic liver function**
- Elevated in both acute and chronic liver disease
- Elevated levels more reflective of general decline than diagnostic tool of therapy endpoint
- **Prothrombin time—marker of hepatocyte synthetic function**
- Increases with decreased synthesis of vitamin K–dependent factors II, VII, IX, X

- Measure of hepatic function, as is albumin—gauge acuity of process

TREATMENT

- Generally supportive
- Fluid/electrolyte/vitamin/nutritional supplementation
- Paracentesis: diagnostic and/or therapeutic
- Correct coagulopathy prior to invasive procedure or active bleeding
- Paracentesis okay without correcting coagulopathy
- Early endoscopic intervention for active upper GI tract bleeding

Clinical syndromes associated with cirrhosis and end-stage liver disease

- **Gastroesophageal varices:** discussed in detail under esophagus
- **Ascites/spontaneous bacterial peritonitis (SBP):** Discussed in "Peritoneum: Spontaneous Bacterial Peritonitis"
- **Hepatorenal syndrome**

SIGNS AND SYMPTOMS

- Development of acute renal failure (without a reversible cause) in patient with preexisting liver disease

DIAGNOSIS

- Laboratory tests reveal new renal failure

TREATMENT

- Search for reversible causes (volume depletion, drug-induced interstitial nephritis, postrenal obstruction, infection)
- Overall prognosis very poor but albumin infusion may improve survival
- **Hepatic encephalopathy**
- Probably results from the accumulation of nitrogenous waste products normally metabolized by the liver

SIGNS AND SYMPTOMS

- Four clinical stages: (1) general apathy; (2) lethargy, drowsiness; (3) stupor; (4) coma
- Common complication following transjugular intrahepatic portosystemic shunt (TIPS) procedure
- Common precipitants: GI tract bleeding, infection

DIAGNOSIS

- Diagnosis of exclusion: must rule out intracranial pathology, hypoglycemia, nutritional deficiencies, electrolyte imbalance, medication side effects, sepsis
- Serum ammonia levels are generally elevated but do not necessarily correlate with severity of encephalopathy

TREATMENT

- Lactulose: traps ammonia in GI tract and excreted in stool
- Neomycin may be beneficial by directly inhibiting bacterial growth and protein metabolism
- Flumazenil may have short-term benefit but no effect on survival or long-term recovery

INFECTIOUS CAUSES OF LIVER DISEASE

Viruses

- About one third of U.S. population immune to hepatitis A virus (HAV)
- Liver failure rare complication of HAV
- Chronic infection in about 6% to 10% of hepatitis B (HBV)
- Chronic liver disease in up to 85% of hepatitis C (HCV)
- Hepatitis D (HDV) infection depends on concomitant or preexisting chronic infection by HBV
- Hepatitis E is enterically spread and responsible for more than 50% of acute viral hepatitis occurring in some developing countries

SIGNS AND SYMPTOMS

- Common symptoms include fever, anorexia, vomiting, abdominal pain, diarrhea, "flu-like" syndrome. Majority of cases do not develop jaundice. Many cases are asymptomatic
- Physical examination findings may include hepatomegaly, scleral jaundice, tenderness in the right upper quadrant (RUQ)
- HAV spread by fecal–oral route and clinically occult commonly in children, whereas adults have more severe and prolonged course
- Common outbreaks for HAV include people exposed to contaminated food or water supplies, day care centers, raw shellfish
- Incubation period generally 30 days for HAV; viremia is of relatively short duration and is most prominent before the onset of symptoms

- Greatest infectivity occurs before the onset of symptoms
- No chronic carrier state for HAV
- HBV generally spread via serum/bodily secretions, with highest rates among IV drug abusers and homosexual men
- HBV onset of clinical symptoms between 60 and 90 days
- Patients with HBV may present with polyarticular arthritis, arthralgias, or dermatitis
- About 1% of patients with HBV will progress to fulminant hepatic failure
- HCV linked to blood transfusions, IVDA, occupational exposure
- HCV most frequent indication for liver transplantation
- HCV clinical symptoms develop within 30 to 90 days
- HDV spread in a manner similar to HBV
- HDV infection with chronic HBV often results in fulminant liver failure

DIAGNOSIS

- Viral hepatitis ought to be reported to the health department
- ALT generally elevated more than AST, with elevations tenfold to 100fold
- Bilirubin generally moderately elevated 5 to 10 mg/dL and typically present days to weeks after symptoms
- Elevated prothrombin time may predict complicated course
  - Note Table 1-1 for serologic markers in hepatitis
- Acute HAV by IgM HAV antibody whereas prior infection determined by IgG antibody
- Acute HBV diagnosed by presence of Hepatitis B surface antigen (HBsAg) and IgM antibody to HBcAg (core antigen)
- Anti-HBcAg antibody is generally the best indicator of prior HBV infection
- Anti-HBsAg antibody is the best marker for immunity to HBV

TABLE 1-1 Serologic Markers in Hepatitis

Serologic Marker	Abbreviation	Interpretation
Antibody to HAV	Anti-HAV	A combination of IgG and IgM antibody defining infection with HAV, acute or chronic
IgM antibody to HAV	Anti-HAV IgM	Antibody to HAV, indicating acute infection
Hepatitis B surface antigen	HBsAg	Surface antigen associated with acute or chronic HBV infection
Hepatitis B e antigen	HBeAg	Antigen associated with active infection, acute or chronic, and indicative of high infectivity
Antibody to B surface antigen	HBsAb	Antibody indicative of acute or past infection or immunization
Antibody to B core antigen	HBcAb	A combination of IgG and IgM antibody defining infection with HBV, acute or past
IgM antibody to B core antigen	HBcAb-IgM	Antibody to B core antigen, indicating acute infection with HBV
Antibody to B e antigen	HBeAb	Antibody to e antigen, possibly representing resolving HBV infection and decreased infectivity
Antibody to HDV	Anti-HDV	Antibody defining infection with HDV; HBsAg should be present
Antibody to HCV	Anti-HCV	A new antibody that defines infection with HCV, acute or past

From Marx JA, Hockberger RS, Walls RM: *Rosen's emergency medicine: concepts and clinical practice*, ed 6, Philadelphia, 2006, Mosby.
HAV, Hepatitis A virus; *HBV*, hepatitis B virus; *HCV*, hepatitis C virus; *HDV*, hepatitis delta virus; *IgG*, immunoglobulin G; *IgM*, immunoglobulin M.

- Anti-HCV antibody defines infection with HCV but may be delayed in onset and remain positive up to 3 months; test does not distinguish between acute and chronic hepatitis C infection
- Anti-HDV antibody defines infection with HDV, and HBsAg should be present

TREATMENT

- Treatment is generally supportive
- Hospital admission for severe fluid and electrolyte abnormalities, persistent vomiting, altered mental status, prolongation of PT 5 seconds beyond normal, immunosuppression, hypoglycemia
- Infected individual with HAV should practice meticulous hygiene and not to return to work (especially if food handler) until jaundice resolves
- Immunoglobulin to HAV should be given to all household and sexual contacts of persons confirmed with HAV, children of day-care facilities and employees caring for children in diapers if one or more cases of HAV develops among staff, or classroom contacts in young children (0.02 mL/kg IM)
- Postexposure prophylaxis for percutaneous and mucous membrane exposure to HBV:
  - In an unvaccinated individual (exposed person): If source person is known HBsAg positive, start HBIG and initiate HB vaccine series; otherwise initiate HB vaccine only
  - In a vaccinated individual (exposed person) with adequate levels of serum antibody to HBsAg—no treatment to exposure is necessary
  - In a vaccinated individual (exposed person) with known inadequate response to vaccination with an exposure from a HBsAg-positive source (or high-risk patient with unknown lab results) give HBIG and initiate revaccination
  - In a vaccinated individual (exposed person) with an unknown antibody response exposed to source with HBsAg-positive, test-exposed individual for antibody to HBsAg; if adequate, no treatment; if inadequate, give HBIG and vaccine booster
  - Effectiveness of HBIG greatest within 24 hours
- No accepted postexposure prophylaxis after exposure to HCV-positive blood, but treatment includes interferon and ribavirin
  - Chronic HCV occurs in up to 85% of patients and patients generally appear clinically well
  - Chronic HCV is leading cause of liver transplantation in the United States

Pyogenic abscess

SIGNS AND SYMPTOMS

- Most commonly associated with biliary tract obstruction or cholangitis
- Subacute onset of high fever, chills, RUQ pain, nausea/vomiting
- Patients generally ill-appearing

DIAGNOSIS

- Generally leukocytosis, elevated alkaline phosphatase, bilirubin >2 mg/dL
- Chest x-ray may reveal right pleural effusion
- CT scan and ultrasound most sensitive diagnostic modalities

TREATMENT

- Broad-spectrum antibiotics covering *Escherichia coli*, *Klebsiella*, *Pseudomonas*, *Enterococcus* species, anaerobic *Streptococci*, and *Bacteroides* species until definite pathogen identified
- Definitive treatment requires drainage

Amebic abscess

SIGNS AND SYMPTOMS

- Amebiasis common worldwide and more common in homosexual men
- *Entamoeba histolytica* most common ameba responsible
- Acute fever, chills, abdominal pain, vomiting; diarrhea is more common in children
- Common complication is rupture into adjacent anatomic structures

DIAGNOSIS

- Leukocytosis, elevated alkaline phosphatase, and aminotransferases
- Ultrasound/CT/magnetic resonance imaging (MRI) useful in diagnosis

TREATMENT

- Supportive therapy with initiation of amebicidal therapy (metronidazole 750 mg three times daily for 7 days)
- Drainage required for refractory/complicated cases

TUMORS

- Hepatocellular carcinoma most common primary hepatic malignancy. More common in underdeveloped areas of world where chronic HBV infection is present. HBV usually related to development of hepatoma in 75% to 90% of cases worldwide. Metastatic cancer to liver much more common in United States from tumors of the GI tract, lung, and breast.

SIGNS AND SYMPTOMS

- Nausea/vomiting, abdominal pain, jaundice, weight loss, cachexia
- Enlarged liver in cirrhotic patient is suggestive of cancer

DIAGNOSIS

- Liver tests often abnormal but nondiagnostic
- Alpha-fetoprotein elevated, but nonspecific
- Ultrasound/CT/MRI identifies tumor with biopsy for definitive diagnosis

TREATMENT

- Supportive emergency department (ED) treatment
- Hepatitis B serologies

Gallbladder and biliary tract

CHOLELITHIASIS

SIGNS AND SYMPTOMS

- Classic patient with gallstones: obese female aged 20 to 40 with upper abdominal pain
- Increased age and pregnancy common risk factors for gallstones
- Cholesterol stones (radiolucent) most common, with pigment stones (radiopaque) second
- RUQ/epigastric pain lasting 2 to 6 hours (more frequently constant as opposed to colicky), often postprandial; associated nausea and vomiting
- Pain not related to meals in up to one third of patients
- Physical examination reveals mild RUQ tenderness
- Radiation of pain to shoulder or around waist

DIAGNOSIS

- Laboratory tests are frequently normal
- Plain film reveals gallstones only 10% to 20% of time
- Consider alternative diagnoses
- Ultrasound is diagnostic modality of choice: may show gallstones but no pericholecystic fluid, gallbladder distension, wall thickening, or sonographic Murphy sign (signs of cholecystitis)

TREATMENT

- Symptomatic treatment with antispasmodic agents, analgesics, and antiemetics
- Definitive treatment includes cholecystectomy, medical dissolution therapy and gallstone lithotripsy

CHOLEDOCHOLITHIASIS

- Gallstones in the common bile duct

SIGNS AND SYMPTOMS

- Presentation is usually similar to that of acute cholecystitis but may be variable and sometimes more subtle
- Jaundice may be present if symptoms longer than 24 hours

DIAGNOSIS

- Elevation in alkaline phosphatase and conjugated bilirubin, consistent with extrahepatic obstruction
- May have increased amylase/lipase
- Dilated common bile duct or intraluminal stone on ultrasound

TREATMENT

- Symptomatic treatment
- Endoscopic sphincterotomy or dilatation to relieve obstruction followed by elective cholecystectomy

CHOLECYSTITIS

SIGNS AND SYMPTOMS

- Similar symptoms as with cholelithiasis plus:
  - Pain typically longer than 6 hours
  - Fever/chills/vomiting/anorexia
  - Signs of systemic toxicity
  - Murphy sign: worsened pain or inspiratory arrest resulting from deep, subcostal palpation on inspiration is about 65% sensitive and 97% specific for cholecystitis
- Acalculous cholecystitis (5% to 10% of patient with cholecystitis) has more rapid and malignant course
  - Patients at higher risk: children (50% to 70% of acute cholecystitis in children), elderly, diabetics, multiple-trauma victim, extensive burns, AIDS

DIAGNOSIS

- Leukocytosis, abnormal liver function studies or lipase levels commonly present
- Ultrasound diagnostic study of choice (Fig. 1-2)
  - Gallstones, gallbladder distension, wall thickening, pericholecystic fluid, sonographic Murphy sign
  - Ultrasound about 94% sensitive and 78% specific for acute cholecystitis
- Nuclear scintigraphy with technetium-99m–labeled iminodiacetic acid (HIDA) scan is 97% sensitive and 90% specific for acute cholecystitis
  - Normal patient will have clearly outlined gallbladder and cystic duct within 1 hour
- Complications of acute cholecystitis include:
  - Gallbladder empyema: complete obstruction of cystic duct with bacterial infection and abscess formation in wall of gallbladder
  - Emphysematous cholecystitis: gangrene of entire gallbladder
    - Comprise less than 1% of patients with cholecystitis

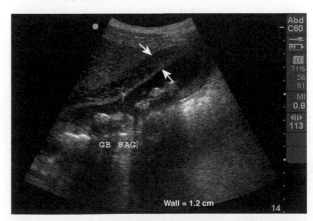

Figure 1-2. Ultrasound of acute cholecystitis. Arrows indicate thickening of gall bladder wall. Stones with shadowing are also visible.

- Patients typically elderly/diabetic and critically ill
- Plain film may show air in gallbladder wall/biliary tree
- Polymicrobial infection is common

TREATMENT

- Supportive care, broad-spectrum antibiotic therapy recommended, surgical treatment (more emergent in acalculous/emphysematous cholecystitis)

CHOLANGITIS

SIGNS AND SYMPTOMS

- Results from complete biliary obstruction in the presence of bacteria
- Common bile duct most common site of obstruction
- Jaundice, fever, RUQ pain, mental confusion, and shock
- Charcot's triad of fever, RUQ pain, jaundice present in only 25% of patients

DIAGNOSIS

- History, physical examination, and ultrasound
- Nuclear scintigraphy may be a more sensitive means to diagnose early obstruction

TREATMENT

- Volume support, broad-spectrum antibiotics, and rapid decompression (surgical or endoscopic) of biliary tree
- Very high mortality rate if untreated or improperly treated

TUMORS

SIGNS AND SYMPTOMS

- Gallbladder malignancy is 5th most common GI cancer, more common in women older than 50 years
  - Symptoms include chronic RUQ pain and jaundice, and examination reveals tenderness in the RUQ
  - Patients with chronic cholecystitis who develop "porcelain gallbladder" have a 25% risk of cancer
- Carcinoma of biliary tract is uncommon
- Extrahepatic bile duct carcinoma is less frequent than gallbladder malignancy and is more common in men
  - Jaundice is the most frequent finding

DIAGNOSIS

- Ultrasound is more sensitive than CT for diagnosing gallbladder carcinoma
- Extrahepatic bile duct carcinoma is suggested by the presence of dilated intrahepatic and extrahepatic bile ducts on sonography

Pancreas

ACUTE PANCREATITIS

SIGNS AND SYMPTOMS

- Cholelithiasis or alcohol abuse are the two most common causes of acute pancreatitis in the United States
  - Community setting, female, age more than 50 more likely cholelithiasis
  - Urban, male, age 35 to 45, more likely from alcohol abuse
- Other causes include many drugs, infection, inflammation, trauma (most common cause in children), scorpion bites, and metabolic disturbances
- Major symptom is midepigastric or left upper quadrant (LUQ) abdominal pain, constant, often radiating to back
- Pain intensity is variable and nausea and vomiting common
- Physical examination generally midepigastric tenderness
- Cullen sign (bluish discoloration around umbilicus) and Grey–Turner sign (bluish discoloration of the flanks) are signs of hemorrhagic pancreatitis
- Wide spectrum of presentation: may present in shock

DIAGNOSIS

- Amylase rises within 6 to 24 hours, peaks at 48 hours, and normalizes in 5 days; amylase has high sensitivity (decreases after a few days) but has low specificity for pancreatitis
- Lipase has higher sensitivity and specificity as compared to amylase
- Amylase/lipase levels do not correlate with severity of disease
- Obstruction series may show sentinel loop of small bowel from localized ileus or colon-cutoff sign, suggesting local colonic ileus
- Ultrasound should be performed within 24 hours of admission to identify gallstones or dilatation of biliary tree
- CT scan indicated for uncertain diagnosis, concern for complication, Ranson score greater than 3, severe disease, fever higher than 102° F
- Prognostic markers such as Ranson criteria are used to predict mortality; the five criteria on admission reflect the degree of local inflammation; the six criteria at 48 hours note the development of systemic complications
- Ranson criteria at admission: age >55 years, **white blood cell** count >16,000 cells/mm^3, **blood glucose** >200 mg/dL, serum **AST** >250 IU/L, serum **LDH** >350 IU/L
- Ranson criteria at 48 hours: serum calcium <8.0 mg/dL, **hematocrit** fall >10%, Po$_2$ <60 mmHg, **BUN** increased by ≥5 mg/dL after IV fluid hydration, negative **base excess** >4 mEq/L, sequestration of fluids >6 L

- APACHE-II score on the day of admission has a high sensitivity and specificity in distinguishing mild from severe pancreatitis; daily scores are determined, and with score <7, survival is likely

TREATMENT

- Treatment is fluid resuscitation, pain control, antiemetics, and limited oral intake
- Decompression indicated via endoscopic sphincterotomy for biliary pancreatitis
- For severe course of pancreatitis, broad-spectrum antibiotics generally warranted
- Many patients will require admission
- Complications include:
  - Pulmonary: pleural effusion, ARDS
  - Metabolic: hypocalcemia, hyperglycemia, hyperlipidemia
  - Other: hemorrhage, renal failure, abscess
  - Pseudocyst may develop in up to 1% to 8% of patients after 4 to 6 weeks, more frequently in alcoholic pancreatitis

CHRONIC PANCREATITIS

SIGNS AND SYMPTOMS

- 70% to 80% of cases from alcohol abuse
- Other causes include malnutrition, hyperparathyroidism, pancreas divisum, trauma, ampullary stenosis, cystic fibrosis
- Clinically significant malabsorption does not occur until more than 90% of pancreatic glandular function is lost
- Hallmark symptom is abdominal pain, but up to 10% of patients may be painless
- Patients generally chronically ill appearing

DIAGNOSIS

- No criterion standard test to distinguish acute from chronic pancreatitis
- Amylase/lipase levels may be elevated but have no prognostic significance; may be normal when pancreatic fibrosis is advanced
- Pancreatic calcifications may be present on plain radiographs
- Ultrasound less useful in chronic pancreatitis
- CT scan may be indicated to identify complications such as abscess or pseudocyst (can occur in up to 25% in chronic pancreatitis)

TREATMENT

- Generally supportive care and cessation of alcohol
- Many patients can be discharged from the ED once complications have been ruled out and adequate pain control accomplished

TUMORS

SIGNS AND SYMPTOMS

- Fourth most common GI cancer, with a 5-year survival rate of 3%
- Risk factors: heavy smoking, chronic alcohol, chronic pancreatitis, diabetes, family history
- Most common is adenocarcinoma at head of pancreas
- Commonly present with weight loss, dull/constant pain in the epigastrium that may radiate to the back, jaundice
- Courvoisier sign: enlarged, palpable, painless gallbladder in the presence of jaundice is most commonly associated with pancreatic cancer

DIAGNOSIS

- Ultrasound may make diagnosis, but CT provides better imaging of the cancer
- Needle biopsy needed to obtain tissue diagnosis

TREATMENT

- Complete resection is only definitive treatment
- Median survival for unresectable tumors about 6 months from time of diagnosis
- ED care focused on treating complications such as bowel obstruction, jaundice, pain management

Peritoneum

SPONTANEOUS BACTERIAL PERITONITIS

- Acute bacterial infection of ascitic fluid (commonly in patients with cirrhosis)
- Portal hypertension causes translocation of bowel flora across bowel wall into the peritoneum
- Empiric antibiotic therapy should cover Gram-negative rods seen in bowel flora
  - Most common cause is *E. coli* followed by *Streptococcus* species

SIGNS AND SYMPTOMS

- Fever (absent in 20%)
- Diffuse abdominal pain in patient with ascites, abdominal tenderness on palpation

DIAGNOSIS

- Made by paracentesis of ascitic fluid
  - Neutrophil count greater than 250 cells/μL is diagnostic
  - Total white cell count greater than 1000 cells/μL is also diagnostic
  - Gram stain of fluid and culture (negative in 30% to 40%)

TREATMENT

- Empirical therapy started in ED based on clinical suspicion before laboratory tests back
- Cefotaxime 2.0 g IV every 8 hours or
- Ampicillin-sulbactam 3.0 g IV every 6 hours

Stomach

GASTRITIS

- Inflammation of gastric mucosa
- *Helicobacter pylori*—most common cause
  - Spiral Gram-negative rod found in gastric antrum
  - 60% to 70% gastric ulcers infected with *H. pylori*
  - Increases risk of peptic ulcer disease and gastric adenocarcinoma
  - More prevalent in lower socioeconomic groups
  - Only a minority of people infected develop gastric ulcers or peptic ulcer disease
  - No practical tests for diagnosis of *H. pylori* in ED
- Other causes
  - Direct toxic effects of agents
    - Aspirin and other NSAIDs, alcohol, iron supplements, corrosive ingestion
  - Ischemia from severe illness
    - Any condition causing hypovolemia or hypotension (shock, burns)

SIGNS AND SYMPTOMS

- Epigastric pain (burning or gnawing in nature)
- Nausea/vomiting

DIAGNOSIS

- Can only be made via endoscopy and biopsy
- No definitive tests in ED
- Must rule out other diagnoses prior to settling on this diagnosis

TREATMENT

- Must treat underlying cause
  - Cessation of alcohol, NSAIDS
  - Treatment of *H. pylori*
- Antacids, H_2 blockers help ease symptoms
- Referral to gastroenterologist for definitive diagnosis

PEPTIC ULCER DISEASE (PUD)

- Formed by exposure of mucosa to imbalance between protective and destructive forces
  - Hydrochloric acid and pepsin (destructive)
  - Bicarbonate and mucus (protective)
- Ulcers commonly found along lesser curvature stomach and first part duodenum
- Pain is visceral, not well defined
- Causes
  - *H. Pylori*
  - NSAIDs, aspirin, prolonged steroid use
  - Cigarette smoking, emotional stress
  - Alcohol is *not* a cause

SIGNS AND SYMPTOMS

- Burning epigastric pain
  - Gastric ulcer pain occurs right after eating
  - Duodenal ulcer pain occurs 3 to 4 hours after eating and is relieved by food
- Nausea and vomiting

DIAGNOSIS

- Definitive diagnosis is via endoscopy
- Generally no radiologic or laboratory test practical for diagnosis in ED
- In elderly patients, must consider myocardial ischemia as cause of epigastric pain

TREATMENT

- Antacids
  - Heal ulcers by buffering gastric acids
- H_2-receptor antagonists
  - Inhibit gastric acid secretion
  - Cimetidine inhibits p450 system, increasing blood levels of warfarin and phenytoin
- Proton-pump inhibitors (PPI)
  - Blocks secretion of acid by inhibiting H^+/K^+ ATPase system (proton pump)
  - Usually used in patients that fail H_2-blocker therapy
- Sucralfate
  - Binds to base of ulcer, protecting it from further damage from acid
  - Causes aluminum absorption, so should not use concurrently with antacids
- Misoprostol
  - Synthetic prostaglandin E_1 (causes secretion of mucus and bicarbonate)
  - *Only* approved for use in ulcers caused by *NSAIDs*
  - Contraindicated in pregnancy
- *H. pylori* treatment
  - Patients with confirmed infections started on triple therapy
    - Clarithromycin, amoxicillin, and omeprazole, or
    - Bismuth subsalicylate, metronidazole, and tetracycline

Complications of peptic ulcer disease

- **Hemorrhage**
  - Most common complication of ulcers is hemorrhage
  - Bleeding ulcer most common cause of upper GI tract bleeding
  - Gastric ulcers more likely to re-bleed than duodenal

SIGNS AND SYMPTOMS

- Nausea/vomiting
- Hematemesis, melena
- Dizziness/weakness if copious amount of blood vomited

DIAGNOSIS

- NG lavage return of bright red blood indicates upper GI tract bleeding, but not source
- Endoscopy confirms diagnosis

TREATMENT

- Two large-bore IV lines
- Cardiac monitor

- Complete blood count, type and crossmatch, coagulation panel
- NG lavage with water until clear
- Administer proton pump inhibitor
- Gastroenterology consult
- Emergent endoscopic evaluation may be necessary
- Surgery or interventional radiology embolization procedure may be required if cannot stop bleeding via endoscopy

- **Perforation**
  - Chemical peritonitis from spilling of gastric/duodenal contents
  - Swift development of bacterial peritonitis

SIGNS AND SYMPTOMS

- Abrupt onset of severe abdominal pain, peritoneal signs on examination
- Posterior duodenal perforations
- Patients will complain of severe pain into back
- No free air on x-ray as perforation will communicate with retroperitoneum

DIAGNOSIS

- Free air on upright chest x-ray (absence of finding does not rule out diagnosis)
- CT scan can confirm diagnosis

TREATMENT

- Two large-bore IV lines, cardiac monitoring
- Complete blood count (CBC), type and crossmatch, coagulation panel
- Broad-spectrum IV antibiotics against Gram-negative rods and anaerobes
- Immediate surgical consult

- **Gastric outlet obstruction**
  - Occurs in 2% of ulcer patients because of edema and scarring of gastric outlet from chronic ulcer disease

SIGNS AND SYMPTOMS

- Abdominal fullness, early satiety, and succussion splash
- Nausea/vomiting leading to hypokalemic, hypochloremic metabolic alkalosis

DIAGNOSIS

- Esophagogastroduodenoscopy can show gastric outlet obstruction

TREATMENT

- IV fluid and electrolyte replacement
- Admission for possible surgical correction

STRUCTURAL DISORDERS

Gastric volvulus

- Occurs when stomach rotates on itself 180 degrees, causing closed loop obstruction

- Usually in patients 40 to 55 years of age and with paraesophageal hernia
- Two thirds of gastric volvulus occurs along long axis of stomach

SIGNS AND SYMPTOMS

- Sudden onset of severe abdominal pain with abdominal distension
- Vomiting
- Inability to pass NG tube

DIAGNOSIS

- Chest x-ray can show enlarged gastric bubble

TREATMENT

- Attempt NG tube placement, which may reduce volvulus
- If unsuccessful, will need endoscopic reduction or surgical correction

Gastric foreign body

- Once in stomach, 80% to 90% of objects pass through entire digestive tract in 7 to 10 days
- Factors preventing passage of foreign body from stomach
  - Length of foreign body (>5 cm may not pass)
  - Diameter of foreign body (>2 cm may not pass)
  - Pyloric stenosis or deformity secondary to damage from peptic ulcers

SIGNS AND SYMPTOMS

- May be asymptomatic
- Abdominal pain, vomiting

DIAGNOSIS AND TREATMENT

- X-ray
  - Can help determine presence and location of foreign body
  - May not see radiolucent objects such as food or wood
- Upper GI series can show bezoar
- Endoscopy or surgical retrieval required for objects that do not pass stomach

Bezoar

- **Phytobezoar** (most common)
  - Seen in food with large amounts of nondigestible dietary fiber
- **Trichobezoar**
  - Result from ingestion of large quantities of hair, carpet fiber
  - Frequently in children, young women, patients with psychiatric disorders
- **Pharmacobezoars**
  - Seen with nonabsorbable antacids and enteric-coated aspirin

TREATMENT

- Endoscopic break-up of bezoar, so smaller parts can pass
- Very large trichobezoars require surgical removal

TUMORS

Adenocarcinoma

- Most common gastric tumor
- Commonly seen in Japan and Korea; less common in North America
- Usually seen between 65 and 75 years of age
- *H. pylori* is the most common cause
- Risks for adenocarcinoma
  - Smoking, lower socioeconomic status
- Fruits and vegetables *protect against* adenocarcinoma

SIGNS AND SYMPTOMS

- Pain, vomiting, weight loss, early satiety
- Left supraclavicular sentinel node (Virchow node)
- Metastatic spread to umbilicus (Sister Mary Joseph nodule)

DIAGNOSIS AND TREATMENT

- Esophagogastroduodenoscopy with biopsy is used to make definitive diagnosis
- Surgical resection is curative and palliative
- Conventional chemotherapy and radiation not helpful

Gastric lymphoma

- 3% to 6% of all gastric malignancies
- 95% of gastric lymphomas are non-Hodgkin lymphoma

SIGNS AND SYMPTOMS

- Pain, weight loss, early satiety, vomiting, upper GI tract bleeding

DIAGNOSIS AND TREATMENT

- Endoscopy with biopsy
- Surgical resection

Small bowel

INFECTIOUS DISORDERS

- Small-bowel bacterial, viral, and parasitic enteritis are included in the "Large Bowel Infectious Disorders" section in Table 1-2.

INFLAMMATORY DISORDERS

Crohn disease (regional enteritis)

- Can involve any part of the GI tract from mouth to anus
- Disease is discontinuous with normal bowel between involved areas (skip lesions)

- The ileum is most commonly involved (terminal ileitis)
- Involves all layers of bowel wall

SIGNS AND SYMPTOMS

- Abdominal cramping and pain
- Tenesmus with loose bowel movements, diarrhea that may be bloody
- Fever
- Extraintestinal manifestations
- *Arthritis*—migratory monarticular or polyarticular
- *Uveitis*—blurred vision, photophobia, pain
- *Erythema nodosum*—on extensor surfaces of arms/legs
- *Hepatobiliary*—cholelithiasis, fatty liver, chronic active hepatitis

DIAGNOSIS

- Definitive diagnosis made by colonoscopy
- Abdominal CT scanning useful in patients with acute symptoms, and to look for complications such as fistula, abscess, and/or obstruction
- Barium examination may demonstrate the "string sign" (Fig. 1-3) because of bowel narrowing from full-thickness involvement of the bowel wall

TREATMENT

- Must focus on complications of disease and rule out other life-threatening causes

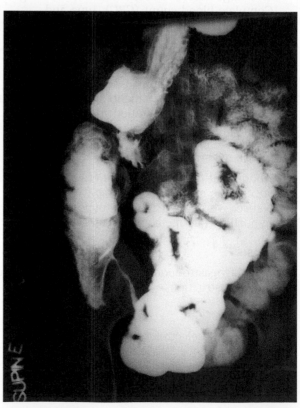

Figure 1-3. Small-bowel contrast study demonstrating "string sign" caused by inflammation and narrowing of the terminal ileum. (From Townsend CM, Jr et al: *Sabiston textbook of surgery*, ed 18, Philadelphia, 2007, Saunders.)

- Admit patients with dehydration, electrolyte disturbances, acute complications
- IV fluid, electrolyte replacement, and analgesics
- Steroids—40 to 60 mg per day (prednisone)
- Sulfasalazine—3 to 4 g per day (or mesalamine)
- Azathioprine—helps to decrease dose of steroids, used in patients with fistulas
- Antibiotics
- For patients with abscess or fistula
  - Metronidazole—efficacious in patients with perianal and fistula disease
  - Surgery for patients with intra-abdominal abscess, fistula, obstruction
- **Complications of Crohn Disease**
  - Abscess
    - Intraperitoneal, intramesenteric, perianal, ischiorectal
    - Patients have fever, abdominal pain, occasional palpable mass
  - Fistula
    - Most common sites are between ileum and sigmoid bowel
    - Can be internal or perianal
  - Intestinal stricture—leads to bowel obstruction
  - Cancer of small and large bowel three times higher in Crohn patients
- **Toxic megacolon**
  - Patients are severely ill appearing, toxic
  - Abdominal examination reveals marked distension and tenderness
  - Non-Crohn causes of toxic megacolon include:
    - Ulcerative colitis
    - Infectious colitis (*Shigella, Salmonella,* etc.)
    - Narcotics

DIAGNOSIS

- X-ray shows greater than 6 cm diameter, air-filled colon (Fig. 1-4)
- Three of the following required
- Fever >101.5° F, HR >120 beats/minute, WBC >10.5, anemia
- One of the following required
- Dehydration, change in mental status, electrolyte abnormality, hypotension

TREATMENT

- IV steroids
- Broad-spectrum antibiotics
- IV fluids and electrolyte replacement
- Surgical colectomy in 24 to 48 hours if no improvement

MOTOR ABNORMALITIES

Small-bowel obstruction

CAUSES

- Adhesions (most common cause)
- Hernia (second most common cause)
  - Incarcerated hernia in inguinal region most likely to cause obstruction

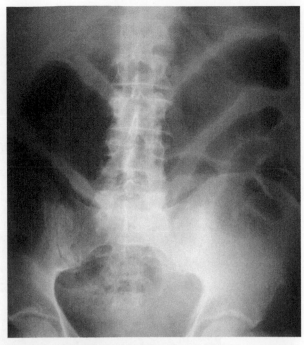

Figure 1-4. Toxic megacolon. The ascending and transverse colon appears gas-filled and dilated with a thickened wall. There is an absence of haustral markings, indicating full-thickness mural inflammation. (From Adam A et al: *Grainger and Allison's diagnostic radiology,* ed 5, Philadelphia, 2008, Churchill Livingstone.)

- Obturator/femoral hernias commonly cause obstruction in women
- Neoplasm (lymphoma, adenocarcinoma)
- Gallstone ileus—obstruction at ileocecal valve
- Inflammatory bowel disease (Crohn)

SIGNS AND SYMPTOMS

- Crampy, spasmodic abdominal pain
- Vomiting with proximal obstruction
- Abdominal distension with distal small-bowel obstructions

DIAGNOSIS

- Abdominal x-ray (obstruction series) (Fig. 1-5)
- Air-fluid levels
- Dilated loops of bowel more central in location
- Can see the plicae circulares that traverse the entire small bowel
- CT scan more sensitive when diagnosis is unclear and shows cut-off point

TREATMENT

- NG tube to remove excess air and bowel contents
- IV fluid and electrolyte replenishment
- Admission and surgery consultation
- Broad-spectrum antibiotic coverage when surgery is planned

Adynamic ileus (paralytic ileus)

- No mechanical obstruction

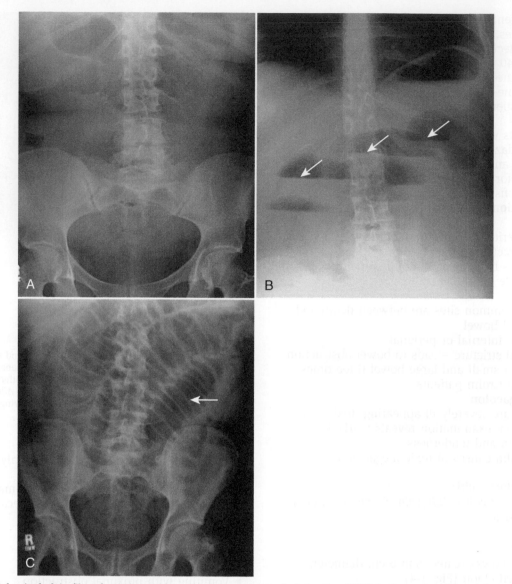

Figure 1-5. Abdominal plain film of a patient with a complete small-bowel obstruction (SBO) in the supine **(A)** and the upright **(B)** positions. The supine abdominal film demonstrates centrally located dilated loops of the small intestine without gas in the colon or rectum. The upright abdominal film demonstrates multiple air-fluid levels *(arrows)*. **C,** An abdominal film of a patient with another high-grade SBO demonstrating markedly dilated small intestine with prominent plica circulares *(arrow)*. (From Feldman M, Friedman LS, Brandt LJ: *Sleisenger and Fordtran's gastrointestinal and liver disease,* ed 8, Philadelphia, 2006, Saunders.)

- Disturbance in gut motility causes failure of passage of bowel contents
- Most commonly seen immediately after surgery
- Other causes include medications, abdominal trauma, hypokalemia, hypomagnesemia, sepsis

TREATMENT

- IV fluids, NG decompression
- Observation with correction of any known cause

STRUCTURAL DISORDERS

Aortoenteric fistula

- Rare but potentially fatal cause of GI tract bleeding (mortality rate of 50%)

- Almost always secondary to previous reconstructive aortoiliac surgery
- Usually have self-limited "herald bleed" followed by massive bleed weeks later
- Upper GI tract endoscopy, CT angiography, and aortography are used for diagnosis
- Quick diagnosis and surgical repair necessary for survival

Intestinal malabsorption

- Defective mucosal absorption of nutrients, vitamins, and minerals
- Patients complain of greasy floating stools, diarrhea, abdominal bloating
- Signs and symptoms particular to vitamin, mineral, and nutrient not being absorbed

- **Vitamin B$_{12}$ malabsorption**
  - Vitamin B$_{12}$ binds to intrinsic factor and is absorbed in the ileum
  - Causes of malabsorption of vitamin B$_{12}$
    - Resection of ileum, decreasing vitamin B$_{12}$ absorbing area
    - Pernicious anemia
      - Autoantibodies destroy parietal cells making intrinsic factor
      - Not enough intrinsic factor leads to vitamin B$_{12}$ malabsorption
      - Associated with gastric atrophy
        - Bacterial overgrowth in intestine (blind loop syndrome)

SIGNS AND SYMPTOMS

- Macrocytic anemia
- Paresthesias in hands and feet, weakness, poor balance/coordination

DIAGNOSIS AND TREATMENT

- Identifying correct underlying cause

Short bowel syndrome

- Occurs after resection of portions of small bowel
- Degree of malabsorption is determined by the length of the remnant intestine

SIGNS AND SYMPTOMS

- Large amounts of watery diarrhea
- Hypovolemia, hyponatremia, and hypokalemia, with vitamin deficiencies

TREATMENT

- IV fluids, electrolyte replenishment, and parenteral nutrition

Meckel diverticulum

- Caused by an incomplete obliteration of the vitelline duct
- In 2% of population and 2 feet from ileocecal junction
- Adults present with obstruction and inflammation, bleeding less common
- Diagnosed via Meckel scan—technetium study
- Treatment includes IV fluids and surgery consult for excision of diverticulum

TUMORS

- Two thirds of small bowel tumors malignant
- Rare, only account for 1% to 2.4% of GI tumors
- More common in men and elderly
- Adenocarcinoma is the most common small-bowel malignancy, followed by carcinoid, lymphoma

SIGNS AND SYMPTOMS

- Signs and symptoms occur late in progression of disease
- Obstruction, vomiting, crampy abdominal pain

DIAGNOSIS

- Small-bowel enteroscopy with biopsy

TREATMENT

- Surgical resection
- Chemotherapy/radiation not shown to cause improvement

VASCULAR INSUFFICIENCY

Mesenteric ischemia/infarction

- Commonly occurs in patients older than age 50
- Especially seen in those with cardiovascular disease
- Early diagnosis and aggressive treatment are absolute key
- Once bowel infarction has occurred, mortality is 70% to 90%

FOUR TYPES OF MESENTERIC ISCHEMIA

- **Mesenteric arterial embolism**
  - Most common form of mesenteric ischemia/infarction
  - Two thirds of cases occur in women
  - Risk factors for embolic occlusion
    - Dysrhythmias—atrial fibrillation being most common
    - Post–myocardial infarction (MI) mural thrombi
    - Rheumatic mitral valve disease
- **Mesenteric arterial thrombus**
  - Superior mesenteric artery diameter commonly decreased by atherosclerosis
  - Occurs in patients with chronic, severe atherosclerosis
  - 50% patients give history of pain after meals (abdominal angina)
- **Mesenteric venous thrombosis**
  - 60% of patients with mesenteric venous thrombosis had prior deep-vein thrombosis (DVT)
  - Patients are typically younger in age
  - Causes
    - Hypercoagulable state
    - Inflammatory process—pancreatitis, diverticulitis
    - Local abdominal trauma
- **Nonocclusive mesenteric ischemia**
  - Pathogenesis multifactorial but final pathway of vasoconstriction common
  - Seen in patients with systemic diseases causing hypotension
  - Causes
    - Congestive heart failure (CHF)
    - Cardiogenic shock
    - Septic shock

SIGNS AND SYMPTOMS

- Severe abdominal pain
- Fever
- *Pain out of proportion to findings on physical examination*

- Guaiac positive stool only in 25% of patients, and is a late finding
- Abdominal distension also late finding

DIAGNOSIS

- Lactate has high sensitivity but *low specificity*
- Elevated lactate and unexplained acidosis suggest mesenteric ischemia in those at risk
- Upright x-ray
  - Done to rule out free air or obstruction, but often normal
- CT scan
  - Can show edema of bowel wall and mesentery, or pneumatosis intestinalis
  - Negative CT scan does not rule out mesenteric ischemia
  - CT angiography has not been studied extensively in mesenteric ischemia
- Angiography
- Criterion standard for diagnosis
- Allows pinpointing of site of obstruction and type of occlusion
- Can provide treatment via papaverine after diagnosis is made

TREATMENT

- Early diagnosis via angiography is absolutely key
- Emergent surgical consultation
- Broad-spectrum antibiotics
- Papaverine—relieves vasoconstriction and used during angiography
- Anticoagulation for mesenteric arterial embolism or venous thrombosis
- Nonocclusive mesenteric ischemia—nonsurgical; treat underlying cause

Large bowel

INFECTIOUS DISORDERS

Pseudomembranous colitis

- Caused by *C. difficile*, an anaerobic Gram-positive bacillus
- Antibiotic use alters GI tract flora, causing *C. difficile* overgrowth
- Vancomycin and metronidazole, which treat the disease, may also cause it
- Diarrhea occurs 5 to 10 days after start of antibiotic course

SIGNS AND SYMPTOMS

- Diarrhea two to six times a day, abdominal cramping
- Fever with leukocytosis

DIAGNOSIS

- Stool testing for *C. difficile* **toxin** (not the organism)

TREATMENT

- Stop offending antibiotic
- 7 to 10 days of metronidazole 500 mg three times a day or vancomycin orally 250 mg four times a day

Bacterial enteritis

- Two types of bacterial enteritis: invasive and enterotoxin mediated
  - Invasive
    - Acts primarily on the large bowel by damaging cell membranes
    - Blood and mucus in stool
    - Invasive bacterial causes of enteritis are summarized in Table 1-2
  - Enterotoxin mediated
    - Toxin acts mostly on small bowel, altering water and electrolyte absorption
    - Watery diarrhea, no blood
    - Enterotoxin mediated causes of enteritis are summarized in Table 1-3

Parasitic infections

- Parasitic causes of gastrointestinal infection are summarized in Table 1-4

Viral enteritis

- Viruses are the most common cause of gastroenteritis
- Two major viruses most commonly accountable for gastroenteritis
  - Norwalk Virus
    - Seen most commonly in adults and older children
    - Cruise ships
  - Rotavirus
    - Seen mostly in young children; associated upper/lower respiratory tract infection
    - Day care centers
- Short incubation periods with explosive start to symptoms
- Can be transmitted via fecal–oral route, but food and water-borne outbreaks are common
- Disease is self-limited, with supportive measures being required
- Meticulous hand washing and hygiene are required for prevention

INFLAMMATORY DISORDERS

Acute appendicitis

- Occurs with obstruction of lumen of appendix
- Retrocecal appendix may refer pain to right flank
- Pregnant patients may have pain in RUQ

SIGNS AND SYMPTOMS

- Classically, pain at the periumbilical region localizes to right lower quadrant

TABLE 1-2   **Invasive Causes of Bacterial Gastroenteritis**

Organism	Duration	Source	Treatment	Symptoms and Key Points
Escherichia coli O157:H7	5-10 days	■ Inadequately cooked beef ■ Unpasteurized milk	■ Supportive, *no antibiotics*	■ Starts as watery diarrhea that becomes bloody ■ Can cause TTP, hemolytic uremic syndrome
Yersinia	1-3 weeks	■ Unpasteurized milk ■ Undercooked pork	■ TMP–SMX or ciprofloxacin for severe cases	■ Fever ■ Watery diarrhea, then bloody ■ Can cause terminal ileitis, which mimics appendicitis
Shigella	4-7 days	■ Contaminated water	■ TMP–SMX or ciprofloxacin	■ Fever, crampy abdominal pain ■ Bloody stools seen in one third ■ Seizures possible in children
Salmonella	4-7 days	■ Eggs ■ Poultry ■ Pet turtles, iguanas	■ TMP–SMX or ciprofloxacin	■ High fever, relative bradycardia ■ Osteomyelitis in sickle cell patients
Campylobacter	2-10 days	■ Milk ■ Water	■ Erythromycin	■ Most common bacterial diarrhea ■ Fever, abdominal pain ■ Can develop Guillain–Barré after infection
Vibrio parahaemolyticus	1-2 days	■ Raw seafood	■ No antibiotics	■ Vomiting, diarrhea ■ Usually in summer months

SMX, sulfamethoxazole; *TMP*, trimethoprim; *TTP*, thrombotic thrombocytopenic purpura.

TABLE 1-3   **Enterotoxin-Mediated Bacterial Gastroenteritis**

Organism	Duration	Source	Treatment	Symptoms and Key Points
Staphylococcus aureus	1-2 days	■ Eggs ■ Mayonnaise ■ Protein-rich food not refrigerated	■ Supportive therapy	■ Very large outbreaks, usually at outdoor events ■ Sudden onset of vomiting
Bacillus cereus	1 day	■ Uncooked rice ■ Fried rice	■ Supportive therapy	■ Heat-stable toxin ■ Onset 1-6 hr after ingestion of rice
Enterotoxigenic *Escherichia coli*	3-10 days	■ Fecal contamination of water or food	■ Supportive therapy ■ Ciprofloxacin will limit course	■ Traveler's diarrhea ■ Common in areas of poor sanitation
Clostridium perfringens	1-2 days	■ Meat ■ poultry	■ Supportive therapy	■ Large outbreaks ■ Watery diarrhea ■ Abdominal cramping
Ciguatera	1-2 weeks	■ Coral reef fish	■ Supportive therapy ■ Mannitol in sick patients	■ Begins with vomiting/diarrhea ■ Toxin caused by dinoflagellate ■ Loose teeth sensation ■ Reversal of hot and cold sensation ■ Paresthesias
Scombroid	1 day	■ Dark-meat fish ■ Tuna, mahi-mahi, bluefish	■ H_1 or H_2 blocker usually causes sudden relief	■ Onset 20-30 min after ingestion of food ■ Facial flushing ■ Vomiting, diarrhea ■ Symptoms due to histamine release
Vibrio cholera	3-7 days	■ Contaminated water	■ Ciprofloxacin in adults ■ TMP–SMX in kids	■ Rice-water diarrhea ■ Severe dehydration

SMX, sulfamethoxazole; *TMP*, trimethoprim.

■ Anorexia, nausea and vomiting
■ Rovsing sign—pain in right lower quadrant with palpation of left lower quadrant
■ Psoas sign—patient feels pain when asked to extend at hip against resistance
■ Obturator sign—pain when hip flexed and externally rotated

■ No one sign or symptom has high sensitivity *and* specificity for appendicitis

DIAGNOSIS

■ 80% to 90% of patients with appendicitis have WBC count above 10,000/mm^3, but not specific

TABLE 1-4 **Parasitic Causes of Gastroenteritis**

Organism	Source	Treatment	Symptoms and Key Points
Entamoeba histolytica	■ Ingestion of cysts in fecally contaminated food or water	■ Iodoquinol ■ Metronidazole in severely ill	■ Prevalence high in patients with AIDS, homosexual men, and travelers ■ Abdominal cramps, bloody diarrhea ■ Liver abscess most common extraintestinal manifestation
Giardia lamblia	■ Ingestion of contaminated water	■ Metronidazole	■ Backpackers' diarrhea ■ Most common cause of water-borne diarrhea outbreaks ■ Duodenal aspiration can give diagnosis
Cryptosporidium	■ Fecal–oral transmission	■ Symptomatic usually ■ No good antibiotics	■ Most common cause of chronic diarrhea in AIDS ■ Profuse watery diarrhea
Isospora belli	■ Fecal–oral transmission	■ TMP–SMX very effective	■ Most commonly seen in AIDS patients ■ Diagnosed by identifying oocysts in stool
Cyclospora	■ Contaminated fresh fruit	■ TMP–SMX	■ Explosive watery diarrhea ■ Sustained fatigue ■ Weight loss in long courses
Strongyloides stercoralis	■ Skin penetration via infected soil, usually on foot	■ Ivermectin	■ Serpiginous urticarial rash ■ Chronic watery diarrhea ■ High mortality in immunocompromised
Necator americanus (Hookworm)	■ Hookworm in soil penetrates bare skin, usually foot	■ Mebendazole	■ Diagnosis made by identifying ova in stool ■ Hypochromic microcytic anemia on labwork
Enterobiasis (Pinworm)	■ Direct transfer of eggs from anus to mouth via fingers	■ Mebendazole	■ Outbreaks in schools, day care centers ■ Pruritus ani ■ Cellophane tape of anus will identify worms

SMX, sulfamethoxazole; *TMP*, trimethoprim.

■ Urinalysis: mild sterile pyuria may be seen in patients with appendicitis
■ CT scan of abdomen/pelvis (Fig. 1-6)
  ■ Sensitivity of 87% to 100% and specificity of 89% to 98%
  ■ Findings are appendix diameter greater than 6 mm, periappendiceal inflammation, abscess

TREATMENT

■ Nothing by mouth (NPO), IV fluids, analgesics
■ Surgery consult for appendectomy
■ When decision made to operate, give prophylactic antibiotics

Radiation colitis

■ Side effect of radiation therapy damaging rapidly dividing intestinal endothelium
■ Occurs in 50% to 75% of patients receiving radiation to the pelvis
■ Acute
  ■ Onset with start of radiation treatment
  ■ Self-limited
■ Chronic
  ■ Can occur up to 2 years after end of radiation therapy

■ Nonspecific and delayed presentation makes diagnosis hard

SIGNS AND SYMPTOMS

■ Abdominal pain, diarrhea, tenesmus
■ Lower GI tract bleeding

DIAGNOSIS

■ Mostly clinical diagnosis based on history and symptoms
■ Endoscopy can reveal pale, friable mucosa

TREATMENT

■ Reduction of daily radiation dose
■ Steroid enemas
■ Symptomatic treatment

Ulcerative colitis

■ Chronic inflammation of colon and rectum
■ Primarily involves mucosa and submucosa, not entire bowel wall
■ Continuous lesion begins in rectum and can spread proximally (no skip lesions)
■ Can form crypt abscesses and mucosal ulceration

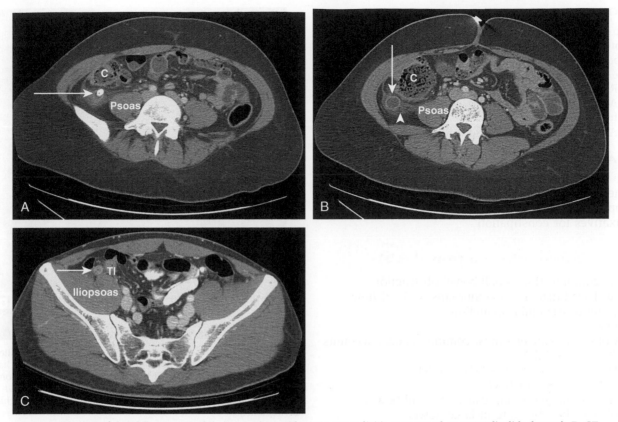

Figure 1-6. A, CT scan of the abdomen or pelvis in a patient with acute appendicitis may reveal an appendicolith *(arrow)*. **B,** CT typically shows a distended appendix *(arrow)* with diffuse wall-thickening and periappendiceal fluid *(arrowhead)*. **C,** The appendix may be described as having mural stratification, referring to the layers of enhancement and edema within the wall *(arrow)*, and this may also referred to as a target sign. *C,* Cecum; *TI,* terminal ileum. (From Townsend CM, Jr et al: *Sabiston textbook of surgery,* ed 18, Philadelphia, 2007, Saunders.)

SIGNS AND SYMPTOMS

- Frequent bowel movements, small volume, loose or diarrheal, tenesmus
- Fever and tachycardia
- Anorexia, weight loss, abdominal pain
- Extraintestinal complications
- Peripheral arthritis, ankylosing spondylitis, uveitis, erythema nodosum
- Complications
  - Toxic megacolon (see Crohn section for details)
  - Massive GI tract bleeding
  - Perirectal fistulas and abscesses (although more common in Crohn)
  - 10- to 30-fold increase in cancer (higher than in Crohn)

DIAGNOSIS

- Laboratory tests are nonspecific
- Barium enema can show changes to bowel wall
- Colonoscopy/sigmoidoscopy for definitive diagnosis

TREATMENT

- Mild to moderate disease
  - Treated as outpatients
  - Prednisone 40 to 60 mg daily
  - Sulfasalazine 1.5 to 2 g per day (or mesalamine)

- Azathioprine, 6-mercaptopurine used in refractory cases
- Severe cases
  - IV steroids
  - IV fluids and electrolyte correction
  - Broad-spectrum antibiotics
  - Eventual elective colectomy for refractory cases
  - Surgical consult for toxic megacolon

MOTOR ABNORMALITIES

Irritable bowel

- Diagnosis of exclusion after more serious etiologies ruled out
- Twice as common in women as men
- Stress is an exacerbating factor
- Anxiety or depression often coexist in patients with irritable bowel

SIGNS AND SYMPTOMS

- Abdominal pain, bloating sensation, constipation, diarrhea
- Pain relieved with defecation
- Fever, rectal bleeding, nocturnal stools are *not* generally seen in irritable bowel syndrome (IBS)

DIAGNOSIS

- No specific physical or laboratory abnormalities
- Rome II criteria for IBS
- Abdominal pain for greater than 12 weeks during the past year *and* two of the following
  - Relief of discomfort with defecation
  - Association of discomfort with altered stool frequency
  - Association of discomfort with altered stool form

TREATMENT

- No curative therapy available
- Therapy directed at symptoms
- Loperamide for diarrhea
- Laxatives for constipation

Large-bowel obstruction (LBO)

- Less common than small-bowel obstruction
- Bowel wall distension compromises blood flow, leading to ischemia, infarction
- Causes
  - Colorectal cancer—most common cause, accounts for 60% of LBO
  - Diverticular disease—20% of LBO
  - Volvulus—5% of LBO
  - Adhesions—common cause of small-bowel obstruction, but rare in large bowel
  - Ogilvie syndrome (pseudo-obstruction)
    - No mechanical obstruction
    - Seen in patients with chronic opioid use, electrolyte disturbance, spine or retroperitoneal trauma

SIGNS AND SYMPTOMS

- Abdominal pain and distention, obstipation, vomiting
- Change in caliber of stool indicates carcinoma as cause

DIAGNOSIS

- X-ray (Fig. 1-7)
  - Will show distended loops of bowel in a peripheral location with haustra, which do not involve the entire diameter of the colon
  - Does not show exact location or cause of obstruction
- CT scan
  - May show cause of obstruction as well as location

TREATMENT

- NPO
- IV fluids and electrolyte replacement
- NG tube insertion
- If bowel perforation suspected, antibiotics should be given
- Surgical consultation
- Ogilvie (pseudo-obstruction)
  - Managed initially with bowel rest, IV fluids, correction of electrolytes

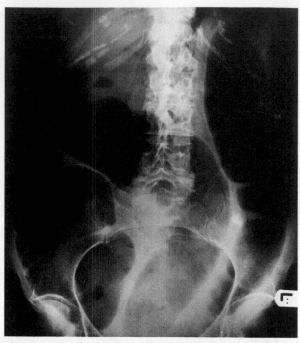

Figure 1-7. Large-bowel obstruction: supine position. Gas-filled, distended large bowel and cecum. Competent ileocecal valve has resulted in no dilation of small bowel. Eighty-four-year-old woman with carcinoma of sigmoid. (From Adam A et al: *Grainger and Allison's diagnostic radiology*, ed 5, Philadelphia, 2008, Churchill Livingstone.)

STRUCTURAL DISORDERS

Diverticular disease

- Most common in middle-aged and elderly patients, and incidence increases with age
- Mostly Western-civilization disease due to low-fiber diets
- Diverticula occur at site of vessel penetration into colon wall (weakest part of wall)
- 85% diverticular disease occurs in left colon/sigmoid

SIGNS AND SYMPTOMS

- Diverticulosis
  - Mostly asymptomatic
  - Painless bleeding
    - Occurs in 3% to 5% of patients with diverticulosis
    - Accounts for 40% of lower GI tract bleeding
- Diverticulitis
  - Typically left lower quadrant pain and tenderness
  - Right-sided diverticulitis presents as right lower quadrant pain (mimicking appendicitis)
  - Nausea/vomiting, low-grade fever
  - Perforations can lead to generalized abdominal pain and peritoneal signs

DIAGNOSIS

- Diverticulosis
  - Generally made on sigmoidoscopy/colonoscopy

- Diverticulitis
  - Abdominal CT scan is the best method for diagnosis
  - Abdominal CT scan will show abscesses or perforation
  - Sigmoidoscopy/colonoscopy limited in acute presentations due to perforation risk

TREATMENT

- Diverticulosis
  - High-fiber diet
  - No evidence that avoidance of nuts, small seeds prevents recurrences
- Diverticulitis
  - Uncomplicated cases in healthy patients can be treated as outpatients
    - Liquid diet
    - Ciprofloxacin 500 mg every 12 hours and metronidazole 500 mg every 6 hours for 7 to 10 days
  - Complicated cases
    - Admit if failed outpatient therapy, cannot tolerate oral medications, poor follow-up
    - IV fluids and bowel rest (NPO)
    - Ciprofloxacin 500 mg every 12 hours IV and metronidazole 500 mg every 6 hours IV
    - Surgical intervention for abscess or perforation

Intussusception in adults

- Rare in adults compared with children
- 80% adult intussusceptions occur in the small bowel
- Most common cause is cancer acting as a lead point for intussusception
- Presents as acute partial obstruction, abdominal pain
- Classic triad of abdominal pain, mass, and heme-positive stool is rare in adults
- Typically found on CT scan
- Treatment is surgical

Volvulus

- Occurs when a loop of bowel twists and obstructs the lumen
- Twisting can compromise vascular supply to bowel, leading to gangrene and perforation
- Two types
  - Sigmoid
    - Elderly, bedridden patients
    - Patients with neurologic/psychiatric disorders
    - Chronic severe constipation increases risk
  - Cecal
    - Because of an incomplete fusion of the cecal mesentery to posterior abdominal wall
    - Seen in younger patients (20 to 30 years of age)

SIGNS AND SYMPTOMS

- Abdominal pain
- Vomiting
- Abdominal distension

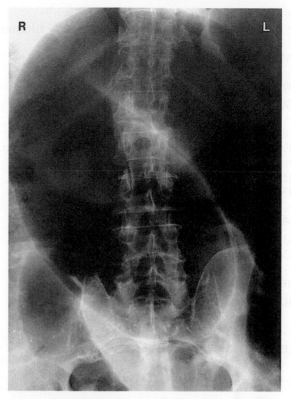

Figure 1-8. Sigmoid volvulus. A plain film of the abdomen shows the massively dilated "inverted U" of colon pointing toward the right upper quadrant. (From Mettler FA, Jr: *Essentials of radiology,* ed 2, Philadelphia, 2005, Saunders.)

DIAGNOSIS

- X-ray (Fig. 1-8)
  - Sigmoid
  - Diagnosis made on plain film 80% of the time
  - Dilated bowel loop in bent inner tube appearance in lower quadrants
- Cecal
  - Diagnosis only made 50% of time on plain film
  - Classic "coffee bean" sign—a large oval gas shadow with a line down the middle representing bowel bent over on itself in the center of the abdomen

TREATMENT

- Sigmoid
  - Endoscopic decompression via rectal tube—recurrence rate is 60%
  - Elective resection recommended at later time
- Cecal
  - Barium enema can be done in attempt to reduce cecal volvulus
  - If enema unsuccessful, surgical reduction required

TUMORS

Colorectal cancer

- Third-most common cancer in men and women
- Risk factors
  - Advanced age

- Diet high in fat, low in fiber
- Inflammatory bowel disease (especially ulcerative colitis)
- Majority of colon cancer is adenocarcinoma

SIGNS AND SYMPTOMS

- 50% present with abdominal pain
- Abdominal distension from cancer, causing obstruction
- Fatigue, shortness of breath, angina secondary to microcytic hypochromic anemia
- Hematochezia
- Decreased stool caliber, constipation

DIAGNOSIS

- CT scan may show mass
- Colonoscopy with biopsy

TREATMENT

- Bowel resection and chemotherapy

Rectum and anus

INFECTIOUS DISORDERS

Perianal/perirectal abscess

- Obstruction of anal crypt and gland leads to abscess formation
- Polymicrobial infection with anaerobes and aerobes
- Usually seen in young men aged 30 to 50
- Complications
  - Chronic infection can lead to fistula formation
  - Deeper-space infections of intersphincteric and ischiorectal spaces

SIGNS AND SYMPTOMS

- Perianal abscesses (*most common* anorectal abscess)
  - Superficial tender mass close to anal verge, posterior midline
  - Can be fluctuant
  - Usually no fever or leukocytosis
- Ischiorectal abscess
  - More lateral than perianal abscesses, on medial aspect of buttocks
  - Large, circumscribed, and indurated
  - Fever and leukocytosis may be present
- Perirectal abscess
  - Few external signs
  - Pain out of proportion to physical findings
  - Deep rectal pain; fluctuance and extreme tenderness on rectal examination

DIAGNOSIS

- Perianal abscess clinically diagnosed by examination
- Endorectal ultrasound or CT abdomen/pelvis with contrast can localize abscesses

TREATMENT

- Perianal abscess
  - Can do incision and drainage in the ED
  - Local anesthesia required, often along with procedural sedation
  - Packing should be inserted with follow-up in 1 to 2 days
  - No antibiotics unless concurrent cellulitis or comorbid diseases such as diabetes, AIDS, or on chemotherapy
- Intersphincteric, perirectal, and ischiorectal abscesses
  - Surgical consultation
  - Incision and drainage in operating room, not in the emergency department

Pilonidal cyst and abscess

- Pilonidal sinus located above the gluteal cleft overlying the distal sacrum/coccyx
- *Always* located midline
- Ingrowing hair causes a foreign-body granuloma reaction
- Usually seen in men under the age of 40

SIGNS AND SYMPTOMS

- Painful fluctuant mass in midline distal sacral region

DIAGNOSIS

- Clinical, no laboratory studies or imaging required

TREATMENT

- Incision and drainage with packing insertion
- Incision and drainage not curative
- Referral to surgeon for excision to prevent recurrence

INFLAMMATORY DISORDERS

Proctitis

- Inflammation of the lining of the rectal mucosa
- Causes
  - STDs via anal intercourse (gonorrhea, chlamydia, herpes)
  - Side effect of radiation
  - Crohn disease

SIGNS AND SYMPTOMS

- Sensation of rectal fullness
- Tenesmus
- Pain in left lower quadrant
- Small bowel movements of mucus and blood

DIAGNOSIS

- First must rule out other more severe disorders
- Sigmoidoscopy will reveal friable bleeding mucosa

TREATMENT

- Must treat underlying cause
- STD: ceftriaxone (gonorrhea), doxycycline (chlamydia), acyclovir (herpes)

- Crohn proctitis: corticosteroid suppositories
- Radiation proctitis: anti-inflammatory agents, botulinum toxin injection

STRUCTURAL DISORDERS

Anal fissure

- Superficial straight line tear in anoderm caused when hard stool expelled
- More than 90% of fissures occur in midline posteriorly
- Fissure not in midline should arouse suspicion for Crohn disease leukemia, HIV, cancer
- Commonly seen in children, young adults, pregnant women

SIGNS AND SYMPTOMS

- Sudden, severe pain with defecation
- Pain subsides between bowel movements
- Bleeding in small amounts is bright red, no melena

DIAGNOSIS

- Suggested by clinical history and physical examination

TREATMENT

- Hot sitz baths
- Eliminating constipation with stool bulking agents, fiber, stool softeners
- Local analgesic ointments; nitroglycerin
- Surgical excision of fissure if healing does not occur

Anal fistula

- Abnormal tract connecting anal canal to skin
- Causes
  - Ischiorectal abscess (most common)
  - Ulcerative colitis/Crohn disease
  - Cancer
  - Tuberculosis
- Goodsall's rule
  - Anterior-opening fistulas following direct course to anal canal
  - Posterior-opening fistulas follow a curving, horseshoe path

SIGNS AND SYMPTOMS

- Recurrent abscess formation and drainage at same site
- Bloody, malodorous discharge

DIAGNOSIS

- Intrarectal ultrasound can identify intersphincteric fistulas
- Fistulography with radiopaque dye

TREATMENT

- Definitive treatment requires surgical excision

Rectal foreign body

- Seen in children, psychiatric patients, and during anal-receptive sexual activities

SIGNS AND SYMPTOMS

- Most patients asymptomatic
- Abdominal pain, fever, rectal bleeding may indicate perforation

DIAGNOSIS

- Based on history, which may be given reluctantly and should be obtained in a sympathetic, nonridiculing manner
- May be able to palpate object on rectal examination
- Flat plate of abdomen and upright chest x-ray; look for free air and location of object

TREATMENT

- Procedural sedation may be required to remove object in the ED
- Sphincter relaxation is required for removal of large objects
- If a vacuum has formed behind the object, a catheter is passed beyond the object and air is injected to relieve the vacuum
- Objects that are large, fragile, have sharp edges, or have migrated proximally will require general anesthesia and removal in operating room

Hemorrhoids

- Hemorrhoids are normal structures that are displaced when support structures deteriorate in the 3rd decade of life
- The incidence of symptomatic hemorrhoids is the same in patients with and without portal hypertension
- Pregnant women are more prone to developing hemorrhoids
- External hemorrhoids
  - Modified squamous epithelium
  - Originate below the dentate line
  - Blood supply from inferior hemorrhoidal plexus
- Internal hemorrhoids
  - Transitional or columnar epithelium
  - Originate above the dentate line
  - Blood supply from superior hemorrhoidal plexus
- Classified by severity (internal)
  - First degree—Do not prolapse
  - Second degree—Prolapse and spontaneous reduce
  - Third degree—Prolapse and require manual reduction
  - Fourth degree—Prolapse and are not reducible; strangulation can occur

SIGNS AND SYMPTOMS

- Internal hemorrhoids
  - Simple internal hemorrhoids are painless and present as painless bright red rectal bleeding with bowel movements; may have pruritus

- Can be palpable on digital rectal exam
- Fourth-degree nonreducible hemorrhoids may become thrombosed
- External hemorrhoids
  - Easily visible externally and bluish-purple in color
  - Thrombosed external hemorrhoids are painful to palpation
  - Also may have slow bleeding

DIAGNOSIS

- Via clinical history and examination
- Can visualize internal hemorrhoids with anoscopy

TREATMENT

- For first- to third-degree internal hemorrhoids
  - Manual reduction of prolapsed hemorrhoids
  - Sitz baths
  - Topical analgesics and/or steroid ointments
  - Stool softeners; bulk fiber supplements
- For fourth-degree internal hemorrhoids
  - Emergent surgery consult in ED
- Thrombosed external hemorrhoids
  - If swelling for more than 48 hours and pain tolerable, can do sitz bath/stool softeners
  - If thrombosis acute (less than 48 hours), very painful
    - Excision of hemorrhoid may be done in the ED
    - Local anesthetic with epinephrine injected into hemorrhoid
    - Elliptical incision made exposing thrombosis
    - Clot is removed and pressure dressing applied

Rectal prolapse (procidentia)

- Seen in the very young and the very old
- Incomplete prolapse if only mucosal layer protrudes
- Complete prolapse if all layers of rectum involved
- Associated with long-standing constipation

SIGNS AND SYMPTOMS

- Red, protruding mass from rectum, especially with bowel movements (Fig. 1-9)
- Fecal incontinence
- Bloody mucoid discharge

DIAGNOSIS

- Clinical history and physical examination
- Concentric circumferential rings of mucosa indicative of prolapse

TREATMENT

- Manual reduction, under procedural sedation if necessary
- Surgical consultation may be necessary
- Emergency resection required if cannot be reduced and bowel viability low

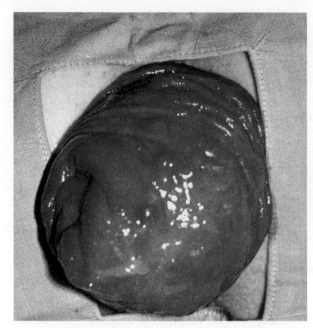

Figure 1-9. Rectal prolapse. (From Townsend CM, Jr et al: *Sabiston textbook of surgery,* ed 18, Philadelphia, 2007, Saunders.)

TUMORS

- Anal canal neoplasms
  - Malignancies proximal to the dentate line
  - Adenocarcinomas, transitional carcinoma, melanoma
  - High malignant potential, metastasize quickly
- Anal margin neoplasms
  - Distal to the dentate line
  - Can be squamous cell carcinoma, basal cell carcinoma, and Paget disease
  - Low malignant potential and slow to metastasize

Spleen

STRUCTURAL DISORDERS

Splenomegaly

CAUSES

- Infectious mononucleosis
- Bacterial endocarditis
- Tuberculosis
- Leukemia, Hodgkin lymphoma
- Hereditary spherocytosis
- Cirrhosis

SIGNS AND SYMPTOMS

- Patients usually asymptomatic, can complain of mild left upper abdominal pain
- Early satiety from gastric displacement by large spleen
- Weakness and pallor if red blood cells are being sequestered in the spleen
- Enlarged spleen on palpation

DIAGNOSIS

- CT may show splenomegaly, infarcts, infiltrative changes

TREATMENT

- Treat underlying cause
- Splenectomy indicated for chronic, severe splenomegaly

IMMUNOLOGIC

- The spleen is the primary site for IgM synthesis
- Functional asplenism
  - Spleen is present but not functioning well
  - Patients are more susceptible to infections from encapsulated organisms such as *Streptococcus pneumoniae, Haemophilus influenzae, Neisseria meningitidis, E. coli, Salmonella*
  - Causes of functional asplenism include sickle cell disease, lupus, sarcoidosis, hereditary spherocytosis
  - Need to be vaccinated against encapsulated organisms
  - Patients should seek prompt evaluation for fever

HEMATOLOGIC

Splenic sequestration

- Sudden enlargement of spleen with drop in hemoglobin due to red blood cells trapped in spleen
- Symptoms can include pallor, tachycardia, hypotension
- Spleen is usually palpable
- Occasionally thrombocytopenia and leukopenia can occur due to sequestration
- Commonly associated with sickle cell anemia
- Treat with IV fluids, which mobilize trapped red blood cells in spleen
- Recurrence of syndrome is common
- On rare occasions, splenectomy is required

PEARLS

- Esophageal foreign bodies are more common in children, and the most common anatomic site of obstruction is the cricopharyngeal narrowing.

- Impacted esophageal food bolus should be removed within 12 hours, whereas a button battery requires immediate removal if lodged in the esophagus.

- Hepatitis A virus spreads by the fecal–oral route and is commonly clinically occult in children, whereas adults have more severe and prolonged course.

- Acute HBV is diagnosed by presence of Hepatitis B surface antigen (HBsAg) and IgM antibody to HBcAg (core antigen).

- Patients commonly suffering from acalculous cholecystitis include children, elderly, diabetics, multiple-trauma victim, extensive burns, and AIDS.

- Charcot triad of fever, right upper quadrant (RUQ) pain, and jaundice is present in only 25% of patients with acute cholangitis.

- Cholelithiasis and alcohol abuse are the two most common causes of acute pancreatitis in the United States.

- Lipase has higher sensitivity and specificity as compared to amylase in pancreatitis.

- Most common cause of upper GI tract bleeding is a bleeding gastric or duodenal ulcer.

- Crohn disease causes skip lesions and can lead to abscesses, fistulas, and strictures.

- Small-bowel obstructions are most commonly caused by adhesions, followed by hernias and cancer.

- Toxic megacolon is a complication of Crohn disease and ulcerative colitis and can be identified on x-ray with greater than 6 cm dilated colon. Patients are toxic in appearance.

- Typhoid fever is caused by salmonella and is marked by high fever, abdominal pain, and relative bradycardia.

- Ciguatera toxin causes the sensation of loose painful teeth, reversal of hot and cold sensation, and paresthesias.

- Ulcerative colitis is a continuous lesion beginning in the rectum and proceeding proximally with no skip lesions and has a higher risk for colon cancer than Crohn disease.

- Most common cause of large bowel obstruction is cancer followed by diverticular disease and volvulus. Adhesions, though a common cause of small-bowel obstructions, are rare in the large bowel.

- Sigmoid volvulus is commonly seen in elderly bedridden patients, whereas cecal volvulus is seen in patients in their 30s.

- Asplenism and functional asplenism leave patients prone to infection from encapsulated organisms.

BIBLIOGRAPHY

Aranda-Michel J, Giannella RA: Acute diarrhea: a practical review, *Am J Med* 106:670–676, 1999.

Ault MJ, Geiderman JM: Hepatitis. In Wolfson AB, Hendey GW, Hendry PL et al (eds): *Harwood-Nuss' clinical practice of emergency medicine,* ed 4, Philadelphia, 2005, Lippincott Williams & Wilkins, pp. 366–373.

Baumgart DC, Sandborn WJ: Inflammatory bowel disease: clinical aspects and established and evolving therapies, *Lancet* 369:1641-1657, 2007.

Brady WJ, Aufderheide TP, Tintinalli JE: Cholecystitis and biliary colic. In Tintinalli JE, Kelen GD, Stapczynski JS (eds): *Emergency medicine: a comprehensive study guide,* ed 6, New York, 2004, McGraw-Hill, pp. 561-566.

Brandt LJ: Vascular lesions of the gastrointestinal tract. In Feldman M, Friedman LS, Brandt LJ (eds): *Sleisenger & Fordtran's gastrointestinal and liver disease,* ed 8, Philadelphia, 2006, Saunders, pp. 757-777.

Brandt LJ, Bjorkman D, Fennerty MB et al: Systematic review on the management of irritable bowel syndrome in North America, *Am J Gastroenterol* 97:S7-S26, 2002.

Broder JS: Hepatic disorders and hepatic failure. In Tintinalli JE, Kelen GD, Stapczynski JS (eds): *Emergency medicine: a comprehensive study guide,* ed 6, New York, 2004, McGraw-Hill, pp. 566-573.

Browning Jeffrey D, Sreenarasimhaiah J: Gallstone disease. In Feldman M, Friedman LS, Brandt LJ (eds): *Sleisenger & Fordtran's gastrointestinal and liver disease,* ed 8, Philadelphia, 2006, Saunders Elsevier, pp. 1387-1418.

Buchman AL: Short bowel syndrome. In Feldman M, Friedman LS, Brandt LJ (eds): *Sleisenger & Fordtran's gastrointestinal and liver disease,* ed 8, Philadelphia, 2006, Saunders Elsevier, pp. 2257-2276.

Burgess BE, Bouzoukis JK: Anorectal disorders. In Tintinalli JE, Kelen GD, Stapczynski JS (eds): *Emergency medicine: a comprehensive study guide,* ed 6, New York, 2004, McGraw-Hill. pp. 539-551.

Cline DM: Hepatic failure and cirrhosis. In Wolfson AB, Hendey GW, Hendry PL et al (eds): *Harwood-Nuss' clinical practice of emergency medicine,* ed 4, Philadelphia, 2005, Lippincott Williams & Wilkins, pp. 374-376.

Coates WC: Anorectum. In Marx JA, Hockberger RS, Walls RM (eds): *Rosen's emergency medicine: concepts and clinical practice,* ed 6, Philadelphia, 2006, Mosby, pp. 1507-1523.

FitzGerald DJ, Pancioli AM: Acute appendicitis. In Tintinalli JE, Kelen GD, Stapczynski JS (eds): *Emergency medicine: a comprehensive study guide,* ed 6, New York, 2004, McGraw-Hill, pp. 520-523.

Gaasch WR, Barish RA: Swallowed foreign bodies. In Tintinalli JE, Kelen GD, Stapczynski JS (eds): *Emergency medicine: a comprehensive study guide,* ed 6, New York, 2004, McGraw-Hill, pp. 513-516.

Garcia-Tsao G: Current management of the complications of cirrhosis and portal hypertension: variceal hemorrhage, ascites, and spontaneous bacterial peritonitis, *Gastroenterology* 120:726-748, 2001.

Godshall D, Mossallam U, Rosenbaum R: Gastric volvulus: case report and review of the literature, *J Emerg Med* 17:837-840, 1999.

Gratton MC, Werman HA: Peptic ulcer disease and gastritis. In Tintinalli JE, Kelen GD, Stapczynski JS (eds): *Emergency medicine: a comprehensive study guide,* ed 6, New York, 2004, McGraw-Hill, pp. 516-520.

Guss DA: Liver and biliary tract. In Marx JA, Hockberger RS, Walls RM (eds): *Rosen's emergency medicine: concepts and clinical practice,* ed 6, Philadelphia, 2006, Mosby, pp. 1402-1425.

Herbert GS, Steele SR: Acute and chronic mesenteric ischemia, *Surg Clin N Am* 87:1115-1134, 2007.

Hogenauer C, Hammer HF: Maldigestion and malabsorption. In Feldman M, Friedman LS, Brandt LJ (eds): *Sleisenger & Fordtran's gastrointestinal and liver disease,* ed 8. Philadelphia, 2006, Saunders Elsevier, pp. 2199-2241.

Houghton J, Wang TC: Tumors of the stomach. In Feldman M, Friedman LS, Brandt LJ (eds): *Sleisenger & Fordtran's gastrointestinal and liver disease,* ed 8, Philadelphia, 2006, Saunders Elsevier, pp. 1139-1170.

Lavoie FW, Becker MH: Hernia in adults and children. In Tintinalli JE, Kelen GD, Stapczynski JS (eds): *Emergency medicine: a comprehensive study guide,* ed 6, New York, 2004, McGraw-Hill, pp. 527-530.

Lowell MJ: Esophagus, stomach, and duodenum. In Marx JA, Hockberger RS, Walls RM (eds): *Rosen's emergency medicine: concepts and clinical practice,* ed 6, Philadelphia, 2006, Mosby, pp. 1382-1401.

Mendelson MH: Esophageal emergencies. In Tintinalli JE, Kelen GD, Stapczynski JS (eds): *Emergency medicine: a comprehensive study guide,* ed 6, New York, 2004, McGraw-Hill, pp. 508-513.

Panacek EA, Diercks D: Upper GI bleeding. In Wolfson AB, Hendey GW, Hendry PL et al (eds): *Harwood-Nuss' clinical practice of emergency medicine,* ed 4, Philadelphia, 2005, Lippincott Williams & Wilkins, pp. 346-349.

Pfau PR, Ginsberg GG: Foreign bodies and bezoars. In Feldman M, Friedman LS, Brandt LJ (eds): *Sleisenger & Fordtran's gastrointestinal and liver disease,* ed 8, Philadelphia, 2006, Saunders Elsevier, pp. 499-513.

Ramakrishnan K, Salinas RC: Peptic ulcer disease, *Am Family Phys* 76:1005-1012, 2007.

Rinnart KJ: Occupational exposures, infection control & standard precautions. In Tintinalli JE, Kelen GD, Stapczynski JS (eds): *Emergency medicine: a comprehensive study guide,* ed 6, New York, 2004, McGraw-Hill, pp. 994-1006.

Rustgi AK: Small intestinal neoplasms. In Feldman M, Friedman LS, Brandt LJ (eds): *Sleisenger & Fordtran's gastrointestinal and liver disease,* ed 8, Philadelphia, 2006, Saunders Elsevier, pp. 2703-2712.

Sands BE: Crohn's disease. In Feldman M, Friedman LS, Brandt LJ (eds): *Sleisenger & Fordtran's gastrointestinal and liver disease,* ed 8, Philadelphia, 2006, Saunders Elsevier, pp. 2459-2498.

Santen SA, Hemphill RR: Pancreas. In Marx JA, Hockberger RS, Walls RM (eds): *Rosen's emergency medicine: concepts and clinical practice,* ed 6, Philadelphia, 2006, Mosby, pp. 1426-1439.

Seaberg DC, Wolfson AB: Pancreatitis. In Wolfson AB, Hendey GW, Hendry PL, et al (eds): *Harwood-Nuss' clinical practice of emergency medicine,* ed 4, Philadelphia, 2005, Lippincott Williams & Wilkins, pp. 383-387.

Seamans CM, Mickiewicz ML: Esophageal disease. In Wolfson AB, Hendey GW, Hendry PL et al (eds): *Harwood-Nuss' clinical practice of emergency medicine,* ed 4, Philadelphia, 2005, Lippincott Williams & Wilkins, pp. 341-345.

Sheth AA, Longo W, Floch MH: Diverticular disease and diverticulitis, *Am J Gastroenterol* 103:1550-1556, 2008.

Torrey SP, Henneman PL: Disorders of the small intestine. In Marx JA, Hockberger RS, Walls RM (eds): *Rosen's emergency medicine: concepts and clinical practice,* ed 6, Philadelphia, 2006, Mosby, pp. 1440-1450.

Vissers RJ, Abu-Laban RB: Acute and chronic pancreatitis. In Tintinalli JE, Kelen GD, Stapczynski JS (eds): *Emergency medicine: a comprehensive study guide,* ed 6, New York, 2004, McGraw-Hill, pp. 573-577.

Werman HA, Mekhjian HS, Rund DA: Ileitis, colitis, and diverticulitis. In Tintinalli JE, Kelen GD, Stapczynski JS (eds): *Emergency medicine: a comprehensive study guide,* ed 6, New York, 2004, McGraw-Hill, pp. 530-539.

Wilson LD: Acute diseases of biliary tract. In Wolfson AB, Hendey GW, Hendry PL et al (eds): *Harwood-Nuss' clinical practice of emergency medicine,* ed 4, Philadelphia, 2005, Lippincott Williams & Wilkins, pp. 362-365.

Wolfe JM, Henneman PL: Acute appendicitis. In Marx JA, Hockberger RS, Walls RM (eds): *Rosen's emergency medicine: concepts and clinical practice,* ed 6, Philadelphia, 2006, Mosby, pp. 1451-1459.

Questions and Answers

1. A 48-year-old man with past medical history of cirrhosis and ascites presents with increasing abdominal size and pain for the past 2 days. He is also complaining of mild shortness of breath. He has not had a fever, vomiting, or diarrhea. On physical examination, his vital signs are temperature (T) = 98.4° F, pulse (P) = 108 bpm, respiratory rate (RR) = 22/min, and blood pressure (BP) = 133/78 mmHg. His lungs are clear to auscultation. His abdomen is distended with diffuse tenderness on palpation. There is no rebound or guarding. You can appreciate a fluid wave. Management and disposition for this condition would be:
   a. discharge on pain medications
   b. paracentesis and discharge of patient to home to wait for culture results of ascites fluid
   c. paracentesis with fluid sent for culture and empiric antibiotic administration
   d. antibiotic administration only if the Gram stain of the ascites fluid is positive

2. A 50-year-old man with no past medical history presents to the emergency department (ED) stating that "a piece of steak is stuck in my throat." His vital signs are normal, and he is in no respiratory distress. He is vomiting his secretions and unable to swallow liquids without vomiting. What is an appropriate course of action for this patient?
   a. discharge the patient with follow-up endoscopy in 48 hours
   b. give the patient an aqueous solution of meat tenderizer
   c. give the patient 1 mg intravenous (IV) glucagon, repeat dose of 2 mg if needed
   d. give the patient 1 mg nifedipine sublingually

3. A 60-year-old alcoholic man presents to the ED 12 hours after multiple episodes of forceful blood-streaked emesis. The patient is complaining of severe chest pain. Vitals: T = 101° F, P = 125 bpm, BP = 90/60 mmHg, RR = 22/min. You are able to palpate subcutaneous air on the chest wall. His electrocardiographic findings are normal and his rectal exam has heme-negative results. Which of the following statements is true regarding this patient's likely diagnosis?
   a. chest x-ray (CXR) is abnormal about 30% of the time
   b. patients are generally well appearing
   c. misdiagnosis is common
   d. treatment includes supportive care and IV antibiotics only

4. What is the most common cause of small-bowel obstruction?
   a. hernia
   b. adhesions
   c. cancer
   d. gallstone ileus

5. What is the most common type of abdominal-wall hernia?
   a. direct inguinal hernia
   b. indirect inguinal hernia
   c. femoral hernia
   d. umbilical hernia

6. A 40-year-old alcoholic man with cirrhosis presents to the ED after vomiting a "bucket full" of blood at home. The patient feels slightly weak and tired, otherwise has no complaints. Vitals: afebrile, HR = 110 bpm, BP = 120/70 mmHg, RR = 16/min. He is nontender on abdominal exam and his rectal exam has heme-negative findings. What treatment option below is *inaccurate* regarding this probable diagnosis?
   a. consider early airway management
   b. octreotide infusion is indicated
   c. no role for broad-spectrum antibiotic therapy
   d. early consultation with gastroenterologist for possible endoscopy

7. Which of the following is correct regarding ingestion of caustic agents?
   a. strong acid ingestion causes liquefaction necrosis of the esophagus
   b. strong alkali ingestion causes coagulation necrosis of the esophagus
   c. household bleach (3% to 6% sodium hypochlorite) is generally not corrosive to the esophagus
   d. passage of a nasogastric tube is indicated

8. Which of the following statements is true regarding foreign body ingestions affecting the esophagus?
   a. the most common site of obstruction in children is the cricopharyngeal narrowing
   b. the most common site of obstruction in adults is the mid-esophagus
   c. the time limit to remove button batteries lodged in the esophagus is 24 hours
   d. sharp-edged foreign bodies are the only indication for endoscopic consultation

9. A 23-year-old woman presents with several weeks of abdominal cramping, diarrhea, and bloody stools. She initially did not have a fever, but has had low-grade fever over the past few

days. She has had weight loss and some pain in her right upper quadrant. She has no complaints of vaginal discharge or dyspareunia. There is no yellowing of the skin or eyes. Physical examination reveals right upper quadrant tenderness. Findings from the pelvic examination are unremarkable. A computer tomographic (CT) scan is ordered, which shows a low-attenuation lesion with rim enhancement in the liver. What does this person have?

a. Fitz–Hugh–Curtis syndrome
b. amebiasis
c. cholangitis
d. schistosomiasis

10. A 72-year-old woman with no past medical history or abdominal surgeries presents to the ED with the complaint of abdominal pain. The pain has been ongoing for the past 2 days and is in the left lower portion of her abdomen. She has had a low-grade fever, some vomiting, and a few episodes of diarrhea. Vital signs are T = 99.8° F, HR = 110 bpm, R = 22/min, and BP = 136/78 mmHg. On examination, the patient has pain localized to the left lower quadrant. Palpation in that region elicits pain with guarding, but there is no rebound. There are no palpable masses in the abdomen or bruits on auscultation. Rectal exam shows brown stool but is heme positive. Pelvic examination is unremarkable. Which of the following is true about this clinical picture?

a. this clinical scenario came about because the patient's diet consists primarily of high-fiber fruits and vegetables
b. this disease does not occur on the right side of the abdomen
c. treatment involves broad-spectrum antibiotic coverage that will provide aerobic and anaerobic coverage
d. ultrasound is the preferred diagnostic study for this disorder in the ED

11. Which of the following tests the synthetic function of the liver?

a. aspartate transaminase (AST)/alanine transaminase (ALT)
b. alkaline phosphatase
c. bilirubin
d. prothrombin time

12. Which of the following statements is true regarding hepatic encephalopathy?

a. patients may present with a mental status range from general apathy to coma
b. serum ammonia levels generally correlate to the severity of encephalopathy
c. gastrointestinal bleeding is an uncommon precipitant for hepatic encephalopathy
d. no medical treatment is indicated in the ED for hepatic encephalopathy

13. After a through history, physical exam, and laboratory results, you diagnose a 30-year-old woman with no known medical problems with probable viral hepatitis. Which of the following is an indication to admit this patient to the hospital?

a. mild fluid and electrolyte abnormalities
b. intractable vomiting
c. AST >1000 units/L
d. prolongation of prothrombin time (PT) beyond 2 seconds of normal

14. A 70-year-old man with a history of hepatic encephalopathy presents to the ED with a change in mental status. He is drowsy but arouses to verbal stimuli. His vital signs are normal and findings from his remaining exam are unremarkable except for slightly icteric sclera and a mildly distended, nontender abdomen. Which of the following statements is true regarding the patient's ED evaluation?

a. a rectal exam for heme-positive stool is indicated
b. a glucose check is unnecessary
c. a CT of the head is never indicated in this type of patient scenario
d. an elevated ammonia level clinches the diagnosis of hepatic encephalopathy

15. Which of the following is a correct description of the bowel changes in Crohn disease?

a. continuous involvement of the bowel with no skip lesions
b. only involves the mucosa and submucosa of the bowel
c. the ileum is involved in a majority of Crohn disease cases
d. weakening of the bowel wall at the insertion of blood vessels

16. A 23-year-old woman presents to the ED concerned about contracting Hepatitis A from work. She works in a day care facility caring for infants in diapers. Four infants and two coworkers have just been diagnosed with Hepatitis A. The patient is asymptomatic. Which of the following statements is true regarding Hepatitis A prophylactic treatment for this patient?

a. immunoglobulin for Hepatitis A should be given to all household contacts of this patient
b. immunoglobulin for Hepatitis A should be given only to sexual contacts of this patient
c. immunoglobulin for Hepatitis A should not be given to this patient
d. immunoglobulin for Hepatitis A is indicated for this patient

17. A 40-year-old obese woman presents to the ED complaining of intermittent, stabbing right upper quadrant pain for the past 2 hours. Her

symptoms started after eating French fries and she admits to similar pain in the past that has usually resolved after 30 minutes. Her vital signs are normal and on exam she has mild RUQ tenderness to palpation but no guarding, rebound, or Murphy sign. Which of the following statements is true regarding this diagnosis?

a. increased age and pregnancy are not risk factors for gallstones
b. cholesterol gallstones are the most common
c. pain is always related to meals
d. pain typically lasts 24 hours

18. Which of the following is true regarding viral hepatitis?

a. hepatitis A commonly causes hepatic failure
b. hepatitis B is related to development of hepatoma in 75% to 90% of cases worldwide
c. hepatitis C rarely causes chronic liver disease
d. hepatitis D infection depends on concomitant or preexisting chronic infection with Hepatitis C virus

19. Which hepatitis virus is classically linked to blood transfusions?

a. hepatitis A
b. hepatitis B
c. hepatitis C
d. hepatitis E

20. Which of the following is true about cecal volvulus?

a. typically seen in patients aged 70 to 80 years
b. patients with neurologic or psychiatric disorders are more prone to getting a cecal volvulus
c. a plain-film radiograph will make the diagnosis more than 95% of the time
d. endoscopy and/or colonoscopy cannot be used to correct cecal volvulus

21. Which of the following is true about perianal/perirectal abscesses?

a. all perianal and perirectal abscesses should be drained in the ED
b. patients with perirectal and intersphincteric abscesses will generally allow a rectal examination to be performed
c. patients with perianal abscesses require antibiotics even if a cellulitis is not present
d. perianal and perirectal abscesses are polymicrobial, with aerobes and anaerobes

22. While working in the ED, one of the new EM nurses accidently sticks herself with a needle from a patient known to have hepatitis B (HBsAg +). The nurse completed one Hepatitis B vaccination series but was recently told she is a nonresponder to the vaccine (inadequate response to vaccination: serum anti-HBs <10 mIU/mL). What is the appropriate treatment?

a. local wound care only and refer to occupational health
b. hepatitis B immune globulin (HBIG) only
c. HBIG and initiate vaccine series
d. initiate vaccine series only

23. Which organism has a predilection for the terminal ileum, and thus may mimic appendicitis?

a. *Yersinia*
b. *Campylobacter*
c. *Salmonella*
d. *Shigella*

24. A 71-year-old woman with past medical history of hypertension and atrial fibrillation presents with 8 hours of severe abdominal pain. The pain is diffuse and not worsened by movement or food. She denies fever, but did have one episode of vomiting. Her last bowel movement was yesterday. Vital signs are T = 100.8° F, P = 116 bpm, R = 22/min, and BP = 121/64 mmHg. On physical examination, the patient is moaning softly. Abdominal examination is significant for a soft abdomen, nondistended with hypoactive bowel sounds, and no abdominal bruits or masses. When you press on the patient's abdomen, it does not elicit a change in response from the patient. She has strong femoral pulses bilaterally and both legs are warm. She has heme-positive stool. What is the correct etiology and diagnosis?

a. mesenteric ischemia secondary to arterial embolism
b. mesenteric ischemia secondary to arterial thrombus
c. mesenteric ischemia secondary to venous thrombus
d. abdominal aortic aneurysm secondary to hypertension
e. abdominal aortic dissection secondary to hypertension

25. Which of the following causes a reversal of hot and cold sensation, loose painful teeth, and perioral paresthesias?

a. *Ciguatera*
b. *Scombroid*
c. *Vibrio cholera*
d. *Giardia lamblia*

26. A 31-year-old woman rushes into your ED complaining of palpitations and diarrhea. She was just with her boyfriend eating at a seafood restaurant. On physical examination, you have an anxious well-developed woman with facial flushing. She is talking in full sentences without retractions or audible wheezing. Lungs are clear to auscultation and abdomen is soft and nontender. Neurologic exam findings are unremarkable. What medication do you want to give this patient?

a. epinephrine
b. diphenhydramine
c. mannitol
d. ciprofloxacin
e. trimethoprim (TMP) / sulfamethoxazole (SMX)

27. What organism causes a serpiginous urticarial rash along with chronic watery diarrhea?

   a. *Enterobius vermicularis*
   b. *Necator americanus*
   c. *Strongyloides stercoralis*
   d. *Dracunculus medinensis*

28. Which of the following groups of patients is *not* at higher risk for acalculous cholecystitis?

   a. middle-aged individuals
   b. AIDS patients
   c. multiple-trauma victim
   d. patient with extensive burns

29. The triad of fever, right upper quadrant pain, and jaundice is classically associated with which condition?

   a. cholelithiasis
   b. acute cholecystitis
   c. cholangitis
   d. pancreatitis

30. A 41-year-old man with a history of gastric ulcers presents to you with the complaint of a dull ache in his epigastrium for 6 weeks now. Food occasionally makes the pain worse. He has not vomited but he feels nauseous. He denies any alcohol or drug use. The patient has seen his physician who did blood tests and had put the patient on three medicines to "clear up an infection," but he had not taken the medicines yet. On physical examination, the patient is well appearing and in no acute distress. He is tender in the epigastric region but not in the right upper quadrant. Otherwise his abdominal exam is unremarkable. The patient is asking you if you can give him details about this infection. Which of the following is a correct statement you can make to the patient?

   a. "Your doctor must have meant inflammation and not infection. You simply need to take Maalox with meals and you will be fine"
   b. "The infection you have does not increase your risk of gastric cancer at all"
   c. "We have tests we can do quickly in the emergency department right now that can diagnose what this infection is"
   d. "60 to 70 percent of gastric ulcers are caused by your infection, but not all people infected develop ulcers"

31. A 48-year-old man presents with acute pancreatitis. Which of the following diagnostic criteria on admission has been identified to predict a worse patient outcome?

a. age >40
b. amylase >300 IU/100 mL
c. white blood cell (WBC) count >16,000/L
d. blood sugar <150 mg/dL
e. lactate dehydrogenase (LDH) <300 IU/L

32. A 55-year-old man presents to the ED with mid-epigastric pain that radiates to his back. The pain is sharp in nature and began about 12 hours ago. He has vomited multiple times and is unable to tolerate his oral pain medications prescribed by his physician for "chronic pancreatitis." Which of the following statements is true regarding chronic pancreatitis?

   a. normal amylase/lipase levels "rule out" chronic pancreatitis
   b. pancreatic calcifications may be present on plain radiographs
   c. up to 40% of patients may present without abdominal pain
   d. clinically significant malabsorption does not occur until >70% of pancreatic glandular function is lost

33. An 82-year-old man presents with severe abdominal distension and pain for the past 36 hours. The patient complains of feculent vomiting. He has not had a bowel movement in 3 days. His past medical history is significant for colon cancer. Vital signs are T = 96.7° F, HR = 110 bpm, RR = 22/min, BP = 145/90 mmHg. On physical examination, the patient looks distressed. Lungs are clear to auscultation and no cardiac murmurs are appreciated. The abdomen is severely distended with tympany, and there is diffuse abdominal tenderness. An obstruction series does not reveal free air, but there are very large dilated loops of bowel in the periphery. Which of the following is correct?

   a. adhesions are the primary cause of this bowel obstruction
   b. a radiograph showing dilated loops of bowel in the periphery with lines not involving the entire diameter of the bowel is consistent with a small bowel obstruction
   c. the patient should be allowed to eat if hungry
   d. severe bowel wall distension in this patient can lead to vascular compromise of the bowel, causing infarction and perforation

34. Which of the following statements regarding pancreatitis is true?

   a. Alcohol abuse and gallstones are the two most common causes of acute pancreatitis in the United States
   b. the absolute level of serum amylase and lipase correlates to the severity of pancreatitis
   c. lipase has a lower specificity as compared to amylase to diagnose acute pancreatitis
   d. there are very few complications associated with acute pancreatitis

35. Which of the following is true about the workup for mesenteric ischemia?

   a. lactate is highly specific but not sensitive for mesenteric ischemia
   b. a negative CT scan of the abdomen/pelvis rules out mesenteric ischemia
   c. angiography is the criterion standard for diagnosis
   d. all patients have occult or frank blood in their stools

36. Which of the following is true about pseudomembranous colitis?

   a. vancomycin and metronidazole do not cause pseudomembranous colitis
   b. it is commonly diagnosed by culturing the stool for *Clostridium difficile*
   c. symptoms occur commonly one to two days after the initiation of an antibiotic
   d. *C. difficile*, which causes pseudomembranous colitis, is an anaerobic Gram-positive bacillus

37. Which of the following is true about anal fissures?

   a. anal fissures that are not midline should arouse suspicion for inflammatory bowel disease and cancer
   b. anal fissures generally occur anterior and laterally
   c. pain is worse between defecations, not during
   d. surgery is never required as fissures will heal with medical management

38. A 46-year-old woman with past medical history significant for Crohn disease presents with large amounts of watery diarrhea, weight loss, and weakness. Two weeks ago, she had portions of the small bowel including the ileum resected. Physical examination reveals a patient who looks tired, with dry mucous membranes. There are no neurologic deficits. Vital signs reveal the patient to be afebrile but tachycardic. What disorder is occurring?

   a. short bowel syndrome
   b. pernicious anemia
   c. ileus
   d. Crohn exacerbation

39. A 32-year-old man with no past medical history presents with a tender area on his lower back for the past 3 days. The patient states that for the past 3 days, this area has been steadily getting larger and progressively more tender. He has not seen any drainage from the site. He denies any IV drug abuse and has no pain with bowel movements. On physical examination, a 4- by 6-cm fluctuant mass is noted in the lower lumbar and presacral region. The mass is in the midline and very tender to the touch. The patient has good rectal tone. Which of the following is true about this fluctuant painful mass?

   a. this is an intersphincteric abscess; therefore, it must be drained in the operating room
   b. recurrence rates after drainage are very low
   c. an ingrowing hair was the nidus for this formation
   d. this is commonly seen in men above the age of 60

40. Parents bring in a healthy 4-year-old into your emergency room with the complaint that "he just won't sit down." He has no past medical history and is not on any medications. He is in day care currently. On examination you have a well-looking 4-year-old who is running around the examination room with one hand rubbing his buttocks. He denies any pain but nods his head vigorously when you ask him if it itches. He has not had any trouble with bowel movements. On examination of the buttocks, you note numerous excoriations and what looks to be bits of white cotton thread. What treatment is indicated for this patient?

   a. no treatment, just observation
   b. hydrocortisone cream
   c. metronidazole
   d. mebendazole

---

1. Answer: c

This patient has a history and exam consistent with *spontaneous bacterial peritonitis (SBP)*. Discharge on pain medications **(a)** would not be appropriate as it would not be treating the underlying cause. Paracentesis and discharge of the patient to home to await culture results **(b)** is unacceptable as the patient's infection must be treated immediately. Gram stains are only positive 30% to 40% of the time, making **(d)** incorrect as patients can have SBP with a negative Gram stain. The correct answer is **(c)**, where a paracentesis is done and empiric antibiotics are started.

2. Answer: c

A *meat bolus* should not remain impacted for longer than 12 hours, and endoscopy is the preferred method of removal **(a)**. The use of proteolytic enzymes such as meat tenderizer is not recommended secondary to the possibility of esophageal perforation **(b)**. IV administration of glucagon **(c)** to relax the esophageal smooth muscle may be successful but a test dose should be given to ensure hypersensitivity does not exist. A follow-up esophagogram should be performed after medical treatment to ensure passage of the food bolus. Ten milligrams of sublingual **(d)** nifedipine may be successful in relieving the obstruction by reducing the lower-esophageal sphincter pressure.

3. Answer: c

Boerhaave syndrome is a full-thickness perforation of the distal esophagus, most commonly on the left side. Patients are generally ill appearing with neck/chest pain and respiratory distress (b). **Misdiagnosis** may occur in up to 50% of cases (c). The CXR is abnormal up to 90% of the time (a) with pleural effusion, pneumomediastinum, pneumothorax, or pneumoperitoneum. Treatment includes supportive care, broad-spectrum antibiotics, and timely operative repair (d).

4. Answer: b

Adhesions (b) caused by multiple abdominal surgeries are the most common cause of small-bowel obstruction. Incarcerated **hernias (a)** are the second most common cause, with **gallstone ileus (d)** being a rare cause. **Cancer (c),** although the most common cause of large-bowel obstructions is not a common cause of small-bowel obstruction.

5. Answer: b

Indirect inguinal hernias are the most common abdominal-wall hernias, occur more frequently in men on the right side and frequently incarcerate and strangulate, particularly in the first year of life (b). **Direct inguinal hernias (a)** are acquired defects, do not pass through the inguinal canal, occur mainly in adults, and rarely incarcerate. **Femoral hernias (c)** occur more commonly in women but much less commonly than inguinal hernias. **Umbilical hernias (d)** occur more commonly in children and frequently spontaneously heal within the first 4 years of life.

6. Answer: c

Esophageal varices develop in up to 60% of patients with chronic liver disease from portal hypertension. Therapy includes supportive treatment for GI bleed (two large-bore IVs, volume resuscitation, correct coagulopathy, transfusion of blood products as needed), consideration of early airway management (a), vasoactive medication such as somatostatin or octreotide (b) (they cause relaxation of mesenteric vascular smooth muscle, reducing portal venous pressure without arterial vasospasm), and empiric antibiotic therapy to cover enteric organisms (c). Balloon tamponade is an option if pharmacologic agents are failing and endoscopy is unavailable. Endoscopic evaluation provides definitive diagnosis and allows for ligation/sclerotherapy (d). Endoscopy has been shown to reduce mortality in some studies.

7. Answer: c

Household bleach is generally not corrosive to the esophagus (c). Strong acid ingestion (a) causes coagulation necrosis, mainly of the esophagus and stomach whereas strong alkali ingestion (b) causes liquefaction necrosis, mainly affecting the esophagus. Blind nasotracheal intubation, passage of a nasogastric tube (d), charcoal, dilution/neutralization therapy should all be avoided in the setting of a caustic ingestion.

8. Answer: a

Pediatric patients account for up to 80% of all cases of foreign body ingestions, and most pediatric obstructions are in the proximal esophagus, specifically at the cricopharyngeal narrowing (a). The majority of adult obstructions occur in the distal esophagus (b). Button batteries lodged in the esophagus should be removed within 6 hours to avoid erosion through the esophageal mucosa (c). The following are indications for endoscopic consultation (d) with regards to foreign body ingestions: sharp or elongated foreign bodies, multiple foreign bodies, button batteries, evidence of perforation, child who ingests a coin that is lodged at the level of the cricopharyngeus muscle, airway compromise, and presence of foreign body for greater than 24 hours.

9. Answer: b

The CT scan finding of a low-attenuation lesion with ring enhancement in the liver is describing a liver abscess. The patient's symptoms of abdominal cramping, diarrhea, and liver abscess are consistent with **amebiasis (b)**. **Fitz–Hugh–Curtis syndrome (a)** is a complication of PID and can cause RUQ pain and "violin strings" of adhesion on the liver, but not a liver abscess. **Cholangitis (c)** is the constellation of fever, right upper quadrant pain, and jaundice. These symptoms do not last for a few weeks and the patients are very sick. **Schistosomiasis (d)** is caused by a flatworm found in the tropics, causes dermatitis at point of entry in the skin, lymphadenopathy, and hepatomegaly. It does not cause liver abscess.

10. Answer: c

The constellation of symptoms including low-grade fever, left lower quadrant pain, vomiting, and heme-positive stools is consistent with the clinical entity of *diverticulitis*. Patients with fiber-deficient diets are prone to diverticulosis and diverticulitis (a). Diverticulitis can occur on the right side, mimicking appendicitis (b). CT of the abdomen/pelvis is the diagnostic study of choice for diverticulitis, not ultrasound (d). Treatment of diverticulitis includes broad-spectrum coverage against aerobes and anaerobes (c). Generally metronidazole and a fluoroquinolone are used.

11. Answer: d

ALT (serum glutamic oxaloacetic transaminase [SGOT])/AST (serum glutamic pyruvic transaminase [SGPT]) (a) are indicators of hepatocellular injury and death. **Alkaline phosphatase (b)** elevation is associated with biliary obstruction and cholestasis—or with bony disease. Hepatocyte catabolic activity is reflected by direct/indirect **bilirubin (c)**. Hepatocyte synthetic function is reflected by **prothrombin time** and albumin (d).

12. Answer: a

Hepatic encephalopathy probably results from the accumulation of nitrogenous waste products normally metabolized by the liver and is a diagnosis of exclusion. Other causes for altered mental status must be ruled out including: intracranial pathology, hypoglycemia, nutritional deficiencies, electrolyte imbalances, medication side effects, and sepsis. There are four stages of hepatic encephalopathy: apathy, lethargy/drowsiness, stupor, and coma (a). Serum ammonia levels do not correlate with the severity of encephalopathy (b). Gastrointestinal bleeding and TIPS procedures are common precipitants of hepatic encephalopathy (c). Medical treatment includes lactulose (d) (traps ammonia in GI tract and excretes in stool), and neomycin (may be beneficial by directly inhibiting bacterial growth and protein metabolism).

13. Answer: b

The treatment for *viral hepatitis* is generally supportive, but the following are indications for admission: severe fluid and electrolyte abnormalities (a), persistent vomiting (b), altered mental status, prolongation of PT beyond 5 seconds of normal (d), immunosuppression, and hypoglycemia. Altered mental status and prolongation of PT are suggestive of potential liver failure.

14. Answer: a

Hepatic encephalopathy is thought to occur secondary to an accumulation of nitrogenous waste products normally metabolized by the liver. Hepatic encephalopathy is a diagnosis of exclusion, and multiple other causes for change in mental status must be excluded even in the setting of an elevated ammonia level (d). Cirrhotic patients have decreased glycogen stores and impaired gluconeogenesis, thereby increasing their risk for hypoglycemia (b). Patients with end-stage liver disease are often coagulopathic and at risk for spontaneous intracranial hemorrhages (c). Other causes of altered mental status must be ruled out, including electrolyte deficiencies, sepsis, and drug side effects. Gastrointestinal bleeding commonly precipitates hepatic encephalopathy; therefore, a GI bleed must be considered in this patient (a).

15. Answer: c

The ileum is the most common portion of bowel involved in *Crohn disease,* which is why another name for the disease is terminal ileitis. Continuous involvement of bowel wall (a) and involvement of only the mucosa and submucosa (b) are features of another type of inflammatory bowel disease: ulcerative colitis. Crohn has skip lesions and involves all layers of the bowel wall. Weakening of the bowel wall at the insertion of blood vessels (d) is seen in diverticulosis.

16. Answer: d

The following individuals should receive *Hepatitis A* immunoglobulin (0.02 mL/kg IM): all household and sexual contacts of persons *confirmed* with HAV (a, b), employees and children of day-care facilities

caring for children in diapers if one or more cases of HAV develops among staff, or only classroom contacts in elementary children (c, d). Infected individual with HAV should practice meticulous hygiene and not return to work (especially if food handler) until jaundice resolves.

17. Answer: b

The classic patient with *biliary colic* is the obese woman aged 20 to 40 years. Increased age and pregnancy (among many other risk factors) are risk factors for the development of gallstones (a). The pain is more frequent than colicky, and is not related to eating in up to 33% of patients (c). The pain typically lasts 2 to 6 hours (d). Prolonged pain should raise the suspicion for cholecystitis. Cholesterol stones are most common, with brown/black pigment stones second most common (b).

18. Answer: b

Hepatitis A is spread by the fecal–oral route and is generally clinically occult in children, and rarely causes liver failure. Common sources include contaminated water/food supplies, day care centers, and raw shellfish. (a), Metastatic cancer to liver is much more common in United States from tumors of the GI tract, lung, and breast, but worldwide, HBV is related to the development of a hepatoma in 75% to 90% of cases (b). Chronic liver disease results in up to 85% of cases of HCV (c). Hepatitis D infection depends on concomitant or preexisting chronic infection with HBV (d).

19. Answer: c

Hepatitis C is classically linked to blood transfusions but also commonly transmitted via intravenous drug abuse (IVDA) and occupational exposure (c). **Hepatitis A** is spread by the fecal–oral route. (a). **Hepatitis B** is generally spread through serum/bodily secretions, with highest rates among drug abusers and homosexual men (b). **Hepatitis E** is enterically spread and is responsible for up to 50% of cases of acute viral hepatitis in some developing countries such as Sudan, Iraq, and Mexico (d).

20. Answer: d

Cecal volvulus is usually treated by attempting barium enema with surgery required if the barium enema fails. The cecal volvulus is too proximal for endoscopic or colonoscopic reduction. Patients with cecal volvulus are typically in their 30s and 40s. Sigmoid volvulus patients are generally in their 70s and 80s (a). Patients with neurologic and psychiatric disorders (b) are associated with a sigmoid volvulus. A plain-film radiograph will make the diagnosis of cecal volvulus only 50% of the time (c).

21. Answer: d

Perianal and perirectal abscesses are generally polymicrobial with aerobes and anaerobes. Perianal abscesses can be drained in the ED; however, perirectal abscesses should be drained in the operating suite **(a)**. Patients with perirectal and intersphincteric abscesses typically will not allow rectal examination secondary to exquisite pain **(b)**. Patients with perianal abscesses do not require antibiotics unless there is an accompanying cellulitis present or the patient is immunocompromised **(c)**.

22. Answer: c

Previously vaccinated workers who are known responders to the Hepatitis B vaccine series and exposed to source HBsAg+ blood/body secretions require no treatment **(a)**. Previously vaccinated workers who are known nonresponders should receive one dose of HBIG and reinitiate the vaccine series if they have not completed a second three-dose vaccine series **(c)**. For individuals who completed a second vaccine series and fail to respond, two doses of HBIG are preferred. Previously vaccinated workers who do not know their antibody response should have their blood tested for antibody to Hepatitis B surface antigen (anti-HBs). If adequate levels, no treatment; otherwise administer HBIG x1 and vaccine booster **(b, d)**.

23. Answer: a

Yersinia can cause fever, watery diarrhea that becomes bloody, and RLQ tenderness that will mimic appendicitis. *Campylobacter* **(b)** is known to cause fever and generalized abdominal pain. *Salmonella* **(c)** can cause typhoid fever with a relative bradycardia and high fever. *Shigella* **(d)** causes a high fever, bloody diarrhea, and febrile seizures in children.

24. Answer: a

This patient has signs and symptoms of *mesenteric ischemia*. She has pain out of proportion to physical findings. She also has the risk factors of increased age and atrial fibrillation that are common in mesenteric ischemia. That makes choices **(d)** and **(e)** incorrect. Abdominal aortic aneurysms classically present with a pulsatile mass or bruit on auscultation. Aortic dissection typically presents with ripping chest pain, and pain can migrate into abdomen as dissection progresses. Typically patients have high blood pressure. With her history of atrial fibrillation, choice **(a)** becomes correct as atrial fibrillation is a significant risk factor for arterial embolism causing mesenteric ischemia. The main arterial thrombus **(b)** risk factor is atherosclerosis, and food can precipitate pain (bowel angina). Venous thrombus **(c)** patients generally have a history of deep-vein thrombosis (DVT) or pulmonary embolism (PE).

25. Answer: a

The reversal of hot and cold sensation, loose painful teeth, paresthesias, vomiting, and diarrhea are characteristic of *Ciguatera,* which is found in coral reef fish. *Scombroid* **(b)** is linked to dark-fleshed fish such as tuna and mackerel and causes flushing, vomiting, and diarrhea. *Vibrio cholera* **(c)** is noted for its rice-water stools, but does not cause

paresthesias. *Giardia lamblia* **(d)** is commonly referred to as backpacker's diarrhea as people who hike or camp and drink water from a stream are at higher risk. Patients with giardiasis commonly have abdominal cramping and diarrhea.

26. Answer: b

This patient's symptoms of palpitations, diarrhea, and facial flushing after eating at a seafood restaurant are consistent with *scombroid toxicity*. The patient most likely ate a dark-meat fish such as tuna or mahi-mahi. Treatment for this is **diphenhydramine (b)** or an H$_2$-blocker. **Epinephrine (a)** is used in anaphylactic reactions, which this patient is not having. **Mannitol (c)** can be used in ciguatera ingestion. **Antibiotics (d)** and **(e)** are not indicated as this is not an infectious etiology.

27. Answer: c

Strongyloides stercoralis causes a serpiginous urticarial rash along with chronic watery diarrhea, especially in patients who are immunocompromised. *Enterobius vermicularis* **(a)** causes extreme pruritus near the anus in children. *Necator americanus* **(b)** is also known as hookworm and causes a hypochromic, microcytic anemia. *Dracunculus medinensis* **(d)** is a long worm that migrates from the gastrointestinal (GI) tract into the skin with complications of cellulitis and abscess.

28. Answer: a

Acalculous cholecystitis accounts for approximately 5% to 10% of patients with acute cholecystitis. Patients at higher risk include children, elderly people, diabetics, multiple-trauma victims, multiple-burn victims, and AIDS patients **(b, c, d)**. Acalculous cholecystitis generally has a more rapid and malignant course.

29. Answer: c

Acute cholangitis (c) results from complete biliary obstruction in the presence of bacteria. Charcot's triad of fever, jaundice, and right upper quadrant (RUQ) pain presents in about 25% of patients with cholangitis. **Cholelithiasis (a)** presents with RUQ/ epigastric pain with nausea/vomiting that resolves in 2 to 6 hours. **Acute cholecystitis** presents with RUQ/ epigastric pain, nausea, vomiting, pain longer than 6 hours, fever, and Murphy sign **(b)**. **Pancreatitis** classically presents with mid-epigastric abdominal pain radiating to the back with associated vomiting **(d)**.

30. Answer: d

This patient has *Helicobacter pylori,* which can cause gastritis and ulcers. The common treatment is to be on "triple therapy," such as clarithromycin, amoxicillin, and omeprazole or bismuth subsalicylate, metronidazole, and tetracycline. Statement **(a)** is incorrect to simply assume the patient does not have an infection and all will be well if he takes Maalox. Statement **(b)** is incorrect as *H. pylori* does increase the risk of gastric adenocarcinoma. There are no quick, practical tests that can be done in the ED to diagnose *H. pylori* (**c**). Statement (**d**) is correct in that 60% to 70% of gastric ulcers are caused by *H. pylori*, but not all infected people develop ulcers.

31. Answer: c

Prognostic markers such as *Ranson criteria* are used to predict mortality in acute pancreatitis. The five criteria on admission reflect the degree of local inflammation: age >55, Blood sugar >200 mg/dL, WBC >16,000/L, AST >250 units/L, and LDH >350 IU/L (**a, c, d, and e**). The six criteria at 48 hours note the development of systemic complications. The absolute level of amylase/lipase does not correlate to severity of disease (**b**).

32. Answer: b

Seventy percent to 80% of cases of *chronic pancreatitis* results from alcohol abuse. Clinically significant malabsorption does not occur until >90% of pancreatic glandular function is lost (**d**). The hallmark symptom is abdominal pain but up to 10% of patients may present without abdominal pain (**c**). No criterion standard test exists to distinguish acute from chronic pancreatitis, and amylase/lipase levels may be normal when pancreatic fibrosis is advanced (**a**). Pancreatic calcifications may be present on plain radiographs (**b**), and a CT scan of the abdomen may be indicated to identify complications such as abscess and pseudocyst (occurs in up to 25% of chronic pancreatitis patients). Treatment involves supportive care and patients may be discharged once complications have been ruled out and adequate pain control is accomplished.

33. Answer: d

The symptoms of this patient are seen in *large-bowel obstructions*. Generally patients with colon cancer are more prone to large-bowel obstructions. Patients will have a severely distended abdomen, and occasionally can have feculent emesis because of the distal location of a large-bowel obstruction. Radiographs will reveal dilated loops of bowel in the periphery with haustra that do not involve the entire diameter of bowel. Small-bowel obstructions will show bowel dilation in the center of the abdomen with lines (plicae circulares) involving the entire bowel diameter (**b**). The most common cause of large-bowel obstructions is cancer while adhesions most commonly cause small-bowel obstruction (**a**). Patients with obstruction must not eat and be NPO (**c**). Large enough bowel distension can cause vascular compromise, leading to bowel infarction and perforation (**d**).

34. Answer: a

Alcohol abuse and gallstones are the two most common causes of *acute pancreatitis* in the United States (**a**). Other causes include drugs, infections, trauma, scorpion bites, metabolic disturbances. The absolute level of serum amylase/lipase does not correlate to the severity of disease (**b**). A few prognostic markers such as Ranson criteria and the Apache-II score are used to predict mortality. Serum lipase has a higher specificity as compared to amylase for pancreatitis (**c**). Complication from pancreatitis include pulmonary effusion, acute respiratory distress syndrome (ARDS), myocardial depression, hypocalcemia, hyperglycemia, hyperlipidemia, coagulopathy, renal failure, abscess, and pseudocyst (**d**).

35. Answer: c

Angiography is the gold standard for diagnosis of *mesenteric ischemia* and treatment can be administered during the procedure via the delivery of papaverine. Lactate (**a**) is sensitive, but is NOT specific for mesenteric ischemia as elevations of lactate can be seen in sepsis. A negative CT scan of the abdomen/pelvis (**b**) does not rule out mesenteric ischemia and surgery consultation with angiography must be sought if suspicion is still high for the diagnosis. Only a quarter of patients have occult blood on testing of their stools in mesenteric ischemia (**d**).

36. Answer: d

Pseudomembranous colitis is caused by *Clostridium difficile*, which is an anaerobic Gram-positive bacillus. Vancomycin and metronidazole, while treatments for pseudomembranous colitis, can also cause it, making (**a**) incorrect. It is commonly diagnosed by detecting the *C. difficile* **toxin** in the stool, not culture of the stool (**b**). Symptoms of diarrhea and abdominal cramping usually occur 5 to 10 days after the initiation of an antibiotic, not 1 to 2 days (**c**).

37. Answer: a

Anal fissures are generally midline and posterior, not anterior and lateral (**b**). Anal fissures that are not midline should raise suspicion for inflammatory bowel diseases such as Crohn disease and cancer (leukemia) (**a**). Pain is worse during defecations and relieved between bowel movements (**c**). Fissures that do not heal require surgery (**d**).

38. Answer: a

The signs and symptoms of copious amounts of watery diarrhea, weight loss, fatigue, and signs of dehydration via the dry mucous membranes and tachycardia are indicative of (**a**) **short-bowel syndrome.** This can occur a few days following resection of small bowel and can last for months. **Pernicious anemia (b)** is incorrect. While the resection of the terminal ileum can lead to vitamin B_{12} malabsorption, pernicious anemia involves autoantibodies destroying the cells that make intrinsic factor necessary for B_{12} absorption. Resection of bowel is not consistent with pernicious anemia. **Ileus (c)** can be seen following surgery, but symptoms of abdominal distension, vomiting, and cramping are common, which are not seen in this patient. **Crohn** exacerbation (d) is also incorrect as abdominal pain and bloody diarrhea are generally seen.

39. Answer: c

This patient has a *pilonidal abscess*. They usually occur in men under the age of 40, making (d) incorrect. They are midline, fluctuant, exquisitely tender, and located in the lower lumbar or presacral area. The symptoms are not consistent with an intersphincteric abscess as the patient has no pain with bowel movements and allowed a rectal examination to occur (a). Recurrence rates are high for pilonidal abscess (b). An ingrown hair is the most common nidus for causing a pilonidal abscess (c).

40. Answer: d

The symptoms of *pruritus ani* in a 4-year-old are consistent of an infection by a pinworm, or *Enterobius vermicularis*. Occasionally, an adult worm can be seen in the anal area via eyesight alone and will appear to be bits of white thread. **Mebendazole (d)** can help eradicate pinworms. The other options, (a, b, c) are not correct and will not help eradicate this infection.

Cardiovascular I

Robert L. Rogers

2

RHYTHM

Rhythm

NORMAL SINUS

- Rate is 60 to 100 beats per minute (bpm)
- Rhythm originates in the sinus node (P before each QRS)

SINUS ARRHYTHMIA (Fig. 2-1)

- Normal variant most commonly due to respiratory variation
- More common with slower heart rates
- Usually requires no therapy

SINUS BRADYCARDIA

- Sinus rhythm with rate <60 bpm
- Seen in asymptomatic patients as well as in disease states such as drug overdose, hypothyroidism, and myocardial infarction
- May be treated with atropine or pacemaker if symptomatic or hemodynamically unstable

SINUS TACHYCARDIA

- Sinus rhythm with rate >100 bpm
- Usually indicative of underlying disease such as fever, toxin, hypovolemia, sepsis, pulmonary embolism, or hyperthyroidism
- Treatment aimed at the underlying cause of the tachycardia

JUNCTIONAL ESCAPE RHYTHM (JUNCTIONAL BRADYCARDIA) (Fig. 2-2)

- Escape rhythm whereby the atrioventricular (AV) node takes over as pacemaker
- Rate usually 40 to 60 bpm
- P waves usually absent (may occur before, during, or after QRS complex)
- Narrow QRS complex unless accompanying intraventricular conduction delay present

VENTRICULAR ESCAPE RHYTHM

- Ectopic focus in the ventricle
- Rate usually 20 to 40 bpm
- P waves absent and QRS complexes wide

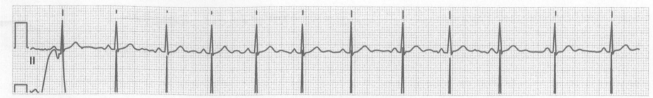

Figure 2-1 Sinus arrhythmia

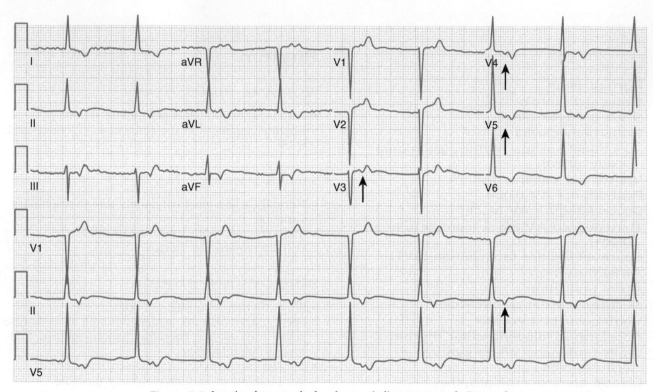

Figure 2-2 Junctional escape rhythm (*arrows* indicates retrograde P waves)

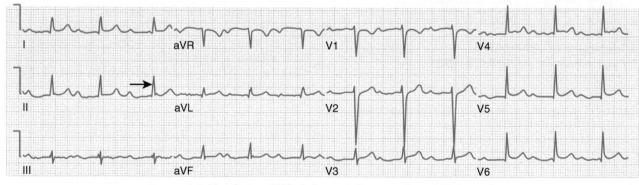

Figure 2-3 First-degree AV block (*arrow* indicates prolonged PR interval)

FIRST-DEGREE AV BLOCK (Fig. 2-3)

- Usually an asymptomatic rhythm
- Characterized by a prolonged PR interval (>0.2 second)
- Causes include AV-blocking medications (e.g., beta-adrenergic blockers, calcium-channel blockers, digoxin)
- Usually requires no specific therapy

SECOND-DEGREE AV BLOCK

Type I (Mobitz I or Wenckebach) (Fig. 2-4)

- Progressively increasing PR interval followed by a nonconducted P wave (P without QRS)
- Associated with inferior myocardial infarction
- Treatment is with atropine or pacemaker if patient is unstable

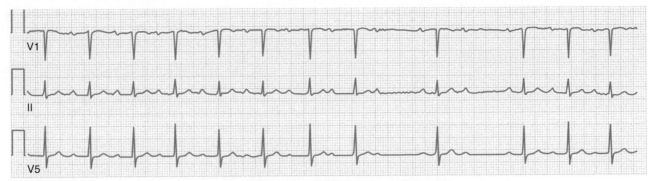

Figure 2-4 Second-degree AV block, type I

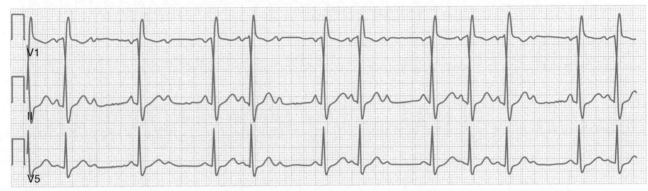

Figure 2-5 Second-degree AV block, type II

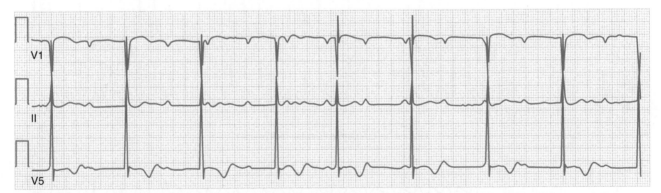

Figure 2-6 Third-degree AV block

- May progress to third-degree AV block but usually resolves

Type II (Mobitz II) (Fig. 2-5)

- Spontaneous development of nonconducted P waves without increasing PR interval
- Associated with anterior myocardial infarction
- More likely to progress to complete heart block
- Pacemaker is treatment of choice

THIRD-DEGREE AV BLOCK
(COMPLETE HEART BLOCK) (Fig. 2-6)

- PP intervals constant; RR intervals constant; PR intervals randomly vary
- Complete AV dissociation—all complete heart block features AV dissociation, but not all AV

dissociation is due to complete heart block (e.g., ventricular tachycardia also features dissociation of atria and ventricles)
- Wide QRS complexes often with anterior myocardial infarction
- Pacemaker is treatment of choice in the setting of MI or hemodynamic instability

SUPRAVENTRICULAR TACHYCARDIA (SVT) (Fig. 2-7)

- Regular, narrow-complex tachycardia
- May see retrograde P waves following the QRS complex
- Usually caused by a reentrant circuit
- QRS complex may be wide if there is a bundle-branch block and may simulate ventricular tachycardia

- Treatment is with vagal maneuvers, adenosine, beta-adrenergic blockers, calcium-channel blockers
- If unstable, treat with synchronized cardioversion

ATRIAL FLUTTER (Fig. 2-8)

- Atrial rate of 250 to 350 (usually about 300) bpm
- Characteristic saw tooth configuration (lead II and V1 best)

- 2:1 conduction (most common) generally produces a ventricular rate of 150 bpm; narrow-complex tachycardia at a rate of 150 is atrial flutter until proven otherwise
- May look like atrial fibrillation, particularly if AV conduction varies
- Treatment of the stable patient is with beta-adrenergic blockers, calcium channel blockers, or digoxin (for rate control)
- Unstable patients should undergo synchronized cardioversion

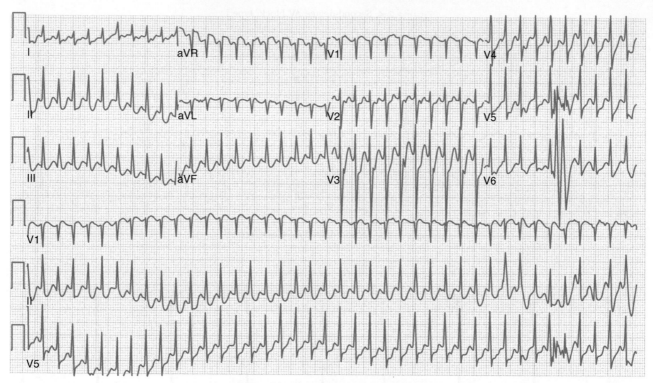

Figure 2-7 Supraventricular tachycardia

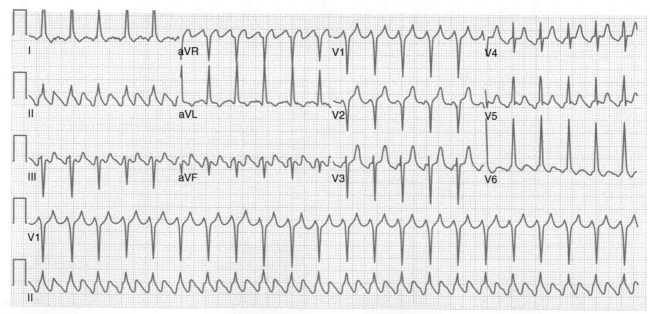

Figure 2-8 Atrial flutter, 2:1 conduction

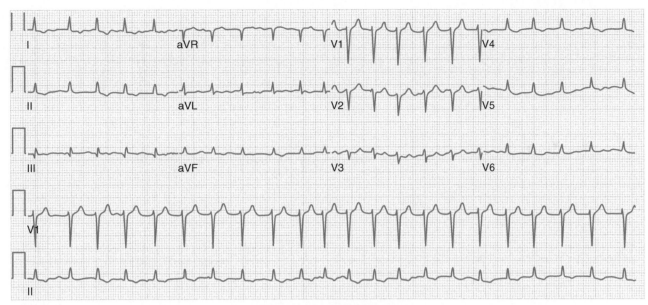

Figure 2-9 Atrial fibrillation

ATRIAL FIBRILLATION (Fig. 2-9)

- Irregularly, irregular rhythm with no identifiable P waves
- Most common chronic arrhythmia
- Chaotic atrial rate (>300 to 350 bpm)
- Causes include hypertension, valvular heart disease, alcohol ("holiday heart"), hyperthyroidism, and coronary artery disease
- Treatment for stable patients centers on rate control, and includes AV nodal blocking drugs like beta-adrenergic blockers, calcium-channel blockers, and digoxin
- Perform cardioversion if the patient is unstable

MULTIFOCAL ATRIAL TACHYCARDIA (Fig. 2-10)

- Characterized by P waves with at least three different morphologies
- Most commonly caused by underlying pulmonary disease (chronic obstructive pulmonary disease)
- Treat underlying condition

VENTRICULAR TACHYCARDIA

- Regular, wide-complex tachyarrhythmia

Monomorphic (Fig. 2-11)

- Regular, wide-complex tachycardia
- Rate always >120 bpm
- Causes include myocardial infarction, drug overdose, hypoxia, and electrolyte abnormalities
- Treatment: (if stable) may administer antiarrhythmic (procainamide, lidocaine, amiodarone) or may elect synchronized cardioversion
- If unstable, immediate cardioversion
- Treatment of underlying cause

Polymorphic (Fig. 2-12)

- Ventricular tachycardia with varying QRS morphologies
- Torsade de pointes is a variant of polymorphic ventricular tachycardia
- Treatment of choice: cardioversion

ACCELERATED IDIOVENTRICULAR RHYTHM (AIVR) (Fig. 2-13)

- A "reperfusion arrhythmia" seen in patients with acute myocardial infarction
- Wide-complex rhythm with a rate between 40 and 120 bpm; rate is generally around 100 bpm
- No specific therapy indicated, as is usually transient
- Key pitfall: avoid treating like ventricular tachycardia
- Antiarrhythmic therapy may precipitate ventricular fibrillation and is contraindicated

WOLFF PARKINSON WHITE SYNDROME ARRHYTHMIAS (Fig. 2-14)

- Presence of accessory bypass tract (bundle of Kent)
- Delta waves (slurred upstroke of QRS complex), short PR interval, and wide QRS
- Patients predisposed to atrial tachycardias, especially supraventricular tachycardia and atrial fibrillation

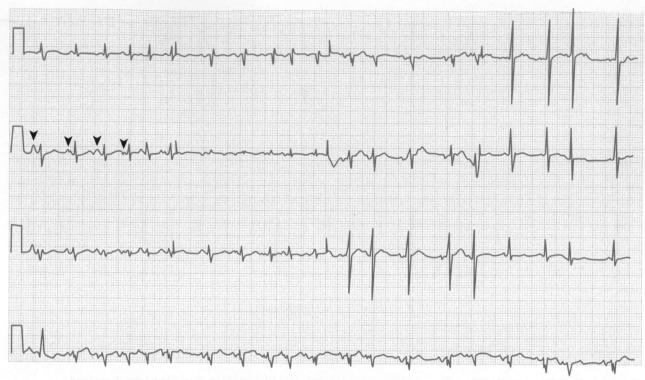

Figure 2-10 Multifocal atrial tachycardia

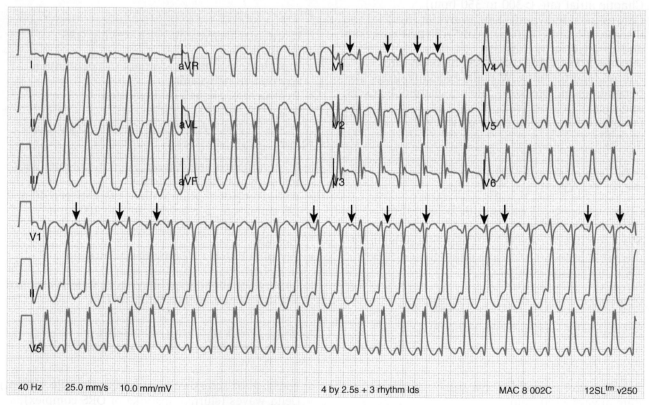

| 40 Hz | 25.0 mm/s | 10.0 mm/mV | | 4 by 2.5s + 3 rhythm lds | MAC 8 002C | 12SL^{tm} v250 |

Figure 2-11 Monomorphic ventricular tachycardia

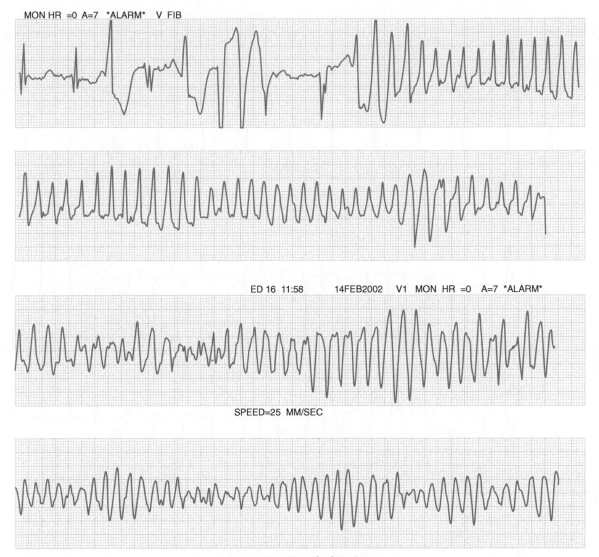

Figure 2-12 Torsade de pointes

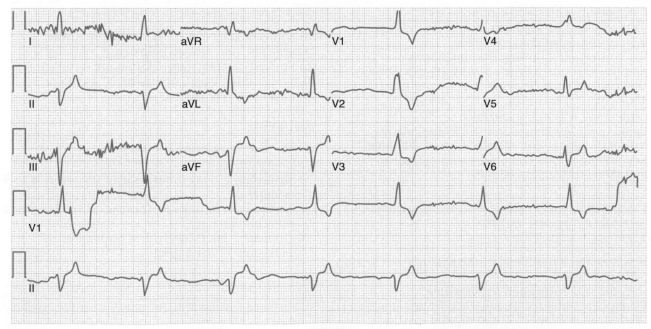

Figure 2-13 Accelerated idioventricular rhythm

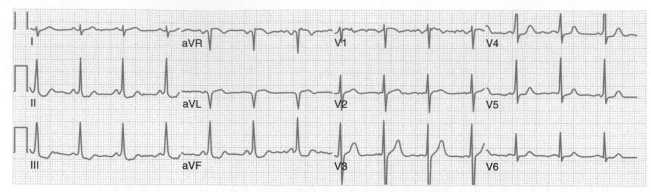

Figure 2-14 Wolff Parkinson White syndrome

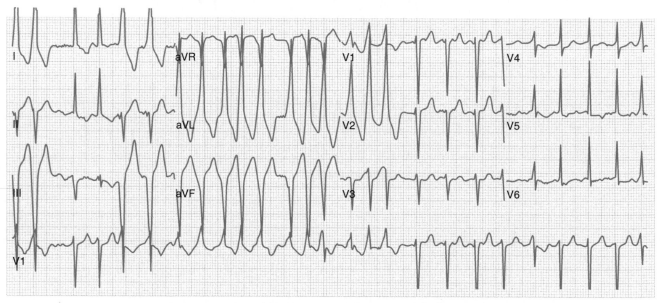

Figure 2-15 Atrial fibrillation in Wolff Parkinson White syndrome

- Can present with narrow-complex SVT (orthodromic) or wide-complex SVT (antidromic), which are treated conventionally
- Key arrhythmia to recognize: *rapid atrial fibrillation in the setting of WPW* (Fig. 2-15)—(1) avoid all AV node blocking drugs when this is suspected; (2) treatment options include cardioversion and procainamide
- Rapid atrial fibrillation and WPW: irregularly, irregular rhythm with rates as high as 300 bpm. Key finding is QRS complexes with changing morphologies/varying widths

CLASSIC ELECTROCARDIOGRAPHIC ASSOCIATIONS WITH UNDERLYING DISEASE

- U waves and hypokalemia (although not pathognomonic)
- Osborne or J waves and hypothermia
- Paroxysmal atrial tachycardia/accelerated junctional rhythm/bidirectional VT and digoxin toxicity

CARDIAC ARREST RHYTHMS

All with simultaneous consideration of airway, oxygenation, and cardiac pulmonary resuscitation (CPR; chest compressions 100/minute; ventilate 8 to 10/minute if intubated; otherwise 30:2 ratio of compressions/ventilations)

Asystole

- "Flat line" in two or more leads
- Pharmacotherapy
  - Epinephrine 1 mg intravenously (IV) every 3 to 5 minutes *or*
  - Vasopressin 40 units IV (instead of 1st/2nd doses epinephrine)
  - Atropine 1 mg IV every 3 to 5 minutes, maximum of 0.4 mg/kg

Pulseless electrical activity (PEA)

- Organized rhythm without pulse; treat underlying cause

- Pharmacotherapy as with asystole; consider atropine for bradycardic PEA
- Consider causes: "6 Hs and 5 Ts"
  - Hypoxia, hypovolemia, hyper/hypokalemia, hypothermia, hydrogen ion (acidosis), hypoglycemia
  - Tamponade, toxin, trauma, tension pneumothorax, thrombosis (pulmonary embolism, myocardial infarction [MI])

Ventricular fibrillation

- Chaotic rhythm with no discernible waves
- Nonperfusing rhythm
- Treatment is immediate defibrillation followed by antiarrhythmics if successful
- Defibrillation: 120-200 J (biphasic) or 360 J (monophasic) followed by 2 minutes of CPR, then repeat as needed
- Vasopressors (same as asystole/PEA)
- Antiarrhythmics
  - Amiodarone 300 mg IV (may repeat 150 mg once)
  - Lidocaine 1 to 1.5 mg/kg IV (repeat half that dose as needed to a maximum of 3 mg/kg)
  - Magnesium 1 to 2 g IV (if suspect torsade)
  - Drugs via endotracheal tube, if no IV/intraosseous (IO) access: "NAVEL" (naloxone, atropine, vasopressin, epinephrine, and lidocaine at 2 to 2.5 times the IV/IO dose)

Acute coronary syndrome/ acute myocardial infarction (AMI)

Acute coronary syndrome—a spectrum of disease characterized by rupture of coronary artery plaques resulting in myocardial ischemia

DIAGNOSIS OF AMI/ACS

- Diagnosis made my history, physical examination, and 12-lead electrocardiogram as well as serum biomarkers
- Initial ECG only diagnostic for AMI 25% to 50% of the time
- Normal ECG does not rule out AMI
- Serial ECGs are recommended to capture evolving changes
- ECG findings in ST segment elevation MI (STEMI): ST segment elevation (STE; usually, not always, convex or domed) in addition to reciprocal ST-segment depression; earliest change may be hyperacute T waves followed by STEMI
- Decision to admit should not be solely based on results of serum biomarkers but the history obtained from the patient
- Serum markers of AMI: CK-MB, myoglobin, and troponin (I or T)
  - **Myoglobin** rises in 1 to 3 hours, peaks in 5 to 7 hours, and remains elevated for <1 day

- **CK-MB** rises in 3 to 10 hours, peaks in about 18 to 24 hours, and remains elevated for 2 to 3 days
- **Troponins** (I and T) rise in 3 to 6 hours, peak in 12 to 18 hours, and stay elevated for up to 7 to 10 days
- Troponin specificity and prognostic value
  - Most specific cardiac marker available
  - Troponin I also elevated in some non-ACS conditions (e.g., myopericarditis, CHF, LVH, blunt cardiac trauma) as well as noncardiac conditions (e.g., pulmonary embolism, pulmonary hypertension, chemotherapy, sepsis, renal insufficiency)
  - Elevated troponins in non-ACS conditions: poorer prognosis

TREATMENT OF AMI/ACS—ED CONSIDERATIONS

- Therapy dictated by point-in-time on ACS continuum; ECG findings
- Aspirin (chewable)—administer 162 to 325 milligrams
- Clopidogrel may be given if the patient is allergic to aspirin
  - Higher doses (e.g., 300-600 mg orally) are given to patients prior to percutaneous coronary intervention (PCI)
  - Antiplatelet agent; works by inhibiting ADP-mediated platelet aggregation
- Glycoprotein receptor antagonists (GP IIb/IIIa receptor antagonists)
  - Intravenous platelet inhibitors generally reserved for patients with ACS and troponin elevation in whom PCI is planned
  - Agents include abciximab, eptifibatide, and tirofiban
- Unfractionated heparin (UFH) indicated for all patients with ACS (STEMI, NSTEMI, unstable angina)
  - Acts as an indirect thrombin inhibitor by promoting the action of antithrombin III and is complementary to the effects of aspirin
- Low-molecular-weight heparin (LMWH; e.g. enoxaparin)
  - An alternative to UFH
- Nitroglycerin
  - Limits infarct size; reduces myocardial oxygen demand
  - May be given sublingually or intravenously
  - Contraindicated in patients with hypotension
  - Contraindicated in patients taking medications for erectile dysfunction (for 24 hours after sildenafil; for 48 hours after tadalafil)
  - May precipitate hypotension in cases of inferior MI complicated by right ventricular infarction; usually responsive to IV fluid bolus
- Beta-adrenergic blockers
  - Current guidelines no longer emphasize administration of these agents in ED
  - May give for tachycardia if necessary; may give orally
  - Avoid in cocaine-induced MI

- Morphine
  - May be given for pain relief but not first-line agent
- Fibrinolysis: many different agents available
  - Streptokinase (SK); tissue plasminogen activator (TPA, Activase, Alteplase); reteplase (RPA, Reptilase, Retavase) and tenecteplase (TNK)
  - All of these agents convert plasminogen to plasmin which then lyses fibrin
  - Indicated when STEMI (at least 1 mm) is present in two contiguous leads OR a new or presumed new left bundle branch block (LBBB) AND history consistent with AMI
  - Not indicated for ST-segment depression or NSTEMI
  - Contraindications are many, and include prior intracerebral hemorrhage, CNS lesions, recent ischemic stroke, active bleeding, aortic dissection, and pericarditis
  - Relative contraindications numerous—include pregnancy, recent trauma, recent internal bleeding (2 to 4 weeks), major surgery <3 weeks, noncompressible vascular punctures, active peptic ulcer, uncontrolled hypertension, and current use of anticoagulants (INR >2 to 3)
  - Complications: bleeding (especially intracerebral).
- Percutaneous coronary intervention
  - According to the American Heart Association (AHA), the preferred reperfusion modality
  - Not all centers have PCI capability and may need to administer thrombolytic therapy prior to transfer to another center

STEMI AND INFARCT TERRITORY

Anterior (Fig. 2-16)

- STE V1–V4
- Reciprocal ST depression inferiorly (possibly)
- STE V1–V6, I, and aVL = anterolateral
- Usually left anterior descending artery lesion
- More likely to develop AV block and CHF

Lateral

- STE I, aVL, V5 and V6
- Usually left circumflex coronary artery or posterior descending coronary artery lesion

Inferior (Fig. 2-17)

- STE II, III, and aVF
- Reciprocal ST depression in aVL, possibly I
- Usually right coronary artery (STE III >II); less commonly left circumflex (STE III = II)
- Association with right ventricular and/or posterior MI

Right ventricular (Fig. 2-18)

- STE in right-sided precordial leads (maximal V4R)
- Right coronary artery
- High risk for hypotension/shock (decreased preload)

Posterior (Fig. 2-19)

- ST depression V1, V2, possibly V3
- Growth of R wave > S wave V2
- STE posterior leads (V8, V9)

Other causes of STE include: pericarditis, myocarditis, bundle branch block, Prinzmetal angina, early repolarization, left ventricular aneurysm (see below), apical left ventricular ballooning syndrome (Takotsubo cardiomyopathy), and Wolff Parkinson White syndrome.

NON–ST-SEGMENT ELEVATION MYOCARDIAL INFARCTION (NSTEMI)

- ECG may be relatively normal or show ST-segment depression with or without inverted T waves; serum biomarkers are positive
- May progress to STEMI
- Treatment options vary and include aggressive anticoagulation and PCI
- Thrombolytic therapy not indicated

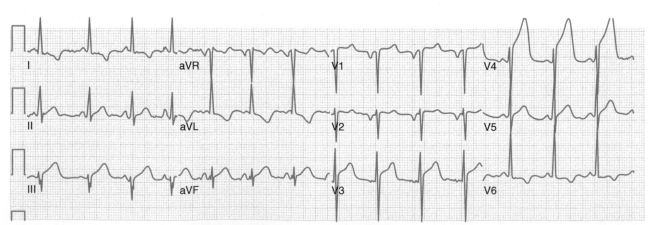

Figure 2-16 Anterior myocardial infarction, acute

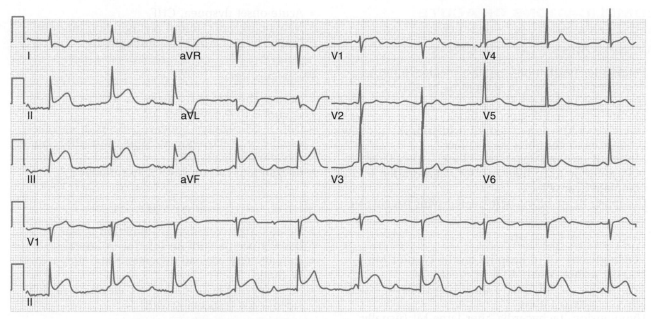

Figure 2-17 Inferior myocardial infarction, acute, with reciprocal ST segment depression

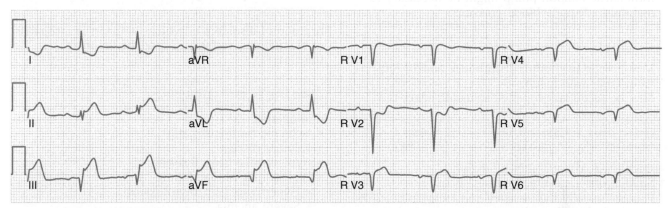

Figure 2-18 Inferior myocardial infarction, acute, with right ventricular involvement (leads RV_1-RV_6 are right-sided)

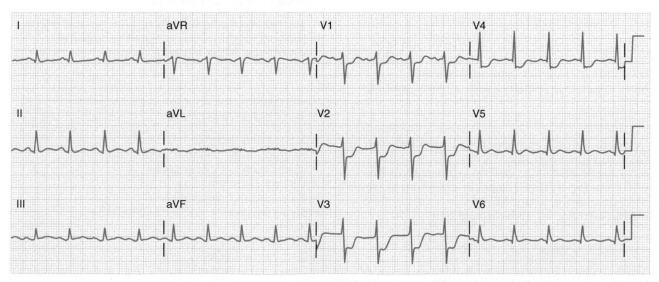

Figure 2-19 Posterior myocardial infarction, acute

COMPLICATIONS OF ACUTE MYOCARDIAL INFARCTION
Arrhythmias and AV block

- Ventricular fibrillation—highest incidence in the first hour after onset of symptoms of AMI
- Ventricular tachycardia
- Mobitz I (second-degree AV block) (Wenckebach)—associated with inferior AMI; rarely progresses to complete heart block
- Mobitz II (second-degree AV block)—associated with anterior AMI; high risk for deterioration into complete heart block
- Complete heart block best treated with pacemaker

Cardiogenic shock

- Leading cause of in-hospital mortality after MI
- Usually occurs when 40% or greater of myocardium is infarcted—most cases due to severe left ventricular failure
- Hypotension, tachycardia after large MI (usually STEMI)
- Treatment involves revascularization
- Intra-aortic balloon pump might be necessary to maintain adequate blood pressure

Congestive heart failure

- May be due to rhythm disturbance and/or left ventricular wall insult
- May be secondary to valvular insufficiency

Free wall rupture (usually fatal, secondary to acute tamponade)

- Occurs 1 to 5 days after infarction
- Sudden onset, severe, "tearing" pain
- Patients usually hypotensive and tachycardic; 20% paradoxical bradycardia
- Diagnosis by echocardiography
- Treatment: immediate surgery

Ventricular septal rupture

- Sudden onset of dyspnea, chest pain, and new holosystolic murmur at the left lower sternal border
- Diagnosis by Doppler echocardiography
- More common in patients with anterior wall MI

Ventricular aneurysm

- Defect in the left ventricular wall (usually) seen in cases of transmural infarction
- Most result from large anterior (transmural) MI
- ECG—characteristic ST-segment elevation; Q waves
- May simulate an acute STEMI
- Diagnosis made by echocardiography

Papillary muscle rupture

- More common in patients with inferoposterior MI
- Usually occurs 3 to 5 days after AMI
- Acute-onset dyspnea, CHF
- New holosystolic mitral regurgitation murmur
- Diagnosis made by echocardiography

Pericarditis

- Occurs after MI in as many as 10% of patients
- Occurs 2 to 4 days after MI
- Diffuse ST-segment concave (scooped) elevation usually with PR-segment depression (PR-segment elevation in lead aVR)
- Intermittent rub on cardiac examination

Right ventricular infarction

- Isolated right ventricular infarction is rare
- Usually occurs with an inferior or lateral wall MI
- Patients very preload-dependent and may require IV fluids
- Most specific ECG finding: ST elevation in right-sided leads (especially V4R)

Congestive Heart Failure (CHF)

A group of disorders in which the heart is incapable of maintaining perfusion for adequate organ function

CAUSES OF CHF

- Idiopathic
- Ischemic cardiomyopathy
- Valvular disease
- Hypertensive heart disease
- High-output cardiac failure
  - Hyperthyroidism/thyrotoxicosis
  - Severe anemia

SYSTOLIC VERSUS DIASTOLIC DYSFUNCTION

- Systolic dysfunction leads to low ejection fraction
- Diastolic dysfunction is related to impaired ventricular filling but with preserved ejection fraction

PRECIPITANTS OF ACUTE EXACERBATIONS

- Myocardial infarction/ischemia
- Acute/chronic valvular dysfunction
- Medication noncompliance
- Dietary indiscretion (salt)
- Endocarditis/myocarditis
- Hypertension
- Anemia
- Hypoxemia
- Tachyarrhythmias
- Acute hemodynamic stress (e.g., infection, trauma, pregnancy)

SIGNS AND SYMPTOMS

- Dyspnea, paroxysmal nocturnal dyspnea (PND), orthopnea, nocturia, cough, weakness and fatigue, anxiety
- Tachypnea, tachycardia, jugular venous distension (JVD), edema, hepatojugular reflux, S3 gallop
- **Chest x-ray findings**
  - Cephalization, pleural effusions, cardiomegaly, Kerley B lines, perihilar, "batwing" infiltrates (especially in acute or "flash" pulmonary edema)
- **Brain-natriuretic peptide (BNP) as a marker of CHF**
  - Released in response to ventricular stretch from volume overload
  - Marker for the presence of CHF
  - BNP released from ventricular myocardium induces smooth muscle relaxation and leads to vasodilatation
  - BNP causes natriuresis and diuresis

DIAGNOSIS

- Often based on clinical findings and chest xray
- Echocardiography
- Incorporation of BNP testing
  - Levels higher than 400 pg/mL highly specific for congestive heart failure
  - BNP levels between 100 to 400 pg/mL are nondiagnostic
  - BNP levels <100 pg/mL effectively rules out CHF

TREATMENT

- Oxygen
- Early application of noninvasive ventilation (CPAP or BiPAP) has been shown to improve outcomes in CPE
- Endotracheal intubation if worsening respiratory fatigue, hypoxemia, or decline in mental status secondary to CO_2 retention
- Nitroglycerin (NTG)
  - At low doses, is a venodilator and reduces preload
  - Increases coronary artery blood flow
  - Given sublingually in a dose of 0.4 mg every 5 to 10 minutes
- Acute afterload reduction—particularly useful if patients have elevated BP
  - Intravenous enalaprilat/sublingual captopril
  - High-dose IV nitroglycerin
  - Nitroprusside
- Diuretics
  - Furosemide
  - Direct venodilator effect
  - Usual starting dose is 40 to 80 mg intravenously
- Morphine sulfate
  - Controversial in current practice
  - Reported to reduce anxiety
  - Many authorities recommend benzodiazepines over morphine

- Hemodynamic treatment: inotropic/vasopressor support
  - Dopamine—preferred agent for persistent shock
  - Dobutamine—an inotrope with vasodilator qualities; indicated if no signs/symptoms of shock are present
  - Amrinone—a phosphodiesterase inhibitor with hemodynamic properties similar to dobutamine
  - Nesiritide—induces a natriuresis and diuresis, but its use is controversial
  - Thrombolytic therapy or PCI is indicated in patients with CPE due to AMI

Cardiomyopathies

DILATED

- Myocardium is dilated and hypertrophied
- Systolic dysfunction
- Most cases idiopathic in nature
- May be caused by chronic cocaine or alcohol toxicity

SIGNS AND SYMPTOMS

- Congestive heart failure

DIAGNOSIS

- ECG: left ventricular hypertrophy; atrial fibrillation and ventricular ectopy common
- Echocardiogram: decreased systolic function and chamber dilatation
- Chest x-ray: classic CHF findings (e.g., cephalization, edema, pleural effusions, cardiomegaly)

TREATMENT

- Diuretic therapy, nitrates, angiotensin-converting enzyme inhibitors (ACEI) beta-adrenergic blockers (not acutely)
- Many patients may require systemic anticoagulation to prevent embolization of mural thrombi
- Many patients will have automated internal cardioverter–defibrillators (AICD) to prevent sudden cardiac death

RESTRICTIVE

- Restrictive filling defect of myocardium
- Decreased diastolic volumes
- Uncommon and causes include: sarcoidosis, amyloidosis, scleroderma, and hemochromatosis

SIGNS AND SYMPTOMS

- Signs and symptoms of CHF

DIAGNOSIS

- Classic finding is low voltage on ECG, defined as QRS amplitude <5 mm in limb and <10 mm in precordial leads
- CXR: Classic findings of CHF

TREATMENT

- Usual therapies for CHF
- Treatment of the underlying causative systemic condition

HYPERTROPHIC

- Resulting from hypertrophy of ventricular myocardium (commonly the septum) without dilatation
- Poor relaxation during diastole (diastolic dysfunction) and therefore poor ventricular filling

SIGNS AND SYMPTOMS

- Exertional dyspnea, syncope, chest pain
- Associated with sudden death
- Characteristic murmur: systolic ejection murmur that increases with Valsalva or standing after squatting; decreases with squatting or passive leg elevation (i.e., *decreased* ventricular filling *increases* the murmur)

DIAGNOSIS

- ECG: large-amplitude QRS complexes
- Similar to findings of LVH
- Narrow but deep Q waves seen best in the anterior, inferior, or lateral leads
- Chest x-ray may be normal
- Diagnosis made by echocardiography

TREATMENT

- Patients with this condition must be instructed not to engage in vigorous activities
- Beta-adrenergic blocker therapy

PEARLS

- Mobitz II (second-degree heart block, type II) is associated with anterior wall myocardial infarction (MI) and is more likely to progress to complete heart block.

- Atrial fibrillation is the most common chronic arrhythmia.

- Accelerated idioventricular rhythm (AIVR) is a "reperfusion rhythm" that is seen as the infarct-related artery is recanalized by thrombolytic therapy.

- Beware atrial fibrillation in the setting of Wolff Parkinson White syndrome (WPW); there is high risk for deterioration into ventricular fibrillation, especially if atrioventricular (AV) nodal blocking medications are given.

- ST-segment depression and large R waves in leads V1 and V2, usually in association with an inferior or lateral ST-segment elevation myocardial infarction (STEMI), is highly suggestive of a posterior wall MI, which deserves urgent reperfusion therapy.

- Highest incidence of ventricular fibrillation is in the first hour after onset of acute-MI symptoms.

- Papillary muscle rupture is more common in patients with an inferior MI and presents as acute-onset dyspnea and new-onset holosystolic murmur.

- Early application of noninvasive ventilation (BiPAP) in patients with acute cardiogenic pulmonary edema has been shown to improve outcomes.

BIBLIOGRAPHY

ACC/AHA: ACC/AHA 2007 Guidelines for the management of patients with unstable angina/non-ST-elevation myocardial infarction, *Circulation* 116:e148–e304, 2007.

Brady WJ, Harrigan RA, Chan TC: Acute coronary syndromes. In Marx JA, Hockberger RS, Walls RM (eds): *Rosen's emergency medicine: concepts and clinical practice*, ed 6, Philadelphia, 2006, Mosby Elsevier, pp. 1154–1198.

ECGs, Nathanson LA, McClennen S, Safran C, Goldberger AL: *ECG Wave-Maven: self-assessment program for students and clinicians* (website). http://ecg.bidmc.harvard.edu.

Chan TC, Brady WJ, Harrigan RA et al (eds): *ECG in emergency medicine and acute care*, Philadelphia, 2005, Elsevier Mosby.

Hollander JE: Acute coronary syndromes: acute myocardial infarction and unstable angina. In Tintinalli JE, Kelen GD, Stapczynski JS (eds): *Emergency medicine: a comprehensive study guide*, ed 6, New York, 2004, McGraw-Hill, pp. 343–351.

Naples RM, Harris JW, Ghaemmaghami CA: Critical care aspects in the management of patients with acute coronary syndromes, *Emerg Med Clin North Am* 26:685–702, 2008.

Niemann JT: The cardiomyopathies, myocarditis, and pericardial disease. In Tintinalli JE, Kelen GD, Stapczynski JS (eds): *Emergency medicine: a comprehensive study guide*, ed 6, New York, 2004, McGraw-Hill, pp. 378–386.

Peacock WF: Congestive heart failure and acute pulmonary edema. In Tintinalli JE, Kelen GD, Stapczynski JS (eds): *Emergency medicine: a comprehensive study guide*, ed 6, New York, 2004, McGraw-Hill, pp. 364–373.

Questions and Answers

1. A 71-year-old woman presents with the acute onset of dyspnea, chest tightness, and diaphoresis 1 hour ago. She has long-standing hypertension and hypothyroidism. She is in obvious distress, sitting upright in bed. Her blood pressure is 187/98 mmHg, her heart rate is 119 bpm, and her respiratory rate if 28/minute. Oxygen saturation is 90% on ambient air. Rales are evident in both lungs, and there is a third heart sound on auscultation of the precordium. The legs show trace pitting pretibial edema. Optimal pharmacotherapy within the first 10 minutes would include oxygen as well as:

a. intravenous enalaprilat and sublingual nitroglycerin
b. aspirin and clopidogrel
c. aspirin and intravenous metoprolol
d. intravenous furosemide and intravenous morphine sulfate

2. A 77-year-old man presents with midsternal chest pressure for 5 hours, waxing and waning, and not made better by antacids at home. He complains of nausea, lightheadedness, and global weakness as well. On physical examination, his heart rate is 77 bpm, his respiratory rate is 22/minute, and his blood pressure is 110/62 mmHg; his oxygen saturation is 99% at the bedside. He is diaphoretic, anxious, and cooperative. His lungs are clear, and his heart examination features a grade II/VI systolic ejection murmur at the left upper sternal border. The first electrocardiogram (ECG) shows 2 to 3 mm of ST-segment elevation in leads II, III, and aVF, with 1 mm ST segment depression in lead aVL. He receives oxygen, aspirin 325 mg orally, followed by nitroglycerin 0.4 mg sublingually. He becomes more anxious, and his blood pressure drops to 67/38 mmHg; his lung and heart examinations are unchanged. Repeat electrocardiography is most likely to show

a. resolution of the inferior ST segment elevation
b. ST-segment elevation in the anterior precordial leads as well
c. ST-segment elevation in leads V3R and V4R
d. resolution of the inferior ST-segment elevation, with new ST-segment depression in the same leads

3. The next most logical treatment intervention for the patient in the previous question would be

a. switch nitroglycerin route of administration to continuous infusion
b. judicious intravenous metoprolol to decrease myocardial oxygen demand
c. bolus of intravenous normal saline solution
d. intravenous enalaprilat for acute afterload reduction
e. dopamine infusion

4. Which of the following arrhythmias is peculiar in the sense that it should not be treated with antiarrhythmic medications?

a. accelerated idioventricular rhythm
b. polymorphic ventricular tachycardia
c. torsade de pointes
d. monomorphic ventricular tachycardia

5. Which of the following complications of acute myocardial infarction presents in the first 3 to 5 days with acute-onset dyspnea, tachypnea, rales on lung examination, and a new holosystolic murmur at the base that radiates to the axilla?

a. free wall rupture
b. papillary muscle rupture
c. ventricular septal rupture
d. cardiac tamponade

6. A 44-year-old man presents with pleuritic central chest pain of 2 days' duration, associated with exertional shortness of breath; the pain is worse when supine and improves with sitting up. Expected ECG findings include

a. diffuse ST-segment depression with PR segment elevation
b. diffuse ST-segment elevation with PR segment elevation
c. diffuse ST-segment elevation with PR segment depression
d. anterior ST-segment elevation with inferior or reciprocal PR segment depression

7. A 59-year-old man with long-standing diabetes mellitus and hypertension presents with precordial chest heaviness and dyspnea at rest for 1 hour. His blood pressure is 145/80 mmHg, his heart rate is 88 bpm, and his respiratory rate is 22/minute. Contraindications to sublingual nitroglycerin therapy include

a. earlier use of nitrates during the day
b. tadalafil taken 30 hours ago
c. ST-segment depression in the inferior leads on ECG
d. clopidogrel taken 24 hours ago

8. Which of the following arrhythmias is associated with the highest risk of deteriorating into complete heart block?

a. first-degree AV block
b. Mobitz I second-degree AV block
c. Mobitz II second-degree AV block
d. sinus arrhythmia

9. Which of the following arrhythmias is most common in clinical practice?

a. atrial fibrillation
b. atrial flutter
c. supraventricular tachycardia
d. Wolff Parkinson White syndrome

10. Multifocal atrial tachycardia is seen most commonly with what group of diseases?

a. coronary artery disease
b. connective tissue disease
c. gastrointestinal disease
d. pulmonary disease

11. Which of the following coronary arteries is most likely occluded in patients with symptoms of acute coronary ischemia and anterior ST-segment elevation in leads I, aVL, and V1–V4 on the ECG?

a. left circumflex
b. left anterior descending
c. posterior descending
d. right coronary artery

12. Which intravenous pharmacologic agent is contraindicated in patients with Wolff Parkinson White (WPW) syndrome and rapid atrial fibrillation?

    a. adenosine
    b. calcium blocker (diltiazem)
    c. metoprolol
    d. all of the above

13. Which of the following cardiac biomarkers stays elevated the longest after acute myocardial infarction?

    a. creatine phosphokinase
    b. MB fraction of creatine phosphokinase
    d. myoglobin
    d. troponin I

14. Which of the following ECG findings is an indication to administer fibrinolytic therapy?

    a. ST-segment depression across V2–V6
    b. R wave > S wave amplitude in leads V1 and V2
    c. new ST-segment elevation >1 mm in two contiguous leads
    d. ST-segment elevation >2 mm in lead III

15. Which of the following is true regarding the murmur of hypertrophic cardiomyopathy?

    a. squatting increases the intensity
    b. Trendelenburg positioning increases the intensity
    c. standing after squatting increases the intensity
    d. standing after squatting decreases the intensity

16. A 21-year-old man presents with palpitations and near syncope while cleaning his apartment. He has no significant medical history, takes no medications, and does not use drugs. There is no history of syncope or near syncope. There is no family history of sudden death or congenital long QT syndrome. He does recall being told he has "WPW." On examination, the patient is awake and alert, but anxious. His heart rate is 200 beats/minute, his respiratory rate is 24/minute, and his blood pressure is 122/58 mmHg. His heart is tachycardic, without murmurs. His lungs are clear.

    The ECG shows a regular, narrow-complex tachycardia, with 1 to 2 mm of up-sloping ST-segment depression diffusely. The most prudent first-line treatment at this point is

    a. immediate defibrillation
    b. intravenous lidocaine
    c. intravenous adenosine
    d. intravenous procainamide

17. An elderly female with a history of hypertension, dyslipidemia, and arthritis presents with diffuse weakness and failure to thrive over the past week. She is compliant with her medications, which include amlodipine, hydrochlorothiazide, valsartan, rosuvastatin, and naproxen. Vital signs are all within normal limits. Her laboratory studies are remarkable for a sodium level of 129 mg/dL and a potassium level of 1.9 mg/dL. Her renal function is normal. Her ECG might reasonably show

    a. short QT interval with diffuse, scooped, ST-segment depression
    b. short PR interval with a delta wave, and a QRS interval of 0.10 second
    c. J waves
    d. U waves

18. When confronted with pulseless electrical activity (PEA), consider which of the following conditions as causative?

    a. hypoxia
    b. hypothermia
    c. hypovolemia
    d. acidosis
    e. all of the above

19. A 55-year-old woman with a history of colon cancer, undergoing chemotherapy, presents with the acute onset of pleuritic left-sided chest pain and shortness of breath for 1 day. There is no fever or purulent sputum. She has no history of cardiopulmonary disease. She describes no calf pain or immobility. Physical examination is remarkable for a normal temperature, a heart rate of 110 bpm, a respiratory rate of 28/minute, and a blood pressure of 144/77 mmHg. Her oxygen saturation is 92% on room air. Chest x-ray is clear. ECG shows sinus tachycardia with nonspecific T-wave changes across the precordium. A CT angiogram reveals a large left-sided pulmonary embolism. Which of the following laboratory values still supports that diagnosis?

    a. mild elevation of troponin I
    b. marked elevation of BNP (>2000 pg/mL)
    c. marked elevation of serum lipase
    d. all of the above

20. An 81-year-old man presents via local emergency medical service (EMS) as a resuscitation-in-progress. He was intubated in the field, and bedside end-tidal carbon dioxide monitoring verifies correct endotracheal tube placement. As he is shifted from the transport stretcher to the emergency department stretcher, his intravenous line is accidentally pulled out. Which of the following drugs can be given via the endotracheal tube, while intravenous access is reestablished?

    a. amiodarone
    b. magnesium
    c. atropine
    d. verapamil

1. Answer: a

The clinical picture here is one of acute congestive heart failure (CHF) with pulmonary edema. The cornerstones of treatment are **oxygenation, preload reduction with nitrates,** and **afterload reduction with angiotensin-converting enzyme (ACE) inhibitors.** Use of a diuretic is reasonable, but to restrict early pharmacotherapy to **furosemide** and **morphine** is not. **Aspirin** is also reasonable, as this patient may be experiencing acute coronary syndrome (ACS); however, **intravenous metoprolol** in the setting of florid pulmonary edema is not recommended—it may remove the compensatory tachycardic response to low cardiac output.

2. Answer: c

In the setting of an inferior acute myocardial infarction (AMI), the drop in blood pressure following administration of nitrates is suggestive of right ventricular involvement. **Acute right ventricular MI** is best detected by the application of right-sided precordial leads; lead V4R is the most sensitive.

3. Answer: c

Although this patient may indeed need vasopressor therapy, these agents do increase myocardial oxygen demand, so **dopamine** would not be the *next* treatment to institute. **Nitroglycerin** would further drop preload, which is already compromised in the case of right ventricular infarction, so it would be contraindicated. **Metoprolol** is also contraindicated in hypotensive patients. **Enalaprilat** is helpful in the management of acute pulmonary edema, but this patient, with hypotension and clear lungs, does not match that clinical picture. Suspected right ventricular ischemia with consequent hypotension should be treated first with preload filling—**intravenous fluid boluses.**

4. Answer: a

Accelerated idioventricular rhythm is a reperfusion rhythm found in patients undergoing percutaneous coronary intervention or who receive fibrinolytic therapy for AMI. The rhythm, an accelerated rhythm of ventricular origin, in most cases indicates recanalization of the infarct-related artery. Treatment of accelerated idioventricular rhythm with antiarrhythmics like lidocaine or amiodarone may precipitate sudden cardiac arrest.

5. Answer: b

Papillary muscle rupture occurs in patients with AMI (more common in inferior or inferoposterior MI) in the first 3 to 5 days. It presents with acute dyspnea, findings of CHF, and a new holosystolic murmur of mitral regurgitation that typically radiates to the axilla. **Free wall rupture** presents with sudden chest pain, dyspnea, and evidence of shock—if the patient survives the event long enough to seek medical care, they likely have tamponade. **Cardiac tamponade** presents with dyspnea, hypotension, clear lungs, and jugular venous distention. The murmur of **ventricular septal rupture** is holosystolic at the left lower sternal border, and patients usually have chest pain and dyspnea.

6. Answer: c

The clinical picture is one of pericarditis, which may occur post-MI or in an isolated fashion. The electrocardiographic hallmark of acute pericarditis is **diffuse ST-segment elevation** that is usually concave or scooped in morphology, with **PR-segment depression,** best seen in Lead II and the anterior precordial leads. This ST-segment elevation may be more evident in some leads than others. **PR-segment elevation** is seen in lead aVR, but not diffusely. **ST-segment depression** is not consistent with pericarditis.

7. Answer: b

Nitrates are contraindicated in patients on **sildenafil, tadalafil, and vardenafil,** due to an association with refractory hypotension and death; tadalafil has the longest half life, so it is not recommended to use nitrates if the patient has ingested that drug within 48 hours. The is no contraindication to nitrate therapy in patients on platelet inhibitors (aspirin, dipyridamole, **clopidogrel,** ticlopidine). ECG findings of **ST-segment depression** do not preclude nitroglycerin therapy.

8. Answer: c

Mobitz II second-degree AV block, although an uncommon complication of AMI, is at the highest risk for progressing into complete heart block. It is associated with anterior wall myocardial infarction. **First-degree AV block** is a benign electrocardiographic finding, as is **sinus arrhythmia** in young, healthy people. **Second-degree AV block of the Mobitz I** variety is more commonly seen with inferior wall MI and rarely progresses to a more serious rhythm disturbance.

9. Answer: a

Atrial fibrillation is the most common chronic arrhythmia. **Wolff Parkinson White syndrome** does not necessarily manifest as an arrhythmia; associated arrhythmias include narrow and wide-complex tachycardia, including atrial fibrillation or flutter.

10. Answer: d

Multifocal atrial tachycardia (MAT) is more common in chronic pulmonary diseases like chronic obstructive pulmonary disease; treatment of the arrhythmia centers on treatment of the underlying condition.

11. Answer: b

ST-segment elevation in leads I, aVL, and V1–V4 is indicative of a **left anterior coronary occlusion** manifesting as an anterolateral MI; alternatively, the elevation may be restricted to leads V1–V4. Occlusion of the **right coronary artery** usually yields ST-segment elevation in the inferior leads, II, III, and aVF. **Posterior infarctions** demonstrate ST-segment depression in the right precordial leads, with a larger-than-normal R wave in leads V1 and V2. **Left circumflex occlusion** may not be apparent on the 12-lead ECG but is classically linked to lateral changes (I, aVL, V5, V6).

12. Answer: d

Rapid atrial fibrillation in the setting of underlying WPW should not be treated with AV nodal blocking agents, so all are incorrect. Nodal blockade may preferentially speed conduction through the bypass tract, which permits more rapid conduction than the AV node—thus the patient's rhythm may deteriorate into ventricular fibrillation. The drug of choice for rapid atrial fibrillation in WPW is procainamide.

13. Answer: d

Myoglobin rises in 1 to 3 hours, peaks in 5 to 7 hours, and remains elevated for <1 day. **Creatine kinase** and its more cardiac-specific **MB** fraction rises in 3 to 10 hours, peaks in about 18 to 24 hours, and remains elevated for 2 to 3 days, **Troponins** (I and T) rise in 3 to 6 hours, peak in 12 to 18 hours, and stay elevated for up to 7 to 10 days.

14. Answer: c

ST-segment depression in the setting of a clinical picture consistent with ACS may signal NSTEMI, or may evolve into a STEMI, but does not in and of itself merit fibrinolysis—unless it is the harbinger of posterior MI (ST segment depression in V1–V3, R > S wave amplitude in lead V2, and ST-segment elevation in posterior leads V8 and V9). **ST-segment elevation,** though not specific for AMI, is suggestive of it in the proper clinical scenario and must occur in **at least two contiguous leads** to qualify for fibrinolytic therapy. **R > S wave amplitude in leads V1 and V2** may be seen with posterior MI, but also may occur with right ventricular hypertrophy, right bundle branch block, Wolff Parkinson White syndrome, muscular dystrophies, and as a normal variant. This finding along with ST-segment depression in the same leads and the proper clinical picture is consistent with acute posterior MI.

15. Answer: c

The murmur of hypertrophic cardiomyopathy is accentuated by decreasing ventricular filling, thus leading to less distention of the left ventricular outflow tract, which serves to increase turbulent flow and thus increase the sound of the murmur. Squatting and Trendelenburg positioning increase

venous return, thus increasing ventricular filling and decreasing the murmur. **Standing after squatting decreases ventricular return, thus causing an accentuation of the murmur.**

16. Answer: c

This is a case of WPW syndrome presenting with a supraventricular tachyarrhythmia—in this case not atrial fibrillation, but a narrow-complex supraventricular tachycardia. The regular, narrow-complex rhythm suggests orthodromic conduction down the AV node, and back up the bypass tract. Thus, AV nodal blockade **(adenosine, metoprolol, diltiazem)** is reasonable, whereas **procainamide** should be reserved for atrial fibrillation in the setting of WPW. Synchronized cardioversion may be necessary if pharmacotherapy fails; if the patient becomes unstable, **defibrillation** should be employed.

17. Answer: d

Evidence of **hypokalemia** on the ECG includes QT-interval prolongation, T-wave changes, and **U waves.** WPW findings are described in choice **b (shortened PR interval, longer QRS width with a delta wave),** and **J (Osborne) waves** are a feature of hypothermia. **Digoxin effect** is described in the first choice—shortened QT interval, sometimes first-degree AV block, nonspecific T-wave changes, and scooped or concave ST-segment depression best seen in those leads where the R waves are tallest.

18. Answer: e

Pulseless electrical activity (PEA) in the resuscitation situation should invoke consideration of the "6 Hs and 5 Ts." These include hypothermia, hypoxia, hypovolemia, hypo/hyperkalemia, hypoglycemia, and hydrogen ion (acidosis), as well as tamponade, tension pneumothorax, thrombosis, toxins, and trauma.

19. Answer: a

Serum **troponin** is rather specific for coronary ischemia but may be elevated in other diseases, such as pulmonary embolism, pulmonary hypertension, congestive heart failure, sepsis, chemotherapy, and myopericarditis. Marked elevations of **BNP** do not suggest pulmonary embolism, nor does the pancreas-specific **lipase** elevation.

20. Answer: c

The mnemonic for medications that can be given down the endotracheal tube, albeit in doses of 2 to 2.5 times normal, is "NAVEL"—**n**aloxone, **a**tropine, **v**asopressin, **e**pinephrine, and **l**idocaine.

Cardiovascular II

Alexander T. Limkakeng, Jr. | Sarah A. Stahmer

3

Arterial circulation

ABDOMINAL AORTIC ANEURYSM

- Localized dilatation of the terminal portion of the abdominal aorta
- 2% to 10% of the population more than 65 years old
- Men greater than women (5:1)

Etiology

- Atherosclerosis
- Deterioration of the arterial media
- Hydraulic factors of wall stress near bifurcations
- Uncoiling and tortuosity (ectasia)
- Rare: syphilis, tuberculosis, connective tissue disorders, trauma, aortic dissection

SIGNS AND SYMPTOMS

- Abdominal pain
- Flank/back pain
- Renal colic is a common misdiagnosis
- Syncope
- Lower-extremity paresthesias/pulse deficit
- Pulsatile abdominal mass
- Abdominal bruit
- Hemodynamic instability: Acute rupture: less than 20% into peritoneum, mostly retroperitoneal; operative mortality 50% to 80% depending on additional risk factors
- Gastrointestinal (GI) bleeding: Aorto-enteric fistula; usually seen in patients after aortic repair
- Asymptomatic: aneurysms greater than 6 cm in diameter are at high risk of rupture

DIAGNOSIS

- Abdominal plain film
  - Visible calcification of the media (85% to 90%)
  - Soft tissue (67%). May overestimate size
  - Loss of one or both psoas margins (75%)
  - Loss of one or both renal outlines (78%)
  - Renal displacement (25%)
  - Change in retroperitoneal flank stripe (19%)
- B-Mode ultrasonography (Fig. 3-1)
  - Noninvasive, painless, inexpensive, rapidly done, reproducible
  - Near 100% sensitivity if the aneurysm can be clearly visualized
  - Accurately measures aneurysmal dimensions
  - Will not reliably identify potential complications
    - Retroperitoneal blood

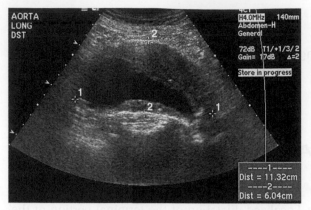

Figure 3-1. Ultrasound image of a 6-cm abdominal aortic aneurysm in the longitudinal plane. Note the large amount of thrombus in the aneurysm. (From Townsend CM, Jr et al: *Sabiston textbook of surgery*, ed 18, Philadelphia, 2007, Saunders.)

- Dissection
  - Involvement of branch arteries
- Angiography
  - *Not useful* for diagnosing the presence or size of aneurysm
  - Mural thrombus may fill lumen and cause nonvisualization
  - Primary indication is for planning surgery in selected patients
  - Helps in assessing renal arteries and associated vascular lesions
- Computed tomography
  - *Criterion standard* in stable patients
  - Contrast shows vascular anatomy
  - Can identify aneurysm, mural thrombus, renal arteries
  - Gas and fat do not interfere
  - Can demonstrate retroperitoneal hemorrhage

TREATMENT

- Ruptured aneurysm
  - Prehospital and emergency department (ED) use of the military antishock trousers (MAST) suit
  - Two large-bore intravenous (IV) lines and rapid IV fluid bolus
  - Type and crossmatch 10 units of blood
  - Vascular surgery consultation for rapid operative control
- Symptomatic unruptured aneurysm
  - Any aneurysm with symptoms should be assumed to be expanding, dissecting, or leaking
  - Blood pressure control
  - Vascular surgery consultation
- Asymptomatic aneurysm
  - Risk of rupture related to size of the aneurysm
  - More than 6 cm in diameter: risk of rupture is significant
  - Any aneurysm more than 4 cm in diameter requires close follow-up

AORTIC DISSECTION

- Transverse tear in the intima of aorta with dissection of blood in the media (outer part)
- Propagation depends on location and shear forces on aorta (dp/dt)
- 1:10,000 hospital admissions
- 90% die in first week if diagnosis is missed
- 70% recover if treated aggressively
- Stanford classification
  - Type A: Any involvement of the ascending aorta
  - Type B: Restricted to the descending aorta
- Debakey classification:
  - Type I: dissection usually begins in ascending aorta and involves the remaining portions of distal aorta
  - Type II: dissection is limited to ascending aorta, and aortic valvular incompetence can occur
  - Type III: dissection arises distal to left subclavian and may extend below diaphragm to the renal and iliac arteries

Risk factors

- Hypertension (90%)
- Marfan syndrome
- Congenital deformity of aortic valve
- Third trimester of pregnancy
- Coarctation of aorta (may be related to hypertension)
- Giant cell arteritis
- Cocaine

SIGNS AND SYMPTOMS

- Sharp, tearing chest pain radiating to back (classic)
- Pain maximal at time of onset
- Syncope
- Congestive heart failure
- Stroke-like symptoms resulting from carotid involvement
- Dysphagia/hoarseness due to recurrent laryngeal nerve involvement
- Abdominal pain/distention resulting from abdominal aorta extension and bowel ischemia
- Lower-extremity pain/paresthesia/pulse deficit if dissection extends there
- Hematuria due to abdominal aorta involvement
- Hypertension
- BP differential between arms
  - May occur in up to 20% of normal subjects
- Pulse deficits in proximal dissection
- Aortic regurgitation murmur (proximal)
- May be painless, especially in the elderly (syncope)

DIAGNOSIS

- Electrocardiogram (ECG)—nonspecific
  - Left ventricular hypertrophy (LVH)/strain
  - Active ischemia
  - Right coronary artery can be involved, mimicking inferior ischemia/infarct

- Chest radiograph—not sensitive; may be normal (12% of cases)
  - Mediastinal widening
  - Apical cap
  - Loss of aortopulmonary artery window
  - Displacement of intimal calcium in aortic wall
  - Left pleural effusion
  - Deviation of the nasogastric tube
- CT chest—with intravenous contrast (Fig. 3-2)
  - Sensitivity: 83% to 100%, specificity 91% to 100%
  - Good screening test in stable patients
  - Visualization of two lumens, intimal flap, hematoma
  - Identifies other causes of mediastinal widening
- Transesophageal echocardiography
  - Fast, portable, no contrast
  - Detects aortic regurgitation
  - Sensitivity 97% to 100%, specificity 68% to 97%
  - Presence of intimal flap or aortic wall thickening
  - Identifies pericardial effusions
  - Invasive
- Magnetic resonance imaging (MRI)
  - Similar to CT but superior in arch vessel involvement
  - Sensitivity 90% to 100%, specificity 98% to 100%
  - Preferable in patients with less acute symptoms or in follow-up
  - Not always readily available
  - Loss of monitoring of patient
- Aortography
  - Traditional criterion standard for identifying dissection

- Hallmark of diagnosis is presence of intimal flap
- Does not reliably identify hemopericardium, intramural hematoma, thrombosed false channel
- Sensitivity 81% to 91%, with specificity 94% to 98%
- Helps plan surgery

COMPLICATIONS

- Rupture of aorta
- Pericardial tamponade resulting from rupture into sac
- Aortic regurgitation
- Congestive heart failure
- Dissection can block coronary arteries—usually right

TREATMENT

- Nitroprusside + beta-adrenergic blocker, or labetalol, intravenously
- Maintain blood pressure at 100 to 110 mmHg systolic
- Ascending aortic dissections—early surgical repair
- Isolated descending aortic dissection—medical management as above

PERIPHERAL ARTERIAL OCCLUSIVE DISEASE

- Blockage of blood flow in a peripheral artery secondary to atherosclerosis, emboli, or atherosclerotic thrombus
- **Embolic etiologies**
  - Heart is most common source (77% to 85%)
  - Myocardial infarction (30%)
  - Atrial fibrillation (34%)
  - Two thirds of emboli enter lower extremity with 50% in ilio-femoral system
  - 15% go to upper extremity, viscera, or aorto-iliac
  - Embolus from atheromatous lesion of abdominal aorta is rare
- **Thrombotic etiologies**
  - Occurs in advanced vascular disease and collaterals often present
  - Final occlusion may be silent
  - Usually not as emergent unless acute thrombus
  - May be hard to differentiate from embolus

SIGNS AND SYMPTOMS

- Embolic—sudden-onset pain
  - Paraesthesia/numbness
  - Poikilothermia/coolness
  - Pallor
  - Pulselessness
  - Paralysis
- Thrombotic
  - Intermittent claudication
  - Pain may be improved by dangling leg over side of bed
  - Claudication that progresses to pain at rest—indication for vascular surgery consult

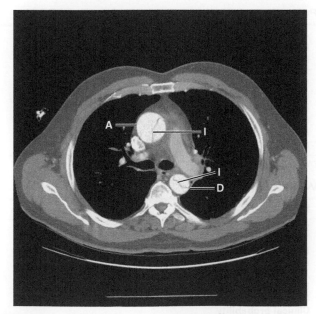

Figure 3-2. Aortic dissection. A contrast medium-enhanced computed tomography scan of the chest at the level of the pulmonary artery shows an intimal flap (I) separating the two lumens of the ascending (A) and the descending (D) thoracic aorta in a type A aortic dissection. (From Goldman L: *Cecil textbook of medicine*, ed 23, Philadelphia, 2007, Saunders.)

- Elderly may just complain of numbness, cold, or color change
- Pulses decreased or absent, bruits over larger vessels
- Trophic signs of ischemia present: decreased hair, thickened nails, subcutaneous atrophy, petechial-like lesions, ischemic ulcers, gangrene
- Capillary refill delayed

DIAGNOSIS

- Segmental blood pressure: measures blood pressure at thigh, knee, and ankle
- Ankle/brachial indices: measure systolic blood pressure at lower extremity and divide by upper-extremity systolic
- Hand-held Doppler device (presence and/or amplitude of pulse flow)
- Doppler ultrasound
- Arteriogram—in consultation with vascular surgery

TREATMENT

- Embolic
  - Heparinization prevents thrombus propagation
  - Early embolectomy
  - Intra-arterial thrombolysis with streptokinase, urokinase or tPA: 50% to 85% reperfusion is an alternative to surgery—superior to systemic lytic therapy
  - Amputation rate related to time gap—onset of symptoms to embolectomy (9.5% vs 20.3% if delayed more than 24 hours)
- Thrombotic
  - Noninvasive testing helps confirm suspicions
  - Arteriography needed if surgery indicated; defines anatomy
  - Medical therapy not very successful: vasodilator drugs do not work
  - Endarterectomy is effective therapy for proximal lesions
  - Vein or graft bypass excellent in superficial femoral artery lesions
  - Intervention angiography with balloon dilation useful in isolated stenosis
  - Sympathectomy only as last resort and must be combined with another procedure
  - Limb salvage can be 62% to 96% if aggressive management

Venous circulation/ thromboembolism

PULMONARY EMBOLISM

- Etiology: Virchow triad
  - Hypercoagulability
  - Stasis
  - Venous injury
- Due to embolism of clot from lower extremity/pelvis
- 300,000 die annually, 15% 3-month mortality even if treated
- Risk factors (see Table)

Venous Thromboembolism Risk Factors

Hereditary
Antithrombin deficiency
Protein C/S deficiency
Factor V Leiden mutation
Acquired
Immobility
Advanced age
Cancer
Surgery
Trauma
Spinal cord injury
Pregnancy/postpartum
Polycythemia vera
Antiphospholipid antibodies
Oral hormones/contraceptives (estrogens)
Chemotherapy
Obesity
Central venous catheters
Immobilization/casts

SIGNS AND SYMPTOMS

- Chest pain: pleuritic; can be very localized
- Hemoptysis
- Dyspnea
- Back pain
- Syncope
- Unilateral leg swelling/symptoms of deep-vein thrombosis (DVT)
- Symptoms can be intermittent, and relatively chronic
- Tachypnea
- Tachycardia—approximately 50% will not have this
- Hypotension
- Hypoxemia

DIAGNOSIS

- Clinical criteria: PERC
- Pretest probability: Wells, Geneva, and Charlotte scores

Pulmonary Embolism Rule-out Criteria (PERC)

Age <50
Pulse <100 beats per minute
Pulse oximetry >94%
No unilateral leg swelling
No hemoptysis
No recent surgery
No prior PE or DVT
No exogenous estrogen use
If meets all of the above criteria, prevalence of PE in low risk population is 1.4%

DVT, Deep-vein thrombosis; *PE*, pulmonary embolism.

Wells Score

Risk Factor	Value
Suspected DVT	3
Tachycardia >100 beats per minute	1.5
Prior DVT/PE	1.5
Immobilization in past 4 weeks	1.5
Active malignancy (or treatment in past 6 months)	1
Hemoptysis	1
PE is most likely diagnosis	3
Clinical probability	
Low (appropriate D-dimer assay is adequate ED screening test)	0-2
Intermediate	3-6
High	>6

DVT, Deep-vein thrombosis; *PE*, pulmonary embolism.

Revised Geneva Score

Risk factor	
Age >65	1
Previous DVT/PE	3
Recent surgery (general anesthesia) /fracture (lower limbs) <1 month	2
Active malignancy <1 year	2
Symptoms	
Unilateral lower limb pain	3
Hemoptysis	2
Clinical signs	
Heart rate 75-94 beats per minute	3
Heart rate ≥95 beats per minute	5
Pain on lower limb deep venous palpation and unilateral edema	4
Clinical probability	
Low	<4
Intermediate	4-10
High	>10

DVT, Deep-vein thrombosis; *PE*, pulmonary embolism.

Charlotte Criteria

For patients with suspicion for PE, which patients are eligible for safe D-dimer rule-out testing?
A. If age ≤50 and HR < systolic blood pressure = safe for D-dimer testing
B. If age >50, go to 4 items below; if yes to any, not safe for D-dimer testing
C. If age ≤50, but HR ≥ systolic blood pressure, go to 4 items below; if yes to any, not safe for D-dimer testing
  1. Unexplained hypoxemia (Pulse oximetry <95%, nonsmoker, no asthma/COPD)
  2. Unilateral leg swelling
  3. Recent surgery (last 4 weeks)
  4. Hemoptysis

HR, Heart rate; *COPD*, chronic obstructive pulmonary disorder.

- ECG
  - Sinus tachycardia most common
  - S1Q3T3 or new right bundle branch block—suggests right heart strain; nonspecific findings, however
  - May be normal; at best is nonspecific
- Chest x-ray (CXR)
  - Cardiomegaly is most common finding
  - Up to 25% may be normal
  - Pleural effusion
  - Atelectasis
  - Pathognomic findings:
    - **Hampton hump:** peripheral, pleural-based, wedge-shaped density
    - **Westermark sign:** paucity of vascular markings in the involved segment/involved lung
- Arterial blood gas
  - Not essential to making the diagnosis
  - Up to 25% will have PaO_2 >80 mmHg
  - Widened alveolar–arterial (A–a) gradient
  - Hypoxia, or A–a gradient has a sensitivity of 90% but a specificity of 15%
- International normalized ratio (INR)—PE can occur even at therapeutic INR
- D-dimer
  - ELISA-based tests have the best sensitivity, 96% to 98%

- Excludes PE in low–intermediate risk patients (see Charlotte Criteria) when negative, require more testing when positive
  - Elevated in infection, cancer, trauma, or other inflammatory states
  - Elevated in pregnant patients but should not exceed 1,000 micrograms/L at any point
- Troponin/ B-natriuretic peptide (BNP)—elevations associated with higher risk in patients diagnosed with PE
- Ventilation–perfusion (V/Q) scan
  - Helpful in patients at the extremes of pretest probability; when the V/Q result is concordant it rules-in or rules-out disease
  - Normal study effectively rules out PE
  - Can do perfusion only in pregnant patients to reduce fetal radiation
- CT angiography
  - Good outcome studies support withholding treatment when negative
  - Can identify alternative diagnoses
  - Can shield abdomen in pregnant patients
  - Controversial whether it causes more radiation exposure to fetus or mother than V/Q
- Pulmonary angiography
  - Criterion standard
  - Can detect subsegmental clot and filling pressures
  - 1% of negative studies had subsequent PEs
- Lower-extremity compression ultrasound
  - An alternative if other imaging is not feasible
  - Treatment is same if positive
  - Not helpful if negative
- Echocardiography
- Check for right ventricular (RV) dysfunction, alternative diagnoses

TREATMENT

- Heparin: low-molecular-weight heparin (LMWH) preferred over unfractionated heparin (UFH) because of more reliable effect, easier administration, lower incidence of major bleeding and heparin-induced thrombocytopenia
- Empiric treatment—should be given if pretest probability is >50%, hypoxemic, or hypotensive, or obese patients that cannot receive imaging
- UFH: bolus 80 units/kg, drip 18 units/kg
- Goal: prothrombin time (PTT) of 55 to 80
- LMWH—monitoring not needed
  - Enoxaparin 1 mg/kg subcutaneous (SC) twice daily or 1.5 mg/kg every day, maximum 180 mg
  - Dalteparin 200 units/kg daily maximum 18,000 units
  - Renally excreted, can have prolonged effect in renal failure
  - Can be partially reversed with protamine
  - Can be monitored with anti-Factor Xa levels
- Thrombin inhibitors
  - For those with contraindications to heparin
  - Monitoring not required except in renal disease
  - Lepirudin: 0.4 mg/kg slow bolus over 15 minutes, drip 0.1 mg/kg/hour

- Warfarin—should be started and continued 3 to 6 months; INR 2 to 3
- Thrombolytics
  - Cardiogenic shock/arrest due to PE
  - Controversial indications:
  - Right ventricular collapse on echocardiogram
  - Troponin positive
  - Significant clot burden on imaging
  - 1% to 3% rate of intracranial hemorrhage
- Vena cava filter
  - When anticoagulation contraindicated
  - Recurrent embolism on adequate anticoagulation

DEEP-VEIN THROMBOSIS

- Similar risk factors as PE
- Associated with fourfold increase with travel longer than 4 hours
- Thrombi form at intimal defects or cusps of deep veins

SIGNS AND SYMPTOMS

- Leg pain/tenderness
- Swelling
- Redness
- Fever can be present
- Phlegmasia cerulea dolens: painful blue severe inflammation representing massive iliofemoral thrombosis, can cause compartment syndrome
- Phlegmasia alba dolens: "milk leg" also represents massive iliofemoral thrombosis with arterial spasm and diminished arterial flow in the leg

DIAGNOSIS

- Pretest probability
  - Wells score (see table)
  - Divides patients into risk of 5%, 33%, and 85%, for low, intermediate, and high risk groups, respectively

Wells Score for Deep-Vein Thrombosis

Feature	Score
Active cancer (ongoing treatment; within 6 months)	+1
Limb immobilization	+1
Bedridden >3 days, or surgery in past 4 weeks	+1
Localized tenderness along deep-venous system	+1
Entire leg swollen	+1
Calf swelling >3 cm difference, measured 10 cm below tibial tuberosity	+1
Pitting edema on symptomatic leg only	+1
Collateral superficial veins (nonvaricose)	+1
Previous DVT documented	+1
Alternative diagnosis as likely or more likely than DVT	−2
Clinical probability	Score
Low	0
Intermediate	1–2
High	≥3

- D-dimer
  - ELISA-based tests have the best sensitivity, 96% to 98%
  - Useful to exclude in low or intermediate-probability patients (Wells score ≤2)
  - Also used in some systems to assess need for follow-up ultrasound studies (follow-up ultrasound recommended when positive)
- Ultrasound
  - Inexpensive, noninvasive, portable
  - Insensitive for calf clots, need follow-up exams to rule out proximal propagation
  - Can identify alternative diagnoses, e.g., Baker's cyst, hematoma, aneurysms, abscesses
  - Follow-up study not needed in low-risk patients, in 1 week for moderate/high-risk patients
- Venography
  - Criterion standard; however, rarely used
  - Slightly more sensitive, but painful and can cause phlebitis/DVT
- Studies for hypercoagulable states should be postponed until resolution of acute clot

TREATMENT

- Same as for PE: LMWH/UFH; warfarin
- Thrombolytics via catheter-directed targeting rarely indicated except for massive iliofemoral thrombosis with low bleeding risk
- Surgical treatment when limb viability threatened by arterial spasm/compartment syndrome

SUPERFICIAL THROMBOPHLEBITIS

- Same risk factors as DVT
- Can occur with intravenous drug abuse
- Saphenous vein common
- 3% extend into DVT; embolization rare

SIGNS AND SYMPTOMS

- Localized pain, redness, warmth, streaking, and "cord" along course of vein

DIAGNOSIS

- Diagnosis of exclusion
- Ultrasound—rules out DVT
  - Follow-up study in 1 week recommended to rule out subsequent extension

TREATMENT

- Warm compresses
- Nonsteroidal anti-inflammatory drugs (NSAIDs)
- Elastic support
- Antibiotics and anticoagulants of no proven benefit unless due to intravenous drug injection
- Severe cases can be treated with bedrest and elevation temporarily, surgical excision of the vein
- Recurrent cases should prompt search for malignancy or hypercoagulable state

Diseases of the myocardium, endocardium, and pericardium

MYOCARDITIS

Etiology

- Infectious
  - Viruses
    - Enteroviruses (Coxsackie A and B, ECHO)
    - Influenza
    - HIV
  - Bacteria
    - Diphtheria toxin
    - Abscess formation (e.g., staphylococcal, enterococcal species)
    - Lyme disease
  - Protozoa
    - Chagas disease: *Trypanosoma cruzi*
    - Toxoplasmosis
    - Trichonosis
- Cardiac transplant rejection
- Giant cell myocarditis
- Peripartum myocarditis
- Toxins (e.g., cocaine, inhalants [toluene], ethanol)
- Systemic illness (e.g., sarcoidosis, systemic lupus erythematosus, Kawasaki disease)
- Medications (e.g., interleukin-2, cyclophosphamides, penicillins, hydrochlorothiazide)

Incidence

- The true incidence of myocarditis is unknown because the majority of cases are asymptomatic
- Involvement of the myocardium has been reported in 1% to 5% of patients with acute viral infections

RISK FACTORS

- Groups at increased risk of virus-induced myocarditis (course may be hyperacute)
  - Young males
  - Pregnant women
  - Children (particularly neonates)
  - Immunocompromised patients

PATHOGENESIS

- Direct viral-induced myocyte damage and post–viral-immune inflammatory reactions
- Inflammatory lesions and the necrotic process may persist for months
- Cytokines such as interleukin-1 and tumor necrosis factor, oxygen free radicals, and microvascular changes as contributory pathogenic factors

SIGNS AND SYMPTOMS

- Prodrome of gastroenteritis, or "flu"-like symptoms
- Cardiac
  - Congestive heart failure: mild to fatal

- Syncope
- Heart block
- Physical examination often reveals direct evidence of cardiac dysfunction in symptomatic patients (e.g., S3 or S4; friction rub)
- Young male with otherwise unexplained cardiac abnormalities of new onset, such as heart failure, arrhythmias, or conduction disturbances
- History of recent upper respiratory infection or enteritis

DIAGNOSIS

- Viral titers
- Chest radiograph
- ECG
  - May be normal
  - Nonspecific ST abnormalities
  - Atrial tachycardia or atrial fibrillation
  - High-grade ventricular arrhythmias
- Echocardiography
  - Dysfunction is generally global
  - Mild impairment in contractility may be evident only when the study is performed at rest and during exercise
- MRI
  - Contrast-enhanced MRI can detect the degree and extent of inflammation
  - Extent of relative myocardial enhancement correlates with clinical status and left ventricular function
- Endomyocardial biopsy
  - Idiopathic cardiomyopathy—50%
  - Myocarditis—10%

TREATMENT

- Symptomatic
- Identify and treat underlying causes

ACUTE PERICARDITIS

- Common causes include idiopathic, infectious, malignancy, drug-induced, connective tissue disease, radiation-induced, postinfarction, uremia, and myxedema

SIGNS AND SYMPTOMS

- Most common symptom is precordial or retrosternal chest pain
- Aggravated by inspiration, movement, swallowing, or the supine position
- Radiates to trapezius ridge
- Relief with leaning forward
- Associated symptoms include
  - Low-grade fever
  - Dyspnea
  - Dysphagia
- Associated signs
  - Resting tachycardia
  - Pulsus paradoxus
  - Jugular venous distention (JVD)
  - Pericardial rub (best heard sitting up, leaning forward)

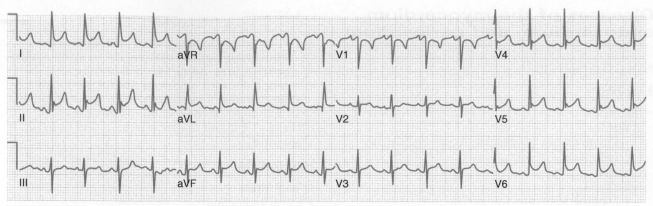

Figure 3-3. Pericarditis. This tracing features several of the characteristic findings of acute pericarditis: *(1)* diffuse, concave upward, ST-segment elevation; *(2)* PR segment depression (seen well in lead II); and *(3)* PR segment elevation in lead aVR.

DIAGNOSIS

- ECG (Fig. 3-3)
- Serial ECGs recorded over a number of days may be diagnostic
- Evolutionary ECG changes have been divided into four stages:
  - Stage 1: Diffuse, concave ST segment elevation, PR segment depression; PR segment elevation in aVR
  - Stage 2: ST segment returns to baseline, decreased T-wave amplitude
  - Stage 3: Isoelectric ST segment, diffuse T-wave inversion
  - Stage 4: Normalization, may retain T-wave inversion

TREATMENT

- Identify and treat the underlying cause of pericarditis
- NSAIDs for 1 to 3 weeks for idiopathic or viral pericarditis
- Colchicine
- Hospitalize those with pericardial effusion or intractable pain

PERICARDIAL EFFUSION AND TAMPONADE

Etiology

- Any process capable of causing pericarditis may produce an effusion big enough to produce signs and symptoms
- Acute tamponade may be seen in the setting of:
  - Blunt or penetrating chest trauma
  - Central venous access or pacemaker placement
  - Within 2 weeks after acute myocardial infarction (MI)
- Subacute tamponade if often due to:
  - Neoplastic involvement of the pericardium
  - Patients on hemodialysis
  - Patients with collagen vascular disease

SIGNS AND SYMPTOMS

- Acute tamponade
  - "Beck's triad"—hypotension, JVD, muffled heart sounds (not always reliable)

- Hypotension in a chest trauma patient
- Pulsus paradoxus
- Subacute tamponade
  - Dyspnea, fatigue, chest tightness
  - Pulsus paradoxus
  - Tachycardia, JVD
  - Pericardial friction rub

DIAGNOSIS

- CXR—nonspecific; may show cardiomegaly without CHF
- ECG—nonspecific; may show decreased voltage, electrical alternans
- Echocardiogram

TREATMENT

- Drainage of pericardial fluid is the only definitive therapy
- Temporizing therapy:
  - Volume expansion
  - Inotropic support (dobutamine, isoproterenol)

INFECTIVE ENDOCARDITIS

Risk factors

- Cardiac valve leaflets susceptible to infection because of limited blood supply
- Most common in patients with damaged valves (e.g., congenital/acquired valvular heart disease; intravenous drug use; hemodialysis)
- Antibodies form in reaction to the foreign antigen and immune complex injury to the basement membrane of the kidneys may result (glomerulonephritis)
- May be acute or subacute depending on
  - Virulence of the organism
  - Susceptibility of the host
  - Intravenous drug use
- Left-sided disease—most common overall
  - Caused by
    - *Streptococcus viridans*
    - *Staphylococcus aureus*
    - Enterococcal species
    - Fungal organisms

- Right-sided disease—usually seen in intravenous drug users (IVDU) (60%)
  - Caused by
    - *Staphylococcus aureus* (75%)
    - *Streptococcus pneumoniae* (20%)
    - Gram-negative organism (4%)
    - Fungal

SIGNS AND SYMPTOMS

- Classic triad of fever, anemia, and a new heart murmur
- Fever, chills, tachycardia, and symptoms of congestive heart failure
- The presence of a murmur alone is sufficient to suspect in febrile patient, particularly IVDU
- More common in left-sided subacute endocarditis:
  - Roth spots
  - Osler nodes (painful)
  - Janeway lesions (painless)
  - Splinter hemorrhages

DIAGNOSIS

- 30% to 40% have neurologic symptoms as a result of embolization
- Pulmonary emboli present as patchy infiltrates on CXR
- 25% to 30% of patients have splenomegaly
- Microscopic hematuria is common (25% to 50%)
- Positive blood cultures
- Echocardiography showing vegetations

TREATMENT

- Three sets of blood cultures from three different sites should be obtained before antibiotics are initiated
- Vancomycin and gentamicin based on local susceptibilities
- Febrile IVDU patients should be admitted

ANTIBIOTIC PROPHYLAXIS FOR INFECTIVE ENDOCARDITIS

- Low-risk patients (dental or minor GI or GY procedure)
  - Amoxicillin 2.0 g orally (1 hour before procedure); or
  - Clindamycin 600 mg orally (1 hour before the procedure); or
  - Azithromycin or clarithromycin 500 mg (1 hour before the procedure)
- High-risk patients
  - Ampicillin 2 g IV plus gentamicin (for GU procedures)
  - Cefazolin 1.0 gm IV or cephalexin 2.0 g PO 1 hr before the procedure (I&D of infected tissue)
- Conditions requiring antibiotic prophylaxis
  - Prosthetic heart valve
  - Endocarditis history
  - Rheumatic heart disease history
  - Congenital heart disease

- Mitral valve prolapse with regurgitation
- Acquired valvular heart disease
- Indications for prophylaxis
  - Teeth cleaning
  - Bronchoscopy (rigid)
  - Endoscopic retrograde cholangiopancreatography (ERCP)
  - Cystoscopy
  - Urethral dilatation

Hypertension

ASYMPTOMATIC HYPERTENSION (HTN)

- Elevated blood pressure (BP) that is not yet leading to significant organ damage. Usually no treatment is required, but treatment can be initiated in the ED in consultation with patient's primary care physician.

SIGNS AND SYMPTOMS

- None except elevated BP

DIAGNOSIS

- Standard blood pressure cuff reading
  - Both arms can be measured and readings averaged
  - Should have more than one measurement
  - Severely elevated readings are highly associated with sustained hypertension on follow-up and should be assumed to represent true hypertension and treated
  - BP threshold that indicates need for ED treatment is unclear
- End-organ workup
  - Controversial
  - Some recommend urinalysis, creatinine test, and ECG for severe HTN (180/110)—although not data-supported—or those with end-organ disease

TREATMENT

- Initiation of treatment in the ED is acceptable, particularly for those with severely elevated BP and/or end-organ damage, but not mandatory if good follow-up is available and only one reading is elevated
- Do not lower blood pressure by more than 30% of the mean arterial pressure
- Follow-up within 1 week for repeat measurement and monitoring of therapy

HYPERTENSIVE URGENCY

- Severe elevation of arterial blood pressure without evidence of vital organ dysfunction in which definitive treatment can be initiated over a period of days. It may progress to a hypertensive emergency or cause cardiovascular, neurological, or renal end-organ damage.

SIGNS AND SYMPTOMS

- May or may not be present; may or may not be related to BP
  - Headache
  - Blurry vision
  - Chest pain
  - Shortness of breath

DIAGNOSIS

- Based on clinical assessment and BP readings

TREATMENT

- Oral therapy recommended
- Follow-up within 1 week for repeat measurement and monitoring of therapy versus observation

HYPERTENSIVE EMERGENCIES

- Severe elevation of arterial blood pressure that represents a threat to life or vital organ function unless treatment is initiated immediately

Etiology (see Table)

Hypertensive Emergencies

Chronic essential HTN
Drugs/medications
Cocaine
Sympathomimetics
SSRIs
Amphetamines
Renovascular HTN
Eclampsia
Renal failure
Postoperative
Pheochromocytoma
CHF
Neuroleptic malignant syndrome
Intracranial hemorrhage
Thromboembolic stroke

CHF, Congestive heart failure; *HTN,* hypertension; *SSRI,* selective serotonin reuptake inhibitor.

- Three organ systems of concern
  - Cardiovascular
    - Increased cardiac workload
    - CHF/pulmonary edema
    - Ischemia/infarct
  - CNS
    - Elevated BP overwhelms normal cerebral autoregulation
    - Transudative leak across capillary bed, arteriolar damage
    - Normal autoregulation fails
    - Intracranial pressures rise
  - Renal
    - Loss of normal autoregulation
    - Worsening renal function
    - Hematuria
    - Cast formation
    - Proteinuria

SIGNS AND SYMPTOMS

- Are myriad, and include
  - Headache, altered mental status, blurred vision, chest pain, dyspnea, nausea, fatigue, weakness
  - Depressed sensorium, seizures, papilledema and other retinal changes, pulmonary edema, JVD, lower-extremity edema

DIAGNOSIS

- CT brain
  - Look for bleeding or stroke, mass lesions
- Chest x-ray
  - Pulmonary edema
- ECG
  - LVH or heart strain
  - Infarction/ischemia
- Urinalysis
  - Proteinuria
  - Hematuria
- Serum creatinine
  - May be elevated
- Troponin
  - May be elevated

TREATMENT

- Should be tailored to cause of hypertension and end organ damage; intravenous agents predominate; mean arterial BP (MAP) should be followed
  - MAP = [diastolic BP + 1/3 (systolic BP − diastolic BP)]

DISEASE STATES OF HYPERTENSIVE EMERGENCY

- Acute cardiac ischemia: Goal is to rapidly reverse ischemia and reduce myocardial oxygen demand
  - Nitroglycerin
  - Beta-adrenergic blockers
- CHF with pulmonary edema: Goal is to reduce afterload, signs and symptoms of CHF; usually can be achieved with 10% to 15% reduction in MAP
  - Nitroglycerin
  - ACE inhibitors
  - Furosemide
  - Nicardipine
- Aortic dissection
  - Esmolol + nitroprusside
  - Labetalol
- CVA: BP management controversial—0% to 25% reduction in MAP over 6 to 12 hours
  - Nicardipine
  - Nitroprusside
  - Labetalol
  - Nimodipine
- Intracranial hemorrhage: BP management controversial
  - Nicardipine
  - Nitroprusside
  - Nimodipine
- Hypertensive encephalopathy—25% reduction in MAP over 2 to 3 hours
  - Nitroprusside

- Nicardipine
- Labetalol
- Pheochromocytoma: Goal is to control paroxysms of BP elevation
  - Phentolamine
  - Nitroprusside
  - Labetalol
- Pre-eclampsia/eclampsia: Goal is to reduce BP to 140/90 mmHg
  - Hydralazine
  - Magnesium
  - Labetalol
- Cocaine-related HTN
  - Nitroglycerin
  - Benzodiazepines
  - Phentolamine for end-organ ischemia refractory to above measures

ANTIHYPERTENSIVE AGENTS

- Nicardipine
  - Dihydropyridine calcium channel blocker
  - More cerebral/coronary vessel–specific
  - Used in CHF, CVA, hypertensive encephalopathy
  - Onset of action is within 1 to 2 minutes, duration is 2 to 5 minutes after drug is stopped
  - Side effects: peripheral edema, flushing, fatigue, headache, lightheadedness
- Nitroprusside
  - Direct arterial and venous vasodilator, decreases preload and afterload
  - Criterion standard of emergent antihypertensive therapy
  - Used in hypertensive encephalopathy, aortic dissection, pulmonary edema
  - Onset of action is within 1 to 2 minutes, duration is 2 to 5 minutes after drug is stopped
  - Side effects: weakness, nausea, tinnitus, dizziness, hypotension, thiocyanate toxicity (particularly in renal patients)
- Nitroglycerin
  - Direct arterial and venous vasodilator, decreases preload and afterload
  - Used in acute myocardial infarction (AMI), CHF, intracranial hemorrhage
  - Onset of action 1 to 2 minutes
  - Side effects: headache, reflex tachycardia, hypersensitivity reactions, orthostatic hypotension
  - Contraindicated with erectile dysfunction agents (e.g., sildenafil)
- Labetalol
  - Competitive, selective alpha1-blocker and competitive, nonselective beta-blocker, with the beta-blocking effect 4-8x more potent
  - Decreases blood pressure by decreasing peripheral resistance
  - Alternative to nitroprusside in hypertensive emergencies
  - Contraindicated when a beta-adrenergic blocker can not be used
  - Onset of action (IV) in 5 to 10 minutes and duration is 3 to 4 hours

- Effective in patients on other antihypertensive medications
- Side effects: nausea, orthostasis, vomiting, flushing, headache, scalp tingling, dizziness—all mild
- Esmolol
  - β-1 selective adrenergic blockade—100 times more activity at β-1 than β-2
  - Used in aortic dissection/aneurysm
  - Onset of action 1 to 2 minutes, lasts up to 20 minutes once stopped
  - Side effects: hypotension, heart block, hypoglycemia, dizziness, headache
- Clonidine
  - Centrally acting α_2-adrenergic agonist that decreases central sympathomimetic activity
  - Onset of action is 30 to 60 min with peak effects in 2 to 4 hours
  - Oral dosing
- Captopril/enalaprilat
  - Angiotensin-converting enzyme inhibitors
  - Onset of action in 15 to 30 minutes, peak effect at 60 minutes (captopril)
  - Oral/sublingual dosing of captopril; IV dosing of enalaprilat

Valvular heart disease

- Vast majority are chronic
- Hypertrophy and dilation of the heart enables cardiac function to be maintained for years before symptoms
- Incompetent valves produce regurgitant flow
- Scarring and stenosis produces restricted or stenotic flow
- Multivalvular disease is common with progression of illness

MITRAL VALVE PROLAPSE

Pathophysiology

- Etiology is unknown, but may be congenital
- 5% to 10% of the population
- Abnormal stretching of the mitral valve during systole
- Most commonly the posterior leaflet of the mitral valve alone prolapses and no regurgitation takes place
- If both leaflets prolapse, regurgitation may occur
- Associated with connective tissue disorders
  - Marfan syndrome
  - Ehler Danlos syndrome
  - Pectus excavatum
  - Severe scoliosis
- Majority are young women

SIGNS AND SYMPTOMS

- Chest pain
- Palpitations
- Dyspnea
- Fatigue
- Auscultatory findings variable

- 20% have classic midsystolic click followed by a late systolic crescendo murmur heard between the apex and the left sternal border
- Maneuvers that reduce the end-diastolic ventricular volume cause the click to move closer to S1
- Click is the result of snapping of the chordae tendineae during prolapse of the mitral valve

DIAGNOSIS

- ECG-nonspecific changes
- Increased risk of endocarditis (when regurgitation is present)
- Associated with neurologic abnormalities, from migraine to CVA
- Rarely arrhythmias, including ventricular tachycardia and sudden cardiac death

TREATMENT

- Beta-adrenergic blockers
- Reassurance

MITRAL STENOSIS

- Rheumatic heart disease still most common cause
  - Delay between rheumatic fever and symptom onset is common (20 years)
  - 85% mortality 20 years after the onset of symptoms without surgery
- Pathophysiology
  - Stenosis of the mitral valve impedes flow from the left atrium to the left ventricle
  - May lead to pulmonary hypertension
  - Left atrial hypertension and eventually left ventricular failure and pulmonary edema develop over time

SIGNS AND SYMPTOMS

- Dyspnea on exertion is the most common presenting symptom (80%)
- Hemoptysis
- Auscultatory findings—palpable diastolic thrill over the apex, loud S1, and opening snap of the mitral valve in early diastole followed by a low-pitched diastolic rumbling/murmur

DIAGNOSIS

- CXR
  - Left atrial enlargement—straightening of the left heart border
- ECG
  - Left atrial hypertrophy
  - Right axis deviation (with pulmonary hypertension)
  - Atrial fibrillation
- Atrial fibrillation is the most common complication (40%)
- Embolism is the most dreaded complication (20%)
- Pulmonary hypertension and pulmonary edema
- Respiratory infections and hemoptysis

TREATMENT

- Medical management of pulmonary hypertension and pulmonary edema
- Management of atrial fibrillation; anticoagulation to prevent embolization
- Valvuloplasty or replacement

MITRAL REGURGITATION

- Acute and chronic mitral regurgitation are two distinct diseases
- Acute mitral regurgitation
  - Usually the result of ischemic heart disease, endocarditis, or trauma
  - Associated with cardiogenic shock
  - Usually the result of rupture of papillary muscle, chordae tendineae, or perforation of the mitral valve
- Chronic mitral regurgitation
  - Most commonly the result of rheumatic heart disease

SIGNS AND SYMPTOMS

- Acute
  - Fulminant CHF without a prior history of heart failure
  - Loud crescendo–decrescendo systolic murmur best heard at the base
- Chronic
  - Palpable left ventricular heave and thrill
  - High-pitched holosystolic murmur best heard at the apex and radiating into the axilla

DIAGNOSIS

- Acute
  - CXR
    - Normal cardiac silhouette with pulmonary edema
  - ECG
    - Absence of LVH and left atrial hypertrophy
    - Possible cardiac ischemia (inferior)
- Chronic
  - ECG
    - Usually has LVH and left atrial enlargement
    - Atrial fibrillation is common
  - CXR
    - Left atrial enlargement
- Complications
  - Arrhythmias/atrial fibrillation
  - Sudden death
  - Cerebral ischemia
  - Endocarditis
  - CHF

TREATMENT

- Acute
- Medical stabilization with afterload reduction
  - Emergent cardiac catheterization
  - Surgical intervention
- Chronic
  - Medical management
  - Surgical consultation as needed

AORTIC STENOSIS

- Most common cause in nonelderly is congenital bicuspid valve (50% of cases)
- Most common cause in elderly is calcific degeneration of the valve cusp

Pathophysiology

- LV outflow obstruction occurs when the valve orifice becomes less than 1.0 cm or when the pressure gradient across the valve exceeds 50 mmHg
- Symptoms occur late in the course of the illness

SIGNS AND SYMPTOMS

- Dyspnea
- Angina
- Exertional syncope
- Low-pitched rasping crescendo–decrescendo systolic murmur heard best at the base and radiating into the carotids
- Soft S2, suggesting minimal valve leaflet mobility
- Paradoxical splitting of S2; S3 and S4 are common
- Carotid pulse is diminished in amplitude (parvus)
- Carotid pulse is slow rising (tardus)
- Hyperdynamic left ventricle with a heave
- Pulse pressure may be reduced

DIAGNOSIS

- ECG
  - LVH
- Left or right bundle branch block
- Complications
  - Sudden death from cardiac arrhythmia
  - Endocarditis
  - CHF
  - Cardiac ischemia

TREATMENT

- Medical management has a limited role after symptoms develop
- Maintain balance between preload/afterload
- Nitrates should be used very cautiously
- Fluids, inotropic agents, and balloon pump are temporizing
- Valvuloplasty/valve replacement is definitive therapy

AORTIC REGURGITATION

Etiology

- Rheumatic heart disease is the most common cause overall
- 20% of all cases are acute
- Acute aortic regurgitation is most commonly associated with
  - Endocarditis
  - Aortic dissection
  - Trauma

SIGNS AND SYMPTOMS

- Dyspnea is the most common presenting symptom (50%)
- Symptoms of pulmonary edema are common
- Auscultatory findings: a high-pitched blowing diastolic murmur heard immediately after the second heart sound
- May be asymptomatic for years
- Signs associated with chronic aortic regurgitation
  - Rapidly rising and falling carotid pulse (Corrigan's or water hammer pulse)
  - Nail pulsations (Quincke sign)
  - Head bobbing with pulse (de Musset sign)
  - To-and-fro murmur over the femoral artery (Duroziez sign)
  - Wide pulse pressure
- Austin Flint murmur (soft diastolic rumble resulting from aortic reflux and impact on mitral valve opening)

DIAGNOSIS

- Complications
  - CHF
  - Embolization
  - Sudden cardiac death

TREATMENT

- Valve replacement
- Medical stabilization with afterload reducers, diuretics, and intra-aortic balloon pump

COMPLICATIONS OF PROSTHETIC VALVES

Pathophysiology

- Two types: mechanical and bioprosthetic
- Mechanical valves require continuous anticoagulation
- Some bioprosthetic valves do not require anticoagulation

Complications

- Systemic embolization is the most common complication with mechanical valves and occurs at 1% per year
- Embolization is less frequent with the bioprosthetic valves
- Endocarditis occurs at the rate of 0.5% per year
- Anemia from hemolysis is common with mechanical valve
- Hemodynamic compromise from new arrhythmia (atrial fibrillation)
- Paravalvular leaks may present with CHF

Cardiac tumors

- Metastatic more common than primary; benign primary tumors more common than malignant primary tumors

ATRIAL MYXOMA

- 40% to 50% of primary cardiac tumors; usually solitary, and the majority arise from the left atrium
- Vast majority are sporadic, but 10% are familial, multiple, and arise from the ventricle as well
- Typically benign
- Prevalence is approximately 0.02%, with 75% occurring in females in all age groups

SIGNS AND SYMPTOMS

- Constitutional symptoms are observed in 50% of patients and include fever, weight loss, arthralgias, and Raynaud phenomenon
- Hemoptysis due to pulmonary edema or infarction is observed in up to 15% of patients
- Symptoms result from mechanical interference with cardiac function or embolization from friable myxomatous tissue
- Obstruction
  - Left-sided obstruction from tumor: dyspnea on exertion, orthopnea, paroxysmal nocturnal dyspnea
  - Right-sided obstruction from tumor: peripheral edema, hepatic enlargement, ascites
  - Dizziness and syncope in 20%
  - Positional symptoms are common
- Embolism site depends on the site of the tumor and presence of an intracardiac shunt
  - Left-sided tumors: visceral ischemia, transient ischemic attacks, stroke, seizures
  - Right-sided tumors: pulmonary embolism, infarction
- Systemic findings may include fever, digital clubbing, petechial rash
- Other physical findings may include
  - Delayed S1 due to tumor obstructing the mitral valve
  - Early diastolic sound, known as tumor plop, due to the impact of the tumor against the atrial wall
- Diastolic rumble from the tumor obstructing the tricuspid or mitral valve
- Patients with familial myxoma may have findings grouped as myxoma syndromes that include myxomas in breast, neural tissue, and spotty pigmentation of the skin; Cushing syndrome

DIAGNOSIS

- Clinical suspicion
- Laboratory studies
  - Elevated ESR and C-reactive protein
  - Leukocytosis
  - Anemia, including hemolytic anemia
- Imaging studies
  - Chest radiograph showing enlarged atrial silhouette or pulmonary edema
  - Echocardiography is usually diagnostic
  - MRI

TREATMENT

- Resection of the tumor is the treatment of choice

PEARLS

- Aortic dissection should be suspected with a patient with sudden, tearing chest pain that radiates to the back or has other known risk factors. Chest CT scan is the ideal test if patient is stable.

- Abdominal aortic aneurysm with symptoms is a surgical emergency until proven otherwise. Bedside ultrasound, preoperative workup, and rapid vascular surgery consult are the mainstays of emergency department management.

- Peripheral arterial disease can be embolic or thrombotic and is characterized by the 6 P's: pain, paraesthesia, poikilothermia, pallor, pulselessness, and paralysis; some are late findings.

- Risk factors for venous thromboembolism center include Virchow triad of stasis, hypercoagulability, and endothelial injury.

- The approach to pulmonary embolism begins with pretest probability assessment. The symptoms and results of chest x-ray, arterial blood gas, and electrocardiogram can be nonspecific. For patients with low to moderate risk by scoring systems, a negative sensitive D-dimer rules out disease. Otherwise, ventilation–perfusion scan or CT angiography should be ordered.

- Duplex ultrasound is the mainstay of diagnosis of deep-vein thrombosis. A repeat ultrasound in 7 days should be ordered in high-risk patients with a negative study.

- Acute myocarditis should be suspected whenever a patient, especially a young male, presents with otherwise unexplained cardiac abnormalities of new onset, such as heart failure, arrhythmias, or conduction disturbances, although the majority of cases have a benign course.

- The vast majority of valvular heart disease is chronic. Hypertrophy and dilation of the heart enables cardiac function to be maintained for years before the development of symptoms. The four valves of the heart and the supporting papillary muscles and chordae tendineae are subject to a limited number of abnormalities. Incompetent valves produce regurgitant flow. Valvular scaring and stenosis produces restricted or stenotic flow. Multivalvular disease is common with progression of illness.

■ The treatment of hypertension is dependent on symptoms and presence or absence of end-organ disease. Asymptomatic patients do not need to be treated and should not have the blood pressure rapidly lowered, although it is reasonable to start medications on patient with severe elevations or other end-organ disease. The choice of treatment for HTN urgency or emergency is dependent on co-morbid conditions.

■ Fever, anemia, and new heart murmur should raise concern for endocarditis, and either fever or murmur alone in an intravenous drug user should also raise concern. Blood cultures should be obtained and antibiotics given.

BIBLIOGRAPHY

Backer HD, Decker L, Ackerson L: Reproducibility of increased blood pressure during an emergency department or urgent care visit, *Ann Emerg Med* 41:507–512, 2003.

Brady WJ, Aufderheide T, Kaplan P: Cardiovascular imaging. In Schwartz D, Residorf EJ (eds): *Emergency radiology*, New York, 2000, McGraw-Hill, pp. 479–508.

Chobanian AV, Bakris GL, Black HR et al: Seventh report of the Joint National Committee on Prevention, Detection, Evaluation, and Treatment of High Blood Pressure, *Hypertension* 42:1206–1252, 2003.

Chopra A: Thrombophlebitis and occlusive arterial disease. In Tintinalli J, Kelen GD, Stapczynski JS (eds): *Emergency medicine: a comprehensive study guide*, ed 6, New York, 2004, McGraw-Hill, pp. 409–417.

Decker WW, Godwin SA, Hess EP, Lenamond CC, Jagoda AS: Clinical policy: critical issues in the evaluation and management of adult patients with asymptomatic hypertension in the emergency department, *Ann Emerg Med* 47:237–249, 2006.

Hagan PG, Nienaber CA, Isselbacher EM et al: The International Registry of Acute Aortic Dissection (IRAD): New insights into an old disease, *JAMA* 283:897–903, 2000.

Januzzi JL, Isselbacher EM, Fattori R et al: Characterizing the young patient with aortic dissection: results from the International Registry of Aortic Dissectioin (IRAD), *J Am Coll Cardiol* 43:665–669, 2004.

Karras DJ, Kruus LK, Cienki JJ et al: Utility of routine testing for patients with asymptomatic severe blood pressure elevation in the emergency department, *Ann Emerg Med* 51:231–239, 2008.

Kline J: Pulmonary embolism. In Tintinalli J, Kelen GD, Stapczynski JS (eds): *Emergency medicine: a comprehensive study guide*, ed 6, New York, 2004, McGraw-Hill, pp. 386–393.

Kline JA, Mitchell AM, Kabrhel C, Richman PB, Courtney DM: Clinical criteria to prevent unnecessary diagnostic testing in emergency department patients with suspected pulmonary embolism, *J Thromb Haemost* 2:1247–1255, 2004.

Kline JA, Courtney DM, Kabrhel C et al: Prospective multicenter evaluation of the pulmonary embolism rule-out criteria, *J Thromb Haemost* 6:772–780, 2008.

Klompas M: Does this patient have an acute thoracic aortic dissection? *JAMA* 287:2262–2272, 2002.

Le Gal G, Righini M, Roy P-M et al: Prediction of pulmonary embolism in the emergency department: the revised geneva score, *Ann Intern Med* 144:165–171, 2006.

Rubins JB: The current approach to the diagnosis of pulmonary embolism: lessons from PIOPED II, *Postgrad Med* 120:1–7, 2008.

Schoepf UJ, Goldhaber SZ, Costello P: Spiral computed tomography for acute pulmonary embolism, *Circulation* 109:2160–2167, 2004.

Shayne PH, Pitts SR: Severely increased blood pressure in the emergency department, *Ann Emerg Med* 41:513–529, 2003.

Spates M, Schwartz DT, Savitt D: Abdominal imaging. In Schwartz D, Residorf EJ (eds): *Emergency radiology*, New York, 2000, McGraw-Hill, pp. 509–554.

Spittell PC, Spittell JA Jr, Joyce JW et al: Clinical features and differential diagnosis of aortic dissection: experience with 236 cases (1980 through 1990), *Mayo Clin Proc* 68:642–651, 1993.

Stein PD, Hull RD, Patel KC et al: D-dimer for the exclusion of acute venous thrombosis and pulmonary embolism: a systematic review, *Ann Intern Med* 140:589–602, 2004.

Stein PD, Woodard PK, Weg JG et al: Diagnostic pathways in acute pulmonary embolism: recommendations of the PIOPED II investigators, *Radiology* 242:15–21, 2007.

Tapson VF: Acute pulmonary embolism, *N Engl J Med* 358:1037–1052, 2008.

Wagner M, Wolford R, Hartfelder B, Schwartz DT: Pulmonary chest radiography. In Schwartz D, Residorf EJ (eds): *Emergency radiology*, New York, 2000, McGraw-Hill, pp. 443–478.

Wells PS, Anderson DR, Rodger M et al: Derivation of a simple clinical model to categorize patients' probability of pulmonary embolism: increasing the models utility with the SimpliRED D-dimer, *Thromb Haemost* 83:416–420, 2000.

Wu M, Chanmugam A: Hypertension. In Tintinalli J, Kelen GD, Stapczynski JS (eds): *Emergency medicine: a comprehensive study guide*, ed 6, New York, 2004, McGraw-Hill, pp. 394–403.

Questions and Answers

1. A 72-year-old man with a history of hypertension presents with sudden-onset left-flank pain and hypotension. On examination, he is noted to be hypotensive, with a blood pressure of 80/40 mmHg, heart rate of 110 bpm, and he has epigastric tenderness as well as left costovertebral angle tenderness. His lower-extremity pulses are palpable. The most appropriate initial diagnostic test for this patient would be:

   a. CT chest
   b. Chest x-ray
   c. Bedside ultrasound
   d. D-dimer
   e. ECG

2. A 65-year-old woman presents with sudden onset of severe, sharp pain in her upper back. Her vital signs are as follows: BP = 160/90 mmHg, HR = 110 bpm, and she is diaphoretic. Her ECG shows nonspecific ST-T wave abnormalities. A chest x-ray shows a widened mediastinum with an apical cap. The best initial treatment to start on this patient would be:

   a. aspirin
   b. beta-adrenergic blockade
   c. heparin
   d. fibrinolytics
   e. ceftriaxone

3. A 21-year-old female basketball player presents after collapsing on the court, complaining of severe back pain. Risk factors that would increase suspicion for thoracic aortic dissection would include all of the following *except:*

   a. bicuspid aortic valve
   b. Marfan syndrome

c. cocaine abuse
d. pregnancy
e. Factor V Leiden

4. A 72-year-old woman presents with a painful, cool foot. Her vital signs reveal an irregular pulse. She states she normally only has pain when she walks great distances but now is having rest pain. Symptoms that would raise concern for a peripheral arterial embolism would include all of the following *except:*

a. pulselessness
b. pyrogenesis (fever)
c. poikilothermia
d. paresthesias
e. pallor

5. 29-year-old man presents with progressive dyspnea on exertion, fatigue, and nocturnal cough for 3 days. He noted a viral syndrome 2 weeks prior. All of the following could provide useful information *except:*

a. D-dimer
b. MRI
c. viral titers
d. echocardiogram
e. ECG

6. 45-year-old man presents with 2 days of chest pain and dyspnea. The patient prefers sitting forward in a tripod position. On examination, the patient is noted to have tachypnea, tachycardia, normal oxygen saturations, jugular venous distention, and clear lung fields. The heart sounds are distant, and there is no murmur, gallop, or rub. Which of the following is the *best* initial test to rule out the most emergent complication of this disease?

a. CBC
b. ECG
c. electrolytes
d. arterial blood gas
e. echocardiogram

7. 29-year-old woman with a history of intravenous drug abuse presents with fever and an abscess in her left antecubital area. On exam she has a 3/6 systolic murmur at the left sternal border, and she reports no history of heart murmur. What is the best treatment?

a. penicillin and clindamycin
b. doxycycline and levofloxacin
c. levofloxacin and erythromycin
d. metronidazole and ciprofloxacin
e. vancomycin and gentamicin

8. Which of the following is *not* a risk factor for thoracic aortic dissection?

a. bicuspid aortic valve
b. coarctation of the aorta
c. cocaine use
d. hypertension
e. leg swelling

9. Which of the following is most concerning for thoracic aortic dissection? Chest pain

a. associated with new neurologic deficits
b. relieved with rest
c. with gradual onset
d. not relieved with nitroglycerin
e. following eating

10. Which statement about the Wells score is *true?*

a. Patients with a high Wells score for PE do not require further testing; they can be simply treated with appropriate anticoagulation.
b. The Wells score identifies risk for acute coronary syndrome.
c. The Wells score is affected by patient age.
d. The Wells score does not take vital signs into account.
e. The Wells score can be combined with a negative D-dimer to exclude PE in low-risk patients.

11. A 16-year-old football player collapses on the field. He regains consciousness, and is transported to the emergency department. His vital signs are BP = 122/80 mmHg, HR = 90 bpm, pulse oximetry = 98% on room air. His cardiac examination reveals an S4, and a soft systolic murmur. A 12-lead ECG shows evidence of left ventricular hypertrophy without ischemia as well as normal intervals. The diagnostic study of choice is:

a. chest radiography
b. echocardiogram
c. CT of his chest
d. cardiac catheterization

12. A 27-year-old woman, 2 weeks postpartum, presents with 2 days of progressive cough, shortness of breath, and difficulty breathing at night. She is sitting upright, tachypneic, with audible wheezing, and her lower extremities demonstrate symmetric pitting edema. She has minimal work of breathing. The intervention that is most likely to help her acute symptomatology is:

a. albuterol 5 mg via nebulizer
b. magnesium sulfate 2 gm IV
c. sublingual, followed by IV, nitroglycerin
d. heliox
e. rapid-sequence intubation

13. The diagnostic study most likely to confirm your clinical diagnosis of the patient above is:

a. CT angiography
b. chest radiography
c. echocardiogram
d. V/Q scan
e. lower-extremity Duplex ultrasonography

14. A 62-year-old woman presents with chest pains that have been accelerating in frequency over the past month, and are now occurring at rest. She is actively complaining of chest pain; her

vital signs are BP = 158/90 mmHg and HR = 110 bpm. She has bi-basilar rales and a 4/6 systolic murmur over the left sternal border with a soft S2, and the murmur is audible over the carotid arteries. An ECG shows sinus tachycardia with ST-segment depression in the precordial leads. The medication that could most likely precipitate cardiovascular collapse in this patient is:

a. nitroglycerin 0.4 mg SL
b. metoprolol 5 mg IV
c. diltiazem 10 mg IV
d. clonidine 0.1 mg orally
e. furosemide 20 mg IV

15. Which of the following is *not* indicated in a case of superficial thrombophlebitis?

a. naproxen
b. warm compresses
c. elastic support stockings
d. warfarin

16. Sinus tachycardia with diffuse ST-segment elevation and PR-segment depression is an electrocardiographic manifestation of

a. pericarditis
b. myocarditis
c. Wolff Parkinson White syndrome
d. hypothermia

17. Sodium nitroprusside

a. is associated with thiocyanate toxicity
b. is contraindicated in patients taking sildenafil
c. is the drug of choice in eclampsia
d. has a gradual onset of action

18. This centrally acting alpha-2 adrenergic agonist has a gradual onset of action (30 to 60 minutes), and is useful as an oral agent for the treatment of hypertension and hypertensive urgencies.

a. captopril
b. valsartan
c. clonidine
d. amlodipine

19. This chest x-ray finding is associated with pulmonary embolism.

a. Westermark sign
b. apical cap
c. deep sulcus sign
d. de Musset sign

20. The Austin Flint murmur is seen with which type of valvular heart disease?

a. mitral stenosis
b. aortic stenosis
c. mitral regurgitation
d. aortic regurgitation

---

1. Answer: c

This patient likely has a *ruptured abdominal aortic aneurysm (AAA)* and needs an emergent vascular

surgery evaluation for operative repair. He is too unstable to go to the CT scanner (**a**). A chest x-ray and ECG (**b, e**) might provide additional usefully information but would not confirm the diagnosis of AAA. The D-dimer (**d**) would not diagnose AAA either.

2. Answer: b

This patient is most likely suffering from *a thoracic aortic dissection.* Beta-adrenergic blockers are needed to reduce the heart rate as well as the shear forces being applied to the aorta. A good agent would be esmolol or labetalol. Nitroprusside is also an acceptable option, but should be used with a beta-adrenergic blocker such as esmolol. Medicines to reduce clotting by inhibiting platelets, the clotting cascade, or thrombin (**a, c, d**) are not helpful and can be dangerous in a patient with an aortic dissection. The patient does not appear to have an infection so ceftriaxone (**e**) is not needed.

3. Answer: e

A **bicuspid aortic valve** and **cocaine** increase the pressure and shear forces distal to the aortic valve leading to risk of dissection (**a, c**). Conditions that affect the elasticity of the connective tissue of the aorta such as **Marfan syndrome** and **pregnancy** (**b, d**) can also lead to dissection. **Factor V Leiden** (**e**) is not a risk factor for dissection but is a risk factor for PE.

4. Answer: b

All of the other answers (**a, c, d, e**) are classic symptoms of peripheral arterial clot.

5. Answer: a

This patient has a history consistent with *myocarditis.* An MRI (**b**) can show the extent of inflammation, whereas viral titers (**c**) can identify the cause of infection. An echocardiogram (**d**) may show global dysfunction, whereas ECG (**e**) may show arrhythmia or nonspecific ECG changes; it is also a good screening test for pericarditis.

6. Answer: e

An echocardiogram (**e**) can most definitively rule out *pericardial effusion with tamponade.* A CBC (**a**) might be elevated from an infectious or inflammatory cause, but is nonspecific. The ECG (**b**) could show electrical alternans or low voltage, but would not definitively rule out tamponade. An electrolyte panel and arterial blood gas (**c, d**) would be nonspecific.

7. Answer: e

None of the other drug combinations (**a, b, c, d**) would cover the correct bacteria concerning for *infectious endocarditis* in an intravenous drug user, most commonly due to staphylococcal species.

8. Answer: e

All of the other answers are risk factors for thoracic aortic dissection.

9. Answer: a

Chest pain with neurologic deficits (a) can occur in *thoracic aortic dissection* due to lack of blood flow down one of the major branches of the aorta from the dissection. Pain relieved with rest (b) is more associated with anginal pain. Pain with gradual onset and not relieved by nitroglycerin (c, d) are nonspecific. Pain after eating can occur (e) with either a GI source of pain or ischemic coronary disease.

10. Answer: e

Patients with a high *Wells score* (a) need a confirmatory test for PE, because the Wells score only establishes pretest probability. The Wells score has not been tested for acute coronary syndrome risk stratification (b) and is not affected by age (c). Tachycardia is one of the Wells criteria (d).

11. Answer: b.

The likely diagnosis is *hypertrophic cardiomyopathy*, and this will be readily demonstrated on echocardiography (b), showing either symmetric or asymmetric ventricular hypertrophy. The likely cause of this patient's collapse is either a primary dysrhythmia or aortic outflow obstruction precipitated by volume depletion and exercise induced–enhanced ventricular contractility.

12. Answer: c

The likely diagnosis is *postpartum cardiomyopathy*. The symptoms are likely due to a dilated cardiomyopathy and congestive heart failure, and probably will respond acutely to preload reduction with nitroglycerin. Because the symptoms are primarily due to fluid overload, treatments aimed at bronchospasm (a, b, d) are less likely to help, and intubation (e) is not necessary.

13. Answer: c

An **echocardiogram** is the best test to diagnose her biventricular failure. A **chest radiograph (b)** will likely show pulmonary edema, so may correctly lead you to initiate appropriate treatment but fail to provide the diagnosis. None of the other tests (a, d, e) are likely to establish the diagnosis.

14. Answer: a

This patient likely has symptomatic *aortic stenosis,* and is dependent on adequate pre-load to maintain her cardiac output and coronary perfusion. Sublingual nitroglycerin (a) will likely result in a precipitous drop in her pre-load and hence hinder her cardiac output, which may adversely compromise perfusion of her coronary vessels, which are just distal to the stenotic aortic valve. None of the other medications (b, c, d, e) are as likely to cause as precipitous a drop in pre-load.

15. Answer: d

Whereas anticoagulation with warfarin (d) is indicated for the treatment of deep-vein thrombosis, it is not known to be helpful in the treatment of the superficial thrombophlebitis. The other selections (a, b, c) are all reasonable in the treatment of this disease entity.

16. Answer: a

These are the classic findings on ECG in the patient with stage I **pericarditis (a)**. **Myocarditis (b)** does not feature specific ECG findings. **Wolff Parkinson White syndrome (c)** typically demonstrates PR interval shortening, QRS complex widening (because of the delta wave), and discordant ST-segment changes. **Hypothermia** may yield Osborne, or J waves, on the ECG—notching of the junction (J point) of the QRS complex and the ST segment.

17. Answer: a

Thiocyanate toxicity (a), especially in patients with renal insufficiency, is a well-recognized side effect of this drug; cyanide is a red cell metabolite that is converted to thiocyanate by the liver, and then excreted by the kidney. Manifestations include tinnitus, blurred vision, delirium, and seizures. **Sildenafil** is contraindicated with nitrate therapy (b). Hydralazine, labetalol, and magnesium infusion are the best agents for **eclampsia (c)**. Nitroprusside has a very rapid onset of action—almost immediate—and a duration that ends shortly after the infusion is interrupted; thus choice **d** is incorrect.

18. Answer: c

Captopril (a) is an angiotensin-converting enzyme inhibitor; **valsartan (b)**, an angiotensin receptor blocker; and **amlodipine (d)** is a dihydropyridine calcium-channel blocker. They are all useful in the treatment of hypertension, but **clonidine** is the only centrally acting alpha-2 adrenergic agonist.

19. Answer: a

Westermark sign (a), found on the chest x-ray, is a paucity of vascular markings in the distribution of the pulmonary embolism; it is sometimes associated with a radiodense area in the adjacent pulmonary artery, representing the clot. An **apical cap (b)** is associated with thoracic aortic dissection. The **deep sulcus sign (c)** is seen with pneumothorax on the supine chest x-ray. Bobbing of the head with each pulse is the **de Musset sign (d)**, seen with severe aortic regurgitation—it is not a radiographic finding.

20. Answer: d

When a regurgitant jet of blood flows back from the aortic valve toward the mitral valve, it can inhibit the opening of the latter, creating the diastolic Austin Flint murmur—because of **aortic regurgitation**, but with a structurally normal mitral valve; thus d, not a, is the correct answer. **Aortic stenosis (b)** and **mitral regurgitation (c)** both cause systolic murmurs: the former classically at the left or right upper sternal border and radiating to the carotids; the latter at the apex and radiating to the axilla.

Cutaneous 4

Matthew L. Tripp | Richard A. Harrigan

DERMATITIS
Atopic
Contact
Psoriasis
Seborrhea

INFECTIONS
Bacterial
Viral
Fungal
Parasitic

MACULOPAPULAR LESIONS
Erythema multiforme
Erythema nodosum
Pityriasis rosea
Urticaria
Drug eruption

BULLOUS
Pemphigus vulgaris
Bullous pemphigoid

CANCEROUS LESIONS
Melanoma
Basal cell carcinoma
Squamous cell carcinoma
Kaposi sarcoma

Dermatitis

ATOPIC

- Associated with allergic disorders (asthma, rhinitis)
- Not itself an allergic condition
- Exact mechanism unknown

SIGNS AND SYMPTOMS

- Acute: vesicular oozing lesions
- Chronic: dry, scaly, hyperpigmented, lichenification
- Intensely pruritic
  - Especially at night, in winter and may be triggered by various stressors
  - Excoriations may become secondarily infected
  - Lichenification develops as a result of repeated scratching
- Distribution: varies by age
  - Infants: extensor surfaces, diaper area, cheeks.
- Onset in 4th to 6th month, improves or resolves by age 3 to 5 years
- Children/adults: flexor surfaces.

TREATMENT

- Symptomatic
  - May include moisturizers, antihistamines, topical corticosteroids, ultraviolet light
- Identify triggers

CONTACT

- Skin reaction to chemical, physical, or biologic irritants
- Delayed hypersensitivity reaction
- Most common irritants
  - Rubber compounds
  - Plants: poison ivy, oak, etc. **(most likely to cause bullae)**
  - Nickel
  - Paraphenylenediamine—found in hair dye

SIGNS AND SYMPTOMS

- Papules, vesicles, bullae on an erythematous base
- Distribution depends on area of contact
- Sparing of mucous membranes

TREATMENT

- Avoidance of triggers
- Wash all contaminated clothes to get rid of persistent oils
- Topical and/or systemic corticosteroids
- Antihistamines

PSORIASIS

- Inherited disorder of overproduction of keratinocyte cells

SIGNS AND SYMPTOMS

- Plaques of erythema, scales, and fissures
- Affected areas: palms, soles of feet, elbows, knees, and scalp

TREATMENT

- Topical steroids, tar preparations, ultraviolet light, methotrexate

SEBORRHEA

- Exact mechanism unknown. May involve the yeast *Pityrosporum ovale*
- Associated with HIV infection

SIGNS AND SYMPTOMS

- Waxy scale in the fold of hair-growing areas of face, scalp, and groin
- May affect any age group
  - Infants: seborrhea of scalp known as "cradle cap"
  - Infants: rarely associated with hair loss (this finding suggests diagnosis of fungal infection)

TREATMENT

- Antidandruff shampoo, ketoconazole (Nizoral) shampoo, topical steroids

Infections

BACTERIAL

Abscess

- 1% to 2% of all emergency department (ED) complaints
- Localized collection of purulent material surrounded by induration, erythema, and/or cellulitis
- Bacterial cause depends on area
- 5% are sterile
- High incidence of community-acquired methicillin-resistant *Staphylococcus aureus* (CA-MRSA)
  - Roughly 59% of abscesses seen in the ED are caused by CA-MRSA (this number is increasing)
- Caused by a break in the skin, blockage of apocrine sweat glands, anal crypts, or Bartholin glands

SIGNS AND SYMPTOMS

- Tender, fluctuant area
- Bedside ultrasound may help delineate pockets of purulent material and differentiate cellulitis from abscess
- Uncomplicated abscess: No cellulitis, fever, or lymphangitis
- Complicated abscess has the above features

TREATMENT

- Incision and drainage with loose packing
- Antibiotic considerations must cover CA-MRSA

- Uncomplicated abscess: doxycycline or trimethoprim/sulfamethoxazole (TMP-SMX) alone, but local resistance patterns may vary. May not need antibiotics.
- Complicated abscess: CA-MRSA and group A streptococcal coverage; cephalexin **plus** TMP-SMX or clindamycin alone or doxycycline alone

Hidradenitis suppurativa

- Chronic inflammation and abscess of the apocrine sweat glands commonly in axilla, groin, and perineal regions
- Female-to-male ratio 3 : 1
- Increased incidence in African American women
- Recurrent and episodic in nature
- Incision and drainage acutely; but may require definitive surgical excision

Cellulitis

- Soft-tissue inflammation secondary to bacterial invasion exacerbated by an exaggerated immune response
- 1% to 3% of hospital visits
- Predisposing factors: elderly, immunocompromised, peripheral vascular disease
- In adults most commonly caused by *S. aureus* or *Streptococcus pyogenes*
- In children *H. influenzae* (vaccination may have decreased incidence)

SIGNS AND SYMPTOMS

- Localized tenderness, erythema, induration, warmth, lymphadenitis, and fever
- Leading-edge aspiration and blood cultures have low diagnostic yield
- "Cobblestoning" on ultrasound

TREATMENT

- Group A streptococcal coverage: cephalexin, dicloxacillin, macrolide antibiotics, amoxicillin-clavulanate
- Consider broader coverage for polymicrobial infection in diabetics

Erysipelas (Fig. 4-1)

- Acute, superficial cellulitis with a sharply demarcated border
- Commonly due to group A streptococcal species and *S. aureus*

SIGNS AND SYMPTOMS

- Abrupt onset of red shiny, hot plaques that may progress to purpura and bullae
- High fevers, rigors, and lymphatic inflammation are common

TREATMENT

- Multiple regimens are reasonable

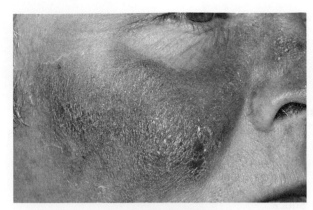

Figure 4-1 Erysipelas

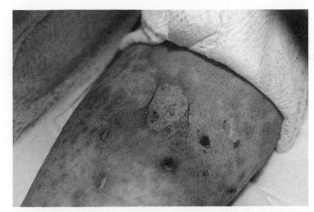

Figure 4-3 Toxic epidermal necrolysis. (From Cohen J, Powderly WG: *Infectious diseases,* ed 2, Philadelphia, 2004, Mosby.)

SIGNS AND SYMPTOMS

- Spares mucous membranes
- Sandpaper skin texture in erythroderma stage
- **Nikolsky sign:** Separation of the skin layers when pressure applied to a blister

TREATMENT

- Broad-spectrum antibiotics
- Supportive care
  - Treatment of secondary infection

Toxic epidermal necrolysis (TEN) (Fig. 4-3)

- Associated with medications: classically TMP-SMX, penicillins, aspirin, nonsteroidal anti-inflammatory drugs (NSAIDs), phenytoin, carbamazepine, allopurinol
- After certain vaccinations: polio, diphtheria (DPT)
- Associated with lymphoma
- As opposed to staphylococcal scalded skin syndrome, separation of the skin in toxic epidermal necrolysis occurs deeper, at the dermo-epidermal junction

SIGNS AND SYMPTOMS

- Mucosal lesions are common and *may precede skin signs*
- Positive Nikolsky sign (separation of the skin layers when pressure applied to a blister)
- Face is the first area involved; anogenital involvement seen
- May cause permanent damage to eyes

TREATMENT

- Identify and discontinue the cause
- Aggressive fluid resuscitation and infection control
- Steroid use remains controversial

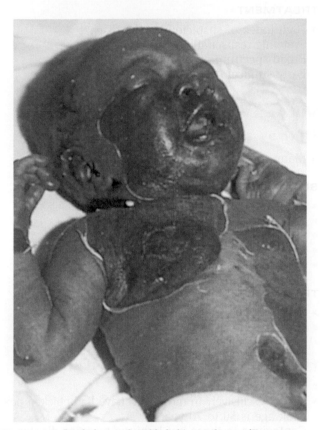

Figure 4-2 Staphylococcal scalded skin syndrome. (From Kliegman RM: *Nelson textbook of pediatrics,* ed 18, Philadelphia, 2007, Saunders.)

Staphylococcal scalded skin syndrome (Fig. 4-2)

- Also known as staphylococcal epidermal necrolysis
- Resulting from exfoliative toxin causing superficial separation of the skin at the stratum corneum, resulting in painful erythema and blistering
- Three phases: erythroderma, exfoliative, desquamation
- Commonly affects children 6 months to 6 years of age
- Mortality is 3% in children and 50% in adults (e.g., immunosuppressed, chronic kidney disease)

Staphylococcal toxic shock syndrome

- Traditionally found in menstruating women using tampons

- Can affect males and females with a focal staph infection

SIGNS AND SYMPTOMS

- Sunburned, sandpaper rash
- Mucosal involvement
- Fever, hypotension, change in mental status and eventual multiorgan dysfunction; headache and diarrhea are prominent complaints

TREATMENT

- Systemic resuscitation
- Broad-spectrum antibiotics
- Removal of the tampon, foreign body/locus of infection

Streptococcal toxic shock syndrome

- Group A streptococcal species *(S. pyogenes)*
- Produce M & T subtype exotoxins that act as a superantigen, triggering a massive immune response
- Often begins with a minor tissue insult

SIGNS AND SYMPTOMS

- Abrupt onset of severe pain and tenderness, commonly in the extremities—characteristic
- May present as acute pelvic, chest, or abdominal pain or as vague systemic symptoms such as fever, chills, and diarrhea
- Progresses to hypotension and multi-organ failure

TREATMENT

- Systemic resuscitation
- Broad-spectrum antibiotics
- Surgical debridement

Impetigo

- Superficial infection caused by group A beta-hemolytic strep
- Most common skin infection in children
- Contagious
- Bullous impetigo—staphylococcal

SIGNS AND SYMPTOMS

- Papules that develop vesicles that rupture and crust in the first 24 hours
- Pruritic, painless lesions that may become confluent
- Crust is characteristically thick and amber or honey colored
- Bullae seen in neonates
- Overall nontoxic appearance
- Negative Nikolsky sign

TREATMENT

- Systemic antibiotics are superior to topical
- Cephalexin +/– TMP-SMX

Necrotizing fasciitis

- Devastating polymicrobial infection; group A streptococcal variant exists
- 10 to 20 cases per 100,000 population
- Mortality 20% to 60%

SIGNS AND SYMPTOMS

- Fever and systemic signs of infection and/or sepsis
- Deep pain *out of proportion to clinical exam findings*
- Numbness of a localized area that progresses to necrotic areas of bullae and purpura
- Shock
- Gas may be seen in tissues on radiographic imaging

TREATMENT

- High index of suspicion for the disease
- Systemic resuscitation
- Broad-spectrum antibiotics
- Early surgical debridement is essential

VIRAL

Herpes simplex virus (HSV)

- Many subtypes. HSV1 causes nongenital lesions

SIGNS AND SYMPTOMS

- Mouth is the most common site
- Children more commonly affected
- Clusters of vesicles that break open and crust
- May be severe enough to restrict oral intake
- Associated with Bell palsy as causative agent

TREATMENT

- Spontaneous resolution in 7 to 14 days
- Antiviral therapy

Herpes zoster virus (HZV) (Fig. 4-4)

- Also known as "shingles"
- Occurs exclusively in those who have had chicken pox
- Peak age is 50 to 70 years
- Contagious to those not immune by prior disease or vaccine
- Involvement of nasociliary branch of 5th cranial nerve: look for **ophthalmic keratitis** (clue: tip of nose involvement—Hutchinson sign)
- **Ramsay Hunt syndrome:** 7th cranial nerve involvement; ear canal and tongue lesions; facial palsy

SIGNS AND SYMPTOMS

- Prodromal pain and/or pruritis in the affected dermatome precedes eruption by 1 to 10 days
- Groups of vesicles on an erythematous base in one or multiple dermatomes

TREATMENT

- Analgesia
- Antiviral therapy. Parenteral for severe cases.
- Consider steroids in the elderly

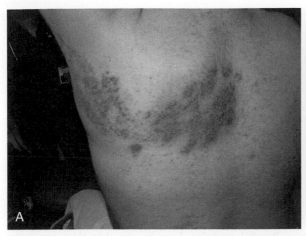
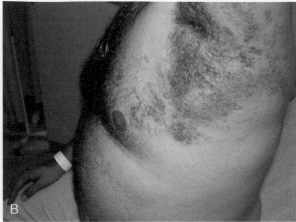

Figure 4-4 Herpes Zoster

FUNGAL

Cutaneous candidiasis

SIGNS AND SYMPTOMS

- Moist areas. Interdigital web spaces, groin, axilla, intergluteal fold and inframammary folds
- Moist red macules rimmed with scale
- Small satellite lesions are common

TREATMENT

- Decrease moisture
- Topical imidazole creams

Tinea

- Superficial fungal infections of the skin caused by various dermatophytes

SIGNS AND SYMPTOMS

- Scaly erythematous plaques, papules, and patches with a sharply demarcated leading edge
- Several forms based on anatomic location

TREATMENT

- Tinea capitis: systemic antifungal agents
- Tinea corporis: topical treatment
- Tinea pedis (athlete's foot) and tinea cruris (jock itch): topical
- Tinea versicolor: often found on chest and trunk; requires antifungal shampoo, topical cream, and occasionally oral agents

PARASITIC

PEDICULOSIS (LICE)

- Head, pubic area, and body

SIGNS AND SYMPTOMS

- Intensely pruritic
- Visible lice and nits
- Body louse is a vector for typhus (*Rickettsia prowazekii*), trench fever (*Rickettsia quinata*) and relapsing fever (*Borrelia recurrentis*)

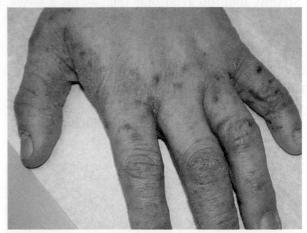

Figure 4-5 Scabies. (From Zaoutis LB, Chiang VW: *Comprehensive pediatric hospital medicine,* Philadelphia, 2007, Elsevier.)

TREATMENT

- Permethrin rinse
- Treatment of close contacts
- Wash all clothing and sheets in hot water

Scabies (Fig. 4-5)

- Infestation with *Sarcoptes scabiei*

SIGNS AND SYMPTOMS

- Intense pruritis, especially at night
- Burrows which appear as fine erythematous linear lesions on the hands, feet, and flexor surfaces of the extremities
- Multiple family members or cohabitants affected

TREATMENT

- Topical scabicides—permethrin, lindane
- Antihistamines for symptomatic relief
- Treatment of household contacts
- Wash all clothes and sheets in hot water

Maculopapular lesions

ERYTHEMA MULTIFORME (Fig. 4-6)

- Acute inflammatory skin disease; pathogenesis unclear
- "Minor" and "major" variants
- Drug exposure, infection (e.g., HSV, mycoplasma), and malignancy are common predisposing factors; many other triggers exist

SIGNS AND SYMPTOMS

- Abrupt onset erythematous macules, papules, vesicles, and bullae in a symmetrical pattern typically on palms and soles. May involve extensor surfaces
- Hallmark is a **target lesion** with three distinct zones of color
- **Stevens Johnson syndrome** (Fig. 4-7) is a severe, occasionally fatal, form accounting for 1% to 15% of cases
  - Characterized by mucous membrane involvement and shock

TREATMENT

- Identify and treat or remove the underlying cause
- Self-limited with spontaneous resolution in 2 to 3 weeks

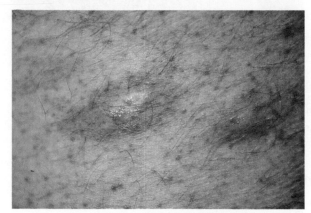

Figure 4-6 Erythema multiforme. (From Rakel RE: *Textbook of family medicine,* ed 7, Philadelphia, 2007, Elsevier.)

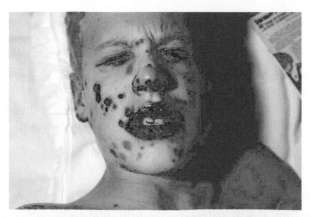

Figure 4-7 Stevens–Johnson syndrome. (From Zaoutis LB, Chiang VW: *Comprehensive pediatric hospital medicine,* Philadelphia, 2007, Elsevier.)

- Intravenous (IV) fluids, steroids, and aggressive supportive care for severe cases
- Management of secondary infections

ERYTHEMA NODOSUM (Fig. 4-8)

- Vasculitis of venules in the subcutaneous tissue
- Associated with various infections, lupus, tuberculosis, sarcoidosis, ulcerative colitis, pregnancy, medications (especially oral contraceptives)
- Female: male ratio 3:1
- Peak at age 30 to 50

SIGNS AND SYMPTOMS

- Painful nodules deep in the skin that are moveable
- Anterior tibia most commonly
- Fever and myalgias

TREATMENT

- Identify and treat or remove the underlying condition or trigger
- Usually self-limited with resolution in 3 to 8 weeks
- High-dose aspirin has been used

PITYRIASIS ROSEA (Fig. 4-9)

- Exact mechanism is unknown
- Children and young adults commonly affected

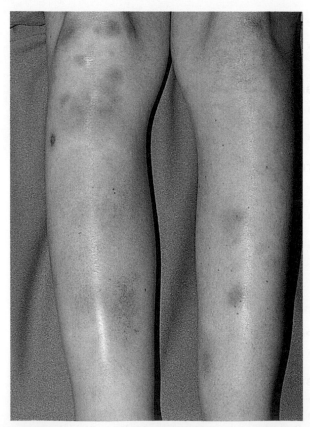

Figure 4-8 Erythema nodosum. (From Kliegman RM: *Nelson textbook of pediatrics,* ed 18, Philadelphia, 2007, Elsevier.)

SIGNS AND SYMPTOMS

- **Herald patch:** 2- to 6-cm lesion that precedes the generalized rash by approximately 7 days
- Followed by multiple pink pigmented papules or plaques on the trunk and extremities in characteristic **Christmas tree** patterns
- Rarely are the mucous membranes involved

TREATMENT

- Antihistamines for symptomatic relief
- Self-limited

URTICARIA

- Usually an allergic trigger; medications, food, plants, infections, exercise, and cold also implicated
- Caused by histamines and other immune modulators

SIGNS AND SYMPTOMS

- Edematous, pale-centered plaques of varied size; may come and go
- Pruritis

TREATMENT

- Trigger identification and avoidance
- Antihistamines and steroids

DRUG ERUPTION

- Urticaria and morbilliform rash are the most common manifestations
- Appear within a week of exposure; semisynthetic penicillin may have a delayed presentation
- Penicillin is the most common offending agent

SIGNS AND SYMPTOMS

- Several forms
  - **Photosensitive:** Generalized erythematous rash. Commonly due to thiazides and tetracyclines
  - **Vasculitic:** Erythematous papules and nodules

- **Fixed:** Recurs at the same anatomic site; sharply demarcated erythema and pruritis

TREATMENT

- Identify and stop the offending agent
- Symptomatic care

Bullous

PEMPHIGUS VULGARIS (Fig. 4-10)

- Exact mechanism unknown. Thought to be autoimmune in nature
- Peak onset at 40 to 60 years
- Mortality 10% to 15%

SIGNS AND SYMPTOMS

- Small fragile fluid-filled bullae
- Mucous membrane involvement in almost all cases
- Variably positive Nikolsky sign
- 50% to 60% of cases have oral lesion *preceding* skin manifestations

TREATMENT

- Pain control and local wound care; secondary infection a concern
- High-dose steroids
- Symptomatic care

BULLOUS PEMPHIGOID

- Disease of the elderly
- Good prognosis

SIGNS AND SYMPTOMS

- Tense blistering lesions
- Intertriginous and flexor surfaces common
- Mucous membrane involvement—less than pemphigus vulgaris, and better tolerated

TREATMENT

- Supportive

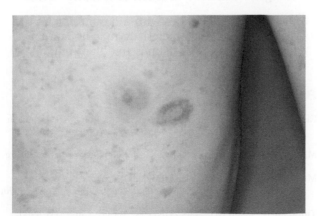

Figure 4-9 Pityriasis rosea. (From Kliegman RM: *Nelson textbook of pediatrics,* ed 18, Philadelphia, 2007, Elsevier.)

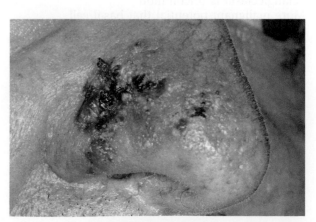

Figure 4-10 Pemphigus vulgaris. (From Regezi JA: *Oral pathology: clinical pathologic correlations,* ed 5, St. Louis, 2008, Saunders.)

Cancerous lesions

MELANOMA (Fig. 4-11)

- Approximately 45,000 cases per year in the United States with 7300 deaths
- Resulting from malignant transformation of melanocytes related to sun exposure

SIGNS AND SYMPTOMS

- Begin as superficial pigmented lesions
- Followed by a period of superficial radial growth without deep penetration
- Progresses into the deeper layers
- Irregular borders with variable pigmentation patterns
- May lack any pigment
- Change in size, color, or bleeding of lesion is often what is noted
- Highly metastatic

TREATMENT

- Prevention is key
- Biopsy for staging (based on depth of invasion)
- Surgical removal

BASAL CELL CARCINOMA

- Malignant transformation of epithelial basal cells

SIGNS AND SYMPTOMS

- Small pearly nodule with telangiectatic vessels
- Slow growing; may develop a central ulcer
- May cause significant local damage

TREATMENT

- Excision
- Radiation therapy

SQUAMOUS CELL CARCINOMA

SIGNS AND SYMPTOMS

- Ulcerated nodule or superficial erosion on skin or lip
- Telangiectasia is uncommon
- More malignant potential that basal cell

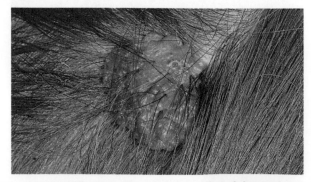

Figure 4-11 Melanoma. (From Habif TP: *Clinical dermatology*, ed 4, Philadelphia, 2004, Mosby.)

TREATMENT

- Excision
- Radiation therapy

KAPOSI SARCOMA

- Associated with HIV infection
- Human herpesvirus 8

SIGNS AND SYMPTOMS

- Large purple macular papular lesions
- May involve internal organs (e.g., GI tract)

TREATMENT

- Surgery, radiation therapy, and chemotherapy

PEARLS

- Dermatology is not a major board exam focus. Review and move on.

- More than 50% of abscesses seen in the ED are caused by CA-MRSA.

- Mucous membrane lesions precede skin signs in toxic epidermal necrosis (TEN).

- Seborrhea is associated with HIV infection in adults.

- Impetigo can manifest as bullae in neonates.

- Toxic epidermal necrolysis and staphylococcal scalded skin syndrome are treated like severe burns. Aggressive fluid resuscitation, infection prevention, and wound care.

- Nikolsky sign: Separation of the epidermis when pressure applied adjacent to a fluid filled bullous lesion. The separation occurs at the dermoepidermal junction in TEN and more superficially at the stratum corneum in staphylococcal scalded skin syndrome.

- Urticaria is a systemic response, often to an allergen; it is not a reaction to a topical irritant.

- Pityriasis rosea begins with a herald patch, followed by the characteristic maculopapular truncal rash in a Christmas tree distribution.

BIBLIOGRAPHY

Faci AS, Braunwald E, Kasper DL, Hauser SL, Longo DL, Jameson JL, Loscalzo J (eds): *Harrison's principles of internal medicine*, ed 17, New York, 2008, McGraw-Hill.

Martin DR (ed): Infectious diseases in emergency medicine, *Emerg Med Clin North Am* 26(2):245–602, 2008.

Marx JA, Hockberger RS, Walls RM (eds): *Rosen's emergency medicine: concepts and clinical practice*, ed 6, Philadelphia, 2006, Mosby.

Tintinalli JE, Kelen GD, Stapczynski JS, Ma OJ, Cline DM (eds): *Emergency medicine: a comprehensive study guide*, ed 6, New York, 2004, McGraw-Hill.

Questions and Answers

1. The dermatitis in newborns referred to as "cradle cap" and rarely associated with hair loss is:
   a. seborrhea
   b. tinea capitis
   c. lichen simplex chronicus
   d. erysipelas

2. A 17-year-old boy presents with complaints of diffuse, intense pruritis. He has no new medications or topical exposures. He has no history of liver or kidney disease. Physical examination reveals anicteric sclera and a normal face and scalp. Scattered excoriations are seen on the torso, most concentrated around the waist-band area and extending into the inguinal creases. Closer inspection of that area reveals faint linear and crescent-shaped lesions with scaling in these areas. Reasonable treatment includes:
   a. psychiatric referral
   b. hydrocortisone cream
   c. antifungal cream
   d. permethrin cream

3. A herald patch is a feature of:
   a. pityriasis rosea
   b. tinea versicolor
   c. drug eruptions
   d. erythema nodosum

4. A positive Nikolsky sign may be seen with:
   a. toxic epidermal necrolysis
   b. staphylococcal scalded skin syndrome
   c. staphylococcal toxic shock syndrome
   d. a and b
   e. b and c

5. A 31-year-old woman presents with complaints of painful changes in the skin of her lower extremities developing over the past 2 days. She recalls no trauma. She has no significant past medical history except for treatment of a MRSA soft tissue infection 3 weeks ago with trimethoprim/sulfamethoxazole, and appendectomy 4 years ago. On physical examination, she is afebrile with normal vital signs. Her skin examination reveals several tender, warm, nodular swellings overlying the pretibial regions of both legs. Her oropharynx is clear. The most likely diagnosis is:
   a. cellulitis
   b. erythema multiforme, minor
   c. erythema nodosum
   d. domestic abuse

6. Cellulitis in the immunocompetent host is most likely due to:

   a. *Staphylococcus aureus* and *Streptococcus pyogenes*
   a. *Staphylococcus aureus* and *Staphylococcus epidermidis*
   b. *Pasteurella multocida* and *Streptococcus pyogenes*
   c. *Escherichia coli* and *Streptococcus pyogenes*

7. A 44-year-old man presents with a painful left posterior thigh soft tissue abscess, with cellulitic changes to the adjacent skin and some lymphangitic streaking. His temperature is 101.1, and his other vital signs are within normal limits. X-rays are unremarkable, and his peripheral leukocyte count is 13,000 cells/mL^3 with 81% segmented neutrophils. In addition to incision and drainage of the abscess, reasonable therapy might include oral:
   a. ciprofloxacin for 7 days
   b. dicloxacillin for 10 days
   c. trimethoprim/sulfamethoxazole (TMP-SMX) for 7 days
   d. vancomycin for 10 days

8. A 66-year-old woman presents with a painful, nonpruritic skin change to her right zygomaxillary region for 2 days, accompanied by malaise and chills. She denies trauma or new topical exposures. Her past history is significant for diabetes mellitus and ulcerative colitis. On physical examination, her temperature is 102.9° F, her heart rate (HR) is 118 bpm, her respiratory rate (RR) is 18/minute, and her blood pressure (BP) is 148/85 mmHg. Her head and neck examination is significant for a raised, warm, tender, erythematous area over her right zygomaxillary region that has a well-demarcated edge to it. There is no meningismus or neck mass. The most likely diagnosis is:
   a. impetigo
   b. urticaria
   c. erythema nodosum
   d. erysipelas

9. Herpes zoster typically:
   a. is painless, but intensely pruritic
   b. does not typically cross the midline of the body
   c. responds to topical antiviral therapy
   d. is the first presentation of varicella zoster (chicken pox) in nonimmunized children

10. A 19-year-old female presents complaining of a rash around her neck, both wrists and her waistband. The affected areas are notable for small vesicles and bullae on an erythematous base in a linear distribution. The rash crosses the midline. She complains of itching but denies fevers or oral lesions. The rash is most likely due to:

a. scabies
b. herpes zoster
c. contact dermatitis
d. psoriasis

11. Unlike older children, impetigo in neonates can present as:

a. confluent honey-colored crusts
b. lichenification
c. papules
d. bullae
e. mucosal lesions

12. A 48-year-old man presents via EMS with a decreased level of consciousness. His vital signs on arrival are a temperature = 101.5° F, HR = 148 bpm, BP = 80/30 mmHg, and RR = 28/minute. His physical examination is notable for a diffuse maculopapular erythematous rash with large bullae. Nikolsky sign is positive. His family states that he was complaining of ulcers in his mouth and a rash on his face the day before. The family tells you that he was recently treated with several antibiotics for a "spider-bite" that had to be drained. Which of the following medications have been identified as causing this condition?

a. TMP-SMX
b. phenytoin
c. aspirin
d. allopurinol
e. all of the above

13. A 17-year-old homeless man presents complaining of diffuse itching for 3 days. He says the itching is worse at night. He denies any fevers or medical problems. He denies allergies or any medications. He smokes cigarettes daily and drinks alcohol and uses intravenous heroin intermittently. His last heroin use was 3 weeks prior. His vital signs are temperature = 97.8° F, HR = 70 bpm, BP = 119/68 mmHg, and RR = 12/minute. On examination, he is a thin disheveled male with multiple areas of chronic excoriation. He has thin linear erythematous rash between his fingers and toes. What is the appropriate treatment for this condition?

a. TMP-SMX and cephalexin
b. intravenous vancomycin
c. permethrin or lindane
d. tar preparations

14. Avoid this antibiotic for treatment of suspected CA-MRSA in a complicated abscess:

a. TMP-SMX
b. clindamycin
c. cephalexin
d. doxycycline

15. A 28-year-old woman presents complaining of intense pain in her left forearm. She denies any medical problems but does admit to using intravenous drugs intermittently. Her last use was 3 days ago in her left arm. She describes the pain as a deep aching sensation from her left elbow to her wrist. She became more concerned today because the middle of her forearm became numb. Her vital signs are temperature = 99.8° F, HR = 104 bpm, BP = 103/60 mmHg, and RR = 22/minute. Examination of her left arm shows a small area of erythema in the left antecubital fossa. Otherwise there is no rash, swelling, or deformity. She has a strong radial pulse and the compartments of the arm feel soft. She complains of severe pain in her forearm when you attempt to range her wrist or elbow. Management of this condition include which of the following?

a. broad-spectrum intravenous antibiotics
b. oral antibiotics and surgical follow-up
c. immediate surgical evaluation and debridement
d. pain control and follow-up with the primary care physician
e. a and c

16. A 42-year-old man presents complaining of an erythematous maculopapular rash on the palms of his hands and the soles of his feet. He also recently noticed a similar rash on his elbows and knees. He saw his regular doctor who tested him for syphilis, which was negative. He has a history of hypertension and gout. His medications include allopurinol and lisinopril. He explains that he completed a course of penicillin for a tooth infection about 2 days before the rash developed. He denies any fevers or oral lesions. Vital signs are temperature = 98.1° F, HR = 78 bpm, BP = 148/80 mmHg, and RR = 12/minute. Physical examination is significant for the rash described above as well as a larger lesion on his lower back with three distinct colorations. The most likely cause of the patient's symptoms is:

a. pityriasis rosea
b. erythema nodosum
c. erythema multiforme
d. psoriasis

17. Erythema multiforme is associated with which of the following?

a. pelvic inflammatory disease
b. systemic lupus erythematosus
c. pregnancy
d. ulcerative colitis
e. herpes simplex virus infection

18. An 86-year-old woman presents from the local nursing home with a complaint of a nonhealing ulcer on her forehead. The patient has a history of hypertension, osteoarthritis, and severe dementia. She is unable to provide any additional history. The nursing home staff notes state that the ulcer has been there for months and has not responded to local wound care measures. Temperature =

97.5° F, HR = 68 bpm, BP = 165/90 mmHg, and RR = 12/minute. Her physical examination is significant for a 6-cm × 8-cm ulcerated erosion on her forehead and nasal bridge with extensive local tissue damage. The remainder of the skin examination reveals several pearly nodules with telangiectasia. This lesion is most likely caused by:

a. herpes zoster
b. melanoma
c. necrotizing fasciitis
d. basal cell carcinoma
e. squamous cell carcinoma

19. Most fixed drug eruptions occur within a week of exposure. A delayed drug eruption is more likely with exposure to:

a. ciprofloxacin
b. semisynthetic penicillin
c. haloperidol
d. chemotherapeutic agents
e. morphine

20. Mortality in necrotizing fasciitis is:

a. 1% to 2%
b. 5%
c. 10% to 15%
d. 20% to 60%
e. 90%

---

1. Answer: a

Seborrheic dermatitis is a common dermatitis seen in all age groups, including infants. When appearing on the scalp, it should be differentiated from **tinea capitis,** a fungal infection with patchy hair loss and hair breakage. **Lichen simplex chronicus** is extremely pruritic, and not common in neonates. **Erysipelas** (see Fig. 4-1) is a bacterial skin infection, characteristically featuring a well-demarcated border of warm red, tender tissue.

2. Answer: d

This is a classic presentation of *scabies* (see Fig. 4-5), which features intense pruritis in regions of involvement, which are typically the hands and feet (web spaces, lateral surfaces), and flexor surfaces of elbows, knees, waist, groin, and genitals. Burrows are the hallmark sign and are described in the case. Skin scrapings yield mites, ova, and fecal material. Treatment is with topical scabicides such as **permethrin** or lindane, as well as eradication of organisms on contact sites (household members, furniture, bedding, etc.). The other topical agents are ineffective; psychiatric referral is here inappropriate.

3. Answer: a

Pityriasis rosea (see Fig. 4-9) is a noncontagious skin eruption that classically begins with a "herald patch" (isolated reddish-brown lesion with a raised border, usually on the torso) followed by the emergence in 1 to 2 weeks of a diffuse, salmon-hued maculopapular

eruption, with a coniferous distribution of the long axes of the eruptions on the back. Mucous membranes may be involved. The herald patch is not a feature of the other skin disorders listed.

4. Answer: d

Nikolsky sign is said to be positive if the examiner places lateral digital pressure on normal skin adjacent to involved skin (bullous lesion) and dislodges the epidermis, resulting in denuded dermis. This is a feature of both **TEN** (see Fig. 4-3) and **staphylococcal scalded skin syndrome** (see Fig. 4-2); **staphylococcal toxic shock** skin changes include a blanching, diffuse erythroderma without pruritis followed by desquamation.

5. Answer: c

Erythema nodosum (see Fig. 4-8) is a vasculitis seen more commonly in women than men, and often involving the pretibial area. Triggers include multiple infectious etiologies, medications (including trimethoprim/sulfamethoxazole), sarcoidosis, inflammatory bowel disease, and pregnancy; often the precipitant is obscure. Patients are clinically nontoxic, with findings of erythematous, tender, nodular swellings—often pretibial in location. **Erythema multiforme** (see Fig. 4-6) is classically associated with target lesions; the nodularity and discrete nature of these lesions, along with a lack of a portal of entry, makes **cellulitis** less likely.

6. Answer: a

Classically, cellulitis is due to Gram-positive organisms, with *S. aureus* and *S. pyogenes* being the most common pathogens; the role that community-acquired MRSA plays in cellulitis remains to be defined. *P. multocida* is linked to dog and cat bites; *E. coli* is uncommon in immunocompetent patients with skin infection.

7. Answer: c

Community-acquired methicillin-resistant *Staphylococcus aureus* (CA-MRSA) has emerged as the leading cause of soft-tissue abscess, and thus reasonable antibiotic therapy would target this pathogen. **Dicloxacillin** would be appropriate for methicillin-sensitive *S. aureus,* but would not be useful in CA-MRSA, and **ciprofloxacin** is not active again MRSA in general. Oral **vancomycin** is not well absorbed from the gastrointestinal tract, so it would not be a possibility. **Trimethoprim/sulfamethoxazole** is the drug of choice among oral agents for CA-MRSA.

8. Answer: d

Urticaria is red, warm, and plaque-like, but it is also pruritic and is not associated with a fever. **Impetigo** is classically associated with infectious lesions that feature golden or amber crusting; it may be painful and pruritic. **Erythema nodosum** (see Fig. 4-8) is red and tender but does not characteristically present with a high fever and is more typically found over the pretibial areas. **Erysipelas** (see Fig. 4-1) fits this clinical case most closely; classically it presented as it does with this woman, on the face, although more recently it occurs on the legs. Streptococcal species are the responsible pathogens. Hallmarks of the disease are high fever and a red, shiny, raised, tender plaque of involved skin.

9. Answer: b

Herpes zoster (see Fig. 4-4) is a dermatomal rash (clusters of vesicles on an erythematous base) caused by reactivation of the varicella zoster virus, and may occur in any age group. It is universally **painful** but may also be pruritic. It is seen in those patients who have had varicella zoster but is not the initial presentation of the disease. Antiviral treatment is with **oral acyclovir** (or **valacyclovir,** or **famciclovir**)—if the agent is initiated within 3 days of the onset of the rash; otherwise, treatment is aimed at pain control. Oral steroids are recommended only in patients more than 50 years of age to decrease the pain of the outbreak.

10. Answer: c

Nickel is a common cause of contact dermatitis and is found in certain types of jewelry, belt buckles, and pant buttons. The distribution of the rash is characteristic of **contact dermatitis.**

11. Answer: d

Impetigo is the most common skin infection seen in children. The typical pattern is that vesicles develop that rupture and crust over in the first 24 hours. The lesions may become confluent and take on a honey-colored crust. They are pruritic but painless and the child is overall well appearing. In neonates, impetigo may present as bullae with a negative Nikolsky sign. Oral lesions are not seen. Oral antibiotics are the mainstay of treatment.

12. Answer: e

The condition described is **toxic epidermal necrolysis** (TEN; see Fig. 4-3). Mucosal membrane involvement often precedes the skin rash. When the rash does appear, it typically begins on the face and then spreads to the rest of the body. Many medications have been implicated, including all of those listed above. It has also been associated with certain vaccinations and lymphoma. Treatment focuses on identifying the offending agent and systemic resuscitation

13. Answer: c

The clinical picture is most consistent with **scabies** infestation (see Fig. 4-5). The linear rash represents burrows formed by *Sarcoptes scabiei.* They typically appear in the hands, feet, and flexor surfaces of the extremities. In addition to topical scabicides, the patient should be instructed to wash all clothes and bedsheets in hot water.

14. Answer: c

Cephalexin, though offering good antibacterial coverage for methicillin-sensitive *Staphylococcus*

aureus, as well as streptococcal species, is not active against CA-MRSA. The other three agents are, as are linezolid and vancomycin. Local resistance patterns vary and the emergency physician (EP) should be cognizant of them.

15. Answer: e

The clinical presentation is worrisome for **necrotizing fasciitis.** The characteristic presentation is pain out of proportion to findings on physical examination, which may be unremarkable except for significant pain. As the disease progresses, areas of numbness may develop as well as bullae and purpura and systemic evidence of sepsis and/or shock. Necrotizing fasciitis is a surgical diagnosis, and suspicion for the disease should prompt immediate surgical consultation and operative exploration. Broad-spectrum antibiotics are indicated but not as an alternative to definitive surgical management.

16. Answer: c

Erythema multiforme (see Fig. 4-6) presents with the characteristic "target lesion," a larger lesion with three distinct areas of coloration. In addition to the target lesion, the rash manifests as a maculopapular erythematous rash often on the palms, soles, and extensor surfaces. **Stevens-Johnson syndrome** (Fig. 4-7) is a more severe form.

17. Answer: e

Erythema multiforme (Fig. 4-6) is associated with many medications and HSV infection. It classically presents with the hallmark "target lesion" and a maculopapular rash on the palms and soles. **Erythema nodosum** (see Fig. 4-8) is associated with lupus, pregnancy, and ulcerative colitis.

18. Answer: d

Basal cell carcinoma is a slow-growing skin cancer that can cause significant local damage. The slow progression of the disease often results in late presentation. The pearly nodular lesion with telangiectasia is characteristic of basal cell carcinoma. It has significantly less malignant potential than either melanoma or squamous cell carcinoma.

19. Answer: b

The majority of drug eruptions occur within 1 week. Penicillin is the most common offender. Delayed reactions, 7 to 20 days, are most commonly seen with the **semisynthetic penicillins.**

20. Answer: d

Necrotizing fasciitis is a life-threatening condition with **a mortality between 20% and 60%.** Classic presentation is pain out of proportion to physical examination findings, requiring a high index of suspicion. As the disease progresses, areas of bullae and purpura can develop. Treatment is surgical, with broad-spectrum antibiotics and systemic resuscitation.

Endocrine-Metabolic/Nutrition

Joel Kravitz

5

Acid–base disorders

ACID–BASE HOMEOSTASIS

- pH is normal, $7.4 - [H^+]$ of 40 nmol/L
  - Range = 7.36–7.44
- While Henderson–Hasselbalch is the better-known equation, the antilog derivation of it, known as the Kassirer–Bleich (K-B) equation, is clinically more useful (Fig. 5-1)

$$[H^+] = 24 \times P_{CO_2}/[HCO_3]$$

- The K-B equation can be used to calculate the concentration of any component of the bicarbonate buffer system
  - Can tell you what the pH should be for any given P_{CO_2} and $[HCO_3]$. This is important as a "quality control" in the emergency department (ED), as most $[HCO_3]$ measurements from the lab are calculated and not measured
- "emia" versus "osis"
  - An acidemia is defined as a state in which the blood pH is <7.36
  - An acidosis is a clinical state that tends to produce an acidemia
    - Sounds the same, but remember that even in an acidemia, a concomitant alkalosis can exist
- *Take home point:* When looking at a blood pH, the pH determines the primary state (e.g., if the pH is less than 7.35, then the acidosis is the primary problem)
- Definition and concept is same for alkalemia and alkalosis but with a pH >7.44
  - Compensation for acidosis and alkalosis—the buffer system
- The bicarbonate–carbonic acid buffer system is the main system and buffers by the following equation:

$$CO_2 \text{ (gas)} \leftrightarrow CO_2 \text{ (aqueous)} + H_2O \leftrightarrow H_2CO_3 \leftrightarrow H^+ + HCO_3^-$$

$$[H+] = 24 * P_{CO_2}/[HCO_3]$$

Figure 5-1. Kassirer–Bleich equation

$$CO_2 \text{ (gas)} \leftrightarrow CO_2 \text{ (aqueous)} + H_2O \leftrightarrow H_2CO_3 \leftrightarrow H^+ + HCO_3^-$$

Figure 5-2. Bicarbonate–carbonic acid buffer system

- This system is open ended (Fig. 5-2)
  - Lungs are able to excrete CO_2 (blood pH can stimulate or decrease ventilatory effort)
  - Kidneys are able to excrete, reabsorb, or regenerate buffer pairs
- The pulmonary compensation is virtually immediate, but the renal compensation takes about 6 hours
  - *Take home point:* Neither system can bring the pH entirely to normal, only toward normal
- Other buffer systems
  - Proteins in the blood—hemoglobin within RBCs
  - Bone contains a large reservoir of bicarbonate and can buffer up to 40% of acute acid loads
  - Potassium: excess H^+ can be moved intracellularly in exchange for K^+ to maintain electroneutrality, with the converse occurring in the course of alkalosis
    - For every 0.1 unit change in arterial pH, an inverse change of 0.2-0.6 mEq/L occurs in the plasma $[K^+]$

A BASIC APPROACH TO ACID–BASE INTERPRETATION

- ABG, anion gap and serum bicarbonate necessary (HCO_3 on the ABG is calculated—the measured value on the electrolyte panel is better for acid–base interpretation)
- pH—determines primary disturbance
  - An increased pH means that alkalosis predominates, and a decreased pH implies a primary acidosis

ACIDOSIS (pH <7.36)

- P_{CO_2} >42: respiratory acidosis
  - $[HCO_3]$ should be high as a metabolic compensation. If not, there is likely an additional metabolic acidosis
- P_{CO_2} 38 to 42: pure metabolic acidosis with no compensation
- P_{CO_2} <38: metabolic acidosis (the low P_{CO_2} is compensatory)

ALKALOSIS (pH >7.44)

- P_{CO_2} >42: metabolic alkalosis (the elevated P_{CO_2} is compensatory)
- P_{CO_2} 38 to 42: metabolic alkalosis without compensation

- P_{CO_2} <38: respiratory alkalosis
  - $[HCO_3]$ should be lower as a metabolic compensation. If not, there is likely an additional metabolic alkalosis

RESPIRATORY ACIDOSIS

- Decrease in pH and an elevation of the P_{CO_2}
  - Chronic compensation: $[HCO_3]$ should increase by 3 to 4 for every 10 mmHg increase in P_{CO_2}
  - If the increase in bicarbonate is greater than expected, a primary metabolic alkalosis is also present

Etiology: "Can't breathe versus won't breathe"

CAN'T BREATHE: LUNG MECHANICS ARE IMPAIRED (CAUSING THE RISE IN P_{CO_2})

- Intrinsic pulmonary disease
  - Asthma
  - Aspiration
  - Inhalational injuries
  - Bronchitis or pneumonia
  - Pulmonary edema
  - Foreign body aspiration
  - Laryngospasm
  - Mechanical ventilation
  - Tracheal/airway edema/stenosis
- Chronic lung disease
  - COPD

WON'T BREATHE: LUNG TISSUE IS WORKING BUT THE ACTUAL ACT OF BREATHING IS IMPAIRED

- Chest wall trauma: flail chest, pneumothorax (tension)
- Neuromuscular impairment
  - Drugs: opioid use and abuse, sedative hypnotics
  - Brainstem or high spinal injury or infarction
  - Neuromuscular disease: myasthenia gravis, Guillain–Barré disease, amyotrophic lateral sclerosis, tetanus, etc.
  - Myopathy: congenital (muscular dystrophy) and acquired (electrolyte disorders, periodic paralysis, etc.)
- Chronically: body habitus affecting respiratory mechanics
  - Kyphoscoliosis
  - Obesity hypoventilation syndrome ("pickwickian syndrome")

Management

- Address the underlying cause
  - In many cases, intubation and mechanical ventilation may be the only option
  - In chronic cases, use only the oxygen needed to maintain P_{O_2}. These patients have acclimatized to a higher P_{CO_2} and thus depend more on a relative hypoxia as their main respiratory drive. Remove

that, and there is a risk of hypoventilation, with an ensuing CO_2 elevation (exactly what you were trying to avoid)

RESPIRATORY ALKALOSIS

- Decrease in P_aCO_2 and an elevated pH
- Chronic compensation: $[HCO_3]$ should decrease by 5 for every 10 mmHg decrease in P_{CO_2}
  - A greater than expected drop in bicarbonate is a primary metabolic acidosis
  - A less than expected decrease means that the compensation has not yet completed or a metabolic alkalosis is lurking in the background

ETIOLOGY

- Central nervous system (CNS) disturbance affecting respiratory center
  - Stroke, infection, tumor
  - Salicylate poisoning has a direct stimulatory effect
- Hypermetabolic state
  - Fever and sepsis
  - Anemia
  - Thyrotoxicosis
- Pulmonary disease
  - Congestive heart failure
  - Pulmonary shunts and ventilation–perfusion (V/Q) mismatches (e.g., pulmonary embolism [PE])
- High altitude (as a compensatory mechanism)
- Pregnancy (even early on, progesterone induces a hyperpnea)
- Hepatic insufficiency
- Psychogenic hyperventilation
- Compensation for metabolic acidosis

MANAGEMENT

- Treat the underlying cause
- In some cases (e.g., pregnancy, high altitude), it is a normal healthy response and the correct option is to not treat the condition

METABOLIC ACIDOSIS

- Check the Anion Gap: $[Na^+] - ([HCO_3] + [Cl^-])$
  - Normal is 12 ± 2 (Table 5-1)

- Winter's formula: Is the respiratory compensation as expected?
  - P_{CO_2} should be $= (1.5 \times [HCO_3]) + 8 \pm 2$
    - P_{CO_2} is higher, there is a concomitant respiratory acidosis
    - P_{CO_2} is lower than the range, there is a concomitant respiratory alkalosis
- Delta gap
  - (Deviation of AG from normal) – (Deviation of $[HCO_3]$ from normal)
  - Delta gap $= (AG - 12) - (24 - bicarb)$
    - In a "pure" high-AG metabolic acidosis, for every 1 mmol/L rise in the anion gap, there should be a 1 mmol/L fall in the bicarbonate
  - Delta gap should be 0 ± 6
    - A delta gap greater than –6 implies a greater loss of bicarbonate than can be accounted for by metabolic acidosis and suggests a concurrent normal anion gap metabolic acidosis, a respiratory alkalosis, or, rarely, a low anion gap state
    - Causes of low anion gap (<6) include paraproteinemias, hypoalbuminemia, lithium toxicity, profound hypercalcemia or hypermagnesemia, bromism (interference with chloride assay), or hyponatremia
- Osmolar gap
  - Measured Osm: $2 \times [Na^+] + (glucose/18) + (BUN/2.8) = 285 - 295$
    - If alcohol is present, then add (blood alcohol level)/5 to the total
    - Measured Osm – calculated Osm should be less than 12 to 15
  - Methanol and ethylene glycol cause an osmolar gap along with the anion gap acidosis
    - Isopropyl alcohol is the exception, as it causes ketosis and an osmolar gap *without* acidosis
- Alcoholic ketoacidosis (AKA)
  - Nausea, vomiting, abdominal pain, usually 12 to 24 hours after patient's last alcohol intake
  - In the metabolism of alcohol, the rate of nicotinamide adenine dinucleotide (NAD) reduction exceeds the rate of NADH oxidation (redox ratio is altered), causing a decrease in the availability of NAD

TABLE 5-1 **Evaluation of the Anion Gap**

Elevated Anion Gap "MUDPILE CATS"		Normal Anion Gap "USED CARP"	
M	Methanol, metformin (rare)	U	Ureterostomy
U	Uremia	S	Small bowel fistula
D	Diabetic ketoacidosis	E	Excess chloride (NaCl, ammonium Cl)
P	Paraldehyde, phenformin	D	Diarrhea
I	Iron, isoniazid		
L	Lactic acidosis	C	Carbonic anhydrase inhibitors, cholestyramine
E	Ethanol, ethylene glycol	A	Addison disease (hypoaldosteronism)
	(ethanol not source of significant metabolic acidosis)	R	Renal tubular acidosis and insufficiency
C	Carbamazepine	P	Pancreatic fistula, Parenteral nutrition
A	Alcoholic ketoacidosis		
T	Toluene		
S	Salicylates, starvation ketoacidosis		

- An NAD-dependent step in the oxidation of fatty acids is then displaced in favor of ketone body formation
- AKA is not a disease of the occasional alcohol drinker—chronic activation of the alcohol dehydrogenase enzyme is needed to maintain the elevated levels of NADH relative to the oxidized NAD form
- Alcohol also induces hypoglycemia (through starvation, depletion of liver glycogen stores because of chronic malnutrition, and inhibition of gluconeogenesis because of alcohol-induced alteration of the NAD/NADH ratio), so insulin levels are low and counter-regulatory hormones are increased, thus promoting lipolysis
- Acetate, an alcohol breakdown product, is converted to ketones
- Vomiting and starvation superimposed on chronic malnutrition also contribute to ketoacidosis
- Treatment is with fluid repletion and glucose (which speeds the normalization of the redox state)—do not forget the thiamine
- Lactic acidosis—two types
  - Type A lactic acidosis is secondary to hypoperfusion or hypoxemia
  - Type B lactic acidosis is associated with systemic diseases such as diabetes, liver disease, and sepsis; ingestion of drugs and toxins (metformin, isoniazid, iron, cyanide, carbon monoxide, hydrogen sulfide); and inborn errors of metabolism

MANAGEMENT

- Treat the underlying cause
- Bicarbonate
  - Not generally used unless pH is lower than 7.0—fix the cause and the pH will correct itself
  - Side effects of bicarbonate
    - Alkalosis by overcorrection
    - Volume overload
    - Paradoxical CNS acidosis
  - HCO_3^- penetration into the CNS across the blood–brain barrier is slow; consequently, HCO_3^- therapy alkalinizes the plasma faster than the CNS
    - Peripheral chemoreceptors slow respiration and CO_2 (which rapidly diffuses across the BBB) will rise intracerebrally
    - CNS becomes more acidotic despite alkalinization of plasma
      - Hypokalemia
      - Bicarbonate in large doses is arrhythmogenic
  - If it must be used, only about half of the bicarbonate deficit should be replaced, and then reassess

METABOLIC ALKALOSIS

- Mainly due to an increase in $[HCO_3]$ resorption, because of either volume, potassium, or chloride depletion

- Causes are subdivided into two groups
  - Saline responsive (urine chloride <10 mEq/L)
    - Because of volume depletion
      - Diuretics
      - Vomiting
      - Gastrointestinal (GI) suctioning
    - Milk–alkali syndrome
    - Cystic fibrosis
  - Saline unresponsive (urine chloride >10 mEq/L)
    - Increased $[Na^+]$ to tubules causes excretion of $[K^+]$ & $[H^+]$, which leads to alkalosis
      - Hyperaldosteronism
- Primary
- Secondary: cirrhosis, congestive heart failure (CHF), renal failure, Bartter's syndrome
  - Severe potassium depletion
  - Massive transfusion—the citrate-containing anticoagulants metabolize to $[HCO_3]$
  - Hypercalcemia (non-parathyroid causes)
- Compensation
  - PCO_2 should rise by 0.6 for every 1 mEq/L increase in $[HCO_3]$
  - PCO_2 cannot rise more than 55 mmHg as a compensatory mechanism—if it is higher, there is an additional respiratory acidosis

MANAGEMENT

- Saline ± KCl suppresses renal acid excretion and promotes excretion of bicarbonate
- KCl serves to reverse the intracellular shift of H^+ seen in cases of mineralocorticoid excess

Electrolyte disturbances

HYPONATREMIA

- Definition: serum Na^+ less than 135 mEq/L
  - Symptoms not often seen at a level greater than 120 mEq/L
- Hypertonic hyponatremia (Osm >295)
  - Translocational hyponatremia results from a shift of water from cells to the extracellular fluid that is driven by solutes confined in the extracellular compartment
    - For example, mannitol, glycerol, hyperglycemia
    - For hyperglycemic states, every 100 mg/dL rise in glucose will cause a decrease in sodium of 1.6 to 1.8 mEq/L
- Isotonic hyponatremia—"pseudohyponatremia"
  - Reduction of the fraction of plasma that is made up of water
    - For example, hyperlipidemia or hyperproteinemia (myeloma)
    - This lab error is avoided by use of alternate measurement techniques
- Hypotonic hyponatremia (Osm <275)
  - Most commonly resulting from impaired renal excretion of water
  - Further subdivided by volume state of patient

- Hypovolemic
  - Renal
    - Diuretic use
    - Osmotic diuresis
    - Adrenal insufficiency
    - Renal tubular acidosis (salt wasting nephropathy)
  - Extrarenal losses
    - GI losses—diarrhea, vomiting
    - Excessive sweating (heat stroke, cystic fibrosis)
    - Third-spacing (burns, peritonitis)
- Euvolemic hyponatremia—mostly by antidiuretic hormone (ADH) suppression
  - Urine Na$^+$ usually >20 mEq/L
  - Syndrome of inappropriate ADH secretion (SIADH)
    - Cancer
    - CNS disorders
    - Pulmonary disorders
  - Medications (either alone or by causing SIADH)
    - Nonsteroidal anti-inflammatory drugs (NSAIDs)
    - Psychiatric medications (phenothiazines, tricyclics, monoamine oxidase [MAO] inhibitors)
    - Chemotherapeutics (colchicines, vincristine, cyclophosphamide)
    - Anticonvulsants (carbamazepine, phenobarbital)
    - Sulfonylureas
  - Pathologic water intoxication
  - Glucocorticoid deficiency (suppresses ADH)
- Hypervolemic
  - Urine Na$^+$ usually >20 mEq/L: renal failure
  - Urine Na$^+$ usually <20 mEq/L: kidney "sees" less fluid
    - Congestive heart failure ("cardiosis")
    - Cirrhosis/liver failure ("cirrhosis")
    - Nephrotic syndrome ("nephrosis")
- Most common causes
  - Adults: diuretic therapy
  - Infants and children: GI losses form diarrhea
- SIADH
  - ADH is a posterior pituitary hormone that is released in response to rises in serum osmolality and decreases in intravascular volume (the latter being the most potent stimulus)
  - ADH enhances renal water reabsorption by increasing tubular water permeability
  - Criteria for SIADH (see list of causes above)
    - Hypotonic hyponatremia
    - Elevated urine osmolality (greater than 200 mOsm/kg)
    - Elevated urinary Na$^+$ greater than 20 mEq/L
    - Euvolemia on clinical examination
    - Correction of deficit with water restriction
    - Normal, renal, adrenal, hepatic, and thyroid function

CLINICAL MANIFESTATIONS

- More conspicuous when the decrease is large or rapid
- Usually asymptomatic at levels greater than 125 mEq/L
- Mainly neurologic
  - Headache, nausea, vomiting, muscle cramps, lethargy, disorientation
  - Seizures, coma, brainstem herniation, and death can occur with severe and rapidly evolving hyponatremia

TREATMENT

- If not severe (less than 100) or unless the patient is actively having neurologic sequelae (i.e. seizures), treatment should be delayed until urinary sodium levels are obtained
- Urinary sodium >20 mEq/L
  - Suggestive of SIADH
  - Water restriction should be initiated—1 to 1.5 L of water per day (intravenous and oral combined)
    - Diuretic can be added for additional effect
    - Underlying cause should be reversed
- Urinary sodium <20 mEq/L and hypovolemic: sodium replacement
  - Rate of correction should be 0.5 to 1.0 mEq/L/hour at most (this may be up to 2.0 mEq/L/hour if patient is having seizures)
    - Too rapid correction can lead to CPM—severe neurologic dysfunction with severe morbidity and high mortality (central pontine myelinolysis)
  - Hypertonic saline—avoid unless patient is actively having seizures
    - Increasing serum sodium by 3 to 7 mEq/L is enough to stop most seizures
- Sodium replacement
  - Calculation of sodium deficit can be done, but it is often easier to approach the problem from the side of the solution administered
  - Formula (Table 5-2) will determine the change in serum sodium caused by the administration of 1 L of a given infusate

TABLE 5-2 **Formula for Use of, and Characteristics of, Infusates in the Treatment of Hyponatremia and Hypernatremia**

Change in serum Na$^+$ = $\dfrac{(\text{Infusate Na}^+ + \text{Infusate K}^+) - \text{Serum Na}^+}{\text{Total body water* } + 1}$

Infusate	Infusate [Na$^+$]
3% NaCl	513 mEq/L
0.9% NaCl (normal)	154
Ringer's lactate	130
0.45% NaCl	77
5% Dextrose	0

*Total body water = 0.6 × body weight in children and adult men
0.5 × body weight in adult women and elderly men
0.45 × body weight in elderly women

- Dividing the change in serum sodium targeted for a given treatment period by the output of this formula determines the volume of infusate required, and hence the rate of infusion
- Formula useful only when the patient needs rapid correction or when the patient is hypovolemic
- For euvolemic (e.g., SIADH) or hypervolemic (e.g., CHF) patients, administration of fluids is counterproductive
- In the hypovolemic patient, once the ECF volume nears restoration, the nonosmotic stimulus to ADH release will cease, causing rapid excretion of dilute urine and correction of hyponatremia at an overly rapid pace
- Therefore, once the initial volume expansion is accomplished, switch to more dilute fluid

HYPERNATREMIA

- Definition: serum Na^+ concentration greater than 150 mEq/L (Table 5-3)

TABLE 5-3 **Causes of Hypernatremia**

Reduced water intake
Disorders of thirst perception
Inability to obtain water (e.g., depressed mentation, intubated patient)
Increased water loss
Gastrointestinal
Vomiting, diarrhea
Nasogastric suctioning
Third-spacing
Renal
  Tubular concentrating defects (loop diuretics, renal disease)
  Osmotic diuresis (e.g., hyperglycemia, mannitol)
  Diabetes insipidus (neurogenic or nephrogenic)
  Relief of urinary obstruction
Dermal (e.g., excessive sweating, severe burns)
Hyperventilation
Gain of sodium
Exogenous sodium intake
Salt tablets
Sodium bicarbonate
Hypertonic saline solutions
Improper formula preparation
Ingestion of sea water
Hypertonic renal dialysate
Increased sodium reabsorption, mainly "hypersteroid" states
Hyperaldosteronism, Cushing's disease, exogenous corticosteroids, congenital adrenal hyperplasia

- Diabetes insipidus (DI) (Table 5-4)
  - Failure of the ADH response at either the central or renal level
  - Urine osmolality is low with higher urinary sodium (greater than 60 mEq/L)
  - DI diagnosis: patient's serum and urine osmolality should not respond to fluid deprivation. Central DI will respond to a small dose of 5 units of subcutaneous vasopressin

CLINICAL MANIFESTATIONS

- Signs and symptoms most prominent when the increase in serum sodium is large (>160 mEq/L) or occurs rapidly
- Infants: characteristic high-pitched cry, restlessness, muscle weakness insomnia, lethargy, and coma
  - Convulsions are typically absent except in cases of inadvertent sodium loading or aggressive rehydration
- Elderly patients generally have few symptoms until the [Na] exceeds 160 mEq/L
- Intense thirst may be present initially but it dissipates as the disorder progresses
- Brain shrinkage from hypernatremia can cause vascular rupture, with cerebral bleeding, subarachnoid hemorrhage, and permanent neurologic damage or death
  - Brain shrinkage is countered by an adaptive response that is initiated promptly and consists of solute gain by the brain ("idiogenic osmoles") that tends to restore lost water

TREATMENT

- Because of the formation of idiogenic osmoles, aggressive treatment of hypernatremic patients with hypotonic fluids may cause cerebral edema, which can lead to coma, convulsions, and death
  - Assume the hypernatremia happens slowly and that idiogenic osmoles are present—correct slowly
- Fluid replacement
  - Hemodynamically unstable: isotonic saline
  - Estimation: Each liter of free water lost will raise the serum sodium by 4 to 5 mEq/L
  - Definitive correction: Use same formula as was used in the treatment of hyponatremia (see Table 5-2) to calculate the change in sodium caused by a liter of infusate and choose an infusate that will lower your sodium by no

TABLE 5-4 **Causes of Diabetes Insipidus (DI)**

Central DI	Nephrogenic DI	Systemic	Drugs
Idiopathic	Congenital renal disorders	Sickle cell disease	Amphotericin
Head trauma	Obstructive uropathy	Sarcoidosis	Phenytoin
Tumors	Renal dysplasia	Amyloidosis	Lithium
Cerebral hemorrhage	Polycystic disease		Aminoglycosides
CNS infections			
Granulomatous disorders (e.g., tuberculosis, sarcoid, Wegener)			Methoxyflurane

more than 10 to 12 mEq/day (same rate as for hyponatremia)
- Correct underlying causes
- Note also that ongoing losses and maintenance fluids need to be added to the rate that is calculated

HYPOKALEMIA

- Definition: K^+ lower than 3.5 mEq/L
- Potassium is mainly an intracellular ion
  - No definite correlation between the plasma K^+ and body K^+ stores
  - In general, a reduction in the plasma K^+ of 1 mEq/L requires the loss of 200 to 400 mEq of K^+
    - Not the case when the cause of hypokalemia is transcellular shifting as in acidosis states
  - Linked to acid–base status
    - Rise in pH of 0.10 causes a drop in K^+ of 0.5 mEq/L

CAUSES (Table 5-5)

- Diuretic use is by far the number one cause (increased sodium delivery to the distal tubule is balanced by potassium excretion)
- Vomiting itself does not cause potassium loss; rather, hypokalemia results from hypovolemia, secondary hyperaldosteronism, and alkalosis
- Diarrhea can cause hypokalemia from K losses in the stool and from secondary hyperaldosteronism

CLINICAL MANIFESTATIONS

- Usually only seen at levels lower than 2.5 mEq/L
- Musculoskeletal:
  - Weakness: seen at K^+ levels <2.5 mEq/L

- Lower extremities are commonly involved first, particularly the quadriceps
- Cranial nerves are rarely involved
- Cramps, paresthesias, tetany, muscle tenderness, and atrophy may also occur
- Involvement of GI smooth muscle can produce a paralytic ileus
- Rhabdomyolysis
- Cardiovascular
  - Hypokalemia enhances automaticity and delays ventricular repolarization, predisposing to reentrant arrhythmias
  - Likelihood of inducing an arrhythmia is enhanced in the settings of coronary ischemia and left ventricular hypertrophy and the use of digitalis
- Electrocardiographic (ECG) changes: due to delayed ventricular repolarization
  - ST depression, decreased amplitude or inversion of the T wave
  - Increased height of the U wave (to >1 mm)
  - Prolongation of the QU interval result
  - When severe, increased amplitude of the P wave, prolongation of the PR interval, and widening of the QRS complex may occur
- Renal: Urine-concentrating problems, nephrogenic diabetes insipidus

TREATMENT

- Oral therapy is preferred whenever possible because the risk of hyperkalemia is significantly less and it is difficult to give large doses of K intravenously because of the required concomitant large fluid volume
  - 20 mEq K^+ every hour until corrected
- Intravenous potassium—reserved for severe cases
  - Usually given as KCl

TABLE 5-5   **Causes of Hypokalemia**

| Decreased Intake | Increased Losses | | | |
	Renal	Gastrointestinal	Skin	Transcellular Shifts
Decreased oral intake	Drugs	Vomiting	Sweating	Alkalosis
Kayexalate	▪ Diuretics #1	Diarrhea	Burns	▪ Diuretics
Malabsorption	▪ Antibiotics	Malabsorptive state	Heat stroke	▪ Vomiting
Clay ingestion (geophagia)	(aminoglycosides, PCNs)	Ileostomy	Febrile illness	▪ Bicarbonate therapy
	▪ Mannitol	Villous adenoma		▪ Hyperventilation
	▪ Lithium	Laxative abuse		Insulin
	Excess steroids			Beta-agonists
	Renal tubular acidosis			Hypokalemic periodic
	Obstructive uropathy			paralysis
	Black licorice ingestion			
	Hyperaldosteronism			
	▪ Primary			
	▪ Secondary			
	▪ CHF			
	▪ Nephrotic syndrome			
	▪ Cirrhosis			
	▪ Dehydration			
	Electrolyte abnormalities			
	▪ Hypomagnesemia			
	▪ Hypercalcemia			

- 10 mEq/hour in a peripheral line, 20 mEq/hour in a central line
  - No more than 40 mEq/hour
- 20 mEq K⁺ will raise the serum potassium by about 0.25 mEq/L
- Avoid dextrose-containing solutions—will promote insulin release and thus drop potassium levels
- Magnesium correction
  - Correction of hypokalemia requires the restoration of magnesium
    - Mg is required for activity of Na–K–ATPase pump

HYPERKALEMIA

- Definition: level higher than 5.5 mEq/L (Table 5-6)

CAUSES

CLINICAL MANIFESTATIONS

- Mainly cardiac
  - ECG changes—predictable pattern of progression, although absolute numbers vary between patients
  - Peaked T waves are generally the first finding seen
    - K⁺ = 5.5 to 7.0 mEq/L: peaked T waves, a shortened QT interval
    - K⁺ = 7.0 to 8.0 mEq/L: QRS complex widens and P wave flattens
    - K⁺ >9.5 mEq/L: widening QRS complex merges with the T wave, producing a sine-wave pattern, followed by ventricular fibrillation

MANAGEMENT

- Cardiac monitoring is essential; any ECG abnormality is an indication to treat
- Calcium: antagonizes potassium at the cardiac membrane and stabilizes
  - Onset in first minute, lasts 1 hour
  - 10 mL of a 10% solution calcium chloride or gluconate (CaCl₂ has more calcium but is sclerosing to peripheral veins) intravenously
  - Does not lower potassium
- Sodium bicarbonate: shifts potassium into cells
  - Onset in 5 minutes, lasts 1 to 2 hours
  - 50 to 100 mEq IV—1 ampule has 44 mEq of HCO₃

- Insulin: shifts potassium intracellularly
  - Onset 30 minutes, lasts 4 hours
  - Regular insulin 10 units
    - Give with 25 to 50 g glucose
- Diuretics: renal potassium excretion
  - Onset about 1 hour, last 4 to 6 hours
  - Furosemide 20 to 40 mg IV
- Albuterol: shifts potassium intracellular by cAMP upregulation
  - Onset 30 minutes, lasts 2 hours
  - Each nebulizer dose will lower potassium by 0.1 to 0.2 mEq/L
- Exchange resins: GI excretion of potassium
  - Onset 1 to 2 hours, lasts 2 to 4 hours
  - *Sodium polystyrene:* 20 to 60 grams in 70% sorbitol orally
    - Rectal enemas of 50 g work in 30 minutes
- Dialysis: most definitive correction by direct potassium removal
  - Onset is dependent on vascular access

HYPOCALCEMIA (Table 5-7)

CALCIUM METABOLISM

- 99% of calcium is found in the mineral component of bone
  - Remainder bound to serum proteins (mainly albumin), anions (phosphate, bicarbonate, citrate, lactate)
  - Less than 0.5% in the free ionized state (the physiologically active form)
- Calcium homeostasis: *falling* serum ionized Ca causes
  - Increased parathyroid hormone (PTH) secretion, which is responsible for increasing release of Ca and phosphate from bone, increasing Ca reabsorption and phosphate excretion in the kidney
  - Increased activated vitamin D formation in the kidney, which leads to increased intestinal absorption of Ca
- Calcium homeostasis: *rising* serum ionized calcium
  - Suppresses PTH production
  - Causes calcitonin release, decreasing osteoclastic activity and enhancing skeletal deposition of calcium

TABLE 5-6 **Causes of Hyperkalemia**

Pseudo-hyperkalemia	Increased intake	Potassium load from cellular injury	Transcellular shifts	Impaired renal excretion
Blood sample hemolysis	High-potassium foods	Hemolysis	Acidosis	Renal failure
Thrombocytosis	Oral K supplements	Rhabdomyolysis	Hypertonicity	Hypoaldosteronism
Leukocytosis	IV K administration	Tumor lysis syndrome	Insulin deficiency	Drugs
Lab error		Burns	Hyperkalemic	▪ NSAIDs
		Crush injuries	periodic paralysis	▪ ACE inhibitors
			Drugs	▪ Heparin
			Digoxin (acute)	▪ Cyclosporine
			Beta-blockers	▪ K-sparing diuretics
			Succinylcholine	Lupus nephritis
				Pseudohypoaldosteronism

TABLE 5-7 **Causes of Hypocalcemia**

Parathyroid hormone insufficiency (hypoparathyroidism)	PTH resistance (pseudohypoparathyroidism)	Calcium chelation	Vitamin D deficiency
Primary hypo-PTH Secondary hypo-PTH ■ Iatrogenic—neck surgery ■ Infiltrative neck disorders ■ Cancer ■ Sepsis ■ Pancreatitis ■ Burns ■ Magnesium derangements ■ Drugs (chemotherapy drugs)	Chronic renal failure	Hyperphosphatemia ■ Renal failure ■ Rhabdomyolysis ■ Tumor lysis syndrome Alkalosis Citrate (massive transfusion) Excess free fatty acids ■ Pancreatitis ■ Diabetic ketoacidosis ■ Alcohol intoxication	Decreased GI absorption ■ Malnutrition (rare) ■ Small bowel disease ■ Biliary disease ■ Pancreatic failure ■ Renal disease (Decreased activation of vitamin D) Anticonvulsants (vitamin D hypercatabolism) ■ Phenytoin ■ Primidone Congenital rickets

■ Acid–base effects
  ■ Acidosis decreases calcium binding to albumin, increasing ionized calcium without affecting the total serum level (alkalosis does the opposite)

CLINICAL MANIFESTATIONS

■ CNS: depression, irritability, confusion, seizures
■ Peripheral nervous system: perioral paresthesias, muscle weakness and cramps, fasciculations, and tetany
  ■ *Chvostek sign:* tapping over the facial nerve causes twitching of the ipsilateral facial muscles
  ■ *Trousseau sign:* carpal spasm in response to inflation of an arm blood pressure cuff to 20 mmHg higher than systolic BP for 3 minutes
■ Cardiovascular: decreased contractility, rarely bradycardia and hypotension
  ■ ECG: QT prolongation
■ Pulmonary: bronchospasm (rarely, laryngospasm)
■ Psychiatric: ranging from anxiety and depression to psychosis and dementia

MANAGEMENT

■ Verify the ionized calcium and check albumin
■ Treat if symptomatic (tetany, seizures, hypotension, or dysrhythmias)
■ Calcium
  ■ Recommended initial dose is 100 to 300 mg of elemental calcium
    ■ 10 mL of 10% Ca-chloride = 360 mg elemental Ca
    ■ 10 mL of 10% Ca-gluconate = 93 mg elemental Ca
  ■ Repeat doses needed after 1 to 2 hours, or an infusion can be started
  ■ Children's dose: 0.5 to 1.0 mL/kg of 10% Ca-gluconate over 5 minutes
  ■ Side effects include hypertension, nausea and vomiting, and flushing
  ■ Calcium should be given cautiously to patients taking digoxin because it may precipitate digoxin-induced cardiotoxicity (so-called "stone heart" from increased inotropy)

■ Calcium can cause severe tissue irritation and necrosis if it extravasates
■ Correct hypomagnesemia as this can cause refractory hypocalcemia
■ Asymptomatic hypocalcemia: treat orally with 1 to 4 g elemental Ca per day

HYPERCALCEMIA

CAUSES—MEET "PAM P. SCHMIDT"

■ P Parathyroidism (hyperparathyroidism—most common cause)
■ A Addison
■ M Multiple myeloma
■ P Paget disease
■ S Sarcoidosis
■ C Cancer (either metastatic or Ca of malignancy)
■ H Hyperthyroidism
■ M Milk-alkali syndrome
■ I Immobilization
■ D Vitamin D excess
■ T Thiazides

CLINICAL MANIFESTATIONS

■ "Bones, stones, abdominal groans, with psychiatric overtones"
■ Neurologic: fatigue, weakness, difficulty concentrating, confusion, lethargy, stupor, coma
■ Cardiovascular: Hypercalcemia causes an increase in vascular tone so BP may be misleadingly normal. Rarely, severe hypercalcemia can cause sinus bradycardia, bundle branch block, AV block
  ■ ECG: QT shortening, PR prolongation, QRS widening
■ Renal: impaired absorption of fluids and electrolytes in the renal tubule with consequent dehydration and can lead to renal failure; also predisposes to renal calculi, nephrocalcinosis, and calcium-induced interstitial nephritis
■ GI: Anorexia, nausea, vomiting, abdominal pain, constipation, ileus. Increased risk of peptic ulcer disease and pancreatitis

MANAGEMENT

- Restoration of intravascular volume with isotonic solution
- Enhancement of renal calcium elimination
  - Saline diuresis
  - Loop diuretics (after volume expansion)
    - AVOID thiazides (enhances calcium absorption)
- Reduction of osteoclastic activity
  - Calcitonin 4 IU/kg SC every 12 hours
    - Works only for first 48 hours
  - Plicamycin and mithramycin
  - Hydrocortisone 200 to 300 mg/day (inhibits vitamin D)
  - Bisphosphonates (inhibit osteoclastic bone resorption)
    - Takes ~48 hours to see effect
    - E.g., Pamidronate 60 to 90 mg over 24 hours
- Treat primary disorder

HYPOPHOSPHATEMIA (Table 5-8)

- Phosphorus handling
  - Primarily intracellular—component of DNA and RNA as well as ATP and 2,3-diphosphoglycerate (2,3-DPG)
  - Major acid–base buffer
  - 80% contained in bone in the form of hydroxyapatite (with calcium)
  - PTH and vitamin D are main regulators, although it is done indirectly—hormone responds primarily to changes in ionized calcium (see "Calcium")
    - PTH releases phosphate from bone into extracellular space
    - PTH inhibits phosphate resorption in kidneys (90% of phosphate is resorbed in proximal tubule)
    - In renal failure, PTH may actually increase phosphorus because of increased intestinal absorption

- Vitamin D enhances intestinal absorption of both phosphate and calcium
- Seen in 2% to 3% of hospitalized patients
- Usually not clinically relevant unless in severe category (<1.0 mg/dL)

CLINICAL MANIFESTATIONS

- Generally not clinically evident unless severe
- Main effects are from phosphate's role in ATP and energy production
- Cardiovascular: myocardial depression, impaired pressor responsiveness
  - Reduced threshold for ventricular arrhythmias
- Pulmonary: Muscle weakness causes respiratory insufficiency
- Musculoskeletal: weakness, myalgias, fatigue, rhabdomyolysis
- Hematologic: impaired 2,3-DPG production, causing left-shift of oxy-hemoglobin dissociation curve and decreased oxygen delivery, hemolysis, leukocyte dysfunction
- Neurologic: weakness, confusion, seizures, coma

MANAGEMENT

- Most mild and moderate cases can be treated with oral supplementation
- Severe—requires IV replacement
  - Because hypokalemia often coexists (as in DKA), KPO_4 is the preferred method
  - Monitor for signs of hypocalcemia

HYPERPHOSPHATEMIA (Table 5-9)

- Definition: levels higher than 5.0 mg/dL
- Rare, as kidneys handle phosphate load well
- Pseudohyperphosphatemia—lab interference caused by proteins or lipids

---

TABLE 5-8 Causes of Hypophosphatemia

Renal losses	Inadequate intake/absorption	Transcellular shifts
Diuretic therapy	Vitamin D deficiency	Respiratory alkalosis
Renal tubular dysfunction	Decreased intake	Salicylate poisoning
Hyperosmolar state (diabetic ketoacidosis)	Phosphate-binding antacids	Neuroleptic malignant syndrome
Hyperparathyroidism	Chronic diarrhea	Sepsis
Hyperaldosteronism		Heatstroke
Steroid use		Hyperglycemia
		Insulin use

TABLE 5-9 Causes of Hyperphosphatemia

Pseudohyperphosphatemia	Renal	Increased load
Paraproteinemia	Renal failure	Cellular injury
Hyperlipidemia	Hypoparathyroidism	Rhabdomyolysis
Hemolysis	Excess vitamin D	Tumor lysis syndrome
Hyperbilirubinemia	Thyrotoxicosis	Hemolysis
		Increased intake
		Phosphate enema/laxative
		IV or oral phosphate administration

CLINICAL MANIFESTATIONS

- Manifestations are those of hypocalcemia—excess phosphate binds serum calcium and precipitates in tissues
  - Hydroxyapatite deposition in cardiac tissue can cause heart block
- Neurologic: Excitability—hyperreflexia, tetany, seizures
- Cardiovascular: myocardial depression

MANAGEMENT

- Supportive care and treatment of hypocalcemia
- Infusion of isotonic saline increases phosphate clearance in patients with normal renal function
- Insulin and dextrose infusion drives phosphate into cells temporarily
- Aluminum antacids are the mainstays of prevention in patients with chronic renal failure
- Hemodialysis should be considered in patients with renal failure when hyperphosphatemia poses a threat to life

HYPOMAGNESEMIA

- Magnesium handling
  - Essential cofactor in many reactions (ATP production, protein synthesis, ion channeling, DNA synthesis, muscular contraction)
  - Only 1% to 2% is extracellular, and one third is bound to albumin
    - Half of total body magnesium is in bone
  - 90% of magnesium is resorbed in the kidney—enhanced by PTH
  - Magnesium is needed for the normal synthesis and release of PTH
- Definition: level lower than 1.8 mg/dL
  - Among most common electrolyte disturbances

CAUSES

- Alcohol abuse—poor nutrition, increased excretion, vomiting, and diarrhea
- Renal losses
  - Diuretic use
  - Renal failure
  - Chronic glomerulonephritis
  - Chronic pyelonephritis
  - Renal transplantation
- GI losses
  - Diarrhea
  - Short gut syndrome
  - Pancreatitis
  - Protein malnutrition
- Endocrine
  - Diabetes mellitus
  - Hyperthyroidism
  - Hypoaldosteronism
  - Hyperparathyroidism
  - Porphyria
- Pregnancy
- Medications
  - Diuretics

- Antibiotics: aminoglycosides, amphotericin
- Chemotherapeutics: cyclosporine, cisplatin
- Beta-agonists

CLINICAL MANIFESTATIONS

- Neuromuscular: muscle weakness, tremor, hyperreflexia, tetany, positive Chvostek and Trousseau signs
- CNS: apathy, irritability, dizziness, seizures, papilledema, coma
- Cardiovascular: supraventricular and ventricular arrhythmias
  - ECG: prolonged PR, QRS, and QT intervals; ST-T segment abnormalities; flattening and widening of the T wave; and presence of U waves—although this is debated as perhaps attributable to concomitant hypokalemia and/or hypocalcemia
- Hypokalemia—because magnesium is needed in the functioning of the Na–K ATPase pump, hypomagnesemia can result in a refractory hypokalemia that potassium administration cannot correct

MANAGEMENT

- In patients with life-threatening conditions (seizures, dysrhythmias) for which hypomagnesemia is the suspected cause, administer 2 to 4 g of magnesium sulfate intravenously over 30 to 60 minutes
- Administer with caution, if at all, to patients with renal failure or AV block
- Adverse effects include bradycardia, AV block, hypotension, respiratory failure

HYPERMAGNESEMIA (Table 5-10)

- Rare, as kidney can handle large magnesium load easily
  - Thus, high magnesium levels are seen almost always in the context of some degree of renal failure

CLINICAL MANIFESTATIONS

- Symptoms correlate with level
- Early: nausea, vomiting, weakness, and flushing
- Hyporeflexia—seen at levels higher than 3.0 mg/dL
  - Loss of deep tendon reflexes greater than 4.0 mg/dL
- Hypotension and ECG changes (QRS widening, QT and PR prolongation, and conduction abnormalities) are seen at 5.0 to 6.0 mg/dL
- Respiratory depression, coma, and complete heart block are seen in severe cases (greater than 9.0 mg/dL)

MANAGEMENT

- Stop all exogenous magnesium
- If symptoms are mild and renal function is normal—observe level

TABLE 5-10 **Causes of Hypermagnesemia**

Impaired renal Mg excretion	Exogenous Mg	Impaired GI elimination	Miscellaneous
Renal failure	Antacids	Bowel obstruction	Rhabdomyolysis
	Laxatives	Colitis	Tumor lysis syndrome
	Cathartics	Chronic constipation	Adrenal insufficiency
	Dialysates	Narcotics	Hyperparathyroidism
		Anticholinergics	Lithium

- Hydration with isotonic fluids and administration of IV furosemide can accelerate magnesium elimination (monitor the potassium carefully)
- In severe cases, IV calcium should be given to directly antagonize the membrane effects of hypermagnesemia and reverse the respiratory depression, hypotension, and cardiac dysrhythmias
- 100 to 200 mg elemental calcium (i.e., one amp of CaCl or two of Ca-gluconate)
  - Repeat boluses or an infusion at 2 to 4 mg/kg/hour may be required
- Consider dialysis for comatose patients or those with respiratory failure, hemodynamic instability, or renal failure

Pituitary disease

- Anterior pituitary makes:
  - Thyroid stimulating hormone (TSH)
  - Adrenocorticotrophic hormone (ACTH)
  - Luteinizing hormone (LH)
  - Follicle-stimulating hormone (FSH)
  - Prolactin
  - Growth hormone (GH)
- Posterior pituitary makes:
  - Antidiuretic hormone (ADH)
  - Oxytocin
- Panhypopituitarism
  - Usually only one or more of the hormones is deficient (complete "panhypopit" is rare)

CAUSES

- Congenital—Kallman syndrome
- Pituitary infiltrative tumors
- Postpartum—Sheehan syndrome
- Infection—tuberculosis, syphilis
- Infiltrative/inflammatory—sarcoidosis, hemochromatosis
- Iatrogenic—surgery, radiation

SYMPTOMS

- Major concerns are adrenal crisis and myxedema coma
- Gonadotropin deficiency is more insidious—amenorrhea, infertility
- In children, morbidity is worse (e.g., GH deficiency)
  - Diagnosis: suspicion, confirmed by hormone levels

- Treatment: hormone supplementation, reverse cause if possible
- Pituitary adenoma
  - Slow-growing, benign tumors in the sella turcica
  - 33% nonfunctioning (i.e., produce no hormone), 25% are prolactinomas, 20% make GH and 10% make ACTH

CLINICAL MANIFESTATIONS

- Enlargement of tumor may be first clue
  - Impingement on optic chiasm—bitemporal visual field loss ("tunnel vision")
  - Blurred or double vision, headache
  - Rarely, tumor may become necrotic or hemorrhage, causing severe headache, visual loss, and meningeal irritation
- If functioning, symptoms of hormone excess
  - Prolactin: Infertility and galactorrhea in women, hypogonadism and impotence in men
  - ACTH: Cushing disease
  - GH: gigantism in children, acromegaly in adults
    - Acromegaly: enlarged facial features, large hands and feet, heart disease, hypertension, arthritis, and amenorrhea/impotence
    - Craniopharyngiomas—most common tumor of pituitary area in children
- May mimic pituitary tumors clinically
- Come from remnants of cells of Ratgke pouch at the junction of the pituitary gland and the infundibulum

DIAGNOSIS

- CT or MRI

TREATMENT

- Depends on size and symptomatology

Adrenal disease (Table 5-11)

- Functions of the adrenal gland are threefold: 3 S's—"salt, sugar, and sex"

HYPERADRENALISM (CUSHING SYNDROME)

CAUSES

- Exogenous (steroid use)—most common
- Adrenal adenomas or carcinoma
- Ectopic ACTH production—pituitary disease
- Adrenal hyperplasia

TABLE 5-11 **Functions of the Adrenal Gland**

Sugar	Salt	Sex
Cortisol (glucocorticoid)	*Aldosterone (mineralocorticoid)*	*Androgens*
Maintains blood glucose Decreases extrahepatic glucose uptake Makes gluconeogenesis precursors Governs distribution of water in body compartments	Increase sodium resorption Induce potassium excretion	Significant in women Men's androgen is mainly produced in testes

CLINICAL MANIFESTATIONS

- Classic appearance—though it may be subtle in milder cases
  - Round face ("moon facies")
  - Central obesity
  - Buffalo hump (pads of fat on back of neck)
  - Skin striae—red or purple (from stretching)
  - Hirsutism (male pattern hair growth)
  - Thin skin
  - Telangiectasia
- Decreased glucose tolerance
- Impotence, infertility, reduced libido
- Hypertension

DIAGNOSIS

- Dexamethasone suppression test (DST)
- 24-hour serum or urine cortisol measurements

TREATMENT

- Remove exogenous steroids (if applicable) or admit to find cause of endogenous steroid production

HYPOADRENALISM

- Adrenal Insufficiency

CAUSES

- Exogenous steroids are most common cause
- *Primary adrenal failure*—deficiency of all corticoid subtypes
  - Idiopathic and autoimmune (Addison disease)— main primary cause
  - Infectious—tubercular, fungal, herpetic, cytomegalovirus
  - Infiltrative— sarcoidosis, lymphoma, hemochromatosis, amyloidosis
- Metastases can be seen often, but they rarely cause symptoms
  - Post adrenalectomy
  - Hemorrhage—stressed glands (e.g., Waterhouse–Friderichsen syndrome)
    - Rarely cause symptoms, as 90% of gland must be affected to produce clinical hypoadrenalism
- *Secondary adrenal failure*—pituitary or hypothalamic ("upstream") dysfunction
  - Glucocorticoid deficiency, not mineralocorticoid
    - ACTH secretion is *depressed*

- Aldosterone levels normal because of the stimulation of the renin–angiotensin system
- Pituitary insufficiency—tumor, infarction, infiltrative (sarcoidosis)
- Hypothalamic insufficiency
- Functional—glucocorticoid administration (this is the **most common cause**)
  - Steroid use for greater than 1 week can put patient at risk

CLINICAL MANIFESTATIONS

- Acute versus chronic *and* primary versus secondary
- Acute adrenal insufficiency is an acute, life-threatening emergency due primarily to cortisol insufficiency (aldosterone to a lesser extent). Occurs when the physiologic demand for these hormones exceeds the capacity of the adrenal glands to produce them (see "Acute Presentations: Adrenal Crisis")
- Chronic adrenal insufficiency develops gradually with subtle signs and symptoms that provide a diagnostic challenge. These patients may be hypotensive but not necessarily in frank shock
- Primary—deficiency of cortisol and aldosterone
  - Nonspecific—general weakness, nausea and vomiting, diarrhea
  - Hypoglycemia (especially with fasting)
  - Hypotension—seen in up to 90% of patients to varying degrees
    - Depressed myocardial contractility
    - Decreased responsiveness to catecholamines
    - Sodium wasting from aldosterone deficiency
  - Abdominal pain in one third of cases
  - Hyperpigmentation of skin—compensatory increase in ACTH and melanocyte-stimulating hormone (MSH) (MSH and ACTH are made from the same precursor)
  - Androgen deficiency—women only
- Secondary—only cortisol deficiency
  - Signs and symptoms of other pituitary–hypothalamic disease (thyroid hormone, growth hormone)
  - Hypoglycemia
  - Androgen deficiency—in both sexes
  - Hyperpigmentation absent
  - Salt and water loss is less

ACUTE PRESENTATIONS: ADRENAL CRISIS

- Causes
  - Abrupt withdrawal of chronic steroids
  - Stress in chronic adrenal insufficiency (adrenals are unable to "step up" to compensate)
  - Sudden massive bilateral adrenal hemorrhage
  - Hypothermia
  - Drugs: morphine, barbiturates
- Clinical manifestations
  - Severely, acutely ill
  - Severe refractory hypotension
    - Severe dehydration
    - Severe circulatory collapse (reduced amount and less responsive to catecholamines)
  - Abdominal pain may mimic an acute abdomen
  - Laboratory findings
    - Hyponatremia—rarely lower than 120 mEq/L
    - Hypoglycemia
    - Hyperkalemia—due to a combination of aldosterone deficiency, acidosis, and decreased glomerular filtration rate
    - Azotemia—from volume contraction
- Treatment
  - Steroid replacement
    - Glucocorticoids—dexamethasone may be given first if diagnosis is uncertain as it will not interfere with cortisol testing (4 mg intravenously with repeat doses to start); if known adrenal insufficiency, hydrocortisone in doses of 200 to 400 mg per day are needed
    - Mineralocorticoids—small doses of fludrocortisone or an equivalent can be added later
    - May be needed if hypotension is refractory to fluids and vasopressors
  - Fluid replacement: patients often profoundly dehydrated; D5NS (5% dextrose in normal saline) is a good choice to replace both salt wasting and hypoglycemia
    - Adequate oral salt intake is important for the patient with Addison disease
  - Treat hyperkalemia as needed
  - ACTH stimulation test
    - Not usually done in the ED
    - Give 0.25 mg of synthetic ACTH (Cortrosyn), and levels of cortisol are drawn at Time 0 and then 1-hour and 6- to 8-hour intervals afterward
  - Rapid screening test is based on the fact that the adrenal response to a single injection of ACTH is maximal within 1 hour
  - Normal persons should respond with a doubling of the baseline cortisol level or an increase of 10 mg/dL
  - Patients with primary adrenal insufficiency show no increase in cortisol levels, whereas those with secondary adrenal failure may show no, or a slight response
    - Used as a screening test, not as a diagnostic test for adrenocortical failure

- A 48-hour ACTH stimulation test confirms the diagnosis and can help differentiate between primary and secondary

PHEOCHROMOCYTOMA

- Tumor of the chromaffin cells of the adrenal medulla, where catecholamines are made and stored
  - 10% occur outside the adrenal
  - Most are benign (except for the effect of the catecholamine production)
- Occasionally associated with neurofibromatosis, von Hippel Lindau disease, and multiple endocrine neoplasias (MENs; see "Tumors")

CLINICAL MANIFESTATIONS

- Paroxysmal occurrence of hypertension, headache, flushing, diarrhea, palpitations, nervousness, and tremor
- On examination, the patient may exhibit fever, tremor, weight loss, postural hypotension, and tachyarrhythmias
  - Diagnosis: 24-hour urine collection for catecholamines (VMA and metanephrines)

TREATMENT

- Alpha-adrenergic blockade (phentolamine) initially
- Removal once medically controlled

Diabetes mellitus and its complications

GLUCOSE HOMEOSTASIS

- In its simplest forms, it is a "tug of war" between two sets of counterregulatory hormones
  - Insulin: anabolic—when energy (i.e., glucose) is more available
    - Increased glucose uptake and usage
    - Promotes glycogen formation
    - Inhibits gluconeogenesis
    - Increases lipogenesis
    - Inhibits triglyceride breakdown
    - Stimulates amino acid uptake in muscle
  - Glucagon (by far main counterregulatory hormone to insulin) catabolic
    - A "call to arms" for energy substrate
    - Growth hormone, catecholamines, and glucocorticoids all have some role in the same functions as glucagon
    - Promotes glycogenolysis and gluconeogenesis
    - Promotes lipolysis and ketone formation
    - Promotes proteolysis for amino acid use in Krebs cycle (catecholamines and glucocorticoids do this as well)

DIABETIC KETOACIDOSIS

- Pathophysiology (Fig. 5-3)
  - Need a combination of a relative insulin deficiency *and* an excess of counterregulatory

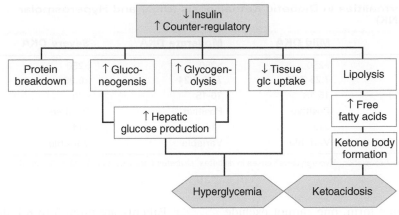

Figure 5-3. Pathophysiology of DKA

hormones (usually brought on by physiologic stress)
- Three fourths of cases have an identifiable cause—poor compliance is most common
- Explains why infection, stroke, and MI are all triggers for DKA
- DKA is, however, the presenting problem for up to one third of new patients with diabetes
- Insulin deficiency itself causes a cellular starvation (of sorts) and induces elevated of levels of counterregulatory hormones
- Hyperglycemia leads to an osmotic diuresis that accounts for the profound dehydration seen in DKA as well as the glucosuria and the losses of electrolytes (notably sodium and potassium)
- Fats are broken down in the liver into 2-carbon entities called ketone bodies whose oxidation cause the ketoacidosis and anion gap seen
  - Two main ketone bodies formed
    - Beta-hydroxybutyrate (BHB) and acetoacetate (ACA)
    - The two exist in equilibrium
- Initially, the more acidic BHB form is preferentially made (Fig. 5-4)
- As acidosis improves, the BHB molecules become converted to ACA
- However, the urine tests for ketones pick up only ACA
- So, ketone urine testing can become more certain with appropriate therapy
- To compensate for the acidosis, potassium is shifted extracellularly as hydrogen ions move into cells
  - The osmotic diuresis causes the potassium to be excreted, resulting in a profound body depletion of potassium (even in the face of an apparently normal serum value)
    - Patients are typically up to 5 mEq/kg deficient in potassium
    - Patients can even have ECG complications of hyperkalemia despite having a total body potassium deficit
- The alteration in mental status seen in DKA patients is a result of both the dehydration and the acidosis

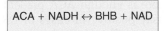

Figure 5-4. Ketone body homeostasis

CLINICAL PRESENTATION

- The 4 P's: polyuria, polydipsia, polyphagia, polyasthenia (weakness)
- Fluid depletion ranges from dehydration to frank shock
- Hyperventilation—often deep and rapid (Kussmaul respirations)
  - Compensation for the acidosis
  - Breath may have a fruity or acetone odor to it
- Nausea/vomiting are common—coffee ground emesis can be seen
- Abdominal pain—DKA is on the differential of the acute abdomen
- Altered mental status—ranging from mild confusion to coma
- Symptoms from the precipitant of the DKA state
  - MI—chest pain, dyspnea
  - Infection—fever, focal symptoms
  - Cerebrovascular accident (CVA)—focal neurologic findings

LABORATORY EVALUATION AND DIAGNOSTICS

- Basic criteria for DKA—elevated glucose greater than 250 mg/dL, acidosis/academia, ketonemia (Table 5-12)
- Finger stick glucose—almost always high
  - Almost always greater than 350 mg/dL
    - 15% have glucose levels lower than 350 mg/dL —called euglycemia DKA—these patient have poor glycogen stores and cannot mount the hyperglycemia (e.g., pregnancy, liver disease, starvation)
- Urine dip/analysis
  - Glucosuria should be universal
  - Ketonuria—almost always present
    - There is some contention that because the urine assay picks up only ACA, and BHB is the

TABLE 5-12 **Lab Abnormalities in Diabetic Ketoacidosis (DKA) and Hyperosmolar Non-Ketotic State (HNK)**

	Mild DKA	Moderate DKA	Severe DKA	HHNK
Plasma glucose (mg/dL)	>250	>250	>250	>600
Plasma pH	7.25-7.30	7.00-7.24	<6.99	>7.30
Serum bicarbonate(mEq/L)	15-18	10-15	<10	>15
Serum/urine ketones	Positive	Positive	Positive	Negative to trace
Anion gap	>12	>14	>14	Normal/variable
Serum osmolarity	Variable	Variable	Variable	>320 mOsm/kg

Adapted from American Diabetes Association: Hyperglycemic crises in diabetes, *Diabetes Care* 27(suppl 1):s94–s102, 2004.

predominant ketone form, one cannot exclude DKA based on urine ketones
- However, the ratio of BHB to ACA is approximately 4:1 in DKA, and most experts agree there is enough ACA present to make the urine assay positive in cases of DKA
- Also, large studies have shown that urine ketone assays carry a sensitivity of 99% for DKA (better than an anion gap or a serum bicarbonate level)
- Electrolytes
  - Low serum bicarbonate suggestive of an acidosis
  - Wide anion gap
  - Potassium is moved extracellularly because of acidosis, so the level may be high despite an actual total body deficiency
  - Sodium may be factitiously low
    - Sodium is lowered about 2 mEq/L for every 100 mg/dL elevation in serum glucose
  - Phosphate and magnesium should be checked as they are often low, although rarely of clinical significance
- Blood gases—although many still use arterial blood gases (ABG), good evidence exists that venous blood gases (VBG) correlate well with ABG to within 0.015 on the pH scale
  - DKA: low pH, low P_{CO_2}, low $[HCO_3]$
  - Caveat: VBG is not as good for picking up mixed acid–base disorders and will not give as accurate an assessment of ventilatory and oxygenation status
- Serum ketones—if there are ketones in the urine and the glucose is elevated with an anion gap, there is minimal need for this
  - Can be considered if urine cannot be obtained for analysis
- ECG
  - Surrogate marker for hyperkalemia (see ECG changes in "Hyperkalemia")
  - May provide insight as to trigger (MI and other causes)
- Other tests to search for possible cause as indicated (CXR, blood cultures, etc.)

MANAGEMENT

- Fluids have supplanted insulin as the lynchpin of therapy

- Patients are often 5 to 8 L deficient and up to 500 mEq of sodium deficient
  - HNK patients can be up to 10 L "dry"
- Normal saline should be used for fluid resuscitation
  - Generally 1 to 2 L to stabilize vital signs and improve end-organ perfusion
- ½ NS should be used for volume repletion
  - Goal is to restore 50% of fluid deficit in the first 8 hours, and the rest over the next 24 hours
- Caveats and complications
  - Cerebral edema
    - Uncommon complication of DKA seen in younger patients
    - Sudden deterioration in first 24 hours of treatment
    - Nonvasogenic edema of brain causing headache and quickly progressing to lethargy coma, respiratory arrest, fixed pupils, and (potentially) death
    - High morbidity and mortality
    - Despite may theories, only overly aggressive hydration has been associated with cerebral edema
    - Can happen even if patients are treated correctly
    - Bottom line: treat the DKA; the morbidity of poorly treated DKA is far greater than the risk of cerebral edema for any individual patient
  - Adding glucose to infusate
    - When the serum glucose level drops lower than 300 mg/dL, glucose should be added to the IV fluids to prevent an overshoot hypoglycemia as a result of insulin administration
    - As well, it is the usage of glucose by the cells that helps to reverse the acidosis, so a steady supply needs to be available
- Insulin
  - Low-dose IV insulin infusion
    - Most will start with a bolus dose of 0.1 U/kg of insulin R, followed by a 0.1 U/kg/hour infusion
    - Goal is slow glucose reduction of about 100 mg/dL/hour
  - Caveat
    - Insulin should be held if the potassium level is lower than 3.3 mEq/L, as insulin will further

- lower potassium, potentially to life-threatening levels as the already low potassium levels shift intracellularly again
  - In this case, hold insulin for 1 hour while infusing 10 to 30 mEq of potassium intravenously and recheck the potassium level
  - Bottom line: see basic metabolic panel (K^+) before starting insulin drip—but institute normal saline fluid resuscitation immediately
- Insulin (with glucose) should be continued until the acidemia has cleared even if the glucose is normal, as the acidosis takes much longer to resolve than the hyperglycemia
- Although SC insulin has a more erratic absorption, some evidence exists that mild DKA patients can be effectively treated with hourly injections based on close glucose monitoring
- Potassium
  - Not to be started until level is known and patient has urine output
  - Body deficit is severe and will worsen as treatment progresses
    - Intracellular stores of potassium are effectively depleted
  - $K^+ < 3.3$ mEq/L: hold insulin, give potassium 10 to 30 mEq and recheck in 1 hour
  - K^+ between 3.3 and 5.0 mEq/L: continue fluid and insulin, but add 20 to 40 mEq/L to the saline infusion and recheck potassium every 1 to 2 hours
  - $K^+ > 5.0$ mEq/L: begin or continue insulin and recheck potassium in 1 to 2 hours
  - Use oral potassium replacement if possible
- Bicarbonate
  - Four well-done studies have revealed no benefit to the use of sodium bicarbonate in the treatment of DKA
  - Current recommendations suggest its use when the pH is less than 6.90, but this is only because no study ever enrolled patients with a pH less than 6.90!
  - Pro argument: Acidosis decreases responsiveness to catecholamines, lowers the threshold for malignant arrhythmias, and increases the work of breathing
  - Con argument: Potential side effects of bicarbonate use
    - Paradoxical CNS acidosis (discussed in "Acid–Base Disorders")
    - Worsening of hypokalemia
    - Evidence shows a delayed recovery of the ketosis
    - Arrhythmogenic in large doses
    - Theoretically may blunt the respiratory compensation for the acidosis
- Phosphate often low, rarely clinically significant
  - No emergency recommendation for phosphate
  - Consider repletion if level is lower than 1.0 mg/dL
  - For replacement, one third of the potassium can be given as K_2PO_4 IV

- Hypophosphatemia can cause hypoxia, lethargy, muscle weakness, impaired cardiac function, and hemolysis when severely depleted
- Magnesium often low, rarely clinically significant
  - Replace if levels are lower than 1.2 mg/dL
- Monitoring and disposition
  - Glucose, check hourly
  - Electrolytes, every 1 to 2 hours depending on stability
  - Most patients will require ICU monitoring, but some milder cases may be appropriate for an intermediate level of care

HYPEROSMOLAR HYPERGLYCEMIC NONKETOTIC STATE

- Many acronyms: HHNK, HNK, HONK
- Similar to DKA in many ways, but description of HHNK is best done by contrasting it against DKA
- Definition: hyperglycemic state with elevated osmolarity and dehydration
- High mortality rate

PATHOPHYSIOLOGY

- Occurs in an almost identical fashion to DKA except:
  - The enzyme which promotes formation and uptake of ketoacids—carnitine palmityl transferase (CPT-1)—is controlled by the ratio of insulin to glucagon in the bloodstream
    - When the ratio tips to one extreme (low insulin and high glucose as in DKA), the enzyme begins the to ketoacid formation process
  - In the HHNK patient, the levels of circulating insulin are sufficient to keep the CPT-1 enzyme inhibited, thus preventing the formation of ketoacids
    - Lipolysis remains inhibited

PRECIPITANTS

- Like DKA, HHNK can be triggered by infection or physiologic stress
- HHNK patients have a different profile than DKA patients
  - Often older
  - Often not on insulin, but often on drugs that inhibit insulin function (thiazides, diuretics, calcium-channel blockers, beta-blockers)
  - Often with poor access to water—nursing home patients, unable to ambulate
  - Elderly patients often have impaired thirst mechanism—by virtue of age or medication—which makes rehydration more problematic
  - Chronic renal or cardiac disease is more common, also impairing effective rehydration

PRESENTATION

- Dehydration is severe; worse than DKA (often up to a 10 liter water deficit)
- Alteration in mental status is usually more severe than DKA patients

- Unlike DKA, HHNK is usually more indolent in onset
  - Laboratory evaluation (see Table 5-12)
- Glucose is often markedly elevated (often greater than 600 mg/dL)
- Serum osmolarity is markedly elevated
  - Calculated osmolarity is 2 (Na$^+$) + (glucose/17) + (BUN/2.8)
- Severe potassium and sodium losses are common
  - Although potassium losses are severe as a result of the osmotic diuresis, the lack of acidosis restricts the loss of intracellular potassium, and so HHNK patients may have a profound hypokalemia on lab testing

TREATMENT

- Principles similar to DKA treatment
- Fluids—similar to those used in DKA
  - NS for volume resuscitation, ½ NS for repletion once stabilized
  - Patient often up to 10 L "dry"
  - Replenish half of the water deficit in the first 8 hours
  - Glucose should be added when the serum glucose level drops lower than 300 mg/dL
- Insulin is *the only major difference* here in the treatment from DKA
  - Use lower doses, as insulin can cause intracellular shifts of electrolytes and water, resulting in cellular edema (cerebral edema) and potentially a worsening of hypovolemia
  - Overly rapid reduction in glucose may slow the osmotic diuresis—this may be the only factor driving the glomerular filtration rate, and an overly rapid correction can worsen renal failure or even precipitate acute tubular necrosis
- Potassium
  - Replace as needed once urine output is established
  - Guidelines similar to those for DKA

HYPOGLYCEMIA

- Definition
  - Low serum glucose level (usually lower than 50 mg/dL)
  - Symptoms consistent with the diagnosis
  - Resolution of symptoms with the administration of glucose
- Frequent problem
  - 7% of all cases of altered mental status presenting to ED
  - 7% of all deaths in insulin-dependent diabetics

PATHOPHYSIOLOGY

- Basic glucose handling
- Most body tissues can use alternate fuels when glucose stores are low (fats, proteins)
- Brain (and formed elements of blood) entirely dependent on glucose as an energy substrate
  - For adult, up to 150 g glucose per day

- Specialized carrier system keeps three times the glucose level in the brain compared to the serum level to ensure supply
- Adequately fed adult has about 24 hours worth of glucose stores to draw on
- Glucose level of ~70 mg/dL is trigger for counterregulatory hormone to provide more glucose; thus, symptoms of hypoglycemia could be seen with a borderline or low-normal glucose level

CAUSES

- Exogenous causes are more common
  - Diabetes—mistakes in therapy, by medication or diet, are the most common cause
    - Includes insulin and oral hypoglycemic agents (OHAs)
  - Alcohol use—alcohol inhibits gluconeogenesis, especially in combination with insulin
  - Medications—nondiabetic medications
    - Beta-blockers impair body's response to hypoglycemia (i.e., less diaphoresis, tremor)—patients less likely to recognize it
    - Salicylates—more in children
    - Barbiturates
    - Antipsychotics
    - Propoxyphene
  - Sepsis
- Endogenous
  - Early diabetes—delay in insulin release, followed by a surge
  - Dumping syndrome—from gastric surgery
    - Rapid gastric emptying (2 to 3 hours postprandial) leads to rapid high levels of carbohydrate in the small intestine, which causes a hyperinsulinemic response
  - Endocrine dysfunction
    - Pancreatic: islet cell tumors, insulinomas
    - Other: pituitary, adrenal, or thyroid insufficiency
  - Clinical states with decreased stored glycogen
    - Prolonged fasting
    - Pregnancy
    - Liver disease
    - Malabsorptive syndromes
  - Factitious—high WBC counts (greater than 50,000 to 60,000)—WBC (formed elements of blood use glucose in the sample tube)
  - Idiopathic ketotic hypoglycemia—diagnosis of exclusion in children

CLINICAL PRESENTATION

- Two groups of symptoms that occur simultaneously
- Neuroglycopenic—results of brain dependence on glucose
  - Mainly alterations in mental status
    - Wide range, from mild confusion to frank coma
  - 10% of hypoglycemic patients will have focal neurologic findings
- Adrenergic—by-product of counterregulatory hormones trying to raise glucose levels
  - Diaphoresis
  - Hypersalivation

- Tremor
- Lightheadedness
- Tachycardia/palpitations
- Hypothermia is not a symptom of hypoglycemia. If present, search for a possible cause
  - Laboratory
- Glucose testing
  - Bedside testing is rapid, but not accurate at extremes
  - Whole blood glucose levels are 15% lower than serum or plasma
    - WBCs continue to use glucose
    - RBCs normally have low intracellular glucose, but equilibration occurs

TREATMENT

- Replacement therapy
  - Oral glucose—preferred whenever possible, as ingestion of food provides fats, proteins
  - IV glucose—1 mL/kg of 50% dextrose will provide a clinical response in almost all cases
    - Infants—high-dose dextrose can sclerose veins; no more than 25% dextrose at 2 mL/kg
      - In newborns—should rarely use more than 10% dextrose
  - Glucagon—1 mg parenterally, 30 to 50 µg in infants
    - Recruits hepatic glycogen stores and induces gluconeogenesis
    - May also induce insulin secretion to a small extent
    - Caveat: must have intact glycogen stores to be effective
  - Octreotide—40 to 100 µg SC/IV
    - Somatostatin analogue
    - Suppresses insulin and glucagon secretion
    - Recent literature shows benefit in treatment of sulfonylurea-induced hypoglycemia
  - Thiamine—100 mg IV
    - IV glucose will cause the patient to use up their thiamine stores and thus theoretically precipitate Wernicke encephalopathy
    - Standard practice is to administer thiamine to patients with altered mental status when starting IV glucose
    - Data have shown that thiamine uptake in the cells is twice as long as glucose uptake
      - Thiamine given will serve as a protection as stores become low

Thyroid disease

- Tetra-iodothyronine (T4) is the main thyroid hormone
  - Converted in periphery to T3 (tri-iodothyronine)—10 times more biologically active than T4
- Responsible for regulation of various cellular processes
  - Vascular tone, ion-channel homeostasis, cellular signal transduction
- Regulation
  - Thyroid function is mainly under influence of TSH from the anterior pituitary
  - TSH levels are controlled by thyrotropin-releasing hormone (TRH) from the hypothalamus and by a negative feedback loop from level of T4 and T3

HYPERTHYROIDISM, THYROTOXICOSIS, AND THYROID STORM

- Hyperthyroidism, thyrotoxicosis, and thyroid storm are a spectrum of the same disease (Table 5-13)
- More common in women
- Causes of hyperthyroidism and thyrotoxicosis

THYROID DISEASE

- Graves disease—by far the most common—80% of all causes
- Toxic adenoma
- Multinodular goiter
- Thyroiditis (see "Thyroiditis")
  - Hashimoto (early on in course)
  - Subacute (de Quervain disease)—painful thyroiditis
- Thyroid cancer (mainly follicular, most other thyroid cancers are "cold")

NONTHYROIDAL DISEASE

- Paraneoplastic TSH stimulation (rare)
- Ectopic thyroid tissue
  - Secondary hyperthyroidism—TSH overproduction
  - Tertiary hyperthyroidism—TRH overproduction

DRUGS

- Factitious hyperthyroidism—from an exogenous source (overdose, fad diets)
- Lithium
- Amiodarone
- Iodine

TABLE 5-13 **Signs and Symptoms of Hyperthyroidism**

Symptoms	Signs
Weakness	Goiter
Fatigue	Lid lag (mainly in Graves disease)
Heat intolerance	Ophthalmopathy (mainly in Graves disease)
Nervousness	Tachycardia
Diaphoresis/increased sweating	Hypertension
Tremor	Tremor
Weight loss (despite eating)	Hyperreflexia
Irregular periods	Warm, moist skin
	Proximal muscle weakness

Thyroid storm

- Rare, but life-threatening
- Severe thyrotoxicosis and storm is typically sudden in onset (coincident with the acute precipitant)
- Symptoms of thyroid storm are same as hyperthyroidism above, BUT
  - Fever
  - Tachycardia out of proportion to the fever
  - CNS disturbance is almost universal in storm and has various manifestations
    - From agitation and manic behavior to obtundation/coma
  - Diarrhea—often heralds impending storm and carries poor prognosis
  - Muscle weakness (usually in the proximal muscle groups) is also very common
  - Jaundice and CHF are considered terminal events and very poor prognostic signs
- Precipitants of thyroid storm
  - Graves disease is still the number one cause
  - Infections—especially pulmonary
  - Vascular—infarction (visceral), pulmonary embolism, stroke
  - Physiologic stress—surgery (not as common a cause now as it used to be), burns, trauma
  - Endocrine—mainly diabetes (insulin-induced hypoglycemia, DKA, HHNK)
  - Iatrogenic
    - Premature withdrawal of antithyroid meds
    - Thyroid hormone overdose
    - Use of iodine contrast in radiologic studies
    - Solutions of KI given to patients with nontoxic goiters
    - Radioactive ^{131}I administration
  - Preeclampsia
  - Drugs—amiodarone, thioridazine
- Diagnosis of thyroid storm
  - No labs distinguish thyrotoxicosis from storm—on the same spectrum
  - Thyroid function tests
    - TSH—usually immeasurably low
    - T4 elevated
    - T3 elevated (not generally done in the ED)
    - Free T4 index—best single test. Measures both the T4 and active T3 in the bloodstream
    - T3 toxicosis is rare but possible and can be missed on standard tests
  - Other lab tests—highly variable

MANAGEMENT

- If suspected—do not wait, start treatment immediately
- Treat the precipitant!
- Supportive care
  - Fever control—acetaminophen cooling
    - No aspirin—displace thyroid hormone from thyroid globulin, and convert T4 to T3
  - Hydration—patients often severely volume depleted

- Correct arrhythmias—propranolol is a good first choice
  - Avoid atropine if possible (parasympathetic effect may accelerate heart rate)
- Steroids—dexamethasone preferred, decreases T4 to T3 conversion peripherally
  - Stress dose—equivalent of 300 mg cortisol per day
  - Rare coexistence of adrenal disease
- Inhibition of thyroid synthesis
  - Propiothiouracil (PTU) 900 to 1200 mg loading dose, followed by 300 to 600 mg daily for 3 to 4 weeks
    - PTU decrease T4 to T3 conversion
  - Methimazole (MMI) 90 to 120 mg load, followed by 30 to 60 mg daily
    - TIP: the dose is 1/10th that of PTU
  - These work within 1 hour, but work maximally in 3 to 4 weeks
  - MMI considered "safe in pregnancy" though literature suggests both are acceptable
  - These drugs inhibit thyroid hormone synthesis, but not release
- Inhibition of thyroid hormone release
  - Preformed hormone can still be released even after synthesis blockade for up to 3 weeks
  - Iodine stops thyroidal release only after synthesis is blocked
    - Give 1 hour after administration of PTU or methimazole (otherwise it is like "adding fuel to fire")
  - IV preparations no longer available
  - Orally; 1% KI 5 drops every 6 hours
    - Ipodate (Orografin)—radiologic contrast also blocks conversion of T4 to T3
    - Not all dyes have this effect
  - Lithium can also inhibit thyroid hormone release, but it is not used generally
- Reduce conversion of T4 to more bioactive T3
  - Propylthiouracil
  - Propranolol
  - Dexamethasone
- Blockade of peripheral hormone effects
  - Propranolol blocks sympathetic drive
    - IV: 1 mg/min, increasing by 1 mg every 10 to 15 minutes to a maximum of 10 mg, can be repeated every 3 to 4 hours
- Effects can be seen in 10 minutes
  - Orally, 20 to 120 mg every 4 to 6 hours, with effects in about 1 hour
  - Esmolol—rapid acting, titratable, does not reduce T4-to-T3 conversion
  - Guanethidine and reserpine deplete catecholamine stores
    - Effects within 6 to 8 hours
    - Not used often because of side effects (hypotension, diarrhea, sedation)

APATHETIC THYROTOXICOSIS

- Also known as "masked hyperthyroidism"
- Differences from typical presentation of thyrotoxicosis
  - Patients are typically older (usually more than 70)

- Symptomatic for a longer time than the usual patients, likely because making the diagnosis is harder
- The typical symptoms of thyrotoxicosis are frequently absent
- Lethargy, depression, muscle weakness, and weight loss are the common symptoms
- The frequent exophthalmos and lid lag are absent; only a droopy lid may be noted
- Symptoms are generally limited to one system—often cardiovascular
  - CHF and atrial fibrillation are common
- Treatment principles are same as for thyroid storm
  - CHF can be treated with digoxin and diuretics (often refractory)
  - Beta-blockers can be used in CHF, but not alone

HYPOTHYROIDISM (Table 5-14)

- More common in women

CAUSES

- Primary hypothyroidism—95% of causes (TSH is high)
  - Iatrogenic—most common cause is overtreatment of hyperthyroidism
    - Ablation, surgery, radiation therapy
  - Infiltrative—sarcoid, amyloid, tuberculosis
  - Autoimmune—Hashimoto thyroiditis (later in disease)
- Secondary hypothyroidism
  - Panhypopituitarism—TSH may be low—pituitary issue
- Tertiary hypothyroidism—TSH low and TRH low—hypothalamic issue

DRUGS/MEDICATIONS

- Amiodarone can cause both hyper- and hypothyroidism
- Lithium
- Antithyroid medications

DIAGNOSIS

- Must be suspected
- Lab testing
  - TSH is best single test—elevated in primary hypothyroidism (which is 95% of all cases)

TABLE 5-14 **Signs and Symptoms of Hypothyroidism**

Symptoms	Signs
Fatigue	Bradycardia
Weight gain	Depressed reflexes—long relaxation phase
Cold intolerance	Cool, dry skin
Depression	Loss of lateral third of eyebrows
Lethargy	Hoarse voice
Constipation	Hypothermia
Paresthesias	Myxedema: dry, waxy, nonpitting swelling
Joint pains	Joint swelling/effusions

- TSH can be normal in cases of pituitary and hypothalamic disease
- T4 is typically low
- T3 is unreliable

TREATMENT

- Thyroid hormone, start at 50 to 100 µg/day
- N.B.: there is a lag between starting thyroid therapy and clinical improvement, usually about 2 weeks

MYXEDEMA COMA

- Rare life-threatening hypothyroid state with a mortality higher than 50%

CAUSES

- List resembles precipitants of thyroid storm
  - Cold exposure—in some form, seen in up to 90% in some series
  - Infection—especially pulmonary
  - CHF
  - Trauma—usually with concomitant cold exposure
  - Stroke
  - Drugs—thiazides, sedatives, lithium, anaesthetics
  - Noncompliance with thyroid meds
  - Hypoglycemia
  - Hemorrhage, especially GI

CLINICAL MANIFESTATIONS

- A misnomer, since most patients are neither myxedematous nor in coma
- Exaggeration of signs and symptoms of hypothyroidism, plus
  - Hypothermia—so common in myxedema coma that a normal temperature (seen in up to 25%) should prompt a search for an infectious trigger
- Myxedema coma is the only hypothermic disease where the temperature correlates with mortality
  - Hypotension not seen in hypothyroidism
  - Altered mental status—coma only at extreme
- Usually slowed cognition and mentation, memory impairment
  - Cerebellar findings (in 40%), although it is not certain why
- Ataxia, positive Romberg sign and nystagmus can all be seen
  - Hypoventilation and hypoxia ± hypercarbia
- Associated lab findings
  - Hyponatremia—as low as 110 mEq/dL
    - Believed to be a combination of dilutional and SIADH
  - Hypoglycemia—rare, and usually mild
  - Mild normochromic normocytic anemia
  - Adrenal insufficiency may be present (Schmidt syndrome)
  - Respiratory acidosis on ABG
  - Thyroid testing shows hypothyroidism but does not correlate with severity

TREATMENT

- Rule out other causes of coma
  - Do not wait for TSH if suspicion is high (e.g., known hypothyroid off medication)
- ICU supportive care
  - Transfusion if hematocrit lower than 30%
  - Hypotension is an ominous sign
    - Fluids, as vasoactive drugs have not been shown to maintain perfusion
- Treat the precipitant if possible
- Stress dose steroids—avoid dexamethasone
  - Schmidt syndrome—adrenal and thyroid insufficiency
- Thyroid hormone administration
  - 500 μg (300 μg/m²)
  - Controversy exists about danger of thyroid replacement
    - Has potential to be harmful to euthyroid patients, especially with heart disease
    - Dose can be dropped in half
    - However, 500 μg only restores 50% of the euthyroid levels, so overtreatment is relatively unlikely
    - Also, use T4 as it is less bioactive and more slowly absorbed
  - Takes 8 hours at minimum to show effect

THYROIDITIS

- DeQuervain thyroiditis
  - Most common cause of a painful thyroid gland
  - Usually a viral trigger—viral illness 1 to 3 weeks prior
  - Clinical—pain is presenting symptom in 90%
    - Diffuse thyroid tenderness, firm to touch
    - Pain worsened by swallowing or head movement
    - 3 to 6 weeks of hyperthyroidism
    - No lid lag or exophthalmos
    - A hypothyroid period of several months follows
  - Diagnosis is mainly *clinical*
    - TSH may be low, but thyroid-binding globulin is always elevated
    - ESR is usually markedly elevated
  - Self-limited disease; treat symptomatically until normalized
- Hashimoto thyroiditis
  - Chronic, autoimmune thyroid disease
  - Often initially hyperthyroid
  - May also have alternating hypo- and hyperthyroid states early on
  - Firm, nontender goiter
  - Associated with Addison disease, diabetes mellitus, celiac disease, hypoparathyroidism, and pernicious anemia

THYROID CANCER

- Most present with a thyroid mass or nodule (though most nodules are not cancerous)
- More common in women
- Four types
  - Papillary and follicular (95%)—97% cure rate if treated appropriately
  - Medullary and anaplastic (5%)—aggressive with poorer prognosis
- Patients are usually euthyroid (i.e., tumors are "cold")

Tumors and paraneoplastic syndromes

- Paraneoplastic syndromes
  - Ectopic hormone production from cancer tissue
  - Common examples
    - SIADH—ADH-like compound released in many lung tumors
    - PTH-like hormone seen in squamous tumors of the head, neck, and lungs
    - ACTH-like peptides seen in small cell lung cancer
- Familial neoplastic syndromes—rare, and hard to remember
  - *Take home point* is that these conditions occasionally "run in packs"
  - Multiple endocrine neoplasia (MEN)
    - MEN 1 (Werner syndrome): hyperfunctioning tumors of the parathyroid glands, pancreas (glucagonoma, VIPoma, insulinoma) and anterior pituitary (prolactinoma)
    - MEN 2A (Sipple syndrome): medullary thyroid cancer, pheochromocytoma, and hyperparathyroidism
    - MEN 2B: medullary thyroid cancer, pheochromocytoma—patients have marfanoid habitus

Nutritional disorders: vitamins

VITAMIN A

- Functions
  - Forms part of visual pigments of retina
  - Maintains bone growth and cellular stability
- Sources—Egg yolk, liver, deeply colored vegetables and fruits (e.g., carrots, squash)
- Deficiency—endemic worldwide
  - Causes—fat soluble, so caused by impaired fat absorption and liver disease
  - Symptoms
    - "Night blindness"—impaired dark vision adaptation
- Seen also with zinc deficiency
  - Second-leading cause of blindness worldwide
  - Susceptibility to infection
- Excess—Hypervitaminosis A—rare; requires large doses over time)
  - Blurred vision
  - Yellow/orange skin pigmentation
  - Hair loss, dry skin
  - Long bone pain (due to hypercalcemia)
  - Pseudotumor cerebri

VITAMIN B$_1$ (THIAMINE)

- Functions
  - Cofactor in Krebs cycle and for glucose uptake into cells
- Sources—meat, whole grains, enriched bread
  - Not stored in the body; must have a steady supply
- Deficiency—tissues that rely on rapid glycolysis—brain, nerve, and muscle
  - Wet beriberi: high-output heart failure resulting from peripheral vasodilation and the formation of AV fistulae as a result of myocardial and muscle weakness
  - Dry beriberi: peripheral nerve dysfunction with myopathy
  - CNS disease: the **Wernicke–Korsakoff** syndrome (thought to be at least in part due to thiamine deficiency; there may be other factors)
    - Wernicke encephalopathy is described by the classic triad of oculomotor abnormalities, ataxia, and global confusion
    - Associated with a 10% to 20% mortality rate
  - Generally the eyes symptoms are first, followed by the ataxia and then the confusion—they resolve in the same order (often some remnant of the confusion remains)
  - Korsakoff psychosis is a disorder of learning and processing new information, characterized by a deficit in short-term memory and confabulation
- Excess-—thiamine is not stored, so not an issue
- Hypoglycemia and thiamine
  - Standard practice is to administer thiamine to comatose or confused patients when starting IV glucose. While it makes sense, as the IV glucose will cause the patient to use up his or her thiamine stores and thus theoretically precipitate Wernicke, data has shown that thiamine uptake in the cells takes twice as long as glucose uptake. Thus, the thiamine you give will not have an immediate effect, but rather will serve as a protection for later if stores become low

VITAMIN B$_2$ (RIBOFLAVIN)

- Functions—Antioxidant—involved in glutathione pathways
  - Aids in metabolism of fats and proteins
- Sources—50% from dairy products
  - Not stored—need a steady intake
- Deficiency—rare
  - Sore mouth, cracked lips, red "magenta" tongue
  - Eczematous lesions to face and genital area
- Excess—not stored, and overdosage is rare

VITAMIN B$_3$ (NIACIN)

- Functions
  - Becomes part of NAD–NADP pathway—in almost all major metabolic pathways
- Sources—ubiquitous in foods, but mainly in poultry meat and fish
  - Can be made from tryptophan, so malnutrition must be severe to be deficient

- Deficiency: Pellagra
  - The 4 Ds of Pellagra
  - Dementia—irritability and even psychosis
  - Dermatitis—glossitis, sore tongue, dark, scaling skin in sun-exposed areas
  - Diarrhea
  - Death
- Excess
  - Nicotinic acid form used in treatment of hyperlipidemia
  - *Niacin flush* seen in large doses—due to histamine release
    - Diffuse skin reddening, itching, and burning
    - Self-limiting and tolerance develops
  - Can cause a reversible hepatitis in large doses

VITAMIN B$_6$ (PYRIDOXINE)

- Functions
  - Forms a coenzyme needed for transamination of amino acids
  - Deficiency rate-limits most biosynthetic pathways
- Sources—meat, vegetables, and whole grains
- Deficiency
  - Isoniazid and penicillamine both remove it from the body (birth control pills also, to a lesser extent)
  - Seizures (decreased GABA synthesis)
  - Anemia
  - Peripheral neuropathy
- Excess
  - Reversible peripheral sensory neuropathy
  - Can cause intestinal inactivation of levodopa; beware in Parkinson's patients

VITAMIN B$_{12}$ (COBALAMIN) AND FOLIC ACID

- The two are intimately connected and should be discussed together
- Functions
  - Together, they transfer one-carbon groups to acceptor molecules in numerous metabolic pathways
    - DNA, RNA synthesis
    - Serine protease function and cysteine formation
  - B$_{12}$, on its own, is needed for myelin synthesis, which is why its deficiency causes neuropathy (whereas folate does not)
- Sources
  - B$_{12}$: From bacterial synthesis—meat or dairy products of animals
    - Requires intestinal intrinsic factor (IF) for absorption
    - No IF: Pernicious anemia
    - True vegans are at risk
  - Folic acid: Leafy greens (though it is lost in cooking)
- Deficiency
  - Megaloblastic anemia
  - B$_{12}$—causes neuropathy—typically years to develop
    - Classically, proprioceptive changes form posterior column disease in the spinal cord

- Folate replacements will not reverse the neuropathy, and if left long enough, they can become permanent. Always check both folate and B_{12} levels in cases of megaloblastic anemia
- Excess: Rarely seen

VITAMIN C (ASCORBIC ACID)

- Functions
  - Strong reducing agent—antioxidant
  - Co-factor for the formation of collagen
- Sources: green vegetables and citrus fruits
- Deficiency—scurvy
  - Malaise, lethargy and weakness
  - Mouth: swollen, bleeding gums
  - Skin: petechiae, corkscrew hairs, poor wound healing
  - Painful joints
  - Iron deficiency and anemia: vitamin C aids in intestinal absorption of iron
- Excess
  - Diarrhea and abdominal cramping
  - Risk of gout and kidney stones

VITAMIN D (CHOLECALCIFEROL)

- Functions
  - Activated version elevates plasma calcium and phosphorus levels and aids in bone mineralization
  - Increases intestinal absorption of calcium
- Sources
  - Can be endogenously made from cholesterol—needs sunlight
    - Skin vitamin D synthesis is less in elderly and dark-skinned people
  - Dietary: enriched milk, egg yolk
- Deficiency
  - Hypocalcemia and hypophosphatemia
    - CNS: depression, irritability, confusion, seizures
    - Peripheral nervous system: muscle cramps, fasciculations, and tetany
  - Chvostek and Trousseau signs
    - Cardiovascular: decreased contractility, rarely bradycardia and hypotension
    - ECG: QT prolongation
    - Pulmonary: bronchospasm (rarely, laryngospasm)
    - Psychiatric: anxiety and depression
- Excess—the only vitamin for which excess carries a considerable risk of death
  - Hypercalcemia and its complications

VITAMIN E (ALPHA-TOCOPHEROL)

- Functions: antioxidant
- Sources: ubiquitous, found in eight forms
- Deficiency: rare in adults
  - Fat soluble; disease of fat malabsorption can cause a deficiency (takes years)
- Excess: No toxicity
  - Antagonizes Vitamin K at high levels

VITAMIN K

- Functions: cofactor for activation of factors II, VII, IX and X in the coagulation cascade
- Sources: dark-green vegetables
  - Also made endogenously by intestinal bacteria (about 50%)
  - Unlike other fat-soluble vitamins, not stored significantly in body
- Deficiency
  - Generally brought on by inhibition by warfarin use
    - Warfarin blocks the vitamin K–dependent enzyme needed for coagulation factor formation
  - Patients on broad-spectrum antibiotics can have the intestinal bacteria killed that make vitamin K
  - Fat-soluble vitamin: liver and or biliary disease will impair its absorption
  - Bleeding is the most common sign
- Excess
  - Large doses of the water-soluble form can cause anemia, liver disease, and mitochondrial myopathies
    - Can also, in large doses, inhibit the coagulative effects of the fat-soluble subtypes

PEARLS

- Always calculate the anion gap—even if all the electrolytes are normal.

- Remember MUDPILE CATS and USED CARP for metabolic acidosis.

- For treating sodium derangements, it is easier to calculate the change in sodium brought about by a liter of a given IV solution, and back-calculate the appropriate treatment:
  Change in serum Na^+ =
  $\{$(infusate Na^+ + infusate K^+) −
  serum Na^+/Total body water + 1$\}$

- Remember PAM P SCHMIDT for causes of hypercalcemia.

- When treating adrenal insufficiency, dexamethasone will not interfere with later cortisol testing but will meet initial therapeutic needs.

- DKA patients with a potassium level lower than 3.3 mEq/L should have their insulin infusion temporarily stopped.

- Presence or absence of urinary ketones has been shown to be more sensitive for DKA than an anion gap.

- When treating thyroid storm, iodide should only be given an hour after propylthiouracil or methimazole.

- Myxedema coma is the only hypothermic condition when temperature correlates inversely with mortality.

- Vitamin D is the only vitamin that when taken in excess, carries a serious threat of death.

BIBLIOGRAPHY

Cooper DS: Antithyroid drugs, *N Engl J Med* 352:905–917, 2005.

Cooper DS: Treatment of thyrotoxicosis. In Braverman LE, Utiger RD (eds): *The thyroid: a fundamental and clinical text*, ed 6, Philadelphia, 1991, Lippincott, pp. 887–916.

Fasano C, O'Malley G, Dominici P et al: Comparison of octreotide and standard therapy alone for the treatment of sulfonylurea-induced hypoglycemia, *Ann Emerg Med* 24:580–581, 2007.

Green SM, Rothrock SG, Ho JD et al: Failure of adjunctive bicarbonate to improve outcome in severe pediatric diabetic ketoacidosis, *Emerg Med* 31:41, 1998.

Kravitz J: Diabetic ketoacidosis: new answers to old questions, *Emerg Med* 39(11):10–15, 2007.

Marx JA, Adams J, Rosen P, Hockberger RS, Walls RM (eds): *Rosen's emergency medicine: clinical concepts and practice*, ed 6, St. Louis, MO, 2005, Mosby Elsevier.

Nicoloff JT: Thyroid storm and myxedema coma, *Med Clin North Am* 69:1005–1019, 1985.

Okuda Y, Adrogue HJ, Field JB, Nohara H, Yamashita K: Counterproductive effects of sodium bicarbonate in diabetic ketoacidosis, *J Clin Endocrinol Metab* 81:314, 1996.

Rowden A, Fasano C: Emergency management of oral hypoglycemic drug toxicity, *Emerg Clin North Am* 25(2):347–356, 2007.

Schwab TM, Hendey G, Soliz T: Screening for ketonemia in patients with diabetes, *Ann Emerg Med* 34(3):342–346, 1999.

Singer PA, Cooper DS, Levy EG et al: Treatment guidelines for patients with hyperthyroidism and hypothyroidism, *JAMA* 273:808–812, 1995.

Tintinalli J, Kelen G, Stapczynski S (eds): *Emergency medicine: a comprehensive study guide*, ed 6, New York, 2004, McGraw-Hill.

Questions and Answers

1. A 55-year-old man is brought by his family to the ED complaining of altered mental status. His family says that his only medical issue is the new discovery of a growing nodule in his neck that is undergoing investigation—he is awaiting the results of a recent neck CT. He has been complaining of aches in his bones all over his body for the past 3 days. He is a former smoker, does not drink alcohol. He has mild hypertension for which he takes hydrochlorothiazide (HCTZ). On examination, the patient is afebrile with a pulse of 88 bpm and a blood pressure of 145/88 mmHg. He is awake, but lethargic and confused, disoriented to time and place. Bedside glucose was measured at 89 mg/dL. His abdomen is diffusely tender with voluntary guarding. He has diffuse muscle weakness with 4/5 strength equally. His ECG shows shortening of the QT interval and prolongation of the PR interval. The next most appropriate therapeutic intervention is:

   a. 40 mg furosemide intravenously and saline diuresis
   b. 10 mL of 10% calcium gluconate intravenously
   c. 3% hypertonic saline intravenously
   d. 60 mg intravenous pamidronate

2. Which of the following clinical conditions causes a metabolic acidosis with a normal anion gap?

   a. diabetic ketoacidosis
   b. pancreatic fistula
   c. methanol toxicity
   d. salicylate poisoning

3. Which of the following ECG changes is generally the first seen in the hyperkalemic patient?

   a. peaked T waves
   b. QRS widening
   c. P-wave flattening
   d. "sine-wave"–like QRS morphology

4. A 34-year-old man is brought to your ED. You recognize the man as a schizophrenic man who presents frequently with alcohol intoxication and suicidal ideations. Today he presents with depressed mental status and deep, rapid respirations. His vital signs are as follows: pulse 115 bpm, blood pressure 125/88 mmHg, respirations of 36/minute, and he is afebrile. His lab results are as follows: sodium 134, potassium 5.1, chloride 98, bicarbonate 8, BUN 25, creatinine 0.9, and a glucose of 120. His arterial blood gas reveals a pH of 7.14, PCO_2 19, PO_2 110 (on room air) and a HCO_3 of 8. This patient has most likely ingested:

   a. isopropyl alcohol
   b. methanol
   c. ethylene glycol
   d. carbonic anhydrase inhibitors

5. Which is the hormone most commonly produced by a pituitary adenoma?

   a. growth hormone (GH)
   b. adrenocorticotrophic hormone (ACTH)
   c. vasopressin
   d. prolactin

6. A 24-year-old man presents to the emergency department (ED) with a depressed mental status. The paramedics inform you that his blood sugar was 40 mg/dL and that his vital signs were as follows: pulse 125 bpm, blood pressure 90/50 mmHg, respirations of 26/minute, and his oral temperature with 37.5° C. His family informs you that he has a history of severe asthma and has been on steroids multiple times in the past 2 months (he is not taking any currently). His respirations are clear with no audible wheezing, and he grimaces and guards when his abdomen is palpated. His laboratory values are as follows: sodium 120, potassium 6.8, glucose 37, bicarbonate 14, BUN 120,

creatinine 3.6. The most appropriate initial medical management of this patient is:

a. intravenous dexamethasone
b. intravenous thyroxine (T4)
c. 3% hypertonic saline
d. antidiuretic hormone (vasopressin)

7. A 55-year-old man is sent to the ED from her primary physician's clinic for evaluation of hypertension, although his blood pressure is 125/85 mmHg when you see him. He has no past medical history, takes no medications, neither smokes nor drinks, and denies any drug use. On review of systems, he describes several episodes over the past 3 months of feeling flushed, diaphoretic, and anxious. He also says that during these episodes, he develops a terrible headache and his heart "feels like it is beating out of my chest." Your examination reveals normal vitals signs and there are no significant abnormalities on physical examination. You contact his primary physician by phone and recommend the patient be treated with:

a. sumatriptan
b. propylthiouracil
c. phentolamine
d. benzodiazepines

8. The only vitamin that, when taken in excess, carries with it a significant risk of death, is:

a. vitamin D
b. vitamin B_1 (thiamine)
c. vitamin C
d. vitamin E

9. A 24-year-old primiparous woman at 36 weeks' gestation is sent down to the ED from the labor and delivery floor for respiratory depression. She suffers from pre-eclampsia and was scheduled for delivery this evening when she became progressively more weak and listless. She is lethargic and complains of diffuse weakness and nausea. She has a pulse of 105 bpm, a blood pressure of 90/50 mmHg and a respiratory rate of 6/minute, with a oxygen saturation of 92% in room air. Your examination reveals flushed skin and diffuse muscle weakness with markedly diminished deep tendon reflexes. What is the next most appropriate course of action?

a. intubation and airway protection
b. dialysis
c. stop her current magnesium infusion
d. immediate CT scan of the head

10. Which is a typical clinical finding of primary hypoadrenalism (i.e., Addison disease)?

a. ophthalmoplegia
b. bronzed or tan skin
c. polyuria
d. galactorrhea

11. Patients with apathetic thyrotoxicosis:

a. are often younger (less than 40 years of age)
b. have a more rapid onset of symptoms
c. frequently have exophthalmos
d. often present with new congestive heart failure (CHF) or atrial fibrillation (A.Fib.) triggered by the thyroid disease

12. A 19-year-old diabetic man is brought in by paramedics with a "high sugar." Family says he has not taken his insulin in 2 days. He is clinically dehydrated, tachycardic at 120 bpm, and is afebrile. His urinalysis shows a high level of glucose and ketones and a low specific gravity. His electrolytes are as follows: sodium 149, potassium 3.8, glucose 576, bicarbonate 6, chloride 105, BUN 30, and creatinine 1.1. His pH on his arterial blood gas is 7.01. Which of the following treatments is *least* appropriate?

a. intravenous infusion of regular insulin at 0.1 units/kg·hr
b. 1 ampule of sodium bicarbonate intravenously
c. intravenous potassium—20 mEq in the first hour
d. 2 L bolus of normal saline intravenously

13. The ingestion of which alcohol causes ketosis with an osmolar gap but does not cause an acidosis?

a. methanol
b. isopropyl alcohol
c. ethanol
d. ethylene glycol

14. After diabetic medications themselves, which drug or medication is the most common cause of hypoglycemia?

a. alcohol
b. beta-blockers
c. propoxyphene
d. salicylates

15. A 35-year-old woman with a history of Graves disease presents to your ED with altered mental status. She has a heart rate of 145 bpm, a blood pressure of 160/95 mmHg, and an oral temperature of 38.3° C. She is confused and noncooperative with your examination, which reveals a prominent goiter, diaphoresis, and proximal muscle weakness. What is the correct order of the correct medications that should be given to this patient?

a. dexamethasone, Lugol iodine, propylthiouracil (PTU), propranolol
b. propranolol, Lugol iodine, PTU, dexamethasone
c. propranolol, PTU, Lugol iodine, acetylsalicylic acid
d. propranolol, PTU, Lugol iodine, dexamethasone

16. A 40-year-old woman is brought to the ED by her family because she is "not acting right." She has a history of schizophrenia and avoids eating fruits because she says they "are all poisoned." Her vital signs are within normal limits. She is unwilling to let you move her on the bed as she says that any movement causes her horrible back pains. You notice pronounced gingival swelling. She has petechiae on the skin and the hairs on her skin are spiraled like a corkscrew. She has no focal or lateralizing neurologic findings. This patient's presentation is most consistent with:

    a. scurvy
    b. dry beriberi
    c. pellagra
    d. B_{12} deficiency

17. Liver or biliary disease will impair the absorption of which of the following vitamins?

    a. vitamin C
    b. vitamin B_1
    c. vitamin B_{12}
    d. vitamin K

18. With respect to the metabolic derangements of diabetic ketoacidosis (DKA):

    a. DKA patients frequently have an overabundance of potassium in the bloodstream
    b. phosphate is often elevated
    c. magnesium is often low, but rarely of clinical significance
    d. the anion gap is usually lower than 12

19. A 65-year-old man is brought from home where he was found unresponsive—no history is available. Paramedics inform you he has been in PEA arrest since they arrived on scene. The patient is pulseless and apneic. A bedside glucose monitor measures 88 mg/dL. Your examination reveals clear lungs when ventilated by bag-valve mask, some moderate pitting pedal edema bilaterally and an arteriovenous fistula with a thrill on the left arm. You notice that the heart monitor bears a striking resemblance to a sine wave (like the ones seen on an oscilloscope). After the airway is secured, the next most appropriate action is to administer intravenous:

    a. tissue plasminogen activator
    b. potassium
    c. calcium
    d. insulin

20. A 23-year-old woman passed out at work just prior to her arrival in the ED. Her boss calls you and says it is the third time she has done this in the past month. She has no past medical history and denies medications, allergies, and drug use. She denies any physical complaints, saying only that she skipped breakfast this morning. She appears in no distress, is well groomed and very thin, but not cachectic. Her pulse is 96 bpm, her respirations are 10/minute, and her blood pressure is 85/45 mmHg (she says she usually "runs in the 90s"); she is afebrile. Her examination reveals some diffuse dental caries and hypertrophic skin changes to the index and ring finger on the right hand with some abrasions on the dorsal aspect of the hand. Her pregnancy test is negative. Her lab results: sodium 138, potassium 2.9, chloride 91, bicarbonate 44, glucose 96, BUN 35, creatinine 1.0. Her arterial blood gases shows a pH of 7.60, PCO_2 52, PO_2 97 (on room air) and an HCO_3 of 43. The next best test to elucidate the cause of her metabolic derangements would be:

    a. urinary sodium level
    b. urinary chloride level
    c. urinary osmolarity
    d. urinary glucose level

---

1. Answer: a

There are several features in this patient to suggest *hypercalcemia* as the most likely diagnosis—bone pain, abdominal pain, and altered mental status are all prominent features. The patient takes HCTZ for his hypertension—thiazides are known to cause hypercalcemia. Lastly, the new diagnosis of a neck mass suggests the possibility of either a hyperparathyroid state or a paraneoplastic syndrome (PTH-like substances are occasionally secreted by squamous cell tumors of the head and neck). Answer **b** would be contraindicated in hypercalcemia, and hypertonic saline **(c)** would be used only in severe hyponatremia—even if this patient were hyponatremic, their clinical status does not support the use of hypertonic saline. Both answers **a** and **d** are options in the treatment of hypercalcemia; however, pamidronate **(d)** requires 24 to 48 hours before it begins to reduce the serum calcium levels. Loop diuretics and saline diuresis **(a)** have a more rapid onset of action in the reduction of calcium levels.

2. Answer: b

Answers **a, c,** and **d** all cause a wide anion-gap metabolic acidosis. Presence of a **pancreatic fistula** **(b)** does not cause the anion gap to widen.

3. Answer: a

Peaked T waves (a) is generally the first abnormality seen on an electrocardiogram in a hyperkalemic patient. Answers **b, c,** and **d** are seen respectively as the *hyperkalemia* worsens, culminating with a sine-wave pattern **(d)**, generally seen at a potassium level greater than 9.5 mEq/L.

4. Answer: b

A proper look at the patient's lab values makes the diagnosis a simple one. A quick calculation of the anion gap reveals that it is wide (134 − (98 + 8) =

28). As well, an analysis of his blood gas reveals a metabolic acidosis with an appropriate compensation (Winter's formula tells us that the CO_2 for this HCO_3 level should be 1.5 (8) + 8 ± 2 = 20 ± 2, so the compensation is appropriate and no other acid base disorder is likely). The presence of wide anion-gap metabolic acidosis eliminates answers **a** and **d,** which do not present this way. **Ethylene glycol** poisoning **(c)** should also present with renal failure, but the patient's creatinine is normal leaving **methanol (b)** as the most likely causative substance from the choices given.

5. Answer: d

Prolactinomas (d) make up 25% of all pituitary adenomas. One third are nonfunctioning (i.e., make no hormones). **Growth hormone-producing adenomas (a)** are second at 20%, followed by **ACTH-producing adenomas (b)** in third place with 10%.

6. Answer: a

The patient's clinical picture is most consistent with an *acute adrenal crisis*—hypotension, tachycardia, hyponatremia, hyperkalemia, hypoglycemia, altered mental status, abdominal pain, and a history of recent steroid use. Intravenous **corticosteroids (a)** should be given as soon as possible. **3% hypertonic saline (c)** should not generally be given unless the patient's hyponatremia is lower than 100 mEq/L or the patient is having a seizure secondary to hyponatremia. There is no clinical or laboratory evidence to definitively support the diagnosis of SIADH **(d).** Myxedema coma is possible in this patient, but hypothermia is almost universally associated with this degree of hypothyroidism, so use of **thyroid hormone (b)** should be withheld until thyroid testing corroborates the diagnosis.

7. Answer: c

A *pheochromocytoma* is a tumor of the chromaffin cells of the adrenal glands that causes episodes of hypertension, diaphoresis, flushing, tremor, tachycardia, anxiety, and headache; patient may appear normal between episodes. While thyroid function testing **(b)** could be part of the evaluation, the patient's clinical presentation does not suggest hyperthyroidism (which does not present episodically). Pheochromocytoma can be confused with certain headache syndromes **(a)** and some psychiatric illnesses **(d).** 90% of pheochromocytomas are in the adrenal glands and almost all are treated by surgical excision, although symptoms are first controlled by alpha-adrenergic blockade, usually phentolamine **(c).**

8. Answer: a

Vitamin D (a) can cause death by virtue of the hypercalcemia it causes—no other vitamin carries a substantial risk of death when taken in excess. **Vitamin B$_1$** (thiamine) **(b)** can lead to beriberi or Wencike–Korsakoff syndrome when deficient.

Vitmain C (c) carries a risk of death from scurvy when it is severely deficient. **Vitamin E (d)** has little adverse effects when either in excess or when deficient.

9. Answer: c

Patients with preeclampsia are routinely placed on infusions of magnesium both before and after delivery for seizure prophylaxis. *Hypermagnesemia* initially presents with nausea, vomiting, and skin flushing, but as levels increase, diffuse muscle weakness develops, with loss of the deep tendon reflexes (which is why OB nurses still carry reflex hammers!). Respiratory depression is the last stage in hypermagnesemia. The first step is to eliminate any possible exogenous source of magnesium **(c).** Intubation **(a)** could be avoided if her clinical status reverses and should be held off at this time. Dialysis **(b)** for hypermagnesemia is reserved for comatose patients or those in respiratory or renal failure.

10. Answer: b

Primary hypoadrenalism causes an increase in ACTH secretion. Melanocyte-stimulating hormone (MSH) is formed from the same precursor as ACTH, and those elevated levels induce the **tanned skin** seen in patients with primary hypoadrenalism **(b).** Secondary hypoadrenalism does not cause bronzing of the skin. **Ophthalmoplegia (a)** is a prominent finding of Graves disease, **polyuria (c)** is seen in diabetes mellitus, and **galactorrhea (d)** is seen in women with a pituitary prolactinoma (not in men).

11. Answer: d

Patients with *apathetic thyrotoxicosis* do not present with typical symptoms of thyrotoxicosis. Patients are typically older (usually over 70) and have been symptomatic for a longer time, likely because making the diagnosis is harder. The typical symptoms of thyrotoxicosis are frequently absent—lethargy, depression, muscle weakness, and weight loss are the common symptoms. The frequent exophthalmos and lid lag are absent. Symptoms are generally limited to one system—often cardiovascular—**CHF** and **atrial fibrillation** are common **(d).**

12. Answer: b

Fluid resuscitation is the mainstay of the treatment of *diabetic ketoacidosis* **(d)**—**saline** should be used for fluid resuscitation until vital signs have stabilized. While bolus dose insulin before the infusion still remains controversial to some, continuous intravenous infusion of **insulin (a)** is recommended to reverse the acidosis. **Potassium** must be carefully monitored—this patient's potassium may appear to be at the low end of the normal spectrum, but in truth these patients suffer a total body depletion of potassium—repletion **(c)** is recommended if the level is lower than 5.0. To date, no study has found an advantage to the use of intravenous **bicarbonate (b)** in the treatment of DKA when the pH is greater than 6.90.

13. Answer: b

Isopropyl alcohol (b) causes an osmolar gap and ketosis without causing an acidosis. **Methanol** and **ethylene glycol (a and d)** both cause a wide anion-gap metabolic acidosis. **Ethyl alcohol (c)** can cause a ketoacidosis in chronic abusers who are also in a state of relative starvation—there is no osmolar gap in alcoholic ketoacidosis.

14. Answer: a

After diabetes medications, **alcohol (a)** is by far the most common drug or medication causing hypoglycemia. Alcohol inhibits gluconeogenesis, especially in combination with insulin. **Beta-blockers (b)** can cause hypoglycemia, but generally do so by blunting the body's response to low glucose levels. **Salicylates (d)** are more prone to causing hypoglycemia in children than adults.

15. Answer: d

By virtue of the history of Graves disease, altered mental status, hyperadrenergic state, and tachycardia out of proportion to the fever, this patient is in *thyroid storm.* **Inorganic iodide** should be given to the patient until approximately 1 hour *after* **PTU** or **methimazole** has been given to stop thyroid synthesis (**a** and **b** are incorrect). **Salicylates (c)** should never be given to patients in thyroid storm as they enhance the conversion of T4 to the more bioactive T3 form and at toxic levels can uncouple oxidative phosphorylation. **Propranolol** is often given to counter the adrenergic effects of the disease, and dexamethasone is given as many patients can suffer concomitant adrenal suppression.

16. Answer: a

This patient presents with almost all the classic signs of **scurvy. Dry beriberi (b)** is a peripheral nerve dysfunction with myopathy due to thiamine deficiency. **Pellagra (c)** is due to niacin deficiency and presents with "the 4 Ds"—dementia, dermatitis, diarrhea, and death. The dermatitis of pellagra is a dark scaling rash in sun-exposed areas. **B$_{12}$ deficiency (d)** presents with proprioceptive neuropathy from posterior column disease in the spinal cord.

17. Answer: d

Vitamins A, D, E and **K (d)** are fat soluble, and their absorption can be impaired by liver or biliary disease. Those in answers **a, b,** and **c** are water-soluble vitamins.

18. Answer: c

Although *DKA* patients have a measured hyperkalemia, they have a total body deficit of potassium. The anion gap is elevated. Both phosphate **(b)** and magnesium **(c)** are often low, but usually neither is clinically significant.

19. Answer: c

Hyperkalemia is among the many possible etiologies of pulseless electrical activity (PEA); in this case, the sine-wave pattern on the heart monitor and the presence of an AV fistula (suggesting the patient is on dialysis) make this the most likely cause of the patient's arrest. Intravenous **calcium (c)** does not lower potassium but is used to stabilize the cardiac cell membranes until definitive reversal of the hyperkalemia can be achieved. **Insulin (d)** is used in the treatment of hyperkalemia but must be given in conjunction with intravenous dextrose (unless the patient is already hyperglycemic). **Thrombolytics (a)** can be considered for other causes of PEA arrest (such as pulmonary embolism or myocardial infarction).

20. Answer: b

The patient has a *metabolic alkalosis,* likely from bulimia nervosa (history of passing out, thin, borderline vitals signs suggesting possible low-grade dehydration, hypertrophic skin, and abrasions to the hand [likely caused by self-induced emesis]). Her primary metabolic derangement is a metabolic alkalosis. The P_{CO_2} should rise by 0.6 for every mEq increase in bicarbonate, or in this case $(44 - 24) \times 0.6 = 12$, so the compensation is complete and no additional acid–base disturbances are apparent. Metabolic alkalosis can be further subdivided into saline-responsive and saline-unresponsive causes. Saline-responsive causes are generally due to volume depletion and can be differentiated by a low **urinary chloride (b),** often lower than 10 mEq/L. Saline unresponsive causes are due to increased sodium delivery to the tubules, causing excretion of potassium and hydrogen ions—urinary chloride is excreted to maintain electric neutrality, so their urinary level is high. **Urinary sodium** levels **(a)** and **urinary osmolarity (c)** are useful in the diagnosis of SIADH, but this patient does not have hyponatremia. **Glycosuria (d)** is unlikely, given the normal glucose level and would not clinically correlate with the patient's findings.

6 Environmental

Michael Greenberg | David Vearrier

Bites and envenomations

ARTHROPODS

Insects

- Most human bites/stings are from insects in the Order Hymenoptera which includes ants, bees, and wasps
- Death may occur from:
  - Anaphylactic reaction in a person with history of previous sting
  - Envenomation to the tongue or throat with local swelling, causing airway compromise
  - Multiple stings, especially in the very young or very old
- Venom varies between species but generally contains proteins/enzymes and may contain acetylcholine, histamine, serotonin, and other biologically active small molecules
  - Because of variations in venom, anaphylaxis to one species does not guarantee the same reaction to another species

SIGNS AND SYMPTOMS

- Local erythema, edema, and pain
- Generalized urticaria
- Anaphylaxis with airway swelling and cardiovascular collapse
- Chest pain following Hymenoptera envenomation has been reported due to myocardial infarction (MI)
- Severe envenomations by hornets have been reported to cause myonecrosis
- Serum sickness may occur 7 to 10 days following envenomation

DIAGNOSIS

- Examination of the sting site for retained stinger
- Thorough physical examination for airway swelling, wheezing, tachypnea, or urticaria
- Cardiac monitor in patients with systemic symptoms to monitor for hypotension
- Consider a period of observation or admission, ECG, and cardiac enzymes as indicated

TREATMENT

- Removal of stinger by scraping it away with a credit card or scalpel blade; grabbing the stinger with forceps may release more venom
- Ice to the area stung and oral antihistamine
- Wheezing should be treated with nebulized albuterol

- Anaphylactic reactions should be treated with an H_1 blocker, H_2 blocker, corticosteroid, and, in severe cases, epinephrine SC or IM
  - Clinician should weigh risks/benefits of epinephrine use carefully in patients with cerebrovascular or coronary artery disease
  - Consider IV epinephrine in life-threatening reactions
  - Terbutaline is an alternative therapy
- All anaphylactic patients should be admitted to an intensive care setting
- Patients with systemic symptoms (e.g., rash) but without anaphylaxis should be given allergist follow-up for skin testing and possible hyposensitization
  - Prescribe epinephrine auto-injector

SPIDERS

- Approximately 50 species in the United States capable of envenomating humans
- Vast majority of envenomations due to the genera *Latrodectus* and *Loxosceles*
  - *Latrodectus* spp.—Black widow spiders (Fig. 6-1)
    - Brown to black; females with red or red-orange hourglass on abdomen
  - *Loxosceles* spp.—Brown recluse spider (Fig. 6-2)
    - Brown with a darker brown violin shape on their dorsal cephalothorax
- Tarantulas in the United States are generally not venomous but may have *urticating hairs,* which they can project from the dorsum of their abdomen at perceived threats

SIGNS AND SYMPTOMS

- *Black widow* envenomation
  - Bite itself is minimally painful and may not be noticed; minimal erythema/edema at the site
  - Within 1 hour, crampy pain starts at the bite site, later becoming generalized; muscle rigidity and generalized pruritis may also be present
  - Systemic symptoms include nausea, vomiting, diaphoresis, dizziness, headache, and shortness of breath
  - Severe envenomation may cause seizures, hypertensive urgency/emergency, or respiratory failure

- Young children are especially vulnerable
- Pregnant women may go into labor
- *Brown recluse* envenomation
  - Bite itself is minimally painful (initially) and may not be noticed
    - Over 3 to 4 hours, vasoconstriction around the bite site gives the appearance of a white ring with increasing pain
    - Later, bleb formation at the site of the bite with outer erythematous ring, bulls-eye in appearance
    - Over hours to days, bleb becomes enlarging necrotic ulcer with extension through subcutaneous fat (Fig. 6-3)
  - Systemic symptoms may include fever, chills, malaise, nausea, and vomiting
- Tarantula urticating hairs can cause local redness, itching, edema, and pain
  - Ocular exposure to urticating hairs causes tearing and eye pain

DIAGNOSIS

- *Black widow* envenomation
  - Hypertension is frequently present
    - Patients with a history of cardiovascular or coronary artery disease are at higher risk for complications

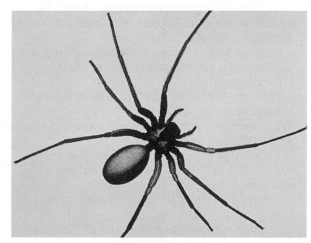

Figure 6-2. Brown recluse spider *(Loxosceles)*. (From Habif TP: *Clinical dermatology,* ed 4, Philadelphia, 2004, Mosby.)

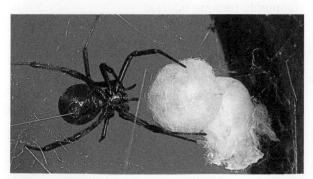

Figure 6-1. Black widow spider *(Latrodectus)*. (From Habif TP: *Clinical dermatology,* ed 4, Philadelphia, 2004, Mosby.)

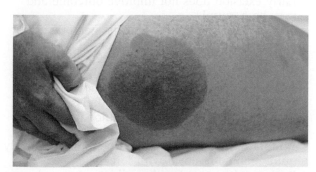

Figure 6-3. Brown recluse spider bite. (From Auerbach PS: *Wilderness medicine,* ed 5, Philadelphia, 2007, Mosby.)

- CSF opening pressure may be elevated
- Abdominal crampiness and stiffness may mimic acute abdomen except that abdomen is not remarkably tender
- ECG may show digoxin-like changes
- Chest pain has been reported to involve myocarditis and ST-elevation MI
- *Brown recluse* envenomation
  - Laboratory studies should include complete blood count, chemistries, and coagulation profile
    - Intravascular hemolysis, pulmonary edema, coagulopathy, and acute renal failure may occur in severe envenomations
- Tarantula urticating hair exposure is based on history
  - Slit lamp examination for retained urticating hairs in cornea or conjunctiva

TREATMENT

- *Black widow* envenomation
  - Tetanus prophylaxis
  - Muscle rigidity/spasm may be relieved with benzodiazepines
  - Calcium, methocarbamol, and dantrolene have been recommended for latrodectism but are likely ineffective
  - Analgesia
  - Hypertensive urgency/emergency should be treated with IV antihypertensive medication
  - Antivenom should be used in:
    - Patients with seizures, hypertensive urgency/emergency, or respiratory failure
    - Pregnant patients
    - The very young or very old with systemic symptoms
  - Antivenom is equine in origin so anaphylaxis and serum sickness may occur
  - Patients with systemic complaints, the very young, and very old should be admitted for monitoring
    - Pregnant patients should be admitted to a unit with fetal monitoring
    - Patients with severe envenomation may require intensive care unit admission
- *Brown recluse* envenomation
  - Tetanus prophylaxis
  - Early excision does not improve outcome and may be harmful
  - Dapsone may limit spread of the necrotic ulcer, though definitive evidence is lacking
  - Antivenom not available in United States
  - If asymptomatic with normal exam after 6 hours of observation, may discharge to home
  - If local or systemic symptoms, admission for monitoring for hemolysis, coagulopathy, pulmonary edema, and renal failure
- Tarantula urticating hairs are barbed and frequently require manual removal with forceps
  - Rash can be treated with antihistamine and topical corticosteroid

- Urticating hairs lodged in the cornea or conjunctiva may be removed in the emergency department with a slit lamp
  - Ophthalmology referral should be provided

MAMMALS

- Dog bites are the most frequent mammalian bite in the United States
  - Approximately 20 fatal dog bites occur yearly, mostly in the very young
  - Most bites are from known dogs (e.g., pet or neighbor's pet)
- Cat bites and rodent bites are common, though less frequent than dog bites
- Less than 2% of bites are from raccoons, monkeys, ferrets, and other mammals

SIGNS AND SYMPTOMS

- Local pain at the site of bite
- Infection of mammalian bites is common and may present with redness, swelling, pain, and purulent discharge
- Cat scratch disease presents with fever, malaise, and painful regional lymphadenopathy 1 to 2 weeks after cat scratch; more common in children

DIAGNOSIS

- Dog bites are typically superficial and do not cause bone or tendon injury
  - Tendon and vascular injuries are more common in police dog bites and with hand bites
  - Small children with bites to the scalp may have perforation of the cranium or depressed skull fracture
    - Wound infection may result in meningitis or brain abscess
  - Rare but dangerous dog bite complication is *Capnocytophaga canimorsus;* it may cause local gangrene, hypotension, renal failure, and disseminated intravascular coagulation; mortality rates of 30% have been reported and the rate may be higher in patients with liver disease, asplenia, or on corticosteroid therapy
  - Wound infections are from a variety of organisms and often polymicrobial
- Cat bites are typically puncture wounds and commonly become infected
  - *Pasteurella multocida* is a typical causative organism
- Cat scratch disease diagnosis is made clinically; *Bartonella henselae* is causative organism
- Human "fight bites" (Fig. 6-4) with closed-fist injury may be complicated by Boxer's fracture (fifth metacarpal), extensor tendon laceration, joint involvement, and *Eikenella corrodens* infection
  - Concern for transmission of bloodborne disease, including Hepatitis B and C and HIV
- *P. multocida* infections following mammalian bites may progress to abscess, osteomyelitis, bacteremia, and bloodborne infections

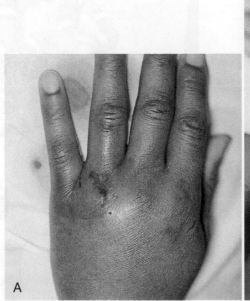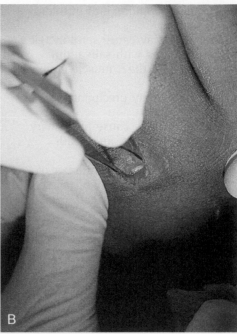

A   B

Figure 6-4. "Fight Bite" or clenched-fist injury. (From Roberts JR, Hedges JR: *Clinical procedures in emergency medicine,* ed 4, Philadelphia, 2004, Saunders.)

TREATMENT

- Thorough decontamination of the wound with wound exploration to evaluate for vascular or tendon injury
- Radiographs as needed to evaluate for fracture or foreign body
- Closure of mammalian bites is controversial because of infection risk
  - Traditionally not closed
  - Bites that are more than 12 hours old, already infected, or are at high risk for infection should be allowed to heal by secondary intention
  - Bites on the hand, lower leg, or feet and cat, human, and monkey bites are at highest risk for infection
- Tetanus prophylaxis
- Prophylactic antibiotics are indicated for human, cat, and monkey bites and in patients with immunocompromise (chronic alcoholics, asplenia, diabetics, patients taking corticosteroids)
  - High risk dog bites should receive prophylactic antibiotics
  - Rodent bites may not require prophylactic antibiotics
  - Amoxicillin-clavulanate is commonly prescribed for outpatient therapy
- Rabies prophylaxis is indicated with skunk, raccoon, bat, carnivore, and fox bites
  - If a bat is found in the room of a sleeping child or adult, prophylaxis is recommended due to the risk of an unnoticed occult bite
  - Dog, cat, and ferret bites should be considered and may depend on if the animal can be observed for 10 days and on the prevalence of rabies in these animals in the area. Local public health guidance should be sought

- Prophylaxis includes human diploid cell vaccine and local infiltration of the wounded area with human rabies immunoglobulin
- Among discharged patients, wound check in 1 to 2 days is recommended
- Cat scratch disease is benign and self-limited; prescribe analgesics and close follow-up
  - Consider antibiotics in immunocompromised patients

MARINE ORGANISMS

- Three main mechanisms of injury: bites, stings, and nematocysts
  - Bites are primarily from cephalopods (squids and octopi)
    - Certain octopus species may be venomous with a toxin similar to tetrodotoxin
  - Stings may be sustained from sea urchins, bony fish, and stingrays
    - All have spines that contain or are coated with venom
    - Bony fishes include zebra fish, scorpion fish, and stonefish
  - Nematocyst injuries are sustained from coelenterates including jellyfish, fire coral, and Portuguese man-of-war
    - Nematocysts are cellular organelles containing venom that are forcefully expelled from specialized cells when chemoreceptors and mechanoreceptors are stimulated

SIGNS AND SYMPTOMS

- Stings frequently cause local burning and pain
  - Retained foreign bodies (spines, stingers, etc.) may precipitate inflammation and infection with

local redness, warmth, swelling, and purulent discharge
- Stingray envenomation may cause serotonergic and cholinergic syndromes with salivation, lacrimation, vomiting, diarrhea, muscle cramping, and fasciculations
  - Severe envenomations may precipitate cardiac dysrhythmia and seizures
- Stonefish envenomation may cause pulmonary edema, cardiovascular collapse, and death
- Nematocysts (Jellyfish, etc.)
  - Symptom severity varies based on number of nematocysts discharged and toxicity of the species
  - Local symptoms include erythema and swelling at the site of envenomation
  - Systemic symptoms may include chills, headache, nausea, vomiting, diarrhea, and muscle cramping
  - Severe envenomations may precipitate angioedema, pulmonary edema, convulsions, and cardiovascular collapse
  - Coelenterate venom is antigenic and allergic reactions are common

DIAGNOSIS

- The diagnosis of octopus envenomation is based primarily on history
- Victims of stings should have radiographs of the affected area and local wound exploration to assess for foreign bodies
- Hemodynamic monitoring for those with systemic symptoms
- The diagnosis of nematocyst envenomation is based primarily on history

TREATMENT

- Allergic and anaphylactic reactions should be treated according to current standard of care
- Tetanus prophylaxis
- Stings may require foreign body removal
  - Stonefish envenomation should be treated with the appropriate antivenom and supportive care
- Nematocyst envenomation
  - Dilute acetic acid (vinegar) should be poured over the envenomated area to inactivate remaining nematocysts
    - Tap water can induce nematocysts to fire as a result of changes in osmotic pressure
  - After inactivation, tentacles can be removed with gloved hands
  - Symptomatic care
  - Systemic symptoms should prompt supportive care
  - Antivenom is available for the box jellyfish, *Chironex fleckeri*, a particularly deadly species

SNAKES

- 45,000 snakebites each year are reported in United States; actual number probably far higher
  - 7000 to 8000 of those are venomous snakes and 5 to 10 deaths occur yearly

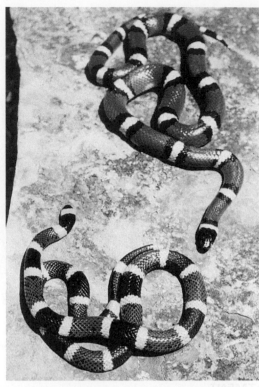

Figure 6-5. Comparison of the Texas coral snake (*Micrurus tener*) with the harmless Mexican milk snake (*Lampropeltis triangulum annulata*). Coral snake (*bottom*) has contiguous red and yellow bands, whereas red and yellow bands of the milk snake are separated by black. (Courtesy of Charles Alfaro; from Auerbach PS: *Wilderness medicine,* ed 5, Philadelphia, 2007, Mosby.)

- Occur more frequently in the Southern United States
- Four venomous snake families, two of which are extinct in the United States
  - Pit vipers are members of Family Viperidae, Subfamily Crotalinae
    - Can be identified by the pit organ between the nostril and eye
    - Include rattlesnakes, sidewinders (Southwestern United States), and cottonmouth (Southeastern United States)
    - Account for 98% of venomous snakebites in the United States
  - Coral snakes are members of Family Elapidae
    - Also includes the yellow-bellied sea snake off the coast of California
    - Mnemonic to differentiate between venomous coral snakes in United States versus nonvenomous king or milk snakes: "Red on yellow, kills a fellow. Red on black, venom lack." (Fig. 6-5)

SIGNS AND SYMPTOMS

- Depends on several factors:
  - Amount of venom injected
    - Venomous snakes only inject venom in 50% to 80% of bites
    - Non-venomous bites called "dry bites"
  - Location of bite

- Elapidae envenomation
  - Neurotoxic
  - Minimal tissue damage/pain
  - First sign of envenomation frequently is ptosis
  - Then weakness, fasciculations, slurred speech, dysphagia
  - Death may occur from weakness or paralysis of muscles of respiration
- Crotalinae envenomation
  - Hematotoxic
  - Local effects are substantial with edema, petechiae, ecchymosis, and bullae (hemorrhagic or serous)
  - Systemic effects may include fever, nausea, vomiting, diaphoresis, perioral tingling, and hypotension
  - Pulmonary edema may occur from increased capillary membrane permeability
  - Death may occur from cardiovascular collapse
- Anaphylactic reactions may occur in persons who have had snakebites in the past

DIAGNOSIS

- A thorough history as to the type of snake
  - Consultation with a herpetologist may be necessary
- Ptosis is often the first sign of Elapidae envenomation
- Local effects are often the first sign of Crotalinae envenomation
  - In Crotalinae bites, evaluate for compartment syndrome
- Cardiac monitoring for any suspected envenomations
- Negative inspiratory flow test for Elapidae envenomations
- Creatine kinase to evaluate for myonecrosis in Crotalinae envenomations
- Evaluate for coagulopathy/disseminated intravascular coagulation in Crotalinae envenomations
- Radiographs and wound exploration of the bite to evaluate for foreign body (e.g., fang)

TREATMENT

- Prehospital care includes calming the victim and immobilization of the extremity
  - Use of an air cast or elastic compression bandage may limit systemic absorption of toxin
    - Can be left on until antivenom given
  - Do NOT use tourniquets that impair arterial flow as they may increase tissue necrosis
- Prophylactic antibiotics are not generally used; amoxicillin/clavulanate may be used for infected bites
- Antivenom administration:
  - Crotalinae antivenom (CroFab) is available and dosing is based on the clinician's opinion of severity of envenomation
    - Made from ovine F_{ab}, so anaphylaxis and serum sickness are less common

- Is polyvalent so effective against all rattlesnake, cottonmouth and copperhead bites
  - Elapidae antivenom (monovalent) is effective for Eastern coral snake bite
    - There is no antivenom for other U.S. species of coral snakes as they are less deadly then the Eastern coral snake
    - Antivenom should be given even in asymptomatic patients bitten by the Eastern coral snake as delay in administration may be detrimental
    - Equine in derivation so anaphylaxis and serum sickness may occur
  - Exotic snake antivenom may be available from zoos with the species in their collection
- Debridement of necrotic wounds should be delayed until coagulopathy resolves
- Fasciotomy as needed for compartment syndrome
- Tetanus prophylaxis
- Crotalinae bites can be observed for 12 hours and discharged if asymptomatic
- Elapidae and exotic snake bites should be admitted to an intensive care setting

Dysbarism

- Dysbarism refers to medical conditions occurring as a result of exposure to increased ambient pressures
- The most common cause of dysbarism is recreational scuba diving
- As a diver descends, the pressure exerted by the surrounding water increases, causing a decrease in volume of air-filled structures (such as the middle ear) and causing more gas to dissolve in body fluids

AIR EMBOLISM

- The most dangerous complication of pulmonary barotrauma
- Second-leading cause of death among recreational divers (first is drowning)
- Mechanism: as a scuba diver ascends, ambient pressure decreases and gas in the lungs expands. If the diver fails to exhale during ascent, pressure in the lung increases and air is pushed into alveolar capillaries
- Other risk factors for air embolism include:
  - Chronic obstructive pulmonary disease: difficulty exhaling
  - Patent foramen ovale: venous gas bubbles that would normally be filtered by the lung can access systemic arterial circulation

SIGNS AND SYMPTOMS

- Vary depending on where the gas embolism lodges but generally rapid onset and occurs within 10 minutes of ascent
- Lodging in the coronary arteries may cause myocardial ischemia or infarction, dysrhythmia, or cardiac arrest

- Lodging in the cerebral circulation may cause stroke
- May present as altered mental state, headache, and seizures
- Pulmonary complaints such as shortness of breath, hemoptysis, or pleuritic chest pain, secondary to related pulmonary barotrauma, are common

DIAGNOSIS

- Divers with loss of consciousness, signs of stroke, or acute coronary syndrome/cardiac dysrhythmias during or within 10 minutes of ascent should be assumed to have an air embolism
- Differential includes:
  - Decompression sickness—more gradual onset, usually within 24 hours of ascent, and usually involves joint pain and skin mottling
  - Contaminated air source—occurs when scuba air tanks are filled too close to a carbon monoxide (CO) source (e.g., gasoline-powered compressor exhaust); presentation with flu-like symptoms; evaluate by obtaining blood gas with co-oximetry

TREATMENT

- Immediate treatment with 100% oxygen by non-rebreather mask
- Expeditious transfer to facility with hyperbaric chamber for recompression therapy
- Supportive measures include:
  - Benzodiazepines for seizure
  - Treat dysrhythmias using standard management
- Use of methylprednisolone in patients with neurological involvement remains controversial

BAROTRAUMA

- Caused by the compression or expansion of air-filled spaces in the body during descent or ascent, respectively
- May affect the external ear, middle ear, inner ear, sinuses, face, lungs, or gastrointestinal (GI) tract

SIGNS AND SYMPTOMS

- Depend on the part of the body affected
- External ear barotrauma—ear pain
- Middle ear barotrauma—ear pain, tympanic membrane (TM) rupture may cause cold-water induced nystagmus and vertigo, and conductive hearing loss
  - Associated facial nerve (CN 7) palsy may be present
- Inner ear barotrauma—ear pain, nystagmus, positional vertigo, tinnitus, and sensorineural hearing loss
- Sinus barotrauma—sinus pain, epistaxis
- Facial barotrauma—subconjunctival hemorrhage, petechiae in the area covered by the mask
- Pulmonary barotrauma—dyspnea, pleuritic chest pain, hemoptysis
- Gastrointestinal barotrauma—eructation or flatulence; abdominal pain or bloating

DIAGNOSIS

- Middle ear barotrauma
  - Serous otitis may be present
  - Examine for TM rupture
  - Examine for associated facial nerve (CN 7) palsy
- Inner ear barotrauma
  - Henneberg test for perilymphatic fistula: insufflate ear canal and assess for nystagmus or vertigo; their presence suggests perilymphatic fistula
- Sinus barotrauma
  - Based on history, examine for subcutaneous emphysema
- Facial barotrauma
  - Diagnosis made based on history and exam
- Pulmonary barotrauma
  - Chest radiograph to evaluate for associated pneumothorax or pneumomediastinum
  - Examine for subcutaneous emphysema
- Gastrointestinal barotrauma
  - Abdomen is generally benign; ruptured viscus or hernia incarceration/strangulation are rare complications

TREATMENT

- Middle ear barotrauma
  - Decongestants if serous otitis media is present
  - Antibiotic prophylaxis if TM is ruptured
  - Prednisone taper may be used if associated facial nerve palsy is present
- Inner ear barotrauma
  - Bed rest for 1 week with elevated head of bed
  - Avoid straining or Valsalva; consider stool softener
  - Decongestants to aid in drainage of perilymph from the middle ear
  - Refer to ENT and to audiologist for audiogram and tympanometric testing
- Sinus barotrauma
  - Treat associated epistaxis if present
  - Decongestants
  - Prophylactic antibiotics may be considered
  - ENT referral
- Facial barotrauma
  - No treatment necessary
- Pulmonary barotrauma
  - Pneumothorax may be treated with pigtail catheter
  - Pneumomediastinum and subcutaneous emphysema may be treated with bed rest; 100% oxygen may speed resolution
  - Alveolar hemorrhage treatment is supportive with supplemental oxygen and intubation as necessary to maintain adequate oxygenation
- Gastrointestinal barotrauma
  - In the absence of hernia or ruptured viscus, course is self-limited and no treatment is necessary

DECOMPRESSION SYNDROME (DCS)

- Gases are more soluble in liquids at higher pressures; while a diver is at depth, more nitrogen dissolves in body fluids; the longer and deeper the dive, the more nitrogen dissolves

- As a diver ascends, nitrogen comes out of solution, forming small bubbles in body fluids/fat
- Nitrogen bubbles then may initiate inflammatory cytokines, inflammatory cascades, and clotting cascades
- Is divided into two types:
  - DCS, Type 1: "The bends"—may affect skin, lymphatics, joints, and skeletal muscles, in isolation or in combination
  - DCS, Type 2: Involves the CNS, vestibulocochlear system, or lungs in addition to systems involved in Type 1

SIGNS AND SYMPTOMS

- Cutaneous symptoms include itching, redness, mottling (cutis marmorata)
- Lymphatic obstruction by nitrogen bubbles may cause edema of the upper or lower extremities
- Joint pain is common; shoulders and elbows most often affected
- In Type 2:
  - Spinal cord DCS may cause
    - Extremity paralysis, numbness, and paresthesias
    - A dermatomal sensory level may occur
    - Cauda equina symptoms may also occur
  - Cerebral DCS (less common than spinal DCS):
    - Headache, visual changes, altered mental status, slurred speech
  - Vestibulocochlear DCS: vertigo, nystagmus
  - Pulmonary DCS: shortness of breath, chest pain, cough
    - May progress to a pulmonary embolus-like picture with cyanosis, hypotension, and right heart strain

DIAGNOSIS

- Based on history
- Inflating a blood pressure cuff over an affected joint may be performed as a diagnostic procedure; pain should decrease as cuff pressure increases
- Computed tomography (CT) or magnetic resonance imaging (MRI) may visualize nitrogen bubbles in cerebral DCS, though obtaining imaging should not delay definitive hyperbaric therapy

TREATMENT

- Immediate treatment with 100% oxygen by non-rebreather mask
- Expeditious transport to a facility with hyperbaric chamber
  - Recompression is the definitive treatment of DCS
- Aspirin may reduce platelet aggregation/thrombosis
- Lidocaine may be of benefit in improving outcome in cerebral DCS, though further study is needed

Electrical and lightning injury

ELECTRICAL

- Mechanism of injury is primarily thermal

- Severity of injury is determined by voltage, current, resistance (of tissues), and how long the victim is in contact with it
  - AC current is more dangerous than DC current as it causes tetany, prolonging the duration of contact with the current
- Two types of electrical burns:
  - Direct electrothermal burns are burns that occur from tissue heating as a current passes through it—typically occur from high-voltage sources
  - Indirect burns are caused by exposure to electrical arcs:
    - Arc burns are from the temperature of the arc itself (typically thousands of degrees)
    - Flash burns are partial-thickness cutaneous burns from electrical current flowing over the skin as it arcs
    - Flame burns are from ignition of clothing or other material in the arc
- Associated blunt-force trauma occurs when the victim is thrown from the current

SIGNS AND SYMPTOMS

- Nature of injuries depends on pathway of the current
  - Thoracic current may cause ventricular fibrillation, asystole, respiratory arrest, and myocardial damage
  - Cerebral current may cause respiratory arrest and seizures
  - Ocular current may cause cataract formation, which may take months to develop
  - "Kissing burns" are pathognomonic for electrical injury: burns in the flexor creases of the arms or legs
- Delayed neurological damage may occur months to years after the initial injury
- Labial artery bleeding is a late complication of electrical burns of the oral commissure, usually related to children chewing on electrical cords (Fig. 6-6)

DIAGNOSIS

- History
- Visual acuity and funduscopic examination
- Plain films and CT scans as needed for blunt-force trauma
  - Posterior shoulder dislocation is classically associated with electrical injury
- ECG to evaluate for arrhythmia and ST-T changes
  - Abnormal ECG should prompt serial cardiac enzymes
- Cardiac monitoring
- Abdominal pain should prompt concern for gallbladder necrosis or mesenteric thrombosis
- Deep burns with muscle necrosis may lead to compartment syndrome and rhabdomyolysis

TREATMENT

- Electrical burns may require fasciotomies rather than escharotomies for deep burns with compartment syndrome

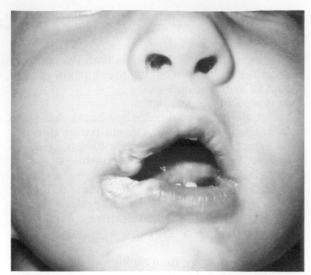

Figure 6-6. Electrical burn of the oral commissure in a child. (From Auerbach PS: *Wilderness medicine,* ed 5, Philadelphia, 2007, Mosby.)

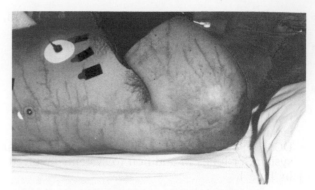

Figure 6-7. Feathering burns due to lightning injury. (From Auerbach PS: *Wilderness medicine,* ed 5, Philadelphia, 2007, Mosby.)

- Cutaneous burns should be treated as with thermal burns, including tetanus prophylaxis and silver sulfadiazine or antibiotic ointment
- Rhabdomyolysis should prompt aggressive fluid resuscitation and alkalinization of the urine to decrease the risk of renal failure
- Patients with significant electrical injuries should be transferred to a burn center
- Patients with low-voltage exposures, no complaints, and a normal physical exam should be provided with outpatient burn center follow-up in case delayed sequelae arise

LIGHTNING

- Estimated to be fatal in 10% of cases
- Causes less burns and thermal tissue damage than electrical injury but causes more cardiac arrest, neurological damage, and autonomic instability
- Four types of lightning strikes
  - In a direct strike, the victim becomes part of the lightning current's path from sky to ground and the current flow passes through the body
  - In a contact injury, the victim is touching an object that is part of the lightning current's path (e.g., tree) and some of the current travels through the victim rather than the object on its way to the ground
  - A splash injury is when the lightning current first hits another object (e.g., tree), then arcs to the victim before entering the ground
  - Ground current occurs when the lightning current has already entered the ground but travels through a person standing in the area where the lightning current dissipates
- Blunt-force trauma occurs from the victim being thrown, from full-body muscle contraction secondary to current and from a blast force

from the rapidly heated air around the lightning current

SIGNS AND SYMPTOMS

- In a direct strike, current enters the body through the eyes, ears, and mouth, causing damage to those structures
- Vascular spasm may cause myocardial ischemia or anterior spinal artery syndrome
  - May also cause *keraunoparalysis:* cyanotic or mottled extremities with numbness and paraplegia that may resolve spontaneously
- Asystole and other dysrhythmias may occur from thoracic current
- Cutaneous burns tend to follow one of four patterns: feathering, linear, punctate, and thermal
  - *Feathering burns* have a fern like pattern and are pathognomonic of lightning injury (Fig. 6-7)

DIAGNOSIS

- Visual acuity and funduscopic examination for ocular injury
- Otoscopy for tympanic membrane rupture and hemotympanum
- ECG to evaluate for arrhythmia and ST-T changes
  - Abnormal ECG should prompt serial cardiac enzymes
- Deep burns are uncommon in lightning injury as lightning tends to flashover the skin
- Plain films and CT scans as needed for blunt-force trauma
- Peripheral nerve damage frequently occurs and may be permanent

TREATMENT

- Lightning-injury victims who do not have cardiorespiratory arrest at the time of injury typically do well
- Patient with ECG changes or altered mental status should be admitted to the hospital for observation
- Asymptomatic patients with normal ECG and normal physical exam may be discharged with ophthalmologic follow-up for delayed cataract formation

High-altitude illness

ACUTE MOUNTAIN SICKNESS (AMS)

- Occurs at elevations above 8000 ft and increases both with elevation and the rapidity of ascent
- Risk factors include pre-existing cardiorespiratory disease and genetic predisposition
- "Tight fit" hypothesis: hypoxemia at altitude increases cerebral blood flow (CBF) and inability to buffer the increase in CBF by a corresponding decrease in CSF leads to mild brain swelling and AMS symptoms

SIGNS AND SYMPTOMS

- Similar to viral syndrome: headache, anorexia, nausea, fatigue, dizziness, insomnia
- Preverbal children may be fussy, have decreased playfulness, poor appetite, or sleep disturbance
- Symptoms begin several hours after ascent, reach their maximum at 24 to 48 hours, and resolve spontaneously over 3 to 4 days

DIAGNOSIS

- Three criteria:
  - A recent increase in altitude and have been at the new altitude for at least several hours
  - Headache
  - One of the following: GI upset, weakness or fatigue, dizziness or lightheadedness, or sleep disturbance

TREATMENT

- Further ascent contraindicated until symptoms resolve
- Supplemental oxygen for headache
- Acetazolamide 250 mg PO twice a day alleviates symptoms and speeds resolution while acetazolamide 125 mg PO twice a day for 3 days starting 24 hours prior to ascent provides prophylaxis against AMS
- Worsening AMS despite intervention requires descent

BAROTRAUMA OF ASCENT

- Caused by the expansion of gas in closed spaces in the body as atmospheric pressure decreases with an ascent
- Most commonly affects the middle ear though the sinuses can also be involved
- Pulmonary barotrauma of ascent occurs only during a rapid ascent while diving and not in high-altitude scenarios

SIGNS AND SYMPTOMS

- Ear pain/pressure, vertigo, and tinnitus with middle ear barotrauma of ascent
- Sinus pain/pressure, epistaxis, subcutaneous emphysema can occur with sinus barotrauma of ascent

DIAGNOSIS

- With middle ear barotrauma of ascent, otoscopic evaluation may reveal TM injection or hemotympanum
- In sinus barotrauma of ascent, the expanding gas in the sinus can result in sinus wall fracture with subcutaneous emphysema, epistaxis, and rarely pneumocephalus
- Patients with sinus barotrauma of ascent and headache should have CT head to evaluate for pneumocephalus

TREATMENT

- Further ascent should be avoided until resolution of symptoms
- Sinus barotrauma can result in facial and CNS infections and patients should be given instructions to return for symptoms of infection

HIGH-ALTITUDE CEREBRAL EDEMA (HACE)

- The least common and most severe form of high-altitude illness

SIGNS AND SYMPTOMS

- Symptom onset is from 12 hours to 9 days after ascent
- Ataxia, seizures, slurred speech, focal neurologic deficits, altered mentation, coma, nausea/vomiting, headache
- Cerebellar signs appear first and onset of ataxia is indication for descent
- Associated retinal hemorrhages may be present
- Transient or long-lasting neurobehavioral sequelae are possible

DIAGNOSIS

- Clinical diagnosis
- Isolated focal neurologic deficit points to TIA/CVA rather than HACE, though HACE treatment should not be delayed by diagnostic testing

TREATMENT

- Immediate descent and high-flow oxygen
- Intubation as indicated for airway protection
- Dexamethasone, mannitol, and furosemide may have adjunctive role but more studies are needed
- With coma, mortality rate >60%

HIGH-ALTITUDE PULMONARY EDEMA (HAPE)

- Most common fatal manifestation of high-altitude illness

SIGNS AND SYMPTOMS

- Gradual onset of symptoms 2 to 4 days after ascent, worse at night

- Dyspnea at rest and cough that progresses from dry to copious clear sputum or hemoptysis
- Fever, tachypnea, tachycardia, and cyanosis
- Rales or rhonchi on auscultation

DIAGNOSIS

- Chest x-ray shows fluffy infiltrates, unilateral or bilateral, with or without pleural effusions
- ECG shows right heart strain and right axis deviation

TREATMENT

- Mild cases may be treated by bed rest with warmed air
- Moderate cases may be treated by bed rest with supplemental oxygen
- Severe cases require immediate descent or portable hyperbaric chamber with high-flow oxygen
- Nifedipine or furosemide may be used as adjunctive treatment

Submersion incidents

COLD WATER IMMERSION

- Abrupt immersion in cold water can induce a cardiac dysrhythmia
- Dysrhythmia may be secondary to vagal stimulation from the cold water, QT prolongation, or from catecholamine release
- Possible dysrhythmias include asystole, ventricular tachycardia, ventricular fibrillation
- Person may drown from resultant syncope while immersed
- The colder the water, the higher the risk for dysrhythmia

SIGNS AND SYMPTOMS

- History is of a patient who lost consciousness after voluntary or accidental sudden immersion in cold water

DIAGNOSIS

- ECG to determine nature of dysrhythmia
- Continuous cardiac monitoring is recommended

TREATMENT

- ACLS protocols for specific dysrhythmia
- In patients with prolonged immersion, treat for hypothermia (see hypothermia section)
- Patients with significant hypothermia (<86° F) may need to be rewarmed before defibrillation will be successful

NEAR DROWNING

- May or may not involve aspiration of water
- Historical distinction between saltwater and freshwater aspiration probably not clinically

relevant as amount of water aspirated not enough to cause electrolyte abnormalities
- Aspiration disturbs functioning of pulmonary surfactant, leading to atelectasis and impaired oxygenation and ventilation
- Diving reflex (in children) and hypothermia can be cardioprotective and neuroprotective in near drowning

SIGNS AND SYMPTOMS

- Respiratory compromise frequently occurs secondary to aspiration with resulting tachypnea, cyanosis, and shortness of breath; wheezes, rales, or rhonchi may be present on examination
- Vomiting of swallowed water occurs with risk for aspiration
- Neurological status and exam is variable
- Cardiac dysrhythmia is common and may be secondary to sudden cold water immersion (see cold water immersion section) or to hypoxemia, acidosis, or hypothermia

DIAGNOSIS

- Differential includes traumatic injury, seizure, cardiac dysrhythmia, hypoglycemia, and alcohol or drug intoxication
- Consider diving injury with spinal trauma and possible need for c-spine precautions
- Laboratory studies may include:
  - ABG to evaluate for hypoxia, hypercarbia, and metabolic or respiratory acidosis
  - Baseline chemistries, cardiac enzymes, and hepatic function profile as renal, cardiac, or hepatic damage may develop
  - Coagulation profile to evaluate for disseminated intravascular coagulation (DIC)
  - Lactate to evaluate for acidosis
- ECG for cardiac dysrhythmias or prolonged QT
- Consider ethanol level and urine drug screen
- Chest x-ray should be obtained for respiratory compromise
- Finger-stick glucose test and CT head for patients with abnormal mental status
- Further imaging may be necessary for trauma

TREATMENT

- Cardiac pulmonary resuscitation (CPR) and advanced cardiac life support (ACLS) as appropriate
- In hypothermic patients, resuscitation should continue until patient is rewarmed ("warm and dead")
- Respiratory support (continuous positive airway pressure [CPAP], bilevel positive airway pressure [BiPAP], or intubation) may be required
- Empiric antibiotics and corticosteroids do not improve outcomes or survival
- Use of hypothermia to improve neurological outcomes is being investigated

Temperature-related illness

HEAT

- Heat illness can be treated as a continuum with a mild case of heat exhaustion representing the mildest form of heat illness, and heat stroke the more severe manifestation

Heat exhaustion

- Water-depletion heat exhaustion results from inadequate replacement of fluid losses, is acute in onset, and generally affects persons engaged in strenuous activities in hot environs
- Salt depletion heat exhaustion results from inadequate replacement of sodium and chloride lost in sweat, is subacute in onset, and generally affects persons inadequately acclimatized to a hot environment

SIGNS AND SYMPTOMS

- Resembles viral illness with headache, fatigue, malaise, weakness, nausea, and vomiting
- Neuropsychiatric symptoms such as cerebellar dysfunction, disorientation, irritability, and agitation may be present but more serious CNS signs (seizures, coma) are absent
- Dizziness and syncope may occur with water depletion heat exhaustion
- Salt depletion heat exhaustion is often accompanied by muscle cramps

DIAGNOSIS

- Temperature may be elevated or normal—temperature above 40° C usually signifies heat stroke
- Chemistry to evaluate for hyponatremia, hypochloremia, and uremia
- Creatine kinase to evaluate for rhabdomyolysis
- Liver function tests: elevated transaminases suggests heat stroke
- Orthostatic vital signs to evaluate fluid status

TREATMENT

- Volume replacement with oral rehydration solution or intravenously with normal saline
- Hypernatremic patients should still be resuscitated with normal saline, as free water can correct the sodium too quickly, leading to cerebral edema
- Healthy patients with normal electrolytes may be discharged to home after fluid replacement, all others should be admitted to an appropriate level of care

Heat stroke

- Heat stroke is a medical emergency
- Classic heat stroke occurs among persons with inadequately cooled residences during summer heat waves and is more common in the poor, elderly, infirm, mentally ill, and alcoholics
- Exertional heat stroke occurs among athletes and military recruits and is often accompanied by rhabdomyolysis and acute renal failure

SIGNS AND SYMPTOMS

- Sweating can be present or absent and is not predictive of heat stroke
- Prodromal period with symptoms similar to heat exhaustion can be present or absent
- Severe CNS dysfunction such as seizures, coma, or delirium

DIAGNOSIS

- Criteria
  - Heat stress that may be exertional or environmental
  - Body core temperature above 40° C
  - CNS dysfunction
- Chemistries, creatine kinase, and liver function tests
  - Elevated transaminases are characteristic of heat stroke and is secondary to splanchnic vasoconstriction
  - Hyponatremia secondary to increased free water intake can mimic exertional heatstroke
- Hypoglycemia occurs secondary to exertion or hepatic dysfunction
- Coagulopathy is common
- Check blood lactate as lactic acidosis may occur secondary to hypotension
- Acute renal failure is more common in exertional (25%) than classic (5%)

TREATMENT

- Immediate cooling is essential to minimize morbidity/mortality
  - Evaporative cooling by spraying patient with water and using fans is easiest
  - Immersion in ice water very effective but difficult to implement
  - Ice packs in the groin, axillae, and on the neck are useful adjuncts
  - Cooling should be discontinued when core temperature is 39° C to avoid overshoot
  - Shivering may be suppressed with benzodiazepines
- Intubation and mechanical ventilation may be necessary for airway protection or respiratory compromise
- Hypotension should be treated with fluids and vasopressors: central venous pressure (CVP) can help determine which should be used
- Benzodiazepines are preferable to barbiturates for seizure control because of hepatic dysfunction impairing metabolism of barbiturates
- Antipyretics are of no value in heatstroke and may be harmful
- Rhabdomyolysis and myoglobinuria should be treated with aggressive hydration and urinary alkalization

COLD

- Cold injuries can be divided into peripheral cold injuries and central hypothermia. Peripheral cold injuries are common because of the human body's homeostatic goal of maintaining core body temperature at the expense of peripheral tissues. Peripheral cold injuries can be divided into freezing (frostbite) and nonfreezing syndromes (frostnip, trench foot, and chilblains).

Frostbite

- Occurs when tissue temperatures fall below 0° C
- Distal extremities such as the nose, ears, digits, and penis are especially at risk
- Tissue damage is mediated by extracellular ice crystal formation, cellular dehydration, microvascular sludging and thrombosis, and ischemia
- Nonviable tissue forms a dry gangrene carapace, though full demarcation between viable and nonviable tissue may take 60 to 90 days

SIGNS AND SYMPTOMS

- Numbness or sensory deficit to light touch, sharp touch, or temperature
- Impaired proprioception resulting in "chunk of wood" or "clumsy" sensation
- Rewarming is accompanied by aching pain that evolves into throbbing pain in 48 to 72 hours, which can last until full demarcation of viable and nonviable tissue (60 to 90 days)
- Frozen tissues appear mottled, violaceous-white, waxy, or pale yellow
- Rapid rewarming results in an initial hyperemia
- Vesicles and large bullae form 6 to 24 hours after rewarming
- Rewarming edema starts within 3 hours and progresses for 48 to 72 hours

DIAGNOSIS

- Historical classification of frostbite into various degrees of severity generally rejected as clinically misleading
- Hallmarks of severity:
  - Inability to roll dermis over bony prominences suggests deep injury while pliable subcutaneous tissues suggest superficial injury
  - Clear bullae are more favorable than hemorrhagic bullae
  - Lack of edema formation after rewarming is ominous as is black eschar

TREATMENT

- Prehospital: remove wet clothing and immobilize and insulate affected areas
- Field rewarming should be avoided because of risk of tissue refreezing
- Crystalloids are helpful for dehydration from cold diuresis and vascular sludging
- Rapid active rewarming in a water bath at 37° C to 40° C on arrival until the area is pliable and distal hyperemia is noted
- Tissue massage increases tissue loss and is to be avoided
- Ketorolac or ibuprofen
- Thawing of large areas may cause "core temperature after-drop," hyperkalemia, and acidemia
- After rewarming, affected areas should be elevated to minimize edema formation
- Be wary of compartment syndrome after rewarming
- Leave blisters and bullae intact
- Consider antibiotic prophylaxis in severe cases
- Tetanus immunization
- Except for the most superficial injuries, patients should be admitted for observation

Frostnip

- Superficial cold insult in which no tissue death occurs
- Tissue temperature falls below 10° C, causing numbness and tingling similar to frostbite but does not reach 0° C

SIGNS AND SYMPTOMS

- Initial signs and symptoms similar to frostbite
- After rewarming, tissue has normal sensation, warmth, and color while pain, edema, and bullae are absent

DIAGNOSIS

- Clinical

TREATMENT

- Rewarming in a 37° to 40° C water bath as for frostbite
- Disposition to home once rewarming completed

Trench foot/Immersion foot

- Nonfreezing injury from prolonged exposure to wet cold above freezing
- Results in neurovascular damage in the absence of ice-crystal formation

SIGNS AND SYMPTOMS

- Numbness or tingling in the feet
- Leg cramping is common
- Cool, pale or cyanotic, and edematous feet
- After rewarming, hyperemic, hyperesthetic feet with or without bullae
- Vasomotor paralysis causes rubor on dependency and pallor on elevation
- Ulceration and liquefaction gangrene can occur in severe cases

DIAGNOSIS

- Clinical

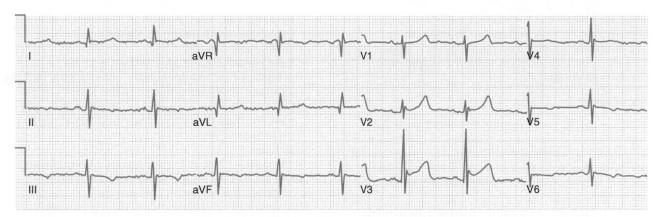

Figure 6-8. Osborn or "J" waves due to hypothermia

TREATMENT

- Rewarming in a 37° to 40° C water bath as for frostbite
- Disposition to home once rewarming completed
- Prolonged sequelae of pain with weight bearing, hyperhydrosis, sensitivity to cold can continue for years

Chilblains (Pernio)

- Nonfreezing injury that occurs after exposure to dry cold
- Young women with a history of Raynaud syndrome are at higher risk
- Pathophysiology is vasculitis and vasospasm

SIGNS AND SYMPTOMS

- Plaques, nodules, and ulcerations develop on the face, dorsum of hands and feet, and pretibial areas
- Pruritis, erythema, and mild edema

DIAGNOSIS

- Clinical

TREATMENT

- Patient to avoid cold exposure
- Disposition to home
- Nifedipine may be used for refractory cases

Hypothermia

- Can be differentiated into mild (32° to 35° C), moderate (28° to 32° C), and severe (<28° C)
- Homeostatic mechanisms such as vasoconstriction, shivering, and metabolic thermogenesis cease at temperatures below 32° C
- The basal metabolic rate *decreases* from 32° to 24° C
- Below 24° C, autonomic, metabolic, and endocrinologic mechanisms for heat conservation are no longer active
- Very young and very old are especially at risk
- Ethanol is the most common cause of heat loss in urban settings

SIGNS AND SYMPTOMS

- Mild hypothermia (32° to 35° C): shivering, hyperventilation, tachypnea, tachycardia, cold diuresis, impaired judgment, amnesia, ataxia, dysarthria, apathy
- Moderate hypothermia (28° to 32° C): stupor, hypoventilation, hyporeflexia, paradoxical undressing, cessation of shivering, dilated minimally responsive pupils
- Severe hypothermia (<28° C): pulmonary edema and apnea, oliguria, hypotension or pulselessness, rigidity, areflexia, coma with fixed dilated pupils
- Cardiovascular effects:
    - ECG: Osborn or J waves (Fig. 6-8) as well as PR, QRS, and QT prolongations
    - Aberrant atrial and junctional rhythms and atrial fibrillation occur <32° C
    - Spontaneous asystole and ventricular fibrillation (VF) occur <25° C
- Central nervous system effects:
    - CNS depression secondary to decreased metabolism
    - Altered electrical activity <33.5° C and flat-line electroencephalogram <20° C
- Renal effects:
    - Cold diuresis occurs regardless of dehydration, excreting large quantity of dilute urine
    - Effect is amplified if patient is intoxicated
- Respiratory effects:
    - Mild hypothermia increases respiratory drive
    - Severe hypothermia causes respiratory depression with hypercarbia and respiratory acidosis
    - Bronchorrhea and noncardiogenic pulmonary edema can occur

DIAGNOSIS

- Evaluate for acidosis
- CBC—hematocrit should rise 2% for every 1° C fall in body temperature, so a normal hematocrit suggests anemia or acute blood loss; normal WBC count does not exclude infection
- Chemistry—hypokalemia common from intracellular shift of potassium

- Creatine kinase to evaluate for rhabdomyolysis
- Liver function tests and lipase to evaluate for ischemic liver damage or pancreatitis if suspected
- TSH and thyroid function tests for suspicion of myxedema coma

TREATMENT

- Severe hypothermia should be treated with ABCs and CPR/ACLS should be initiated as necessary
- VF should be defibrillated, but if it is unsuccessful then future shocks should be avoided until the patient is rewarmed as defibrillation is generally unsuccessful <30° C
- Passive external rewarming—blankets to insulate the patient and prevent further heat loss—can be used to treat mild hypothermia (32° to 35° C)
- Active external rewarming—most commonly forced air systems like the Bair Hugger or less commonly water baths at 40° C—should be used in moderate hypothermia in conjunction with active core rewarming
- Active core rewarming constitutes several different therapies
  - Heated humidified oxygen via mask or ventilator
  - IV fluids should be heated to 40° C before infusion
  - Peritoneal or thoracic lavage with 40° C fluid should be used in severely hypothermic or unstable patients
  - Thoracotomy and mediastinal irrigation and direct myocardial lavage can be considered in severely hypothermic patients in cardiac arrest
  - Extracorporeal blood rewarming via cardiopulmonary bypass, continuous arteriovenous rewarming, extracorporeal venovenous rewarming, and hemodialysis have been used in severely hypothermic patients
- Antibiotics should be administered empirically in children <3 months old and in the elderly for presumed sepsis
- Patients with mild hypothermia (32° to 35° C) may be discharged to home after rewarming while all others should be admitted to an appropriate level of care

Radiation emergencies

- Exposure to radiation may occur occupationally in research, health care, or nuclear industries
- Large-scale radiation exposure may occur with nuclear weapon detonation or dirty bomb (conventional bombs that release radioactive material into the environment) detonation, or civilian nuclear power plant disasters
- Radon gas may seep into buildings from surrounding soil resulting in radiation exposure; uranium miners are particularly at risk
- Different types of radiation exist:
  - Alpha particles are helium nuclei. They are unable to penetrate the body externally and may be dangerous only if they are produced after ingestion or inhalation of the radioactive substances
  - Beta particles are high-energy electrons or positrons that may penetrate up to 8 mm into the skin and may cause burns of the skin
  - Gamma rays are high-energy photons that may pass through the whole body and are thought to be primarily responsible for acute radiation sickness
- Beta particles and gamma rays may be measured using a Geiger counter, while alpha particles cannot be detected with this device
- The quantity of radiation to which a person is exposed can be expressed in several ways:
  - One Gray (Gy) is one Joule of radiation absorbed per kilogram of tissue
  - Radiation absorbed dose (rad) is another unit; One Gray = 100 rad
  - Roentgen equivalent man (rem) is a third unit; 1 rem = 1 rad = 0.01 Gray

SIGNS AND SYMPTOMS

- Symptoms vary considerably with the absorbed radiation dose
- Tissues with higher cell turnover rates are most affected
- Generally, the higher the dose of absorbed radiation, the sooner the onset of symptoms
- Gastrointestinal: nausea and vomiting; fever and bloody diarrhea generally signify a supralethal dose of radiation
- Hematopoietic: fever, infection, petechiae, and bleeding may occur several days to weeks after exposure
- CNS: headache, altered mental status, vertigo, and tinnitus may occur immediately after a supralethal dose of absorbed radiation
- Isolated beta-particle exposure may cause local injury to skin similar to thermal burns

DIAGNOSIS

- Lymphocyte count 48 hours after exposure is the earliest indicator to approximate the dose of radiation absorbed with lower lymphocyte counts corresponding to higher radiation doses
- Neutropenia and thrombocytopenia typically occur days later, with the lowest value being reached 8 to 30 days after exposure
- Radiation burns to the skin may be delayed in onset

TREATMENT

- Decontamination should be performed prehospital if possible to avoid ED contamination
  - Contaminated patients should enter ED through a separate decontamination entrance
  - Patients should be disrobed and exposed skin washed with soap and water
  - Hair may need to be cut and nails trimmed/cleaned

- Wounds should be thoroughly irrigated to minimize contamination with radioactive materials
- Clothing and wash-water should be disposed of as radioactive waste
- Health care providers performing decontamination should wear disposable gowns, gloves, and shoe covers to minimize contamination
- The hospital radiation safety officer should be notified and will monitor decontamination and radiation exposure of facility and staff
- In a mass-casualty scenario, triaging of patients may be necessary
  - Patients with immediate CNS involvement invariably die and should be kept comfortable
- Patients exposed to radioactive iodine should be treated with potassium iodide to reduce thyroid uptake of radioactive iodine
- Ingestion of radioactive lead should be treated with a chelating agent such as calcium disodium edetate or penicillamine
- GI decontamination with activated charcoal or cathartics may be considered in radionuclide ingestions
- With inhaled radionuclides, bronchopulmonary lavage should be considered
- Supportive treatment includes:
  - Hemorrhage from thrombocytopenia should be treated with platelets
  - Anemia does not usually require transfusion
  - IVF to replace GI losses
  - Consider prophylactic antibiotics for bloody diarrhea
  - Radiation burns to the skin should be treated as thermal burns
  - Surgery, if necessary, should be performed early before electrolyte and hematopoietic derangements occur

PEARLS

- Hymenoptera (ants, bees, and wasps) stings should be examined for stinger removal; allergic and anaphylactic reactions are common.
- *Latrodectus* spp. (Black widow spider) bites have minimal local symptoms with risk of systemic symptoms including seizures, hypertensive urgency/emergency, respiratory failure, and preterm labor.
- Antivenom is available for severe envenomations.
- *Loxosceles* spp. (Brown recluse spider) bites may involve severe local reactions, with necrotic ulcers extending through subcutaneous fat; hemolysis, pulmonary edema, coagulopathy, and renal failure are possible systemic complications.

- A rare but feared complication of dog bites is *Capnocytophaga canimorsus* with high mortality rates.
- Cat bites are frequently infected with *Pasteurella multocida;* cat scratch disease is from *Bartonella henselae.*
- Human "fight bites" often become infected with *Eikenella corrodens* and may involve boxer's fracture, extensor tendon laceration, and joint involvement.
- Stinger envenomation should prompt radiographs for foreign bodies; stonefish envenomation is particularly dangerous and antivenom is available.
- Nematocyst envenomation should be treated with dilute acetic acid (vinegar) prior to removal to avoid further nematocyst discharge during tentacle removal.
- Crotalinae envenomation may cause cardiovascular collapse and pulmonary edema and should be treated with antivenom if symptomatic.
- Elapidae envenomation may cause ptosis and respiratory paralysis and should be admitted and treated with antivenom even if asymptomatic.
- Air embolism presents with cerebrovascular or acute coronary-like symptoms with rapid onset within 10 minutes of ascent and should be treated with recompression therapy.
- Middle ear barotrauma is the most common form of barotrauma.
- Facial barotrauma occurs when mask pressure is not equalized during descent, presents with subconjunctival hemorrhage and petechiae in the area of the mask, and resolves spontaneously.
- Decompression sickness typically causes joint pain and pruritis though neurologic and pulmonary derangements may also occur, is gradual in onset, and should be treated with recompression therapy.
- Electrical injuries may cause compartment syndrome and rhabdomyolysis requiring fasciotomy and urinary alkalinization.
- Two pathognomonic signs of lightning injury are keraunoparalysis and feathering burns.
- Acute mountain sickness presents with viral-like symptoms following ascent to elevation and can be treated with acetazolamide (can also be used for prophylaxis).

- High-altitude cerebral edema first presents hours to days after ascent with cerebellar signs (e.g., ataxia) and should prompt immediate descent and high-flow oxygen. Long-term neuropsychiatric sequelae and death have been reported.

- High-altitude pulmonary edema occurs 2 to 4 days after ascent; treat with bed rest and supplemental oxygen; severe or refractory cases require descent; nifedipine or furosemide may be helpful.

- Sudden cold-water immersion can induce asystole, ventricular tachycardia, or ventricular fibrillation.

- Water aspiration during near drowning disturbs pulmonary surfactant function with respiratory compromise that may require intubation and mechanical ventilation.

- Heat exhaustion presents with viral-like symptoms, and patients should be tested for hypernatremia, uremia, and rhabdomyolysis.

- Heat stroke is a medical emergency with temperature above 40° C and seizures, coma, or delirium; evaporative cooling measures should be initiated immediately.

- Frostbite should be rewarmed in 37° C to 40° C water bath; rewarming of large areas can cause core temperature after-drop, hyperkalemia, and acidosis.

- Trench foot is caused by prolonged exposure to wet cold above freezing temperature and does not involve tissue destruction.

- Chilblains/Pernio are erythematous plaques on the face, dorsum of hands/feet, and pretibial areas after cold exposure.

- J or Osborn waves are suggestive of hypothermia.

- The earliest indicator of dose of radiation absorbed is the lymphocyte count 48 hours after exposure.

- Early GI symptoms are a marker of severe radiation exposure.

- Patients exposed to radioactive iodine should be treated with potassium iodide to decrease thyroid uptake of the radioactive species.

BIBLIOGRAPHY

Bessen HA: Hypothermia. In Tintinalli JE, Gabor DK, Staphczynski S (eds): *Tintinalli's emergency medicine: a comprehensive study guide*, ed 6, New York, 2004, McGraw-Hill.

Catlett CL, Piggott PL: Radiation injuries. In Tintinalli JE, Gabor DK, Staphczynski S (eds): *Tintinalli's emergency medicine: a comprehensive study guide*, ed 6, New York, 2004, McGraw-Hill.

Causey AL, Nichter MA: Near-drowning. In Tintinalli JE, Gabor DK, Staphczynski S (eds): *Tintinalli's emergency medicine: a comprehensive study guide*, ed 6, New York, 2004, McGraw-Hill.

Clark RF, Schneir AB: Arthropod bites and stings. In Tintinalli JE, Gabor DK, Staphczynski S (eds): *Tintinalli's emergency medicine: a comprehensive study guide*, ed 6, New York, 2004, McGraw-Hill.

Danzi DF: Accidental hypothermia. In Marx JA, Hockberger RS, Walls RM (eds): *Rosen's emergency medicine: concepts and clinical practice*, ed 6, Philadelphia, 2006, Mosby.

Danzi DF: Frostbite. In Marx JA, Hockberger RS, Walls RM (eds): *Rosen's emergency medicine: concepts and clinical practice*, ed 6, Philadelphia, 2006, Mosby.

Dart RC, Daly FFS: Reptile bites. In Tintinalli JE, Gabor DK, Staphczynski S (eds): *Tintinalli's emergency medicine: a comprehensive study guide*, ed 6, New York, 2004, McGraw-Hill.

Fish RM: Electrical injuries. In Tintinalli JE, Gabor DK, Staphczynski S (eds): *Tintinalli's emergency medicine: a comprehensive study guide*, ed 6, New York, 2004, McGraw-Hill.

Fish RM: Lightning injuries. In Tintinalli JE, Gabor DK, Staphczynski S (eds): *Tintinalli's emergency medicine: a comprehensive study guide*, ed 6, New York, 2004, McGraw-Hill.

Hackett PH: High-altitude medical problems. In Tintinalli JE, Gabor DK, Staphczynski S (eds): *Tintinalli's emergency medicine: a comprehensive study guide*, ed 6, New York, 2004, McGraw-Hill.

Isbister GK, Caldicott DG: Trauma and envenomations from marine fauna. In Tintinalli JE, Gabor DK, Staphczynski S (eds): *Tintinalli's emergency medicine: a comprehensive study guide*, ed 6, New York, 2004, McGraw-Hill.

Knaut AL, Feldhaus KM: Submersion. In Marx JA, Hockberger RS, Walls RM (eds): *Rosen's emergency medicine: concepts and clinical practice*, ed 6, Philadelphia, 2006, Mosby.

Markovchick V: Radiation injuries. In Marx JA, Hockberger RS, Walls RM (eds): *Rosen's emergency medicine: concepts and clinical practice*, ed 6, Philadelphia, 2006, Mosby.

Nomura JT, Sato RL, Ahern RM, Snow JL, Kuwaye TT, Yamamoto LG: A randomized paired comparison trial of cutaneous treatments for acute jellyfish (Carybdea alata) stings, *Am J Emerg Med* 20(7):624–626, 2002.

Otten EJ: Venomous animal injuries. In Marx JA, Hockberger RS, Walls RM (eds): *Rosen's emergency medicine: concepts and clinical practice*, ed 6, Philadelphia, 2006, Mosby.

Price TG, Cooper MA: Electrical and lightning injuries. In Marx JA, Hockberger RS, Walls RM (eds): *Rosen's emergency medicine: concepts and clinical practice*, ed 6, Philadelphia, 2006, Mosby.

Rabold MB: Frostbite and other localized cold-related injuries. In Tintinalli JE, Gabor DK, Staphczynski S, Ma OJ, Cline DM (eds): *Tintinalli's emergency medicine: a comprehensive study guide*, ed 6, New York, 2004, McGraw-Hill.

Shockley LW: Scuba diving and dysbarism. In Marx JA, Hockberger RS, Walls RM (eds): *Rosen's emergency medicine: concepts and clinical practice*, ed 6, Philadelphia, 2006, Mosby.

Snyder B, Neuman T: Dysbarism and complications of diving. In Tintinalli JE, Gabor DK, Staphczynski S (eds): *Tintinalli's emergency medicine: a comprehensive study guide*, ed 6, New York, 2004, McGraw-Hill.

Vicario S: Heat illness. In Marx JA, Hockberger RS, Walls RM (eds): *Rosen's emergency medicine: concepts and clinical practice*, ed 6, Philadelphia, 2006, Mosby.

Walker JS, Hogan DE: Heat emergencies. In Tintinalli JE, Gabor DK, Staphczynski S (eds): *Tintinalli's emergency medicine: a comprehensive study guide*, ed 6, New York, 2004, McGraw-Hill.

Weber EJ: Mammalian bites. In Marx JA, Hockberger RS, Walls RM (eds): *Rosen's emergency medicine: concepts and clinical practice*, ed 6, Philadelphia, 2006, Mosby.

Yaron M, Honigman B: High-altitude medicine. In Marx JA, Hockberger RS, Walls RM (eds): *Rosen's emergency medicine: concepts and clinical practice*, ed 6, Philadelphia, 2006, Mosby.

Zafren K, Thurman J, Storrow AB: Environmental conditions. In Knoop KJ, Stack LB, Storrow AB (eds): *Atlas of emergency medicine*, ed 2, Spain, 2002, McGraw-Hill.

Questions and Answers

1. A 44-year-old man is brought in by paramedics. He was found walking in a city park barefoot and talking to himself. The ambient temperature outside is –5° C and the ground is covered in snow. History is limited by the patient's inappropriate answers. Vital signs are temp = 96.5° F, heart rate (HR) = 95 bpm, blood pressure (BP) = 137/72 mmHg, respiratory rate (RR) = 14/minute. Examination of the patient's feet reveals violaceous skin to the level of the ankles. Clear bullae are present. Dorsalis pedis (DP) and posterior tibialis (PT) pulses cannot be palpated. Several hours after rewarming in a warm water bath, edema formation is minimal though DP and PT pulses are now palpable. Which of the following clinical findings in this patient is most indicative of severe injury?

   a. absence of edema several hours after rewarming
   b. absent pulses prior to rewarming
   c. clear bullae
   d. temperature of 96.5° F
   e. violaceous skin

2. For which of the following venomous creatures is antivenom available in the United States?

   a. Crotalinae subfamily
   b. *Latrodectus mactans*
   c. *Loxosceles reclusa*
   d. a and b
   e. all of the above

3. Rapid-onset mental status change within several minutes of ascent after scuba diving is most characteristic of:

   a. air embolism
   b. decompression sickness
   c. hemorrhagic stroke
   d. inner ear barotrauma
   e. thrombotic stroke

4. A 33-year-old man with no past medical history presents with a chief complaint of snakebite. He was walking through tall grass when he felt a sudden sharp pain in his left calf. While running away he glimpsed a snake through the tall grass but is unable to provide details. He has minimal pain at the site of the bite. Vital signs are BP = 145/90 mmHg, HR = 65 bpm, RR = 14/minute, Temp = 99.4° F. Pulse oximetry is performed and is 98%. Physical examination reveals an anxious man who is in no distress. The site of the snakebite has two puncture wounds but is otherwise unremarkable. Neurological examination reveals bilateral ptosis, with normal sensation and strength in all four extremities. Which of the following is the most appropriate management of this patient?

   a. Crotalinae antivenom should be administered if he develops shortness of breath
   b. Crotalinae antivenom should be administered immediately
   c. Elapidae antivenom should be administered if he develops shortness of breath
   d. Elapidae antivenom should be administered immediately
   e. no antivenom is indicated

5. A 27-year-old female electrician is brought in by paramedics with complaint of electrical injury. She states that she accidentally touched a high-voltage wire with her right hand without protective rubber gloves. She complains of right upper extremity pain. Physical examination reveals erythema and edema on the dorsum of her right hand and forearm with an area of blistering on the dorsum of her right hand. No circumferential cutaneous burns are present. Neurological examination is significant for decreased fine touch sensation diffusely on the right forearm and hand. Volar compartment pressure is 23 mmHg. Dorsal compartment pressure is 52 mmHg. Which of the following is the most appropriate next step in management of this patient?

   a. debridement of the blistered area on her right hand
   b. dressing the burn with silver sulfadiazine and sterile nonadherent bandages
   c. escharotomy
   d. fasciotomy
   e. referral to a burn center

6. Which of the following is the *least* likely in lightning strike?

   a. blunt trauma
   b. current hitting another object then jumping to a person before entering the ground
   c. deep burns from internal current
   d. dysrhythmia or cardiac arrest from thoracic current
   e. temporary paralysis of the legs

7. Which of the following is *least* likely in a near-drowning victim?

   a. atelectasis from pulmonary surfactant dysfunction

b. cervical spine fracture from shallow water diving

c. electrolyte abnormalities from aspiration of large quantities of saltwater

d. elevated lactate from anaerobic metabolism

e. respiratory acidosis from impaired ventilation

8. A 33-year-old man comes in with complaint of diffuse joint pains, myalgias, malaise, and pruritis. He denies any numbness, weakness, or paresthesias. He went scuba diving the previous day. Vital signs are Temp = 97.9° F, HR = 82 bpm, BP = 112/84 mmHg, RR = 12/minute. Physical examination is remarkable for skin mottling. Which of the following is the appropriate definitive treatment for this patient?

a. diphenhydramine 50 mg PO every 6 hours for 3 days and then as needed

b. ibuprofen 600 mg every 8 hours for 3 days and then as needed

c. observation in the emergency department for 6 hours

d. 100% oxygen by non-rebreather mask

e. recompression therapy

9. A 59-year-old man presents with complaint of bilateral foot pain. The pain is described as tingling in nature. He states that he is homeless and walks several miles per day. He has only one pair of shoes, which are too small for his feet. Social history is positive for nicotine and heavy daily alcohol use. On examination, his feet are cold to the touch, pale, and edematous. After warming the feet, they are erythematous when in a dependent position and become pale when raised while the patient is supine. Which of the following put the patient at risk for his condition?

a. walking several miles daily

b. heavy daily alcohol use

c. nicotine use

d. poorly fitting shoes

e. wet, nonfreezing cold

10. Which of the following regarding heat exhaustion is correct?

a. core temperature is usually above 105° F

b. muscle cramps are associated with water-depletion heat exhaustion

c. salt depletion heat exhaustion is common among athletes

d. symptoms frequently resemble viral syndrome

e. water depletion heat exhaustion takes days to develop

11. An 87-year-old woman is found obtunded in her home by neighbors. Her past medical history includes multi-infarct dementia, hypertension, and myocardial infarction. In the emergency department she has a tonic–clonic seizure that lasts one minute and resolves spontaneously. Vital signs are Temp = 106.3° F, HR = 85 bpm, BP = 167/79 mmHg, RR = 12/minute. Pulse oximetry is 98% on room air. Finger stick blood glucose is 65 mg/dL. Laboratory studies are remarkable for an AST of 507 and ALT of 835. Which of the following is the most likely cause of the patient's change in mental status?

a. cerebrovascular accident

b. hepatic encephalopathy

c. heat stroke

d. sepsis

e. hypoglycemia

12. Which of the following is true regarding cold injury?

a. extent of damage becomes apparent after rewarming

b. field rewarming should be initiated immediately

c. hemorrhagic bullae indicate a more favorable outcome than clear bullae

d. rewarming fluids should be 45° C or above

e. rewarming typically causes severe pain

13. Which of the following is *not* a risk factor for chilblains?

a. dry cold exposure

b. eczema

c. female gender

d. Raynaud syndrome

e. young age

14. A 27-year-old woman presents with a complaint of left leg pain. She had been swimming in the ocean earlier today when she felt a stinging sensation on her left leg. She immediately exited the water. The pain has been gradually increasing and is described as sharp and tingling. On examination, her left leg has linear erythematous, edematous lesions. Several jellyfish tentacles are still adhering to her leg. Which of the following interventions would *increase* patient discomfort while removing the jellyfish tentacles?

a. applying baking soda to the tentacles prior to removal

b. washing the tentacles with dilute acetic acid prior to removal

c. washing the tentacles with isopropyl alcohol prior to removal

d. washing the tentacles with sterile water prior to removal

e. wearing sterile latex gloves during tentacle removal

15. Complications typically should be expected from damage to which of the following cell lines by acute radiation exposure?

a. platelets

b. erythrocytes

c. leukocytes

d. a and b

e. a and c

16. A 6-month-old female infant is brought in by her parents after they found a brown spider in her crib. On further questioning, the father states that it did appear to have a darker brown pattern on its back. Examination of the infant reveals a small red edematous lesion of the right thigh consistent with spider bite. Which of the following is the most likely complication of this spider bite?
    a. compartment syndrome with rhabdomyolysis
    b. necrotic ulcer
    c. pulmonary edema
    d. respiratory paralysis
    e. severe hypertension

17. Human fight bites are associated with infection by which organism?
    a. *Bartonella henselae*
    b. *Capnocytophaga canimorsus*
    c. *Eikenella corrodens*
    d. *Pasteurella multocida*
    e. *Streptobacillus moniliformis*

18. A 40-year-old female worker at a nuclear power plant was exposed to ionizing radiation in an industrial accident. After appropriate on-scene decontamination, she is brought in by paramedics. Her only complaint at this time is mild nausea. Vital signs are normal. Physical examination is unremarkable and rectal exam shows brown, heme-negative stool. Which of the laboratory tests will give the earliest estimate of the amount of radiation she absorbed?
    a. eosinophil count
    b. erythrocyte count
    c. lymphocyte count
    d. neutrophil count
    e. platelet count

19. A 35-year-old male mountaineer develops shortness of breath and cough 2 days after arriving at a high-elevation base camp (5,380 meters above sea level). He denies any recent sick contacts. He smokes cigarettes. Vital signs are Temp = 97.5° F, BP = 132/77 mmHg, HR = 105 bpm, RR = 28/minute. Pulmonary auscultation is significant for rales bilaterally. An ECG obtained at base camp shows right heart strain and right axis deviation. Which of the following best describes his prognosis?
    a. this infectious condition is benign and will resolve spontaneously
    b. this is a chronic condition that can be controlled with medications
    c. this is a potentially fatal rapidly evolving condition
    d. this is a chronically progressive condition that can only be resolved with lung transplantation
    e. this condition will resolve only if he stops smoking cigarettes

20. Hypertensive urgency/emergency is associated with which of the following envenomations?
    a. black widow spider envenomation
    b. brown recluse spider envenomation
    c. Eastern coral snake envenomation
    d. pit viper envenomation
    e. Portuguese man-of-war envenomation

---

1. Answer: a
Absence of edema after rewarming or the formation of a black eschar are ominous signs related to *frostbite*. **Clear bullae** are preferable to hemorrhagic bullae, and **violaceous skin** is typical of frostbite. Pulses may return after rewarming, and the **core temperature of 96.5° F** is indicative of mild hypothermia.

2. Answer: d
Antivenom is available for **Crotalinae (pit vipers)** and *Latrodectus* **(black widow spiders)**. No antivenom is available for *Loxosceles* **(brown recluse spider)**.

3. Answer: a
Air embolism most often occurs immediately after ascent. **Decompression sickness** develops more slowly, and **inner ear barotrauma** alone should not cause altered mental status. **Hemorrhagic** or **thrombotic stroke** are much less likely given the timing of onset.

4. Answer: d
The ptosis is a sign of neurotoxic envenomation, and points to a *coral snake (Elapid) bite*. In coral snake bites, antivenom should be administered immediately, in contrast to Crotaline bites, where the administration of antivenom is decided based on clinical and laboratory parameters.

5. Answer: d
The elevated pressure in the dorsal compartment is indicative of *compartment syndrome,* and should be treated with **fasciotomy. Escharotomy** will not be helpful, as no circumferential burns are present. **Debridement of the blistered area** is not necessary, and **dressing of the burn** can be delayed until the compartment syndrome is treated. **Referral to a burn center** should not delay the performance of a fasciotomy.

6. Answer: c
Deep burns do not commonly occur, as lightning usually flashes over the skin. **Blunt trauma** may occur from the victim being thrown. **Splash injury** occurs when the lightning hits another object, then arcs to the victim. **Dysrhythmia and cardiac arrest** may occur with lightning injury, as may **keraunoparalysis** (cyanotic or mottled extremities with numbness and paraplegia that may resolve spontaneously).

7. Answer: c

a, b, d, and **e** are all reasonable possibilities in the near-drowning victim. However, **electrolyte abnormalities** do not typically occur, as the amount of water aspirated is generally not sufficient to cause this.

8. Answer: e

These physical findings are typical of *decompression syndrome (DCS)*. The definitive treatment is **recompression therapy. Oxygen** by non-rebreather mask is appropriate until recompression can be accomplished.

9. Answer: e

This patient's presentation is typical of *trench foot* because of prolonged exposure to wet, nonfreezing cold.

10. Answer: d

The early symptoms of heat exhaustion typically resemble a **viral syndrome. Core temperatures greater than 105° F** typically are a sign of heat stroke. **Muscle cramps** are most commonly associated with salt depletion heat exhaustion, which typically occurs in patients who are poorly acclimatized to new environs. **Water-depletion heat exhaustion** is more common among athletes, and generally occurs soon after or during strenuous activity in hot environs.

11. Answer: c

This presentation is typical of **heat stroke,** manifested in this case by mental status change/seizure, severely elevated core temperature, hypoglycemia, and transaminase elevation. Immediate action should be taken to cool this patient, and this should not be delayed in order to obtain neuroimaging. The possibility of **sepsis** may be pursued in this patient but should not delay rewarming.

12. Answer: e

Severe pain usually occurs with rewarming. The **extent of damage** may not be apparent for hours to days. **Field rewarming** should be avoided because of the risk of re-freezing. Wet clothing should be removed and the area should be immobilized and insulated. Clear bullae are more favorable than **hemorrhagic bullae. Rewarming fluids** should be **37° to 40° C,** as higher temperatures may cause thermal injury.

13. Answer: b

Chilblains (pernio) generally occur after **dry cold** exposure, and are characteristically seen in **young women** with **Raynaud syndrome.**

14. Answer: d

The application of **hypotonic sterile water** may cause further firing of nematocysts, and will increase patient discomfort. **Gloves** should be worn during tentacle removal, and the most appropriate action would be to wash the tentacles with **dilute acetic acid** in order to inactivate nematocysts prior to tentacle removal.

15. Answer: e

Damage to **platelet** lines may lead to hemorrhage and may require the transfusion of platelets. **Leukocyte** line damage increases the risk of infection, and prophylactic antibiotics may be warranted in some patients. **Anemia** related to radiation injury is rarely severe, and rarely requires transfusion.

16. Answer: b

This history is most consistent with a *brown recluse spider bite*. These bites frequently **ulcerate** and become **necrotic** over time. **Compartment syndrome** is most likely with pit viper envenomation, **Pulmonary edema** and **respiratory paralysis** are not associated with brown recluse bite. **Severe hypertension** is generally associated with black widow spider bite.

17. Answer: c

Eikenella corrodens is a typical infectious organism associated with fight bites. *Bartonella* is the causative organism in cat scratch disease. *Capnocytophaga* is a rare and severe complication of dog bite, most frequently occurring in asplenic or functionally asplenic patients. *Pasteurella* is a common organism related to infected cat bites, and *Streptobacillus moniliformis* is commonly associated with rat-bite fever.

18. Answer: c

The lymphocyte count is the best early predictor of the severity of radiation exposure.

19. Answer: c

This presentation is typical of *high-altitude pulmonary edema*. Ascent must be stopped in all cases. Severe cases should be treated with immediate descent or with a portable hyperbaric chamber followed by descent. Symptomatic relief may be gained with furosemide or nifedipine. Less severe cases may be treated with bed rest and oxygen therapy.

20. Answer: a

Severe hypertension is most commonly associated with **black widow spider envenomation. Brown recluse envenomation generally** causes severe local effects. **Eastern coral snake** venom is neurotoxic, and **pit viper** envenomation is generally hematotoxic. Coelenterate envenomation by the potentially fatal **Portuguese man-of-war** may lead to cardiovascular collapse.

Head, Eyes, Ears, Nose, and Throat (HEENT)

Jennifer A. Oman

Ear

FOREIGN BODY

SIGNS AND SYMPTOMS

- Severe ear pain or pressure

DIAGNOSIS

- Visual inspection: thorough examination and visualization of the complete tympanic membrane is mandatory

TREATMENT

- Inability to visualize the entire canal, contact of the foreign body with the tympanic membrane, or the presence of perforation mandates consultation
- Conscious sedation or general anesthesia may be necessary for safe removal of foreign bodies medial to the bony isthmus
- Cerumen loops, a right angle hook, or alligator forceps are frequently the instruments of choice for removal
- Live objects:
  - Should be drowned with 2% lidocaine solution or viscous lidocaine, which immediately paralyzes the bug and provides modest topical anesthesia
  - Liquid can then be suctioned out with butterfly tubing and the insect removed with gentle suction or forceps under direct visualization
  - Care must be taken to ensure that no debris of the insect remains in the canal
- Irrigation with room-temperature water for small nonorganic particles
  - Irrigation should not be used unless the tympanic membrane can be completely visualized and free of perforation
- Complete inspection of the ear canal after the foreign body is removed to exclude more significant injury to the canal, tympanic membranes, and ossicles
- Topical antibiotics considered if there was serious cutaneous damage or if organic matter

CERUMEN IMPACTION

SIGNS AND SYMPTOMS

- Decreased hearing, sensation of pressure or fullness in ear, dizziness, pain, tinnitus
- Associated with use of cotton tip applicators

DIAGNOSIS

- Direct visualization

TREATMENT

- Cerumen loop
- When cerumen is completely occluding—soften first
- Irrigation with body-temperature irrigant—flexible 18-gauge catheter in the distal cartilaginous canal with gentle pulsatile flow directed along the superior portion of the external auditory canal
  - Irrigation of the canal causes a temporary redness of the tympanic membrane—subsequent diagnosis of otitis media should be made with caution
- Most common complication is iatrogenic perforation of tympanic membrane during irrigation of the ear
  - Predisposing factors include previous ear surgery, current otitis media, severe otitis externa
- When determining if perforation occurred, pay attention to symptoms of sudden hearing loss, severe otalgia, and vertigo rather than signs of visualization
- If perforation
  - Reassurance, analgesia, otolaryngologic referral within 1 to 2 weeks
  - Prophylactic antibiotics are not necessary
  - If injury to the ossicles is suspected, immediate consultation is required

LABYRINTHITIS

- Infection may be viral or bacterial
- Unusual, but can occur from otitis media, or cholesteatoma may erode into the inner ear
- Antecedents for bacterial labyrinthitis include otitis media with fistula, meningitis, mastoiditis, and dermoid tumor

SIGNS AND SYMPTOMS

- Sudden onset of vertigo, associated hearing loss, middle ear findings

DIAGNOSIS

- Clinical diagnosis

TREATMENT

- Symptomatic treatment, antibiotics if presumed bacterial
- Referral to otolaryngology for possible admission and possible surgical drainage

MASTOIDITIS

- Serious complication of otitis media
- Infection spreads from the middle ear to the mastoid air cells via the aditus ad antrum
  - When this opening is blocked, the mastoid cavity becomes a closed space and the mastoid air cells become filled with fluid and inflamed

- Infection that spreads through venous channels to the overlying periosteum is referred to as acute mastoiditis with periostitis

SIGNS AND SYMPTOMS

- Symptoms of otitis media
- Postauricular erythema and tenderness
- Auricular protrusion secondary to periosteal elevation over the mastoid complex
- Bezold abscess: abscess of the lateral aspect of the neck inferior to the mastoid tip

DIAGNOSIS

- Made by history and physical examination
- Mastoid radiographs may be helpful, showing mastoid clouding or CT scan

TREATMENT

- Requires admission and IV antibiotics, tympanocentesis and myringotomy
- Cefuroxime 1 g every 8 hours or Imipenem 500 mg every 6 hours (intravenously)
- Urgent otolaryngologic consultation

MÉNIÈRE DISEASE

- Increased endolymph within the cochlea and the labyrinth
- First attack is usually in patients in their 5th decade, or elderly
- Occurs equally in men and women
- Usually unilateral initially but can become bilateral over time

SIGNS AND SYMPTOMS

- Sudden onset of vertigo—duration ranges from 20 minutes to 12 hours—associated with nausea, vomiting, and diaphoresis
- Frequency of attacks can range from several times per week to several times per month
- Roaring tinnitus, diminished hearing, sensation of fullness in the ear
- Between attacks, the patient is usually well although deafness may persist

DIAGNOSIS

- Diagnosis suspected by history and physical examination in the emergency department (ED)
- Confirmed by the introduction of glycerol—a positive test is heralded by temporary improvement in postural control as well as a decrease in vertigo

TREATMENT

- Managed by otolaryngology
- Managed symptomatically by antihistamines as well as diuretics
- No drug treatment improves hearing
- Salt-restricted diet is recommended

OTITIS EXTERNA

- Inflammation of the external auditory canal and the auricle
- Diffuse and malignant types
  - Acute diffuse otitis externa

SIGNS AND SYMPTOMS

- Pruritis, pain, and tenderness of the external auditory canal
- Erythema and edema of the external auditory canal
- Purulent otorrhea and crusting of the external auditory canal
- Severe pain with mastication or movement of the peri-auricular skin
- Hearing impairment
- Lateral protrusion of the auricle
- Common organisms are *Pseudomonas* and *Staphylococcus aureus*—polymicrobial and anaerobic not uncommon
- Otomycosis—10% of cases; higher percentage found in tropical climates, diabetes, HIV, or immunocompromised patients; most otomycosis is caused by aspergillus or candida and may have a black, blue, green, or yellow discoloration to the external auditory canal
- Noninfectious causes—dermatitis from topical meds or hearing aids, seborrhea, and psoriasis

DIAGNOSIS

- History and physical examination make the diagnosis

TREATMENT

- Analgesia, cleaning of the canal, acidifying agents, topical antimicrobials, and sometimes steroids
- Cleansing done with irrigation and Frazier tip suction by a physician
- Theoretical risk of both auditory and vestibular toxicity with aminoglycosides (neomycin), polymyxin, and acetic acid preparations
  - In the presence of an intact tympanic membrane, the risk of systemic absorption of aminoglycoside is negligible
- Nontoxic oto-topical antibiotics (e.g., ciprofloxacin otic) should be considered first-line if unknown integrity or perforation of tympanic membrane, or tympanostomy tubes
- Oral antibiotic therapy reserved for febrile patients and those with peri-auricular extension
- Specific treatment of otomycosis is clotrimazole
- Follow-up if worse or no improvement in 1 week

MALIGNANT OTITIS EXTERNA

- Begins as simple otitis externa, then spreads to deeper tissues
- Variable extension of infection to skull base
- Caused by *Pseudomonas aeruginosa* >90%
- Spectrum of disease—when it is limited to the soft tissue and cartilage, it is called necrotizing otitis externa

- Involvement of the temporal bone or skull base is called skull-based osteomyelitis

SIGNS AND SYMPTOMS

- Typical patient is elderly diabetic or patient with immunocompromise
- Otalgia and edema and erythema of the external auditory canal, with or without otorrhea
- Otalgia may be out of proportion for routine otitis externa
- Cranial nerve involvement is a serious sign
- Parotitis may be present
- Trismus indicates involvement of the masseter muscle or temporomandibular joint
- Examine for facial palsy and hoarseness or dysphagia
  - 7th cranial nerve is usually the first affected
  - Dysfunction of the 9th, 10th, or 11th cranial nerves implies more extensive disease
  - Lateral or sigmoid sinus thrombosis and meningitis are possible complications
- Patients with AIDS and malignant otitis externa tend to be younger, have etiologic organisms other than *Pseudomonas*, and tend to have a worse prognosis than patients without AIDS

DIAGNOSIS

- History and physical examination
- Determine the extent of progression of the disease by identifying involvement of nearby structures

TREATMENT

- Admission
- Aminoglycoside and antipseudomonal penicillin or cephalosporin or quinolone
- Emergent otolaryngology consultation

OTITIS MEDIA

- Primarily a disease of infancy and childhood with prevalence peak in preschool years
- Decreasing incidence after childhood related to Eustachian tube anatomy—angle and length both increase, promoting drainage
- Microbiology
  - *Streptococcus pneumoniae, Haemophilus influenzae,* and *Moraxella catarrhalis*
  - Predominant organisms in chronic otitis media are *S. aureus, P. aeruginosa,* and anaerobic bacteria
  - Viruses play a role in that they may promote bacterial superinfection

SIGNS AND SYMPTOMS

- Otalgia with or without fever
- Otorrhea and hearing loss are variably present, while tinnitus, vertigo, and nystagmus are uncommon

DIAGNOSIS

- Visual inspection
- The tympanic membrane is retracted or bulging

- May be red in color, indicating inflammation, or it may be yellow/white as a result of middle ear effusion
- Pneumatic otoscopy demonstrates impaired mobility
- Facial nerve should always be assessed because of its proximity to the middle ear

TREATMENT

- No guidelines for adults
- Amoxicillin is first choice, but 10% of cases are caused by resistant strains
- For otitis media unresponsive to initial therapy after 72 hours, cefuroxime or amoxicillin–clavulanate may be given
- Pain continues for 8 to 24 hours after the initiation of antibiotics

TYMPANIC MEMBRANE PERFORATION

- Direct trauma or indirect trauma
- Assess for injury to the ossicles if traumatic

SIGNS AND SYMPTOMS

- History of trauma—direct or indirect
- Presence of sensorineural hearing loss, nystagmus, or significant vestibular symptoms suggest the possibility of perilymphatic leak

DIAGNOSIS

- Visual diagnosis

TREATMENT

- Clean perforations do not need antibiotics
- No water in ear
- If contaminated situation—antibiotics
- Reexamine in 10 days
- From otitis media—think resistant streptococcal or staphylococcal species
  - Treat with a topical and oral antibiotic

Eye

EXTERNAL EYE

Blepharitis

- Irritation and inflammation of the lid margin
- Staphylococcal infection causes ulcerative lesions
- Chronic infection

SIGNS AND SYMPTOMS

- Ulcerative appearance to lids
- Irritation, burning, itching; eyes may appear "red-rimmed"
- Scaling is dry and eyelashes fall out easily
- Poor hygiene causes seborrheic blepharitis, with scaling and build-up leading to inflammation

DIAGNOSIS

- Eye examination—absence of disturbance in visual acuity, foreign body, or corneal lesions should be noted

TREATMENT

- Chronic staphylococcal blepharitis may lead to conjunctivitis or keratitis of the lower third of the cornea—start anti-staphylococcal antibiotic drops
- Seborrheic blepharitis does not require antibiotic treatment
  - Remove scaling with cotton-tip applicator and mild soap
- Follow-up in 3 to 5 days if on antibiotic treatment

DISORDERS OF THE LACRIMAL SYSTEM

Dacryocystitis

- Occurs in infants and persons older than 40 years
- Can occur in all age groups after trauma or after fungal infection

SIGNS AND SYMPTOMS

- Inflammation, pain, swelling, and localized tenderness over lacrimal sac below medial canthus
- Profuse tearing and purulent discharge from the lacrimal duct

DIAGNOSIS

- Physical examination

TREATMENT

- Antibiotic eye drops and oral agents
- Follow-up with ophthalmology if unsuccessful

Dacryoadenitis

- Acute inflammation of the lacrimal gland
- Acutely may be caused by gonorrhea in the adult
- Chronic may be related to sarcoidosis, tuberculosis, leukemia, and lymphosarcoma

SIGNS AND SYMPTOMS

- Presentation similar to dacryocystitis

DIAGNOSIS

- History and physical examination

TREATMENT

- Systemic antibiotic treatment if bacterial etiology
- If the gland is extremely enlarged, ophthalmologic consultation for I and D

INFLAMMATION OF THE EYELIDS

Chalazion

- *Chronic* inflammation of a meibomian or Zeis gland

SIGNS AND SYMPTOMS

- Local swelling to the eyelid, pain is generally minimal or absent

DIAGNOSIS

- Physical examination

TREATMENT

- Warm compresses

Hordeolum

- *Acute* infection of a meibomian or Zeis gland

SIGNS AND SYMPTOMS

- Differs from a chalazion in that pain is primary symptom
- Lid margin is erythematous and swollen

DIAGNOSIS

- Physical examination

TREATMENT

- Warm compresses, topical erythromycin ointment, consistent lid hygiene

CONJUNCTIVA

Conjunctivitis

- Inflammation of the bulbar and palpebral conjunctiva due to bacterial, viral, allergic, or toxic causes; look for bulbar and palpebral erythema/injection, diffuse (not just perilimbic) involvement, and improvement of symptoms with application of topical anesthetics as signs suggestive of conjunctivitis; marked pain and photophobia should be absent in simple conjunctivitis

Viral conjunctivitis

- Most common cause of conjunctivitis
- Commonly adenovirus, coxsackievirus, enterovirus
- Commonly presents in the setting of viral syndromes
- Mild morning eye crusting

SIGNS AND SYMPTOMS

- Redness, itching, irritation, and foreign body sensation
- May present with preauricular adenopathy

DIAGNOSIS

- Clinical

TREATMENT

- Symptomatic with cool compresses
- Hand washing and contact precautions

Bacterial conjunctivitis

- Commonly *S. pneumoniae, H. influenzae, S. aureus, M. catarrhalis,* or *Neisseria gonorrhoeae*
- Complications: corneal ulcer, corneal perforation, and keratitis

SIGNS AND SYMPTOMS

- Routine bacterial conjunctivitis
  - Conjunctival erythema and edema, foreign body sensation
  - Drainage and morning eye crusting
- Gonococcal (GC) conjunctivitis
  - Dramatic increase in symptoms
  - Large amount of purulent discharge

DIAGNOSIS

- Clinical
- Visual loss, photophobia are absent
- Cultures only indicated if suspected GC, treatment failures, very severe symptoms

TREATMENT

- Routine bacterial conjunctivitis
  - Warm compresses
  - Topical antibiotics—many choices
  - Avoid neomycin because of common hypersensitivity reactions
- GC conjunctivitis—mild cases
  - Outpatient management with close (1 day) ophthalmology follow-up
  - Saline irrigation of the conjunctiva, Ceftriaxone 1 g IM single dose, topical erythromycin
  - Concomitant treatment for suspected *Chlamydia trachomatis* with oral doxycycline or azithromycin
- GC conjunctivitis—moderate and severe cases
  - Admission and an ophthalmologic consult

Ophthalmia neonatorum

- Conjunctivitis that occurs in the first month of life
- Most common causes: *C. trachomatis, N. gonorrhoeae,* and chemical conjunctivitis due to antibiotic ointment administration at birth
- Infectious causes are acquired in transit through birth canal

SIGNS AND SYMPTOMS

- Conjunctival erythema and edema
- Discharge

DIAGNOSIS

- Gram stain and culture
- Mainly based on timing of onset from birth
  - **1 to 2 days:** typically chemical—symptoms should be mild or investigate other causes
  - **2 to 4 days:** typically GC—look for signs of systemic involvement
  - **5 to 14 days:** typically chlamydia

TREATMENT

- Chemical
  - Consider other causes; management is expectant
- GC
  - GC with no signs of systemic involvement
    - Ceftriaxone IM or IV, topical polymyxin B/ bacitracin ointment, and saline washes
  - GC with signs of systemic involvement
    - Ophthalmologic consultation
    - Consider hospitalization, blood and cerebrospinal fluid (CSF) analysis
  - All patients should be treated for chlamydia (see below), as concomitant infection is possible
    - Topical and oral erythromycin for 14 days

Other conjunctivitis

- Allergic conjunctivitis: due to environmental agents or cosmetics
- Chemical conjunctivitis: due to topical medication or environmental exposures

SIGNS AND SYMPTOMS

- Itching, tearing, and redness
- Often bilateral in cases of allergic conjunctivitis

DIAGNOSIS

- Clinical

TREATMENT

- Artificial tears, cool compresses
- In allergic cases, consider topical ocular decongestants or ocular antihistamine/ vasoconstrictor combinations

CORNEA

Pterygium

- Raised, wedge-shaped growth of fibrovascular tissue extending from the conjunctiva onto the cornea (Fig. 7-1)

SIGNS AND SYMPTOMS

- Many are asymptomatic, but may cause redness, itching, and irritation
- Can grow over the central cornea, affecting vision

DIAGNOSIS

- Clinical

TREATMENT

- Recommend protection from sunlight, dust, and wind
- Nonemergent follow-up with ophthalmologist

Pinguecula

- Yellowish growth on the conjunctiva, on the nasal side near the cornea (Fig. 7-2)
- Benign growth thought to be caused by exposure to UV light

SIGNS AND SYMPTOMS

- Most are asymptomatic, but may present with dry eyes, irritation, or conjunctival inflammation

DIAGNOSIS

- Clinical (naked eye or slit lamp)

TREATMENT

- Usually none needed, but artificial tears and/or a topical NSAID may be used for inflammation

Superficial punctate keratitis

- Multiple punctate corneal epithelial defects (Fig. 7-3)
- Multiple causes—viral, bacterial, chemical (due to chemical exposure or topical medicines), contact lenses, or due to UV exposure without protection (welding, sunlamps)

SIGNS AND SYMPTOMS

- Pain (may be severe), photophobia, redness, tearing, foreign body sensation, possible blurred vision

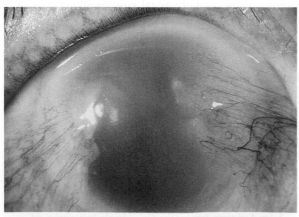

Figure 7-1. Double pterygium. Note both nasal and temporal pterygia in a 57-year-old farmer. (From Yanoff M, Duker JS: *Ophthalmology*, ed 3, Philadelphia, 2008, Mosby.)

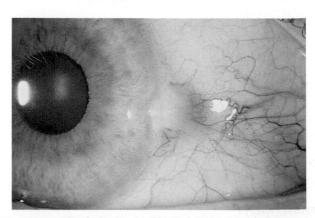

Figure 7-2. Nasal pinguecula. Elevated conjunctival lesion encroaches on nasal limbus. (From Yanoff M, Duker JS: *Ophthalmology*, ed 3, Philadelphia, 2008, Mosby.)

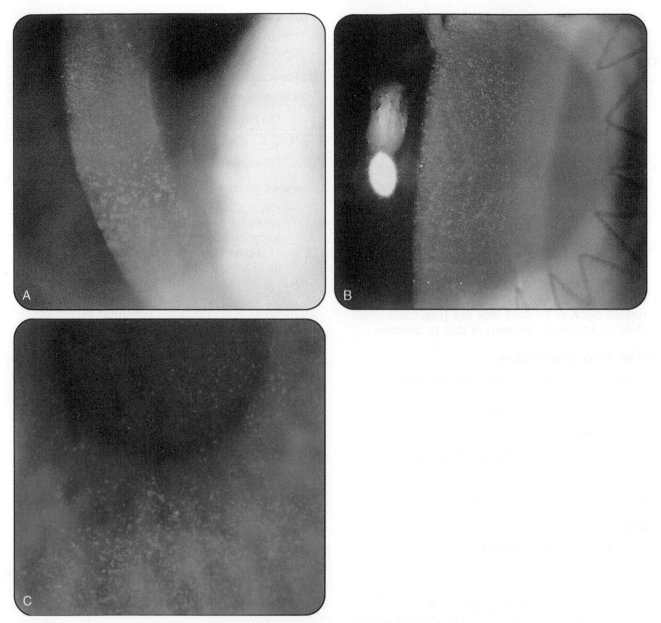

Figure 7-3. Signs of superficial punctate keratitis.

DIAGNOSIS

- History—contact lens use, chemical/topical medicine exposure, UV exposure without proper protective eyewear
- Physical—fluorescein staining and visualization with slit lamp/Wood lamp

TREATMENT

- Viral or chemical (except herpes simplex or zoster)—artificial tears, analgesia, lubricating ointments, discontinue eye drops in chemical causes
- Herpetic—ophthalmologic consultation is warranted
- Bacterial—antibiotic ointment, consider cycloplegic, analgesia
- UV—antibiotic ointment, cycloplegic, analgesia (may require narcotics)

- Contact lens–associated—discontinue lenses, topical tobramycin or fluoroquinolone
- All patients should have close ophthalmologic follow-up

Corneal Abrasion

SIGNS AND SYMPTOMS

- Eye pain, photophobia, tearing
- May result from trauma or contact lens wear

DIAGNOSIS

- Corneal epithelial defect is best seen with fluorescein and a slit lamp exam
- Eyelid should be everted and inspected for foreign bodies

- Examine the cornea for possible full-thickness injury and asses the anterior chamber with the slit lamp

TREATMENT

- Adequate and persistent cycloplegia is essential for controlling pain
- If an abrasion is larger than 2 mm or very painful, consider a cycloplegic agent
- Abrasions from organic sources or potential fungal infections should not be patched
- Abrasions related to contact lens wear should not be patched
- Patients with contact lens wear—consider *Pseudomonas*

Corneal ulcer (Fig. 7-4)

- Corneal defect that is generally superinfected by bacteria, a virus, or a fungus
- Initial insult may be mechanical due to injury, foreign body, or contact lens use (especially when sleeping in contact lenses), or due to infection

SIGNS AND SYMPTOMS

- Pain, foreign body sensation, tearing, and photophobia
- White "spot" on the cornea

DIAGNOSIS

- History—suspect with history of lens use, herpes simplex or zoster infection, trauma
- Physical—appearance of white "spot" on cornea, fluorescein uptake on examination

TREATMENT

- Immediate ophthalmologic referral

Herpetic infection

- Herpes simplex: primary or reactivation
- Herpes zoster: activation on ophthalmic branch of trigeminal nerve

SIGNS AND SYMPTOMS

- Foreign body sensation, tearing, photophobia, possible blurred vision

DIAGNOSIS

HERPES SIMPLEX

- Physical findings may include superficial punctate keratitis, corneal ulceration, or dendrites noted on examination (Fig. 7-5)
- Patients may have herpetic vesicles on eye lid

HERPES ZOSTER

- Physical findings may include dermatomal vesicular rash on face
- *Hutchinson sign* (vesicular rash includes the tip of the nose due to nasociliary nerve involvement) may be present

TREATMENT

- Emergent ophthalmologic consultation
- Topical antivirals, consider cycloplegic and systemic antiviral in conjunction with consultant

Ocular chemical burn

- Severity of injury depends on concentration and duration of exposure
- Acid injury—coagulation necrosis with limited depth of injury limited
- Alkaline injury—liquefaction necrosis with deep and ongoing damage

SIGNS AND SYMPTOMS

- Eye pain
- History of chemical irritant splashed into eye

DIAGNOSIS

- Visual diagnosis along with appropriate history

TREATMENT

- Immediate copious irrigation especially in chemical exposure until pH testing returns to normal

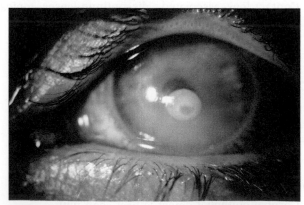

Figure 7-4. This corneal ulcer caused by *Pseudomonas aeruginosa* occurred in a young man who wore decorative contact lenses without professional supervision. (From Yanoff M, Duker JS: *Ophthalmology,* ed 3, Philadelphia, 2008, Mosby.)

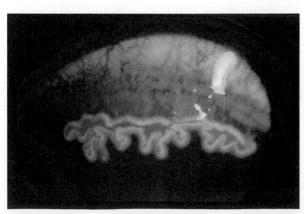

Figure 7-5. Dendrite. (From Yanoff M, Duker JS: *Ophthalmology,* ed 3, Philadelphia, 2008, Mosby.)

- Acid injury—irrigation to pH 7, follow-up with ophthalmology in 24 hours
- Alkali injury—continue irrigation until pH normal and remains normal for 30 minutes after irrigation stopped; ophthalmology consultation in ED

Corneal foreign bodies

- History consistent with high-velocity ocular impact (e.g., grinding, sawing, hammering) should alert you to the possibility of penetrating injury

SIGNS AND SYMPTOMS

- Pain, profuse tearing, foreign body sensation, conjunctival injection

DIAGNOSIS

- History along with slit lamp examination

TREATMENT

- Should be removed under the best magnification available
- Cornea should be inspected with optical sectioning to assess depth of penetration prior to removal
- Full-thickness corneal foreign bodies should not be removed in the ED and require an ophthalmology consult
- Metallic foreign bodies can create rust rings that are toxic to the corneal tissue
- If a rust ring (Fig. 7-6) is present, it is not necessary to remove all the rust aggressively in the ED, as more usually needs to be removed the next day

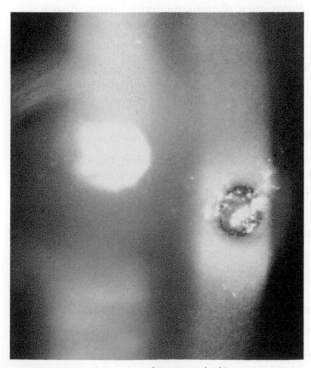

Figure 7-6. Corneal rust ring after removal of iron-containing foreign body demonstrated by slit-lamp examination. (From Marx JA et al: *Rosen's emergency medicine: concepts and clinical practice,* ed 6, Philadelphia, 2006, Mosby.)

- The deeper the stromal involvement, the higher the risk of corneal scarring
- No emergency department drill burring should take place if the rust ring is located in the visual axis owing to the risk of scarring
- Removal, if not done in the ED, should be performed within 24 hours
- Once foreign body removed, treat resultant corneal abrasion

ANTERIOR POLE

Glaucoma

- Increase in the resistance to aqueous outflow due to the malfunction of the trabecular meshwork
- Risk factors include trauma, inflammation, age, ischemia

Open-angle glaucoma

SIGNS AND SYMPTOMS

- Bilateral
- Insidious onset
- Late onset—decreased vision and aching of eyes

DIAGNOSIS

- Eye examination including measurement of intraocular pressure

TREATMENT

- Pilocarpine, acetazolamide, timolol
- Ophthalmologic consultation for eventual surgical correction

Acute closed angle glaucoma

- Sudden increase in intraocular pressure

SIGNS AND SYMPTOMS

- Severe localized pain to the eye or orbit, or headache
- Triggered by entering a darkened area or after going to sleep, emotional upset, or starting sympathomimetic or anticholinergic medication
- Amount of visual loss is variable
- "Halo" vision, nausea and vomiting, photophobia
- Conjunctival hyperemia, corneal edema, and fixed, mid-dilated pupil (Fig. 7-7)
- Anterior chamber angle decreased; intraocular pressures are high (>50 mmHg)

DIAGNOSIS

- Eye examination with slit lamp and eye pressure measurement

TREATMENT

- Immediate consultation with ophthalmologist
- Pilocarpine eye drops 1% to 2%, 1 drop every 15 minutes for two doses
- Topical timolol 0.5%

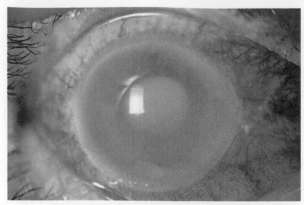

Figure 7-7. Acute angle-closure glaucoma. (From Yanoff M, Duker JS: *Ophthalmology,* ed 3, Philadelphia, 2008, Mosby.)

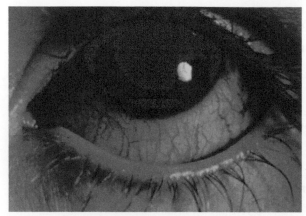

Figure 7-8. Small hyphema layering out in the inferior portion of the anterior chamber. (From Marx JA et al: *Rosen's emergency medicine: concepts and clinical practice,* ed 6, Philadelphia, 2006, Mosby.)

- Acetazolamide 250 to 500 mg IV
- Mannitol 1 to 2 mg/kg over 45 minutes
- Surgical treatment is definitive therapy

Hyphema (Fig. 7-8)

SIGNS AND SYMPTOMS

- Blood in the anterior chamber
- Traumatic or spontaneous
- From trauma—usually the result of a ruptured iris root vessel
- Spontaneous—often related to sickle cell disease

DIAGNOSIS

- History and physical examination
- Measure intraocular pressure if globe is intact

TREATMENT

- ED management consists of assessing concomitant injury and managing rises in intra-ocular pressure (IOP)
  - Head should be elevated
  - Pupil should be dilated

- Pupillary dilation does not compromise angle and aqueous outflow in normal individuals
- If IOP greater than 30 mmHg treat as glaucoma with timolol and acetazolamide
  - In patients with sickle cell disease, acetazolamide should be avoided
- Rebleeding can occur at 3 to 5 days later in up to 30%—more in sickle cell disease
- Admit if unable to follow closely as outpatient or large hyphema
- Outpatient if hyphema size one-third or less of anterior chamber
- Elevate the patient's head
- Administer 1% atropine 3 times daily
- Administer prednisolone acetate 1 drop 4 times daily
- Ophthalmology consult

Iritis

SIGNS AND SYMPTOMS

- Blunt trauma
- Inflammatory reaction in the anterior chamber
- Unilateral red eye and have pain, photophobia, and blurred vision
- Pupillary constrictor spasm may leave the pupil smaller than the contralateral side
- Cells and flare in the anterior chamber

DIAGNOSIS

- History and eye examination with slit lamp demonstrating cells and flare in the anterior chamber
- Consensual photophobia with increased pain in affected eye when light shined in unaffected eye

TREATMENT

- Treatment is long-acting mydriatic and cycloplegic drops and ophthalmologic referral

Purulent endophthalmitis

Infection by Staphylococcus, Streptococcus, or Bacillus species involving the anterior and posterior chamber of the eye and the vitreous chambers
- Often posttraumatic or postsurgical

SIGNS AND SYMPTOMS

- Pain, vision loss, and decreased visual acuity
- Chemosis and hyperemia of the conjunctiva
- Infected chambers appear hazy or opaque

DIAGNOSIS

- Clinical history and physical examination

TREATMENT

- Intraocular and intravenous antibiotics
- Admission and emergent ophthalmologic consultation

POSTERIOR POLE

Choroiditis/chorioretinitis

Inflammation of the vascular layer between the retina and the sclera that can be seen in patients with herpes zoster infection, posterior uveitis, or other inflammatory diseases.

SIGNS AND SYMPTOMS

- Unilateral blurred vision
- Floaters, eye redness, mild pain, photophobia

DIAGNOSIS

- History and eye examination
- Funduscopic examination shows inflammatory lesions of the retina, mild disc edema, and neovascularization of the choroid plexus

TREATMENT

- If herpes zoster is suspected, admit for IV acyclovir and steroid therapy
- If inflammatory cause, consultation and oral steroid therapy may improve symptoms

Optic neuritis

Etiologies include multiple sclerosis, viral infections, and inflammatory diseases of the eye, leading to subacute vision loss.

SIGNS AND SYMPTOMS

- Unilateral loss of visual acuity over hours to days
- Pain with movement of the eye
- Decreased color vision
- Possible antecedent viral infection

DIAGNOSIS

- History and physical examination, funduscopic examination may demonstrate papilledema/hyperemia
- CBC, erythrocyte sedimentation rate, RPR, CT or MRI of the orbits and brain may help discern etiology

TREATMENT

- Intravenous steroids
- Ophthalmologic consultation and admission

Papilledema

Visual loss due to optic disc swelling related to increased intracranial pressure

SIGNS AND SYMPTOMS

- Episodic transient loss of vision, which may be positional
  - Bilateral, transient, may be recurrent

DIAGNOSIS

- Complete history and physical examination
- CT or MRI emergently

- If CT or MRI is normal, lumbar puncture with opening pressure should be performed

TREATMENT

- Specific therapy depends on the etiology of increased intracranial pressure

Retinal detachment

SIGNS AND SYMPTOMS

- Light flashes, dark floating specks, or a curtain-like visual field deficit
- Peripheral or central vision loss depending on location of detachment
- History of antecedent trauma (may be temporally distant), prior retinal surgery or detachment

DIAGNOSIS

- Complete history and physical examination
- If history is consistent with retinal detachment, ophthalmology should be consulted for indirect ophthalmoscopy, which can visualize a far greater portion of the retina

TREATMENT

- Immediate ophthalmologic consultation, treatment is surgical

Vitreous hemorrhage

SIGNS AND SYMPTOMS

- Painless, unilateral visual loss
- May start as sudden appearance of black spots
- Mild afferent papillary defect on examination
- Absent red reflex if severe due to blood in the posterior pole of eye blocking the fundus

DIAGNOSIS

- History and physical examination

TREATMENT

- Admission possible, ophthalmologic consultation
- Bed rest, elevate head of bed
- Avoid antiplatelet medications

Retinal vascular occlusion

CENTRAL RETINAL ARTERY OCCLUSION
(Fig. 7-9)

SIGNS AND SYMPTOMS

- Unilateral painless severe visual loss over seconds
- Often a history of significant atherosclerotic disease
- Relative afferent papillary defect
- Funduscopic examination reveals pale retina with a cherry-red spot in the center of the fovea
- Branch retinal artery occlusions may also occur

DIAGNOSIS

- Complete eye examination and complete history and physical examination

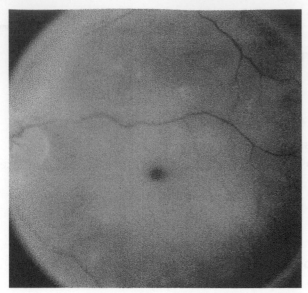

Figure 7-9. Central retinal artery occlusion. Note cherry-red spot (fovea). (From Marx JA et al: *Rosen's emergency medicine: concepts and clinical practice*, ed 6, Philadelphia, 2006, Mosby.)

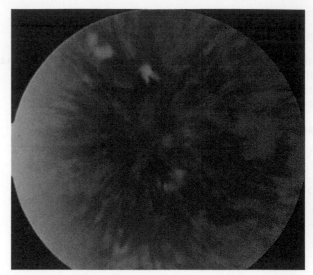

Figure 7-10. Central retinal vein occlusion. (From Marx JA et al: *Rosen's emergency medicine: concepts and clinical practice*, ed 6, Philadelphia, 2006, Mosby.)

TREATMENT

- Massage globe
- Acetazolamide 250 to 500 mg IV
- Blood draw for CBC, ESR, and coagulation studies
- Immediate ophthalmologic consultation
- If the ESR is elevated, high-dose steroids should be started in the ED
- Visual outcomes are generally poor

CENTRAL RETINAL VEIN OCCLUSION
(Fig. 7-10)

SIGNS AND SYMPTOMS

- Acute, unilateral painless loss of vision, usually over minutes
- Relative pupillary defect may or may not be present
- Funduscopic examination shows diffuse retinal hemorrhages in all quadrants of the retina, dilated and tortuous retinal veins, cotton wool spots, optic disc edema, and retinal edema
- Described as "blood and thunder" appearance of the fundus
- Branch retinal vein occlusion may occur, with findings restricted to a portion of the fundus

DIAGNOSIS

- Complete history and physical examination

TREATMENT

- Blood draw for CBC, ESR, coagulation studies
- Ophthalmologic consultation for close follow-up, visual outcomes are often poor
- Correct underlying medical disorders and lower intraocular pressure if indicated

ORBIT

Cellulitis

PRESEPTAL (PERIORBITAL) CELLULITIS

- Is a pre-ocular superficial cellulitis that has not breached the orbital septum

SIGNS AND SYMPTOMS

- Eyelids become edematous, warm and red
- The eye itself is not involved, with acuity and pupillary reaction maintained and full ocular motility preserved
- The offending agent is often a streptococcal or staphylococcal organism

DIAGNOSIS

- Diagnosis made by history and physical examination

TREATMENT

- Oral amoxicillin–clavulanate, many other appropriate antibiotics
- Ensure no restriction of ocular motility, no proptosis, no pain with eye movement and preserved pupillary response and acuity—otherwise must consider postseptal cellulitis

POSTSEPTAL (ORBITAL) CELLULITIS

- Serious orbital infection deep to the orbital septum
- *S. aureus* is the most common pathogen *Haemophilus* and mucormycosis should be considered in diabetics and immunocompromised patients
- Polymicrobial infection is common
- Orbital extension of paranasal sinus infection—ethmoid sinusitis is the most frequent source

SIGNS AND SYMPTOMS

- Eye pain, fever
- Extraocular motility impairment, proptosis may be present
- Decreased visual acuity is a late finding
- Cavernous sinus thrombosis may occur simultaneously

DIAGNOSIS

- History and physical examination
- Orbit and sinus CT should be performed with and without contrast

TREATMENT

- Intravenous antibiotics are mandatory—many appropriate options exist, including ceftriaxone, cefotaxime, and piperacillin/tazobactam; staphylococcal coverage should be provided, with coverage for MRSA if this is a concern
- Admission, immediate ophthalmologic consultation

CAVERNOUS SINUS THROMBOSIS

- Uncommon in the antibiotic era, may be a late complication of sinus, facial, or ear infection, or may be due to noninfectious causes
- Associated with 30% mortality and extremely high neurologic and ophthalmologic complication rate; complete recovery is rare
- 5% of ophthalmoplegias are secondary to involvement of the cavernous sinuses
- Manipulated nostril furuncle is the precipitant etiology in 25% of cases
- Most patients are previously healthy—those with diabetes or immunocompromised at higher risk
- Aseptic a result of space-occupying lesions—parasellar lesions, carotid cavernous fistula, cavernous sinus aneurysm
- Primary tumors are meningiomas, pituitary tumors, and neurofibromas
- Malignant tumors are usually nasopharyngeal, pulmonary, prostatic, or breast metastatic neoplasms
- Less commonly, hypercoagulable states may be the underlying etiology

SIGNS AND SYMPTOMS

- Noninfectious causes usually lack systemic signs or symptoms, and may present with only ophthalmoplegia or diplopia
- Early: fever, chills, malaise, retro-orbital pain and headache; venous stasis will result in periorbital edema, swelling of eyelids, and chemosis
- Late: with progression of the disease, ophthalmologic signs more prominent
  - Lateral gaze palsy is the most common and the earliest ophthalmologic sign, followed by generalized ophthalmoplegia
  - Intraocular pressure usually elevated
  - Presence of a sluggish or fixed and dilated pupil is a late sign
  - Visual acuity significantly decreased
  - Corneal reflex abnormal
  - Painful diplopia, papilledema, retinal hemorrhages
- Stiff neck and signs of meningismus may be present
- Generalized seizures and hemiparesis will commonly develop
- Progression of the infection and involvement of the contralateral cavernous sinus
- Sepsis, delirium, and shock will follow

DIAGNOSIS

- Clinical suspicion with subsequent laboratory tests, CT with contrast or MRI/MRA of brain and orbits, and lumbar puncture if necessary
- Ophthalmoplegia with sinusitis or other mid facial infection must be considered
- Involvement of the contralateral eye is considered pathognomonic
- If lumbar puncture performed, findings will suggest bacterial meningitis
  - Elevated pressure of CSF
  - Increased WBC and protein and decreased glucose
- Blood culture must be obtained and may reveal the causative pathogen

TREATMENT

- Broad-spectrum antibiotics are the mainstay, anticoagulation, and surgery in selected cases

Nose

EPISTAXIS

- Blood supply to nasal mucosa from branches of the carotid artery

Anterior epistaxis

SIGNS AND SYMPTOMS

- Usually younger patients, usually unilateral
- Majority originate from Kiesselbach plexus
- Nasal mucosa dry/cracking from environment, local irritation
- Special consideration—patient or family history of bleeding disorders, anticoagulant or antiplatelet use
- Osler–Weber–Rendu or hereditary telangiectasia may be the cause of recurrent nosebleeds

DIAGNOSIS

- Bleeding site usually easily visible on examination
- Rarely require ENT consultation
- Laboratory tests not warranted unless suspicion for anemia or coagulopathy

TREATMENT

- Direct pressure, vasoconstrictors
- Cautery with silver nitrate sticks if direct visualization of bleeding
  - Thermal and electrical cautery to be avoided

- Anterior nasal packing if unable to stop bleeding or see site of bleeding
  - Prophylaxis against staphylococcal or streptococcal infections (with cephalexin, amoxicillin–clavulanate, clindamycin, or trimethoprim–sulfamethoxazole) if packing placed
  - Remove nasal packing in 2 to 3 days
  - Complications include dislodgement, persistent bleeding, sinusitis, septal necrosis, toxic shock

Posterior epistaxis

- Posterior to the inferior turbinate most common site of posterior bleeding

SIGNS AND SYMPTOMS

- More common in older patients
- Profuse bleeding, with sensation of blood in/down back of throat
- Blood may reflux to unaffected side and present as a bilateral nosebleed

DIAGNOSIS

- IV access and laboratory tests (CBC, coagulation studies, type and screen) often warranted
- Clinical diagnosis

TREATMENT

- Direct pressure ineffective
- Posterior packing
  - Must pack anterior nasal cavity when posterior pack placed to prevent anterior nasal cavity clot formation and aspiration risk
  - Possible complications of posterior nasal packing are many, including cardiac dysrhythmias, cardiac arrest, accidental dislodgement into the airway, or hypoxia
- Admission with airway and cardiac monitoring
- If packing by the consultant is ineffective, arterial ligation or embolization may be necessary

NASAL FOREIGN BODIES

- Generally occur in children

SIGNS AND SYMPTOMS

- Sensation of unilateral nasal obstruction
- Persistent foul-smelling rhinorrhea or persistent unilateral epistaxis

DIAGNOSIS

- Direct visualization

TREATMENT

- Removal includes preparing nasal mucosa with vasoconstrictors and analgesics
- Removal techniques include:
  - Positive pressure with puff of air into mouth by caregiver while occluding unobstructed nare with finger

- Removal by suction catheter or grabbing object with alligator forceps
- Passing a curette or fogarty catheter beyond object and withdrawing the curette/catheter and object

SINUSITIS

- Acute sinusitis is acute inflammation of the paranasal sinuses of less than 3 weeks' duration
- Most sinusitis is viral
- Common bacterial agents include *S. pneumoniae, H. influenzae,* and *M. catarrhalis*
- Immunocompromised patients may also have opportunistic bacteria or fungi as causative agents in addition to usual pathogens
- Chronic sinusitis results from unresolved acute sinusitis of more than 3 weeks' duration and is polymicrobial

SIGNS AND SYMPTOMS

ACUTE BACTERIAL SINUSITIS

- Symptoms for 7 days or more, sinus pain or tenderness in the face/teeth, purulent nasal secretions
- Ethmoid sinusitis causes dull, aching sensation behind the eye
  - Can spread to the orbit, retro-orbital area, and the CNS
- Headache aggravated by bending forward, sneezing, or coughing
- Tenderness to palpation or percussion over the involved sinus
- Nasal cavity may have swollen, erythematous mucosa with purulent exudates from the ostia

DIAGNOSIS

- Radiography not indicated for routine cases
- CT if diagnosis unclear or if patient immunocompromised
- Cultures not routinely recommended but can consider in immunocompromised patients

TREATMENT

- Less than 7 days' duration—treat symptoms only
  - Nasal decongestant sprays for less than 5 days, oral decongestant
  - Consider steroid nasal spray
- Antibiotics should not be used unless symptoms persist beyond 7 days despite symptomatic care or unless symptoms are severe regardless of duration
- Amoxicillin, trimethoprim–sulfamethoxazole, cefuroxime, azithromycin, many others
- Complications
  - *Pott's puffy tumor*—doughy edematous forehead from bony destruction of frontal sinus
  - Extension from ethmoid sinusitis can cause *orbital* or *preseptal cellulitis*
  - Paranasal sinus infection can spread to the venous or lymphatic system causing *cavernous sinus thrombosis*

- If complication suspected, then emergent CT/MRI, intravenous antibiotics, and consultation with specialist

Oropharynx/throat

DENTALGIA (ODONTALGIA)

- Multiple causes: dental caries, cracked tooth or split root syndrome, postextraction pain

DENTAL CARIES

SIGNS AND SYMPTOMS

- Variable history of sudden- or gradual-onset pain
- Sharp/dull throbbing pain, may have temperature/position-related sensitivity
- Most cases can identify tooth causing pain, occasionally generalized pain
- Pain referred to temporal region, ear, eye, neck and sometimes the opposite jaw

DIAGNOSIS

- Visual inspection

TREATMENT

- Symptomatic; dental referral

ROOT CANAL PAIN

SIGNS AND SYMPTOMS

- Pain after oral surgery and root canal
- Swelling in the socket may cause the tooth to be elevated slightly

DIAGNOSIS

- Visual inspection

TREATMENT

- Referral back to dentist or endodontist

CRACKED TOOTH

SIGNS AND SYMPTOMS

- Pain with chewing or forced closure

DIAGNOSIS

- History and physical examination

TREATMENT

- Symptomatic pain relief and referral back to dentist

DRY SOCKET (POSTEXTRACTION ALVEOLAR OSTEITIS)

- Pathophysiology involves premature loss of the healing blood clot from the socket, with localized infection of the bone

SIGNS AND SYMPTOMS

- Pain-free interval after tooth extraction and then sudden onset of excruciating pain and foul odor in mouth 2 to 4 days postextraction

DIAGNOSIS

- History and physical examination

TREATMENT

- Anesthetic nerve block, gentle irrigation of socket and packing of the socket with medicated dental dressing, oral pain medication
- Oral antibiotics: penicillin VK 500 mg three times a day
- No attempt should be made to cause bleeding in the socket—associated with high incidence of osteomyelitis
- Follow up daily with dentist

PERIAPICAL ABSCESS

- In adults, most dental pain is due to periapical pathology—periapical granuloma or periradicular periodontitis most common periapical abscess

SIGNS AND SYMPTOMS

- Headache, sinus pain, eye pain, jaw pain, or neck pain, or localized to a single tooth
- Small swelling of the gingiva with a draining fistula may help identify tooth
- Erosion of periapical abscess through cortical bone and subperiosteal extension results in intraoral swelling or facial swelling and fluctuance

DIAGNOSIS

- Visual inspection

TREATMENT

- Penicillin VK 250 to 500 mg four times a day or clindamycin 300 mg three times a day
- Pain medication
- Incision and drainage of intraoral fluctuance ("pointing abscess")
- Prompt referral to dentist

DISEASES OF THE ORAL SOFT TISSUE

Ludwig angina

- Infection of the submental, sublingual, and submandibular spaces causing elevation and posterior displacement of the tongue and tense "brawny" induration of soft tissue between the hyoid bone and the genu of the mandible

SIGNS AND SYMPTOMS

- Usually patients with poor dental hygiene, dysphagia, odynophagia, trismus, and edema of the upper midline neck and marked floor of the mouth edema

- Second and third molars usually the odontogenic cause
- Bilateral submandibular space and lingual space infection
- Rapidly spreading cellulitis, brawny induration of suprahyoid region, and elevation of the tongue
- Tongue can be rapidly displaced, leading to airway compromise
- Early signs and symptoms of imminent airway collapse may be subtle and many patients will require awake fiberoptic intubation
- Stridor, difficulty managing secretions, anxiety, and cyanosis are late signs and require emergency airway management
- Involvement of the epiglottis is not uncommon
- Airway emergency

DIAGNOSIS

- Clinical diagnosis

TREATMENT

- IV high-dose penicillin and metronidazole
- Clindamycin if penicillin allergic
- Immediate oral maxillofacial or ENT consultation

Stomatitis

- Causes: aphthous, herpes simplex, varicella zoster, herpangina, coxsackie virus

Herpes stomatitis

SIGNS AND SYMPTOMS

- Prodrome of burning or tingling
- Acute painful ulceration of the gingiva and mucosal surfaces, fever, and lymphadenopathy
- Vesicular lesions appear and rupture after 1 to 2 days, leaving ulcers that heal over 1 to 2 weeks

DIAGNOSIS

- Visual diagnosis
- May send culture if first episode

TREATMENT

- Symptomatic
- May use antivirals (e.g., acyclovir) if during prodromal phase

Varicella-zoster stomatitis

SIGNS AND SYMPTOMS

- Common involvement of the mucosa and precedes the skin lesions
- Zoster along the distribution of the trigeminal nerve
- 1- to 4-day prodrome of headache, toothache, vesicular eruptions unilaterally
- Lesions lasting 7 to 10 days

DIAGNOSIS

- Visual diagnosis along with history

TREATMENT

- Symptomatic
- May use antivirals (e.g., acyclovir) if during prodromal phase
- Isolated intraoral lesion may also occur with involvement of the ophthalmologic branch of trigeminal nerve—requires urgent ophthalmologic consultation

Herpangina

- Coxsackie virus group A (most common)
- Summer and autumn

SIGNS AND SYMPTOMS

- Sudden-onset high fever, sore throat, malaise, headache—then an eruption of oral vesicles
- Vesicles rupture leaving ulcerations
- Lasts 7 to 10 days

DIAGNOSIS

- Clinical diagnosis

TREATMENT

- Supportive

Hand, foot, and mouth disease (Coxsackie virus)

SIGNS AND SYMPTOMS

- Few small vesicles on the tongue, gingiva, soft palate, buccal mucosa
- Also involves hands (palmar), feet (plantar), and buttocks to varying degrees
- Fever is of short duration

DIAGNOSIS

- Clinical diagnosis

TREATMENT

- Supportive

Oral candidiasis

- Infection by *Candida albicans*

SIGNS AND SYMPTOMS

- Patches of gray or white friable material covering an erythematous base on the buccal mucosa, gingiva, tongue, palate, or tonsils
- Fissures or crust at the corners of the mouth may be present
- AIDS-defining illness, and immunosuppression should be considered in the absence of dentures, inhaled steroids, or antibiotic use

DIAGNOSIS

- Clinical diagnosis and the ability to scrape off the gray or white friable material exposing an erythematous base

TREATMENT

- Clotrimazole troches dissolved in the mouth five times daily
- If topical therapy is not effective or if chronic oral candidiasis, oral ketoconazole, itraconazole, or fluconazole can be used
- Dentures should be soaked overnight in a dilute sodium hypochlorite solution

DISEASES OF THE SALIVARY GLAND

Sialolithiasis

- Found most commonly between 30 and 50 years of age; rare in children
- Most common gland affected is submandibular/submaxillary in 80% to 95% of cases

SIGNS AND SYMPTOMS

- Pain and swelling of the gland, frequently rapid onset
- Most common viral pathogen is mumps
- *S. aureus, Streptococcus viridans, S. pneumoniae,* and *H. influenzae* predominate in bacterial infections

DIAGNOSIS

- Stones confirmed by palpation or purulent discharge from the glandular duct with massage
- Ultrasound can be helpful

TREATMENT

- Treatment is antibiotics, moist heat, massage, sialogogues, hydration
- Follow-up within 24 hours should be arranged for stones not removed in the emergency department and 4 to 5 days otherwise

Suppurative parotitis

- Potentially fatal in patients with compromised salivary flow
- Caused by retrograde migration of oral bacteria into the salivary ducts and parenchyma

SIGNS AND SYMPTOMS

- Onset is rapid
- Skin over the parotid is red and tender, overlies angle of mandible
- Pus may be expressed from the Stenson duct
- Fever and trismus
- Predisposing factors: recent anesthesia, dehydration, prematurity or advanced age, sialolithiasis and oral neoplasms, salivary duct strictures, tracheostomy, and ductal foreign body
- Medications that can cause either systemic dehydration or decrease salivary flow—e.g., diuretics, antihistamines, tricyclic antidepressants, phenothiazines, beta-adrenergic blockers, and barbiturates

- Caused usually by *S. aureus*—less often by *S. pneumoniae, Streptococcus pyogenes,* and *H. influenzae* or anaerobes such as *Bacteriodies* species
- Severe chronic illness also a predisposing factor
  - HIV, hepatic failure, malnutrition, depression, anorexia/bulimia, hyperuricemia

DIAGNOSIS

- Clinical
- Differentiate from cellulitis by drainage from the Stenson duct
- Imaging not needed unless the patient fails to improve after 48 hours of treatment
- CT or ultrasound if abscess suspected

TREATMENT

- Emergent ENT consultation
- Amoxicillin–clavulanate, ampicillin–sulbactam
- In immunocompromised—treat *Escherichia coli, Pseudomonas*
- Cultures of Stenson duct drainage can guide therapy
- Optimize salivary flow
- Outpatient treatment appropriate—if not sick, able to take oral liquids, oral antibiotics, otherwise inpatient admission

FOREIGN BODIES OF THE OROPHARYNX AND THROAT

SIGNS AND SYMPTOMS

- Asymptomatic or dysphagia, odynophagia, drooling, and wheezing and cough

DIAGNOSIS

- Visual inspection, history, lateral soft-tissue neck radiography, CT if necessary

TREATMENT

- Airway management
- Emergent ENT consultation for removal

GINGIVAL AND PERIODONTAL DISORDERS

Gingivostomatitis

- Stomatitis caused by herpes simplex-1 virus (discussed under stomatitis) or acute necrotizing ulcerative gingivostomatitis

Acute necrotizing ulcerative gingivostomatitis (ANUG) (Fig. 7-11)

SIGNS AND SYMPTOMS

- Anaerobic infection
- Secondary signs include fetid breath, pseudo-membrane formation, wooden teeth sensation,

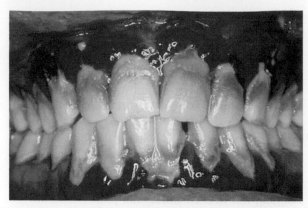

Figure 7-11. Necrotizing ulcerative gingivitis in a cigarette smoker. (From Little JW et al: *Dental management of the medically compromised patient,* ed 7, Philadelphia, 2007, Mosby.)

metallic taste, tooth mobility, lymphadenopathy, fever, malaise
- Opportunistic infection in immunocompromised

DIAGNOSIS

- Visual inspection
- Diagnostic triad of pain, ulcerated or punched-out interdental papillae, gingival bleeding

TREATMENT

- Chlorhexidine rinses and metronidazole or penicillin

PHARYNGITIS/TONSILLITIS

- Viral, bacterial, or fungal etiology

Viral pharyngitis

SIGNS AND SYMPTOMS

- Vesicular or petechial pattern on the soft palate and tonsils
- Associated with rhinorrhea
- Usually no tonsillar exudates or lymphadenopathy

DIAGNOSIS

- Tests not indicated unless caused by influenza, infectious mononucleosis, acute retroviral syndrome

TREATMENT

- Treatment is supportive

Streptococcal pharyngitis

- Group A beta hemolytic *Streptococcus* causative organism

SIGNS AND SYMPTOMS

- Incubation of 2 to 5 days
- Sore throat, odynophagia, chills, fever

- Headache, nausea, and vomiting common
- Marked erythema of the tonsils and tonsillar pillars, tonsillar exudates, enlarged and tender cervical lymph nodes, uvular edema
- Fever, myalgia, and malaise, but no rhinorrhea
- CDC criteria: tonsillar exudates, tender anterior cervical lymph node, absence of cough, history of fever

DIAGNOSIS

- Clinical diagnosis
- Rapid streptococcal testing
- Culture

TREATMENT

- Culture if suspecting other bacterial causes such as *N. gonorrhoeae,* or *Corynebacterium diphtheriae*—gray adherent membrane to tonsillar or pharyngeal surface may extend to the uvula soft palate, larynx
- CDC criteria for treatment of streptococcal pharyngitis:
  - No antibiotic treatment if one criterion
  - If two to three criteria, treatment based on rapid streptococcal testing results
    - Treat with penicillin for 10 days, or oral second-generation cephalosporin—or macrolide (but macrolide resistance increasing) if all 4 CDC criteria

Fungal pharyngitis

- *C. albicans*

SIGNS AND SYMPTOMS

- Whitish exudates that can be scraped off to reveal an erythematous base
- May have candidal infection in other parts of oropharynx simultaneously

DIAGNOSIS

- Visual diagnosis combined with the ability to scrape gray or white discharge from erythematous mucosa

TREATMENT

- Nystatin oral suspension 4 to 6 mL swish and swallow four times a day, or clotrimazole troches dissolved in mouth five times daily for 5 to 7 days

PERITONSILLAR ABSCESS

- Most frequently occurring deep space infection of the head and neck
- Collection of purulent material between the tonsillar capsule and the superior constrictor and the palatopharyngeal muscle
- Rick factors include chronic tonsillitis, multiple trials of oral antibiotics, previous peritonsillar abscess

- Most common between 2nd and 3rd decades and can be bilateral

SIGNS AND SYMPTOMS

- Fever, malaise, "hot potato" voice, sore throat, odynophagia, dysphagia, and otalgia
- Signs include trismus, inferior and medial displacement of the infected tonsils, contralateral displacement of the uvula, palatal edema, tender cervical adenopathy, drooling dehydration

DIAGNOSIS

- Visual diagnosis
- Differential diagnosis includes peritonsillar cellulitis, infectious mononucleosis, herpes simplex tonsillitis, retropharyngeal abscess, epiglottis, neoplasm, foreign body, internal carotid artery aneurysm

TREATMENT

- Treatment by needle aspiration or incision and drainage
- The needle should be introduced lateral to the tonsil approximately halfway between the base of the uvula and the maxillary alveolar ridge; the needle should be inserted no more than 1 cm because the internal carotid artery usually lies laterally and posteriorly to the posterior edge of the tonsil
  - Complications of needle aspiration of a peritonsillar abscess include airway obstruction, rupture of the abscess, bleeding, cavernous sinus thrombosis, epiglottitis, endocarditis, septicemia, retropharyngeal abscess, mediastinitis
- Following needle aspiration, antibiotics for 10 days—high-dose penicillin VK or clindamycin
- Follow-up is needed 24 hours after aspiration
- If not improving, consider reaspiration, ENT consultation

Larynx/trachea

EPIGLOTTITIS

- Most cases in adults since the *H. influenzae* vaccine
- Causative organisms—*H. influenzae, Streptococcus* species, *Staphylococcus* species, viruses, fungi although most frequently no organism can be isolated

SIGNS AND SYMPTOMS

- Typical history is 1- to 2-day history of worsening dysphagia, odynophagia, and dyspnea, particularly in the supine position
- Symptoms include fever, tachycardia, cervical adenopathy, drooling, and pain, with gentle palpation of the larynx and upper trachea
- Stridor is primarily inspiratory, and is softer and lower than in croup

- Patients often position themselves sitting up, leaning forward, mouth open, head extended and panting
- Thick oropharyngeal secretions are commonly present with little or no cough

DIAGNOSIS

- Diagnosis is made by history, clinical examination, radiographs, and laryngoscopy
- Lateral soft tissue cervical radiographs demonstrate obliteration of the vallecula, swelling of the aryepiglottic folds, edema of the prevertebral and retropharyngeal soft tissues and ballooning of the hypopharynx; the epiglottis appears enlarged and thumb-shaped (Fig. 7-12)
- Direct fiberoptic visualization can confirm the diagnosis in adults—should be done with caution because of sudden unpredictable airway obstruction

TREATMENT

- Immediate ENT consultation
- Definitive airway planning
- Humidified oxygen, IV hydration
- Cardiac monitoring and pulse oximetry
- Intravenous antibiotics—cefotaxime ceftriaxone, ampicillin–sulbactam
- In adults requiring airway management—awake fiberoptic intubation in the operating theater—ENT prepared for immediate awake tracheostomy or cricothyroidotomy
- In the ED, endotracheal intubation may be performed if absolutely necessary, but difficult airway preparation necessary
- Consider steroids as in severe pharyngitis for reduction of airway edema

LARYNGITIS

SIGNS AND SYMPTOMS

- Hoarseness and aphonia
- Usually caused by upper respiratory tract infection
- In up to 10% of cases, bacteria such as streptococcal organisms or diphtheria may be responsible

DIAGNOSIS

- Clinical diagnosis, consider epiglottitis

TREATMENT

- Symptomatic treatment, consider steroids
- Antibiotics not needed unless a bacterial cause suspected

RETROPHARYNGEAL ABSCESS

- Space that extends from the skull base to the tracheal bifurcation contains lymph nodes that drain the nasopharynx, adenoids, and posterior nasal sinuses—more common in children
- A retropharyngeal abscess in adults is generally the direct extension of purulent debris from a neighboring soft tissue source (e.g., oropharynx)

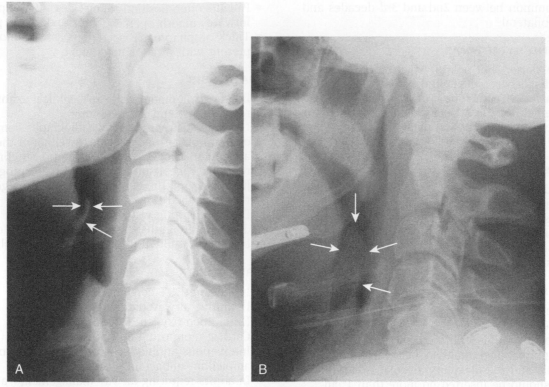

Figure 7-12. Normal epiglottis and epiglottitis. The normal epiglottis is well seen on the lateral soft tissue view of the neck (**A**) as a delicate curved structure. In a patient with epiglottitis (**B**), the epiglottis is swollen and significantly reduces the diameter of the airway. (From Mettler FA, Jr: *Essentials of radiology,* ed 2, Philadelphia, 2005, Saunders.)

SIGNS AND SYMPTOMS

- Fever, dysphagia, neck pain, limitation of cervical motion, cervical lymphadenopathy, sore throat, poor oral intake, muffled "hot potato" voice, respiratory distress
- Stridor and neck edema are likely in children but not in adults
- The intense pain and swelling associated with a retropharyngeal abscess can lead to inflammatory torticollis toward the affected side

DIAGNOSIS

- Cultures are usually polymicrobial—most common anaerobic species are *S. viridans* and *S. pyogenes.* Most staph species are B-lactamase producing, *Bacteroides* and *Peptostreptococcus* are most commonly islolated anaerobes
- Contrast-enhanced CT of the neck
- Lateral soft tissue of neck can be misleading, especially in children—even a small degree of flexion causes bowing of the posterior wall of the pharynx

TREATMENT

- Immediate ENT consultation
- Intravenous hydration and broad-spectrum antibiotic treatment should be initiated
- Complications include extension into the mediastinum and upper airway asphyxia from direct pressure or sudden rupture of the abscess

TEMPOROMANDIBULAR JOINT PAIN (TMJ)

- Articular surfaces are separated by the articular cartilage, which assists the hinge action between the mandibular condyle and the disk and the gliding action between the disk and the temporal bone
- The masseter, temporalis, and medial pterygoid muscles close the mandible (lateral pterygoid serves to open the jaw)
- The jaw is opened by forward traction on the mandibular neck by the lower portion of the lateral pterygoid with assistance from the digastric, mylohyoid, and geniohyoid muscles
- Chronic TMJ pain probably results from variety of causes (neuromuscular disturbance, trauma, congenital issues, dental problems, or systemic disease)

SIGNS AND SYMPTOMS

- No significant correlation between occlusal parameters or bruxism
- Degenerative joint disease may result from chronic internal derangement or systemic disease
- Pain may be localized to one of the muscles of mastication; masseter is most common

DIAGNOSIS

- Clinical
- Physical findings include limitation in the range of motion of the mandible

- Isolated clicking without pain or other dysfunction—not necessarily TMJ
- Palpate the muscles of mastication to find areas of tenderness, induration, or swelling
- No acute need for radiographs—best evaluated by outpatient MRI

TREATMENT

- Symptomatic pain treatment

HEENT cancers

ORAL CANCER

- Squamous cell carcinoma in more than 90%
- Rest are usually lymphomas, Kaposi sarcomas, and melanoma
- Extrinsic factors include tobacco use, especially chewing tobacco or snuff, excessive alcohol consumption, and sunlight exposure
- Intrinsic factors include general malnutrition and chronic iron-deficiency anemia
- Oral candidiasis, immunosuppressive states, and oncogenic viruses may play some role

SIGNS AND SYMPTOMS

- Common morphologic presentations—exophytic, or ulcerative with irregular surfaces, malignant leukoplakia (white lesions that do not scrape off)
- Posterior–lateral border of tongue most common location
- Frequently painless

DIAGNOSIS

- Biopsy

TREATMENT

- Lesions that do not respond to palliative treatment in 10 to 14 days warrant biopsy
- Discharge home unless toxic or serious extension beyond the sinus cavity

NECK TUMORS

- Relatively common finding
- Oral, head, and neck cancer accounts for 3% of all cancers

SIGNS AND SYMPTOMS

- Risk factors include alcohol and tobacco use, viruses such as herpes, sunlight exposure, genetics, diet, exposure to dust, and inhalational exposure
- Dysphagia, odynophagia, otalgia, stridor, changes in speech, and globus sensation
- Referred ear pain is an ominous sign and is presumed to be caused by cancerous lesion
- Hoarseness is usually a late symptom

DIAGNOSIS

- Physical examination

TREATMENT

- Hoarseness for more than 2 weeks should be investigated with fiberoptic examination
- Chest radiographs may be helpful in identifying associated lung masses
- Referral for imaging and/or biopsy
- Any airway symptoms should lead to prompt ENT consultation

PEARLS

- Clean perforations of the tympanic membrane do not need topical antibiotics.

- Hordeolum—pain; chalazion—no pain.

- *Hutchinson sign* in herpes zoster—vesicular rash includes the tip of the nose due to nasociliary nerve involvement.

- Hyphema can be spontaneous in sickle cell disease.

- Avoid carbonic anhydrase inhibitors for increased pressure with sickle cell hyphema—the lower pH can increase sickling, clog outflow, and paradoxically raise the pressure.

- Cherry red spot—central retinal artery occlusion.

- Blood and thunder fundus—central retinal vein occlusion.

- Lateral gaze palsy—most common/earliest ophthalmologic sign of cavernous sinus thrombosis.

- Pott's puffy tumor—soft tissue swelling with pitting edema over frontal region; reflects frontal sinusitis with frontal bone osteomyelitis.

- Severe sore throat with relatively benign appearing oropharynx—consider advanced diagnostic adjuncts (e.g., nasopharyngolaryngoscopy) to rule-out other serious disorders (e.g., epiglottitis).

BIBLIOGRAPHY

Alexander JL, Samadi RR, Burton J: Nose/sinus. In Aghababian R, Allison EJ, Boyer EW, Braen GR, Manno MM, Moorhead JC, Volturo GA (eds): *Essentials of emergency medicine*, ed 1, Sudbury, 2006, Jones and Bartlett, p. 228.

Amsterdam JT: Oral medicine. In Marx JA, Hockberger RS, Walls RM (eds): *Rosen's emergency medicine: concepts and clinical practice*, ed 6, Philadelphia, 2006, Mosby, p. 892.

Beaudeau RW: Oral and dental emergencies. In Tintinalli JE, Kelen GD, Stapczynski JS (eds): *Emergency medicine: a comprehensive study guide*, ed 6, New York, 2004, McGraw-Hill, p. 1482.

Brunette DD: Ophthalmology. In Marx JA, Hockberger RS, Walls RM (eds): *Rosen's emergency medicine: concepts and clinical practice*, ed 6, Philadelphia, 2006, Mosby, p. 1044.

Deflitch CJ: Throat and oropharynx. In Aghababian R, Allison EJ, Boyer EW, Braen GR, Manno MM, Moorhead JC, Volturo GA (eds): *Essentials of emergency medicine*, ed 1, Sudbury, 2006, Jones and Bartlett, p. 237.

Gilbert DN, Moellering RC, Eliopoulos GM et al (eds): *The sanford guide to antimicrobial therapy 2009*, ed 39, Sperryville, Va, 2009, Antimicrobial Therapy Inc.

Haddon R, Peacock WF: Face and jaw emergencies. In Tintinalli JE, Kelen GD, Stapczynski JS (eds): *Emergency medicine: a comprehensive study guide*, ed 6, New York, 2004, McGraw-Hill, p. 1471.

Leaming JM: External eye. In Aghababian R, Allison EJ, Boyer EW, Braen GR, Manno MM, Moorhead JC, Volturo GA (eds): *Essentials of emergency medicine*, ed 1, Sudbury, 2006, Jones and Bartlett, p. 242.

Lee L: Disorders of the external ear. In Aghababian R, Allison EJ, Boyer EW, Braen GR, Manno MM, Moorhead JC, Volturo GA (eds): *Essentials of emergency medicine*, ed 1, Sudbury, Mass, 2006, Jones and Bartlett, p. 223.

Mitchell JD: Ocular emergencies. In Tintinalli JE, Kelen GD, Stapczynski JS (eds): *Emergency medicine: a comprehensive study guide*, ed 6, New York, 2004, McGraw-Hill, p. 1449.

Pfaff JP, Moore GP: Otolaryngology. In Marx JA, Hockberger RS, Walls RM (eds): *Rosen's emergency medicine: concepts and clinical practice*, ed 6, Philadelphia, 2006, Mosby, p. 928.

Rubin MA, Gonzales R, Sande MA: Pharyngitis, sinusitis, otitis, and other upper respiratory tract infections. In: Fauci AS, Braunwald E, Kasper DL et al (eds): *Harrison's principles of internal medicine*, ed 17, New York, 2008, McGraw Hill, pp. 205–214.

Tintinalli A, Lucchesi M: Common disorders of the external, middle and inner ear. In Tintinalli JE, Kelen GD, Stapczynski JS (eds): *Emergency medicine: a comprehensive study guide*, ed 6, New York, 2004, McGraw-Hill, p. 1464.

Waters TA, Peacock WF: Nasal emergencies and sinusitis. In Tintinalli JE, Kelen GD, Stapczynski JS (eds): *Emergency medicine: a comprehensive study guide*, ed 6, New York, 2004, McGraw-Hill, p. 1476.

Questions and Answers

1. An 8-day-old child is brought into the emergency department by her parents. The child has had eye discharge for the last day, as well as redness of the eye. The most appropriate management of this patient includes:

   a. no culture, administer ceftriaxone IM
   b. culture the discharge, administer ceftriaxone IM
   c. culture the discharge, prescribe topical erythromycin
   d. culture the discharge, prescribe topical and oral erythromycin
   e. no culture, prescribe oral erythromycin

2. A 24-year-old welder presents to the emergency department complaining of severe eye pain and photophobia several hours after finishing his work. He reports that he forgot to bring his eye protection to work that day. The findings most likely to be seen on fluorescein examination of the eyes are:

   a. dendrites
   b. a single, large area of fluorescein uptake in one eye
   c. multiple punctate corneal epithelial defects bilaterally
   d. wedge-shaped growth of fibrovascular tissue extending from the conjunctiva onto the cornea
   e. yellowish growth on the conjunctiva on the nasal side near the cornea

3. A vesicular rash that includes the tip of the nose may be a sign of which of the following?

   a. ocular involvement with herpes simplex infection
   b. corneal ulceration
   c. gonococcal conjunctivitis
   d. complications of contact lens use
   e. ocular involvement of herpes zoster infection

4. A 35-year-old woman presents to the emergency department with 6 days of face and dental pain and purulent nasal drainage. The patient does not have any other medical history and has no allergies to medication. The most appropriate therapy for this patient is:

   a. symptomatic treatment with a humidifier
   b. a 7-day course of trimethoprim–sulfamethoxazole
   c. pain medication, and a 7-day course of trimethoprim–sulfamethoxazole
   d. symptomatic treatment with nasal decongestant spray
   e. symptomatic treatment with nasal decongestant spray and a 5-day course of amoxicillin

5. A 21-year-old man presents in obvious distress 2 weeks after cracking a molar, with stridor, dysphagia, odynophagia, trismus, and edema of the midline neck and tongue. The most appropriate management of this patient includes:

   a. IV penicillin, attempt at orotracheal intubation with rapid sequence induction
   b. emergent otolaryngology consultation, IV clindamycin
   c. IV clindamycin and admission to the ICU
   d. IV pain medication, IV clindamycin and admission the ICU
   e. IV penicillin and awake fiberoptic intubation

6. An 80-year-old woman presents with 2 days of fever, and erythema and tenderness over her parotid gland. Which of the following is true regarding this patient's illness?

   a. involvement of the Wharton ducts is common
   b. *Pseudomonas aeruginosa* is a causative agent
   c. recent anesthesia is a risk factor
   d. treatment consists of antihistamines, heat, and massage
   e. aspiration by needle is usually needed

7. An 18-year-old man presents with 1 to 2 days of worsening dysphagia, odynophagia, and dyspnea which seems to worsen on laying supine. He is noted to have inspiratory stridor and drooling. He is tender over his larynx with gentle palpation. Appropriate steps in the management of this patient include:

   a. evaluation of the supraglottic region with a fiberoptic scope, IV hydration, IV antibiotics
   b. prolonged examination of the posterior pharynx, and humidified oxygen
   c. IV hydration, IV steroids, emergent ENT consultation, ultrasound of the posterior pharynx
   d. emergent rapid sequence intubation, IV antibiotics, IV hydration, IV steroids
   e. antibiotics and steroids orally, nebulized epinephrine

8. Which of the following is true regarding retropharyngeal abscess?

   a. the retropharyngeal space ends at the base of the neck
   b. the infection is commonly due to streptococcal species
   c. tenderness over the larynx is common
   d. stridor and neck edema are common in adults
   e. contrast-enhanced CT is the gold standard for diagnosis

9. A 65-year-old man presents with unilateral roaring tinnitus, and sudden vertigo of 20 minutes duration associated with nausea, vomiting, and diaphoresis. What would be the next most appropriate step?

   a. obtain a head CT
   b. obtain an MRI
   c. IV diphenhydramine
   d. IV diazepam
   e. neurology consultation

10. A 72-year-old woman presents with sudden-onset painless vision loss of her left eye. On funduscopic examination, her fundus is noted to be pale with a cherry-red fovea. Which of the following is the best immediate treatment?

    a. ocular massage
    b. IV acetazolamide
    c. IV mannitol
    d. ophthalmologic consultation
    e. IV thrombolytics

11. Which of the following best describes choroiditis?

    a. inflammation of the stromal layer between the retina and sclera
    b. can be seen in patients with herpes zoster
    c. sudden vision loss
    d. lack of eye redness
    e. lack of photophobia

12. Which of the following best describes the symptoms seen in retinal detachment?

    a. light flashes, dark floating specks, curtain-like visual field defect, peripheral or central vision loss
    b. light flashes, floaters, curtain-like visual field defect, peripheral vision loss only
    c. blinding light, eye pain, central vision loss
    d. light flashes, eye pain, curtain-like visual field defect
    e. light flashes, floaters, eye pain, curtain-like visual field defect

13. A 24-year-old without previous medical history or allergies presents with redness and swelling to the left eyelid for 7 days. On examination, there is marked swelling and redness of both the upper and lower left eyelids. The patient is noted to have a temperature of 38.0° C. There are no vision changes, extra-ocular movements are intact without significant pain, and pupillary response to light is brisk. Which of the following is the most appropriate treatment?

    a. emergent ophthalmologic consultation
    b. admission to the hospital for IV piperacillin-tazobactam
    c. lid hygiene with mild soap and water
    d. erythromycin ophthalmic ointment and lid hygiene with mild soap and water
    e. outpatient treatment with amoxicillin–clavulanate

14. The following is true of posterior epistaxis:

    a. usually originates from Kiesselbach plexus
    b. usually unilateral in bleeding from nares
    c. usually in younger patients
    d. usually a result of dry nasal mucosa
    e. bleeding is more profuse than in anterior epistaxis

15. A 55-year-old man with coronary artery disease and a recent myocardial infarction presents with sudden complete painless vision loss in his right eye. The expected finding on funduscopic exam is:

    a. whitening of the retina with a cherry-red spot in the center of the fovea
    b. blood in the posterior pole of the eye blocking the fundus
    c. diffuse retinal hemorrhages in all quadrants of the retina, dilated and tortuous retinal veins, cotton wool spots, optic disc edema, and retinal edema
    d. a normal funduscopic exam
    e. papilledema

16. In what disease is Bezold abscess seen?

    a. otitis media
    b. otitis externa
    c. mastoiditis
    d. sinusitis
    e. orbital cellulitis

17. Which of the following diseases or disease processes is most likely linked to the formation of a cavernous sinus thrombosis?
    a. abscess of the posterior neck
    b. otitis media
    c. manipulation of a nostril furuncle
    d. retained foreign body of the nose
    e. foreign body of the ear

18. A 65-year-old woman walks into a movie theater and has sudden-onset pain in her right eye. Her vision is decreased, and she sees "halos" around objects. Which option is the definitive treatment for the patient's condition?
    a. ocular massage
    b. pilocarpine and acetazolamide
    c. timolol and acetazolamide
    d. pilocarpine and timolol and acetazolamide
    e. ophthalmologic surgery

19. Which statement best describes the symptoms of labyrinthitis?
    a. vertigo and otitis externa
    b. vertigo with hearing loss
    c. roaring tinnitus and vertigo
    d. ophthalmoplegia and vertigo
    e. dental pain and vertigo

20. A 48-year-old patient presents with a neck mass of 2 weeks' duration. Which of the following symptoms is most predictive that the mass is cancerous?
    a. referred ear pain
    b. dysphagia
    c. odynophagia
    d. stridor
    e. feeling of a "lump in the throat"

---

1. Answer: d

Ophthalmia neonatorum refers to conjunctivitis that occurs in the first month of life. Most commonly, this is due to hypersensitivity to ointments administered after birth if it occurs in the first 2 days. From days 2 through 4, it is most commonly due to gonorrhea. From days 5 to 14, it is most commonly due to chlamydia acquired in transit through the birth canal. All patients with ophthalmia neonatorum should have the discharge cultured (thus **a** and **e** are incorrect). Ceftriaxone is the treatment for gonococcal conjunctivitis **(b)**. Because of the age at presentation, this child likely has chlamydial conjunctivitis, and the appropriate treatment is **both topical and oral antibiotics (c)**. All children with ophthalmia neonatorum should have close follow-up with an ophthalmologist.

2. Answer: c

This patient has a presentation that is typical of *superficial punctate keratitis* **(c)**, which demonstrates

multiple punctate corneal epithelial defects on fluorescein examination. **Dendrites** are characteristic of herpes simplex infection **(a)**. **A single large area of fluorescein uptake** is commonly seen with corneal abrasions **(b)**. A wedge-shaped growth of fibrovascular tissue extending onto the conjunctiva is known as a **pterygium (d)**, and **pinguecula** are yellowish growths on the nasal side of the conjunctiva **(e)**.

3. Answer: e

A dermatomal vesicular rash that includes the tip of the nose is known as the *Hutchinson sign*. This signals possible **ocular involvement due to herpes zoster** involving branches of the nasociliary nerve. **Herpes simplex infection** is diagnosed when **dendrites** are seen after corneal staining **(a)**. **Corneal ulceration (b)** appears as a white "spot" on the cornea. **Gonococcal conjunctivitis (c)** presents like other conjunctivitis, but with exaggerated symptoms and physical findings. Contact lens use **(d)** is associated with many complications, including corneal abrasion and ulceration, but not with a vesicular rash.

4. Answer: d

Acute sinusitis may present with sinus pain and tenderness in the face and teeth and purulent nasal secretions of more than 7 days' duration. Treatment mainly consists of **nasal decongestant sprays** (for less than 5 days of symptoms) and the possible addition of a **steroid nasal spray. Antibiotics** should be considered only if symptom duration is longer than 7 days, underlying immunocompromise, or severe symptoms regardless of duration.

5. Answer: e

Ludwig angina is characterized by the presence of rapidly spreading cellulitis of the subhyoid region and the tongue, leading to symptoms of dysphagia, odynophagia, trismus, and edema of the tongue and airway compromise. Stridor, difficulty managing secretions, anxiety, and cyanosis are late signs and require emergent airway management. Imminent airway collapse may be rapid and require **awake fiberoptic intubation (e)**. Emergent consultation of otolaryngology or maxillofacial surgery is warranted. **IV clindamycin** or **IV penicillin** may be used to treat the underlying infection.

6. Answer: c

Suppurative parotitis is caused by retrograde migration of bacteria into the parotid gland. Pus may be expressed or seen coming from the Stenson duct. Predisposing factors are recent anesthesia, advanced age, and dehydration **(c)**. Treatment is usually IV antibiotics and optimization of salivary flow and usually requires hospital admission; however, if the patient appears well, outpatient treatment may be appropriate. Emergent consultation with otolaryngology is warranted.

7. Answer: a

Most cases of *epiglottitis* are in adults since the *H. Influenzae* vaccine. Symptoms are rapid onset over 1 to 2 days and include dysphagia, odynophagia, and dyspnea, particularly in the supine position. Symptoms include tachycardia, fever, cervical adenopathy, drooling, and pain with palpation of the larynx and upper trachea. Direct fiberoptic visualization can confirm the diagnosis and the need for intubation in adults. If the patient's condition requires emergent intubation, endotracheal intubation should be attempted but alternative methods should be considered in advance in the event of a difficult intubation and failure of endotracheal intubation. IV cefuroxime, ceftriaxone, or ampicillin-sulbactam is recommended. Humidified oxygen may decrease the risk for sudden airway blockage due to secretions.

8. Answer: e

The **retropharyngeal space** extends from the skull **base to the bifurcation of the trachea.** *Retropharyngeal abscess* is characterized by fever, dysphagia, neck pain, limitation of cervical motion, cervical adenopathy, muffled voice, and respiratory distress. Stridor and neck edema are not common findings in adults. The **infection is usually polymicrobial** with both aerobic and anaerobic bacteria. **Contrast-enhanced CT is the criterion standard for diagnosis.**

9. Answer: c

Ménière disease can affect patients aged 65 or over and occurs equally in men and women. Although usually unilateral symptoms occur initially, both ears may be affected over time. Onset of vertigo is sudden, and duration ranges from 20 minutes to 12 hours and is associated with nausea, vomiting, and diaphoresis. Other associated symptoms include roaring tinnitus, diminished hearing, and fullness in the ear. **Antihistamines** are used for symptomatic management. No drug improves hearing.

10. Answer: a

Central retinal artery occlusion is characterized by acute-onset sudden dramatic painless vision loss and may progress over seconds. First line of treatment is to attempt to break up the clot with **ocular massage. Ophthalmology should be urgently consulted (d),** but ocular massage should be attempted while awaiting consultation.

11. Answer: b

Choroiditis and *chorioretinitis* are diseases characterized by inflammation of the vascular layer in between the retina and the sclera. It may be seen in patients with **herpes zoster infection,** posterior uveitis, or other inflammatory diseases. Signs and symptoms usually include unilateral blurred vision, the presence of floaters, mild pain, and photophobia. Funduscopic examination will show inflammatory lesions of the retina, mild disc edema, and neovascularization of the choroid plexus. Treatment consists of acyclovir if caused by herpes zoster infection or steroid therapy.

12. Answer: a

Retinal detachment is characterized by **light flashes, dark floating specks, curtain-like visual field defect, or peripheral or central vision loss.** Treatment is urgent consultation with ophthalmologist especially if the detachment is near the macula.

13. Answer: e

The patient has *preseptal cellulitis.* This condition is characterized by lack of involvement of visual acuity and papillary reaction and ocular movement without pain; the presence of these symptoms implies a deeper infection or postseptal cellulitis. Treatment of preseptal cellulitis is generally outpatient antibiotic treatment to cover *S. aureus.*

14. Answer: e

Posterior nose bleeds are more common in older patients. There is frequently a sensation of blood in or going down the back of the throat. **Bleeding is more profuse** than in anterior epistaxis and labs tests to identify anemia are frequently warranted. Although unilateral, blood may reflux to the other side so that it appears to be bilateral and identification of the affected side may be difficult. Direct pressure is ineffective and treatment consists of posterior packing along with anterior packing to prevent clot formation and aspiration risk. These patients with posterior packing are admitted to the hospital for cardio-respiratory monitoring.

15. Answer: a

The patient is at high risk for a *central retinal artery occlusion (CRAO)* because of his atherosclerotic history. CRAO presents as **sudden and acute painless, severe vision loss.** Other processes that cause painless vision loss that is acute are vitreous hemorrhage **(b)** and central retinal vein occlusion **(c).** The characteristic finding of CRAO on funduscopic exam is **whitening or a pale retina with a cherry-red spot** in the center of the fovea.

16. Answer: c

Bezold abscess is seen in **mastoiditis.** It is an abscess that is located at the lateral aspect of the neck inferior to the mastoid tip.

17. Answer: c

Cavernous sinus thrombosis is a medical emergency in which one of the cavernous sinuses located at the base of the skull posterior to the orbits becomes infected from a face, sinus, or ear infection. In as many of 25% of cases, a **manipulated nasal furuncle** is the precipitant etiology. Aseptic cavernous sinus thrombosis can occur in the setting of a space-occupying lesion involving the cavernous sinuses and the parasellar region, including tumors, carotid-cavernous sinus fistula, cavernous sinus aneurysm, and internal carotid aneurysm.

18. Answer: e

Acute closed-angle glaucoma represents an acute increase in intraocular pressure. Symptoms include sudden pain and decrease in vision after entering a dark area. "Halo" vision is also commonly described as a symptom in acute-angle closure glaucoma. There may be nausea, vomiting, headache, and photophobia associated with the pain and decrease vision. Intraocular pressure is frequently >50 mmHg and a mid-position, fixed pupil may be present on exam. Temporizing treatment consists of **pilocarpine, timolol, acetazolamide,** and **mannitol** but **definitive treatment is surgical. Ocular massage (a)** is used in the treatment of central retinal artery occlusion.

19. Answer: b

Labyrinthitis is an infection that may be bacterial or viral. Occasionally, it may occur from otitis media or a cholesteatoma. Hallmarks of the disease include **sudden-onset vertigo** with **associated hearing loss** and middle ear findings. Treatment should include antibiotics if middle ear findings are present and referral to an otorhinolaryngologist.

20. Answer: a

Oral, head, and neck cancer accounts for 3% of all cancers. Risk factors include alcohol and tobacco use, viruses such as herpes, sunlight exposure, genetics, diet, exposure to dust, and inhalational exposure. **Dysphagia, odynophagia, otalgia, stridor, speech disorders,** and a **"lump in the throat"** sensation **(b-e)** are common presenting symptoms with neck masses, with hoarseness usually occurring late. **Referred ear pain (a)** is an ominous sign and is presumed to be caused by a cancerous lesion.

Hematologic

8

Edward H. Seibert | Bernard Lopez

BLOOD TRANSFUSIONS—COMPLICATIONS
Acute
Delayed
HEMOSTATIC DISORDERS
Thrombus formation
Coagulation defects
LYMPHOMAS
Hodgkin lymphoma
Non-Hodgkin lymphoma (NHL)
PANCYTOPENIA
RED BLOOD CELL DISORDERS
Anemias
Polycythemia
Methemoglobinemia
WHITE BLOOD CELL DISORDERS
Leukemias
Multiple myeloma
COMPLICATIONS OF HEMATOLOGIC MALIGNANCIES
Hyperviscosity syndrome
Neutropenic fever
Spinal cord compression
Superior vena cava (SVC) syndrome
Acute tumor lysis syndrome
Hypercalcemia
Pericardial effusion

Blood transfusions—complications

ACUTE
Hemolytic

- **Intravascular** (acute intravascular hemolytic transfusion reaction)
  - Typically due to ABO incompatibility from clerical error
  - Caused by intravascular lysis of donor RBCs

SIGNS AND SYMPTOMS
- Sudden-onset fever, chills, headache, flushing, low back pain, nausea, vomiting, dyspnea, tachycardia, and hypotension (may progress to shock) shortly after start of transfusion
- Hemoglobinuria, hemoglobinemia

DIAGNOSIS
- Check paperwork for clerical error
- Send donor bag back to blood bank—consider culture
- Direct Coombs test on recipient's blood drawn post-transfusion (will detect host antibodies to donor RBCs within the recipient's circulation, unless donor cells have already been destroyed)
- Directly inspect recipient's plasma—if red, suspect hemoglobinemia
- Directly inspect patient's urine—if red, suspect hemoglobinuria
- CBC, chemistries, liver panel, coagulation profile, haptoglobin, lactate dehydrogenase (LDH)

TREATMENT
- Immediately stop transfusion
- Intravenous fluids (IVFs) through new tubing
- Consider furosemide or mannitol

Febrile nonhemolytic

- Typically seen in patients with multiple prior transfusions, or multiparous women (prior exposure to WBC and platelet antigens)

SIGNS AND SYMPTOMS
- Fever, chills shortly after start of transfusion

DIAGNOSIS
- Same workup as for acute intravascular hemolytic reaction (which must be excluded)
- Diagnosis can be made only when hemolytic reaction ruled out

TREATMENT

- Immediately stop transfusion
- IVF through new tubing
- Antipyretic
- Future transfusions may have to be leukoreduced

Allergic

SIGNS AND SYMPTOMS

- Mild—pruritus, urticaria
- Severe—bronchospasm, anaphylaxis

DIAGNOSIS

- Mild allergic reaction—no workup needed
- Severe allergic reaction—same workup as for acute intravascular hemolytic reaction (must be excluded)

TREATMENT

- Mild allergic reaction—temporarily stop transfusion—if patient responds to antihistamine, it may be resumed
- Severe allergic reaction—immediately stop transfusion, antihistamine, steroids, epinephrine, IVF

Transfusion-related acute lung injury

- Noncardiogenic pulmonary edema

SIGNS AND SYMPTOMS

- Develop within 1 to 6 hours of start of infusion
- Dyspnea
- Hypoxia, fever, hypotension, tachypnea, diffuse pulmonary infiltrates

DIAGNOSIS

- Chest x-ray (CXR)
- Can be difficult to differentiate from hypervolemia, but usually results from infusion volume that would be insufficient to produce fluid overload
- Same workup as for acute intravascular hemolytic reaction (which must be excluded)

TREATMENT

- Immediately stop transfusion
- Oxygen
- May require CPAP/BiPAP or intubation

Hypervolemic

- Can be prevented by transfusing 1 unit over 4 hours and administering diuretic
- Can be difficult to distinguish from other acute transfusion reactions initially, and therefore may require a workup to exclude acute intravascular hemolysis

Septic

- From bacterial contamination of stored blood (can be gram-positive or gram-negative)

SIGNS AND SYMPTOMS

- High fever, rigors, shock

DIAGNOSIS

- Same workup as for acute intravascular hemolytic reaction (which must be excluded) with a culture of the unused donor blood

TREATMENT

- Immediately stop transfusion
- Broad-spectrum antibiotics
- IVF

Massive transfusion

- Can cause:
  - Hypocalcemia and hypomagnesemia from chelation by citrate preservative
  - Hyperkalemia or hypokalemia
  - Coagulopathy
  - Hypothermia

DELAYED

Hemolytic

- Extravascular (delayed extravascular hemolytic transfusion reaction)
  - Can be acute, but more often delayed—does not typically present as an emergency (like acute intravascular hemolytic transfusion reaction)
  - Caused by antibodies reacting to non-ABO antigens
  - Antibody-coated donor RBCs are removed from the circulation by the spleen and liver before they are lysed, resulting in extravascular hemolysis (therefore no hemoglobinemia or hemoglobinuria)

SIGNS AND SYMPTOMS

- Typically asymptomatic, but may have fever

DIAGNOSIS

- Same workup as for acute intravascular hemolytic reaction
- Indirect hyperbilirubinemia, positive Direct Coombs test, falling hematocrit or hematocrit that does not rise as expected

TREATMENT

- Stop transfusion if acute
- Consider IVF
- Typically, no treatment necessary

Transfusion-associated graft-versus-host disease

- Donor lymphocytes recognize the immunocompromised recipient as foreign and attack host tissues

SIGNS AND SYMPTOMS

- Onset usually 4 to 10 days after transfusion
- Fever, nausea, vomiting, rash, diarrhea

DIAGNOSIS

- Same workup as for acute intravascular hemolytic reaction
- Can develop abnormal liver panel, pancytopenia

TREATMENT

- Typically fatal—no effective treatment (except stem cell transplant if suitable donor can be found in time)
- Can be prevented by irradiating donor blood prior to transfusing immunocompromised patients

Disease transmission

- Risk of contracting disease from blood transfusion:
  - HIV—1 in 2 million
  - Hepatitis B—1 in 137,000
  - Hepatitis C—1 in 1 million

Hemostatic disorders

THROMBUS FORMATION

- Thrombus forms when damage to the endothelium causes collagen and tissue factor to be exposed to flowing blood
- Exposed collagen causes adherence and activation of platelets, which then recruit more platelets
- Adhesion of platelets to the exposed collagen relies on von Willebrand factor
- Tissue factor activates the coagulation cascade that generates thrombin
- Thrombin converts fibrinogen to fibrin, which polymerizes to form long strands that cross-link to form insoluble clot with entrapped platelets and RBCs
- Thrombin also triggers the release of t-PA from endothelial cells, which activates plasmin
- Plasmin (as well as other proteins, including anti-thrombin III and proteins C and S) cause fibrinolysis, which regulates the process of hemostasis

COAGULATION DEFECTS

Warfarin overdose

- Warfarin inhibits synthesis of vitamin K–dependent clotting factors (II,VII, IX, X)

SIGNS AND SYMPTOMS

- Bleeding in patient on warfarin
- Abnormal PT/INR found during routine monitoring

DIAGNOSIS

- Elevated PT/INR in patient on warfarin

TREATMENT

- No bleeding
  - INR <5—lower or omit warfarin dose
  - INR = 5 to 9—omit next one to two warfarin doses or omit one dose and administer vitamin K orally (1 to 2.5 mg)
  - INR >9—omit warfarin, oral vitamin K (2.5 to 5 mg)
- Serious bleeding (and elevated INR, regardless of magnitude)
  - Vitamin K 10 mg by slow intravenous (IV) infusion
    - Anaphylaxis has been reported
  - Fresh frozen plasma (FFP) (start with 4 to 6 units), prothrombin complex concentrate (factor IX complex, Profilnine), or recombinant factor VIIa (NovoSeven)—the latter two factor concentrates correct coagulopathy more rapidly, but are associated with an increased risk for thromboembolic events
- In general, avoid subcutaneous administration of vitamin K

Heparin overdose

- Heparin activates antithrombin III
  - Coagulopathy from heparin can be reversed with protamine (1 mg IV neutralizes 100 units of heparin)
    - Protamine can also be used to as an antidote to low-molecular-weight heparin (LMWH), but will not reverse it completely

Liver disease

- Liver synthesizes nearly all clotting factors
- Coagulopathy can be corrected with vitamin K (if patient is vitamin K deficient) and FFP (or recombinant factor VIIa), but only if the patient is actively bleeding or requires an invasive procedure—elevated PT/INR do not correlate well with risk of bleeding in patients with liver disease

Hemophilias

- Hemophilia A and B—caused by sex-linked recessive inheritance of gene, which produces defective factor VIII (hemophilia A) or factor IX (hemophilia B)
- Hemophilia A is more common, but they are clinically indistinguishable from one another
- In both, the PTT is elevated
- Degree of clinical severity corresponds to the activity level of the deficient factor relative to normal
  - <1%—severe—frequent spontaneous bleeding into joints and soft tissues
  - 1% to 5%—moderate—occasional spontaneous bleeding into joints and soft tissues, excessive bleeding with surgery or trauma
  - >5%—mild—no spontaneous bleeding, excessive bleeding with surgery or trauma

SIGNS AND SYMPTOMS

- The vast majority of patients who are seen in the ED have a known diagnosis and are presenting

with complications of trauma or spontaneous bleeding
- Intra-articular and intramuscular bleeds are the most common complications in patients with moderate and severe hemophilia

DIAGNOSIS

- Typically already known

TREATMENT

- Replacement dosing of deficient factor is based on presenting complaint
  - For minor bleeding—replacement to 25% (of normal)
  - For severe bleeding—replacement to 50%
  - For life-threatening bleeding—replacement to 100%
  - For factor VIII, 1 U/kg raises the plasma level by 2%
  - For factor IX, 1 U/kg raises the plasma level by 1%
  - In the ED, it should be assumed that the hemophilia patient's baseline plasma level is zero
- Replacement factor is either recombinant or derived from human plasma (FFP, cryoprecipitate, concentrate—can be intermediate-purity, high-purity, or ultrapure)
  - Recombinant and highly purified factor concentrates greatly diminish or negate the risk of viral transmission
- DDAVP is the preferred initial therapy for bleeding in patients with mild to moderate hemophilia A (before factor replacement)—causes release of factor VIII and von Willebrand factor from endothelial cells
- Arthrocentesis is generally not indicated for hemarthrosis
- Any head trauma should warrant factor replacement to 50% activity level, evaluation with head CT, and admission for observation for at least 24 hours

von Willebrand disease

- Patients with von Willebrand disease are more likely to have mucocutaneous bleeding and less likely to have hemarthrosis than hemophiliacs
- Bleeding episodes are treated with factor VIII-VWF concentrate (Humate-P)—cryoprecipitate can be used if this is not available
- DDAVP is only effective in one of the three types of von Willebrand disease and should only be used in consultation with a hematologist (when treating bleeding in von Willebrand disease)

Disseminated intervascular coagulation (DIC)

- Caused by a variety of different medical disorders: infection, obstetrical complications, malignancies, traumatic injury, burns, heat stroke
- Results from loss of regulatory mechanisms of hemostasis

- Thrombin is overproduced, which promotes clotting
- Fibrin can obstruct small vessels, causing tissue ischemia and RBC destruction
- Coagulation factors and platelets are consumed, which promotes bleeding

SIGNS AND SYMPTOMS

- Bleeding
- Organ dysfunction
- May have laboratory abnormalities only, without overt clinical signs

DIAGNOSIS

- CBC—thrombocytopenia, possibly anemia
- Peripheral blood smear—schistocytes (may be seen, but not always)
- PT, PTT—prolonged
- D-dimer—elevated
- Fibrinogen level—decreased

TREATMENT

- If bleeding predominates—FFP or cryoprecipitate, platelet transfusion as needed
- If thrombosis predominates (which happens more commonly in patients with chronic DIC)—consider heparin (generally not appropriate for acute DIC)

Platelet disorders

- Thrombocytopenia (decreased platelets)—can be due to decreased production, splenic sequestration, increased destruction (drugs, infection, idiopathic thrombocytopenic purpura [ITP], DIC, thrombotic thrombocytopenic purpura [TTP]), or dilution (from massive blood transfusion)
- Thrombotic microangiopathies—include TTP and Hemolytic uremic syndrome (HUS) (which are very similar and difficult to distinguish from one another), characterized by formation of platelet-rich thrombi in end arterioles and capillaries

TTP

- Classic pentad (present in 40% of patients with TTP)
  - Microangiopathic hemolytic anemia
  - Thrombocytopenia
  - Neurologic symptoms
  - Fever
  - Renal dysfunction (usually mild)
- More common triad (in 75% of patients on presentation)
  - Microangiopathic hemolytic anemia
  - Neurologic symptoms
  - Thrombocytopenic purpura

SIGNS AND SYMPTOMS

- More common in women, adults in the 4th decade of life
- 40% have URI or flu-like symptoms prior to presentation
- Fatigue, malaise

- Fever
- Neurologic symptoms—headache, confusion, somnolence, seizures, stroke, coma

DIAGNOSIS

- Peripheral blood smear—schistocytes
- CBC—anemia, severe thrombocytopenia
- LDH—markedly elevated due to ischemia and hemolysis
- Elevated creatinine
- PT/PTT typically normal
- Urinalysis—hematuria, proteinuria, casts

TREATMENT

- Plasma exchange—very effective
- Platelet transfusion is relatively contraindicated (can cause sudden clinical deterioration from increased thrombus formation)
- Steroids and/or splenectomy are treatment options only for patients that haven't responded to plasma exchange

HEMOLYTIC UREMIC SYNDROME (HUS)

SIGNS AND SYMPTOMS

- Similar to TTP except that neurologic symptoms are less severe, and renal dysfunction is more severe
- "Typical" or "childhood" HUS follows an acute episode of bloody diarrhea (most commonly *Escherichia coli* O157:H7)—typically in children under 5 years old, but can also occur in adults

DIAGNOSIS

- Same as above
- Thrombocytopenia not as severe
- Anuric renal failure more common (60% of patients require hemodialysis)

TREATMENT

- Plasma exchange (not as effective as with TTP)
- Avoid platelet transfusion (as with TTP)

DRUG-INDUCED

- Heparin-induced thrombocytopenia (HIT)
  - More common with unfractionated heparin, but can also occur with LMWH
  - Caused by a heparin-dependent antibody that activates platelets

SIGNS AND SYMPTOMS

- Occurs 5 to 7 days after initiation of heparin therapy
- 50% of patients develop thrombosis (venous or arterial), which can be life and limb-threatening

DIAGNOSIS

- CBC—moderate thrombocytopenia, drop in platelet count by 50%
- HIT antibodies can be detected in serum (often present without thrombocytopenia or clinical manifestations, however)

TREATMENT

- Discontinue and avoid any future treatment with unfractionated heparin or LMWH
- Avoid warfarin and other oral anticoagulants in patients with active HIT and DVT—can progress to venous limb gangrene
- Many different medications can cause drug-induced immune thrombocytopenia

IDIOPATHIC (AUTOIMMUNE) THROMBOCYTOPENIC PURPURA (ITP)

- Acute form—seen in children 2 to 6 years old, preceded by viral prodrome, typically self-limited with complete remission in 90%, treatment is supportive
- Chronic form—seen in adult females

SIGNS AND SYMPTOMS

- Easy bruising, prolonged menses, mucosal bleeding
- Petechiae, purpura

DIAGNOSIS

- CBC—thrombocytopenia
- Inpatient evaluation to rule out other causes

TREATMENT

- Steroids
- Splenectomy or immunosuppressive therapy in refractory cases
- Platelet transfusion only if serious bleeding
- IVIG is indicated for children with intracranial hemorrhage from ITP (which is a rare complication)

Lymphomas

HODGKIN LYMPHOMA

SIGNS AND SYMPTOMS

- Lymphadenopathy—mostly above the diaphragm (lower neck and supraclavicular)
- Can have chest pressure, cough, or dyspnea from large mediastinal mass
- B symptoms—weight loss, fever, night sweats
  - Can present with B symptoms alone, without peripheral adenopathy

DIAGNOSIS

- Lymph node biopsy showing Reed–Sternberg cells

TREATMENT

- Chemotherapy/radiation

NON-HODGKIN LYMPHOMA (NHL)

- Proliferation of lymphoid cells arising from lymph nodes or lymphatic tissue in organs other than

bone marrow (lymphocytic leukemia if arises from bone marrow)
- Types—B-Cell lymphomas, T-Cell and NK-Cell lymphomas
- Can be indolent or aggressive

SIGNS AND SYMPTOMS
- Vary depending on type/subtype

DIAGNOSIS
- Biopsy

TREATMENT
- Chemotherapy/radiation depending on type/subtype

Pancytopenia

- Anemia, neutropenia, and thrombocytopenia
- Pancytopenia with cellular bone marrow—can be caused by primary bone marrow diseases (myelodysplasia, myelofibrosis, some leukemias and lymphomas) or certain systemic diseases (SLE, hypersplenism, overwhelming infection, alcohol, tuberculosis, sarcoidosis, vitamin B_{12} and folate deficiencies)
- Aplastic anemia = pancytopenia with hypocellular bone marrow
  - Acquired—stem cells in bone marrow damaged by drugs, radiation, viruses, chemicals or immune-mediated processes
  - Inherited—Fanconi's anemia, dyskeratosis congenita

SIGNS AND SYMPTOMS
- Bleeding and easy bruising
- Fatigue, malaise, shortness of breath from anemia
- Infection

DIAGNOSIS
- CBC and reticulocyte count
- Bone marrow biopsy

TREATMENT
- Immediate therapy depends on severity of anemia/neutropenia/thrombocytopenia, and whether or not complications are present
- Bone marrow transplant

Red blood cell disorders

ANEMIAS
Aplastic anemia

- Normocytic (normal MCV) anemia with low reticulocyte count
- In RBC aplasia, only the red blood cell line fails
- See above

Sickle cell disease

- Caused by inherited mutated hemoglobin (HbS)
- When the gene for HbS is inherited from one parent, and the gene for normal hemoglobin (HbA) inherited from the other, the patient has sickle cell trait, which is generally asymptomatic and does not present with painful crises
- When the gene for HbS is present in combination with the gene for HbC or beta-thalassemia, the patient has sickle cell disease, which is characterized by chronic hemolytic anemia and recurrent painful crises
- Patients rarely present to the ED with undiagnosed sickle cell disease, but those with known disease frequently present with the following manifestations

VASO-OCCLUSIVE CRISIS (ACUTE PAINFUL EPISODE)
SIGNS AND SYMPTOMS
- Pain in the extremities, chest, abdomen or back
- Can be triggered by infection
- Important to distinguish "typical crisis pain" from more life threatening illness

DIAGNOSIS
- No lab test can distinguish whether or not the patient is experiencing a vaso-occlusive crisis

TREATMENT
- Analgesia

ACUTE CHEST SYNDROME
- Defined by a new infiltrate on chest x-ray associated with one or more of the following symptoms: fever, cough, sputum production, tachypnea, dyspnea, shortness of breath, or new-onset hypoxia
- Can be caused by pulmonary vaso-occlusion, fat embolism (from bone marrow ischemia or infarction), hypoventilation (from rib/sternal bone infarct or narcotics), pulmonary edema, infection (by atypical and typical bacteria that cause pneumonia or respiratory viruses), venous thromboembolism (from fibrin clot), aspiration

SIGNS AND SYMPTOMS
- Fever and cough are the most common presenting complaints for children
- In adults, fever and chest pain are the most common presenting complaints, but up to half of adults develop acute chest syndrome 2 to 3 days into a hospitalization for acute pain crisis or some other reason
- May be hypoxic

DIAGNOSIS
- Initial CXR can be normal in up to half of cases

TREATMENT

- Supportive care
- Empiric antibiotics (third- or fourth-generation cephalosporin and macrolide)
- Exchange transfusion in severe cases

SPLENIC SEQUESTRATION

- Etiology is unknown

SIGNS AND SYMPTOMS

- Typically occurs in infants (as young as a few weeks of age)
- Tender, enlarged spleen
- Signs of hypovolemia or shock
- May present with concurrent infection

DIAGNOSIS

- Acute worsening of anemia with persistent reticulocytosis and tender and enlarged spleen

TREATMENT

- Intravenous fluids
- Blood transfusion
- Tends to recur and patients may need splenectomy after the acute episode has resolved

APLASTIC CRISIS

- Characterized by an abrupt fall in hemoglobin with low reticulocyte count (<2%)
- Can be caused by many different types of infections (human parvovirus B19 is the most common cause in children)) or folate deficiency
- Usually transient and resolves spontaneously within a few days
- Treated with blood transfusion if patient is severely anemic or has cardiorespiratory symptoms

INFECTION

- Sickle cell patients have functional asplenia, as well as other mechanisms which make them more prone to infection
  - Cerebrovascular attack (CVA)
  - Priapism

Hemolytic anemia

- Caused by destruction of RBCs
- Can be intravascular or extravascular
  - Intravascular
    - Hemolysis occurs directly within the circulation
    - Tends to be a more acute process than extravascular hemolysis
    - Fragmented RBCs (schistocytes or schizocytes) seen on peripheral blood smear
  - Extravascular
    - Hemolysis occurs after the RBC has been removed from the circulation by the spleen or liver
    - Spherocytes seen on peripheral blood smear

- Can be classified as intrinsic (pathology intrinsic to the RBC) or extrinsic (an outside process affecting a normal RBC)
  - Intrinsic—due to enzyme defect (pyruvate kinase deficiency, G-6-PD deficiency), membrane abnormality or hemoglobin abnormality (sickle cell disease, thalassemia)
    - G-6-PD deficiency—exposure to certain drugs (aspirin, antimalarials, sulfa drugs, nitrofurantoin, phenazopyridine), foods (fava beans), or infection triggers acute hemolysis that is typically self-limited
- Anemia is rarely severe enough to require blood transfusion
- Discontinue precipitating agent (and counsel patient on future avoidance)
  - Extrinsic—further classified into autoimmune or nonimmune etiologies
  - Causes of extrinsic nonimmune hemolytic anemias
    - RBC fragmentation
      - Microangiopathy
        - HUS/TTP
        - HELLP syndrome
      - Cardiac abnormality
        - Prosthetic heart valve
      - Arteriovenous malformation
    - Hypersplenism
    - Infection
      - Malaria
    - Drugs
    - Toxins
      - Lead
      - Copper
    - Spider and snake bites
    - Heat

SIGNS AND SYMPTOMS

- Vary depending on disease process
- Symptoms related to anemia
- Jaundice
- Hepatosplenomegaly

DIAGNOSIS

- Peripheral blood smear—schistocytes, spherocytes
- Reticulocyte count—should be elevated to compensate for RBC destruction
- Haptoglobin—binds free hemoglobin, levels are *decreased* when saturated during hemolysis
- Bilirubin—elevated (but not markedly elevated)—direct or indirect
- LDH—released when RBC is destroyed and therefore elevated
- Plasma free and urine hemoglobin
- Direct and indirect Coomb test—90% of autoimmune hemolytic anemias have a positive direct Coomb test

TREATMENT

- Varies depending on disease process

Hypochromic microcytic anemia (low MCV)

- Can be caused by insufficient iron, insufficient globin (thalassemia), insufficient porphyrin (sideroblastic anemia, lead toxicity), or chronic disease
- Iron deficiency

SIGNS AND SYMPTOMS

- Fatigue, malaise, dyspnea, lightheadedness, headache, weakness

DIAGNOSIS

- Serum iron level—low
- Total iron-binding capacity (TIBC)—high
- Serum ferritin level—low

TREATMENT

- Iron supplements
- Recommend outpatient evaluation for source of iron deficiency

Anemia of chronic disease

SIGNS AND SYMPTOMS

- Same as above

DIAGNOSIS

- Often normocytic (normal MCV)
- Serum iron level—low
- TIBC—low
- Serum ferritin level—normal or elevated

TREATMENT

- Evaluation for underlying cause

Macrocytic anemia (high MCV)

- Megaloblastic anemia is caused by impaired DNA synthesis and is the most important cause of macrocytic anemia
- Caused by **folate** (found in green vegetables, cereals, and fruit) or **vitamin B$_{12}$** (found in meat) deficiency

SIGNS AND SYMPTOMS

- Yellow skin, petechiae, mucosal bleeding, infection, typical anemia symptoms, sore mouth or tongue, diarrhea, weight loss
- Patients with B$_{12}$ deficiency can have paresthesias and ataxia

DIAGNOSIS

- Vitamin B$_{12}$ and folate levels

TREATMENT

- Folate or B$_{12}$ replacement depending on deficiency

POLYCYTHEMIA

Increased red blood cells (hematocrit >51% in men, and >48% in women is abnormal and requires further evaluation)

- Apparent polycythemia—hematocrit appears elevated as a result of a decrease in plasma volume (dehydration)
- Secondary polycythemia—resulting from appropriately (from hypoxia) or inappropriately increased erythropoietin
- Polycythemia vera—characterized by overproduction of RBCs (as well as leukocytosis, thrombocytosis, and splenomegaly)
    - Can progress to myelofibrosis or acute leukemia

SIGNS AND SYMPTOMS

- Headaches, weakness, pruritus, dizziness, excessive sweating, visual disturbances, paresthesias, weight loss, joint pain
- Ruddy complexion, hepatomegaly, splenomegaly, hypertension
- Thrombosis—acute myocardial infarction, ischemic stroke, peripheral arterial thrombosis, venous thrombosis or embolism, superficial thrombophlebitis
- Hemorrhage

DIAGNOSIS

- CBC—erythrocytosis, leukocytosis, thrombocytosis
- Diagnosis confirmed by hematologic studies outside scope of EP practice

TREATMENT

- Phlebotomy

METHEMOGLOBINEMIA

- Occurs when there is overproduction or decreased reduction of methemoglobin
- Methemoglobin is hemoglobin with oxidized iron moieties—usually maintained by methemoglobin reductase as <1% of total hemoglobin
- Acquired methemoglobinemia—discussed elsewhere (see Chapter 17, Toxicologic I)
- Congenital methemoglobinemia—from inherited enzyme deficiency

SIGNS AND SYMPTOMS

- Cyanosis
- Patients with congenital methemoglobinemia are otherwise asymptomatic

DIAGNOSIS

- Cyanosis with normal oxygen saturation
- Co-oximetry

TREATMENT

- Patients with congenital methemoglobinemia generally do not require treatment
- If the patient is symptomatic, they are more likely to have an acute toxic methemoglobinemia and require treatment with methylene blue

White blood cell disorders

LEUKEMIA

- Uncontrolled proliferation of undifferentiated hematopoietic stem cells

Lymphocytic

- From progenitors of lymphocytes

ACUTE (ALL)

- Most common malignancy in children under 15 years of age (also occurs in adults—bimodal)

SIGNS AND SYMPTOMS

- Mostly related to anemia, neutropenia, and thrombocytopenia caused by uncontrolled proliferation of abnormal cells crowding out normal cells in the bone marrow
- Fatigue, malaise, dyspnea, dizziness, bleeding, bruising, fever
- Bacterial infection in approximately one third of patients at the time of presentation
- Extremity and joint pain in children from leukemic infiltration
- Pallor, ecchymoses, petechiae, lymphadenopathy, hepatosplenomegaly
- Can present with cranial nerve abnormalities if central nervous system involvement
- Can present with mediastinal mass causing wheezing, stridor, pericardial effusion, or superior vena cava syndrome

DIAGNOSIS

- Abnormal CBC (anemia, thrombocytopenia, neutropenia or leukocytosis, leukemic blast cells)
  - A small percentage of patients can have "aleukemic" leukemias with a normal WBC count and no blasts in peripheral blood
- Bone marrow biopsy

TREATMENT

- Chemotherapy

CHRONIC (CLL)

- Most common type of leukemia in patients more than 50 years old

SIGNS AND SYMPTOMS

- Fatigue and lymph node enlargement, but often asymptomatic—progressing to anemia, thrombocytopenia, and neutropenia
- Infections—particularly respiratory tract

DIAGNOSIS

- Abnormal CBC (absolute lymphocyte count >5000 cells/mm)

TREATMENT

- Monitor
- Treat infections
- Chemotherapy

Myelogenous

- From progenitors of RBCs, non-lymphocytic WBCs, platelets

ACUTE (AML)

SIGNS AND SYMPTOMS

- Similar to ALL

DIAGNOSIS

- Abnormal CBC (anemia, thrombocytopenia, neutropenia or leukocytosis, blasts)
- Bone marrow biopsy

TREATMENT

- Chemotherapy

CHRONIC (CML)

SIGNS AND SYMPTOMS

- Fatigue, anorexia, weight loss, but typically asymptomatic at time of presentation
- Rarely—bleeding (from thrombocytopenia or platelet dysfunction), thrombosis (from thrombocytosis or marked leukocytosis), gouty arthritis, priapism
- Splenomegaly
- Progresses from chronic to accelerated to blastic-phase (>30% blasts in bone marrow and/or blood—resembles acute leukemia, also referred to as blast crisis)

DIAGNOSIS

- Abnormal CBC (neutrophilic leukocytosis, elevated basophils and eosinophils, thrombocytosis more common than thrombocytopenia)
- Philadelphia chromosome (positive or negative)

TREATMENT

- Chemotherapy

MULTIPLE MYELOMA

- Abnormal proliferation of plasma cells leads to monoclonal gammopathy of uncertain significance (MGUS), which progresses to multiple myeloma with the onset of end-organ damage

SIGNS AND SYMPTOMS

- Fatigue (typically from anemia)
- Bone pain (from osteolytic lesions and/or pathologic fractures)

DIAGNOSIS

- Hypercalcemia
- Elevated creatinine

- Bone marrow biopsy: >10% plasma cells
- Serum and/or urine protein electrophoresis (SPEP or UPEP)—monoclonal (M) protein

TREATMENT

- Chemotherapy
- Plasmapheresis for hyperviscosity syndrome
  - 2-unit phlebotomy with normal saline fluid replacement as a temporizing measure in comatose patients
- Normal saline and corticosteroids for hypercalcemia (add pamidronate if insufficient response)

Complications of hematologic malignancies

HYPERVISCOSITY SYNDROME

- Can result from:
  - Elevated, abnormal serum proteins
- Waldenstrom macroglobulinemia
- Less commonly multiple myeloma

SIGNS AND SYMPTOMS

- Neurologic and visual symptoms are most common
  - Headache, dizziness, tinnitus, decreased hearing, impaired mentation (including coma), peripheral neuropathy, blurry vision, visual loss due to retinal vein thrombosis or retinal hemorrhage
- Bleeding
  - Epistaxis, ecchymoses, oozing from mucosa, GI bleed
- CHF—from expanded plasma volume

DIAGNOSIS

- Clinical suspicion
- SPEP/UPEP

TREATMENT

- Plasmapheresis or plasma exchange, chemotherapy

Leukostasis

- Sludging of leukocytes in the microcirculation from very high leukocyte count or high myeloblast or lymphoblast count
- Acute leukemias
- Less commonly chronic leukemias and high-grade NHL

SIGNS AND SYMPTOMS

- Headache, coma, focal neurologic deficits from intracranial hemorrhage
- Acute respiratory failure (with bilateral infiltrates on CXR)

DIAGNOSIS

- Leukocytosis, high blast count

TREATMENT

- Leukapheresis, hydroxyurea, chemotherapy

Erythrocytosis

- Polycythemia vera

SIGNS AND SYMPTOMS

- Stroke, myocardial infarction, peripheral artery occlusion, venous thrombosis

DIAGNOSIS

- Elevated hematocrit

TREATMENT

- Phlebotomy or erythrocytapheresis

NEUTROPENIC FEVER

- ANC (absolute neutrophil count) calculated by multiplying the WBC count by the fraction of the manual differential composed of bands and neutrophils

SIGNS AND SYMPTOMS

- Fever

DIAGNOSIS

- ANC <500 cells/mm or ANC <1000 cells/mm with expected decrease to <500 cells/mm defines neutropenia

TREATMENT

- IV antibiotics following blood and urine cultures
  - Ceftazidime or cefepime ± an aminoglycoside or meropenem
  - Add vancomycin if indwelling catheter present or patient is MRSA-colonized

SPINAL CORD COMPRESSION

- Can be caused by lymphoma, metastatic disease, or primary tumor

SIGNS AND SYMPTOMS

- Back pain
- Weakness
- Numbness
- Autonomic (bowel, bladder, sexual) dysfunction

DIAGNOSIS

- Magnetic resonance imaging (MRI)
- High-resolution CT or CT myelogram if MRI contraindicated

TREATMENT

- Dexamethasone
- Radiation therapy
- Surgery only if etiology is unclear and a tissue diagnosis is needed or if the spine is unstable

SUPERIOR VENA CAVA (SVC) SYNDROME

- Can be caused by lymphoma
- Tumor obstructs the superior vena cava, causing venous hypertension

SIGNS AND SYMPTOMS

- Periorbital edema, conjunctival edema, and facial swelling which are more obvious in the morning and gradually disappear later in the day are early signs
- SOB, cough, dyspnea, chest pain, tachypnea
- Swelling of the face, trunk, and upper extremities
- Distension of thoracic and neck veins
- Cyanosis

DIAGNOSIS

- CXR
- Chest CT with IV contrast

TREATMENT

- Radiation therapy

ACUTE TUMOR LYSIS SYNDROME

- Most commonly seen following chemotherapy for hematologic malignancies
- Lysed cells release intracellular contents into the extracellular space resulting in metabolic derangement

SIGNS AND SYMPTOMS

- Related to metabolic abnormality

Hyperuricemia

- Nausea, vomiting, anorexia
- Acute renal failure due to precipitation of uric acid crystals in the renal tubules

Hyperphosphatemia

- Nausea, vomiting, diarrhea, lethargy, seizures
- Binds with calcium causing calcium-phosphate crystals to precipitate with resultant nephrocalcinosis (and renal impairment) and hypocalcemia

Hypocalcemia

- Cramping, tetany, arrhythmia

Hyperkalemia

- Nausea, vomiting, anorexia, diarrhea
- Muscle weakness, cramps, paresthesia
- Arrhythmia, heart block, asystole

Acute renal failure

DIAGNOSIS

- Characteristic laboratory abnormalities in appropriate setting

TREATMENT

- Monitor for arrhythmia
- IVF
- Alkalizing urine to promote uric acid excretion no longer recommended because it can exacerbate hypocalcemia and hyperphosphatemia
- Allopurinol
- Hemodialysis indicated for:
  - Serum potassium >6 mEq
  - Serum uric acid >10 mg/dL
  - Serum creatinine >10 mg/dL
  - Serum phosphorus >10 mg/dL or rapidly rising
  - Volume overload
  - Symptomatic hypocalcemia

HYPERCALCEMIA (SEE CHAPTER 5, ENDOCRINE–METABOLIC NUTRITION)

PERICARDIAL EFFUSION (SEE CHAPTER 3, CARDIOVASCULAR II)

PEARLS

- The first step in managing any acute transfusion reaction is to stop the transfusion.

- The management of hemarthrosis in a hemophiliac involves factor replacement, not arthrocentesis.

- Hemophiliacs with even minor head trauma require factor replacement, evaluation with a head CT, and admission for observation.

- Desmopressin acetate (DDAVP) is the preferred initial treatment for bleeding in a patient with mild to moderate hemophilia A.

- Avoid platelet transfusions in patients with thrombotic thrombocytopenic purpura (TTP).

- LMWH is less likely than unfractionated heparin to cause heparin-induced thrombocytopenia (HIT), but once a patient has had HIT, they should never again receive either type of heparin therapy.

BIBLIOGRAPHY

Ansel J, Hirsh J, Hylek E, et al: Pharmacology and management of the vitamin K antagonists, *Chest* 133(6):160S, 2008.

Bakdash S, Yazer MH: What every physician should know about transfusion medicine, *Can Med Assoc J* 177:141, 2007.

Benz EJ: Hemoglobin variants associated with hemolytic anemia, altered oxygen affinity, and methemoglobinemias. In Hoffman (ed): *Hematology: basic principles and practice*, ed 4, Philadelphia, 2005, Churchill Livingstone.

Caldwell SH, Hoffman M, Lisman T et al: Coagulation disorders and hemostasis in liver disease: pathophysiology and critical assessment of current management, *Hepatology* 44(4):1039, 2006.

Campana D, Ching-Hon P: Childhood leukemia. In Abeloff (ed): *Abeloff's clinical oncology*, ed 4, Philadelphia, 2008, Churchill Livingstone.

Furie B, Furie BC: Mechanisms of thrombus formation, *N Engl J Med* 359:938, 2008.

Gregg XT, Prchal JT: Red blood cell enzymopathies. In Hoffman (ed): *Hematology: basic principles and practice*, ed 4, Philadelphia, 2005, Churchill Livingstone.

Grever MR, Andritsos LE, Lozanski G: Chronic lymphoid leukemia. In Abeloff (ed): *Abeloff's clinical oncology*, ed 4, Philadelphia, 2008, Churchill Livingstone.

Hamilton GC, Janz TG: Hematology and oncology: In Marx JA, Hockberger RS, Walls RM (eds): *Rosen's emergency medicine: concepts and clinical practice*, ed 4, Philadelphia, 2006, Mosby.

Hochberg J, Cairo MS, Coccia PF: Tumor lysis syndrome. In Abeloff (ed): *Abeloff's clinical oncology*, ed 4, Philadelphia, 2008, Churchill Livingstone.

Hoelzer D, Gokbuget N: Acute lymphocytic leukemia in adults. In Abeloff (ed): *Abeloff's clinical oncology*, ed 4, Philadelphia, 2008, Churchill Livingstone.

Hoffman G: Blood and blood components. In Marx JA, Hockberger RS, Walls RM (eds): *Rosen's emergency medicine: concepts and clinical practice*, ed 6, Philadelphia, 2006, Mosby.

Hoffman R, Baker KR, Prchal JT: The polycythemias. In Hoffman (ed): *Hematology: basic principles and practice*, ed 4, Philadelphia, 2005, Churchill Livingstone.

Horning SJ: Hodgkin's lymphoma. In Abeloff (ed): *Abeloff's clinical oncology*, ed 4, Philadelphia, 2008, Churchill Livingstone.

Janz TG, Hamilton GC: Disorders of hemostasis. In Marx JA, Hockberger RS, Walls RM (eds): *Rosen's emergency medicine: concepts and clinical practice*, ed 4, Philadelphia, 2006, Mosby.

Johnson CS: The acute chest syndrome, *Hematol Oncol Clin N Am* 19:857, 2005.

Kantarjian H, Cortes J: Chronic myeloid leukemia. In Abeloff (ed): *Abeloff's clinical oncology*, ed 4, Philadelphia, 2008, Churchill Livingstone.

Leukemia and Lymphoma Society (website). Available at: http://www.leukemia-lymphoma.org.

Liebman HA, Weltz IC: Disseminated intravascular coagulation. In Hoffman (ed): *Hematology: basic principles and practice*, ed 4, Philadelphia, 2005, Churchill Livingstone.

Lozier JN, Kessler CM: Clinical aspects and therapy of hemophilia. In Hoffman (ed): *Hematology: basic principles and practice*, ed 4, Philadelphia, 2005, Churchill Livingstone.

Manno CS, Larson PJ: Transfusion therapy for coagulation factor deficiencies. In Hoffman (ed): *Hematology: basic principles and practice*, ed 4, Philadelphia, 2005, Churchill Livingstone.

McCrae KR, Sadler JE, Cines D: Thrombocytopenic purpura and the hemolytic uremic syndrome. In Hoffman (ed): *Hematology: basic principles and practice*, ed 4, Philadelphia, 2005, Churchill Livingstone.

Nkwuo N, Schamban N, Borenstein M: Selected oncologic emergencies. In Marx JA, Hockberger RS, Walls RM (eds): *Rosen's emergency medicine: concepts and clinical practice*, ed 6, Philadelphia, 2006, Mosby.

Rajkumar SV, Dispenzieri A: Multiple myeloma and related disorders. In Abeloff (ed): *Abeloff's clinical oncology*, ed 4, Philadelphia, 2008, Churchill Livingstone.

Saunthararajah Y, Vichinsky EP, Embury SH: Sickle cell disease. In Hoffman (ed): *Hematology: basic principles and practice*, ed 4, Philadelphia, 2005, Churchill Livingstone.

Schrier SL, Reid EG: Extrinsic nonimmune hemolytic anemias. In Hoffman (ed): *Hematology: basic principles and practice*, ed 4, Philadelphia, 2005, Churchill Livingstone.

Warkentin TE, Kelton JG: Thrombocytopenia due to platelet destruction and hypersplenism. In Hoffman (ed): *Hematology: basic principles and practice*, ed 4, Philadelphia, 2005, Churchill Livingstone.

Weitz JI: Anticoagulant and fibrinolytic drugs. In Hoffman (ed): *Hematology: basic principles and practice*, ed 4, Philadelphia, 2005, Churchill Livingstone.

White GC, Sadler JC: von Willebrand disease. In Hoffman (ed): *Hematology: basic principles and practice*, ed 4, Philadelphia, 2005, Churchill Livingstone.

Wilson WH, Armitage JO: Non-Hodgkin's lymphoma. In Abeloff (ed): *Abeloff's clinical oncology*, ed 4, Philadelphia, 2008, Churchill Livingstone.

Wu YY, Snyder EL: Transfusion reactions. In Hoffman (ed): *Hematology: basic principles and practice*, ed 4, Philadelphia, 2005, Churchill Livingstone.

Zarkovic M, Kwaan HC: Correction of hyperviscosity by apheresis, *Semi Thromb Hemost* 29(5):535, 2003.

Questions and Answers

1. A patient receiving a blood transfusion in the ED develops sudden-onset fever, chills, headache, and nausea within minutes of the start of the transfusion. The transfusion is stopped immediately. The blood bank is notified, and a workup initiated to determine the cause of the reaction. A direct Coomb test performed on the patient's blood is positive, and the patient subsequently develops red urine. What is the most likely cause of the patient's symptoms?

    a. allergic reaction
    b. bacterial contamination of donor blood
    c. hypervolemia
    d. clerical error
    e. hypocalcemia

2. A 50-year-old woman on warfarin for a deep vein thrombosis is told to go to the ED because of an elevated INR found during routine outpatient monitoring. Labs in the ED confirm that her INR

is 8. She has a stable hemoglobin and is asymptomatic. What would be the most appropriate management of her coagulopathy?

    a. hold warfarin, administer vitamin K 2.5 mg orally
    b. hold warfarin, administer vitamin K 5 mg subcutaneously
    c. hold warfarin, administer vitamin K 5 mg subcutaneously
    d. hold warfarin, administer vitamin K 10 mg slow IV infusion
    e. hold warfarin, administer vitamin K 10 mg slow IV infusion, administer 4 units FFP

3. A 70-year-old man presents with bright-red rectal bleeding. He is hypotensive and seems slightly confused. His list of medications includes warfarin and he has an INR of 4 in the ED. What is the most appropriate management of his coagulopathy?

a. hold warfarin, administer vitamin K 2.5 mg orally
b. hold warfarin, administer vitamin K 5 mg subcutaneously
c. hold warfarin, administer vitamin K 5 mg subcutaneously
d. hold warfarin, administer vitamin K 10 mg slow IV infusion
e. hold warfarin, administer vitamin K 10 mg slow IV infusion, administer 4 units FFP

4. Of the following, which is the most common presenting complaint in a patient with hemophilia?

a. intracranial hemorrhage
b. epistaxis
c. bleeding into joints or muscles
d. gastrointestinal bleeding
e. nonhealing wounds

5. A 28-year-old male with hemophilia presents to the ED a few hours after slipping in a store and hitting his head on metal shelving. He denies losing consciousness after the fall, and does not have a headache. What is the most appropriate management of this patient?

a. perform a thorough neurologic examination and discharge home if normal
b. order a head CT even if the neurologic examination is normal and discharge the patient home if it is negative
c. order a head CT, give replacement factor, discharge the patient home if the head CT is negative
d. initiate factor replacement, order a head CT, admit the patient for observation
e. consult a neurosurgeon immediately or arrange transfer to an ED with a neurosurgeon on-call, replace factor, order a head CT

6. A 24-year-old female with mild hemophilia A presents to the ED with bleeding from her gums following wisdom tooth extraction. What is the most appropriate initial therapy?

a. DDAVP
b. factor IX concentrate
c. recombinant factor VIII
d. platelet transfusion
e. FFP

7. Which of the following laboratory abnormalities would you expect to see in a patient with disseminated intravascular coagulation (DIC)?

a. elevated fibrinogen levels, prolonged PT/PTT, anemia
b. elevated D-dimer, prolonged PT/PTT, thrombocytopenia
c. prolonged PT, normal PTT, schistocytes
d. blast cells on peripheral blood smear
e. elevated fibrinogen levels, elevated D-dimer, elevated haptoglobin

8. A 35-year-old woman presents to the ED with fever, headache, malaise, and mild confusion. Her CBC reveals anemia and a platelet count of 20,000. Her peripheral blood smear demonstrates schistocytes. A head CT was ordered and is negative, as is her urine pregnancy test. Her history and physical examination reveals a purpuric rash, but no active bleeding. What is the next step in her management?

a. platelet transfusion
b. lumbar puncture
c. consult surgery for emergent splenectomy
d. plasma exchange
e. chemotherapy

9. A patient with a known history of heparin-induced thrombocytopenia (HIT) that occurred 3 years ago after receiving subcutaneous unfractionated heparin for deep vein thrombosis prophylaxis following orthopedic surgery presents to the ED after being diagnosed with a deep vein thrombosis at an outpatient radiology site. The most appropriate treatment for this patient would be:

a. admit for IV unfractionated heparin
b. discharge home with subcutaneous low-molecular-weight heparin (LMWH)
c. administer subcutaneous LMWH and admit to monitor platelet count
d. warfarin without unfractionated heparin or LMWH
e. IV lepirudin

10. A well-appearing 4-year-old is brought to the ED by his parents who report that he seems to be covered in bruises and had an episode of epistaxis that resolved spontaneously. He had an episode of fever, cough, and rhinorrhea a few weeks prior, but had recovered completely. On physical examination, he is noted to have multiple areas of ecchymosis and petechiae. His vital signs are normal as is the rest of his physical examination. His platelet count is 35,000. RBC and WBC counts, creatinine, urinalysis, and coagulation studies are normal. What is his most likely diagnosis?

a. TTP (thrombotic thrombocytopenic purpura)
b. ITP (idiopathic thrombocytopenic purpura)
c. ALL (acute lymphocytic leukemia)
d. DIC (disseminated intravascular coagulation)
e. HSP (Henoch–Schönlein purpura)

11. A 32-year-old man with sickle cell disease presents to the ED with cough, fever, chest, and extremity pain. A chest x-ray reveals a right lower lobe infiltrate. He is treated with ceftriaxone and azithromycin, but despite proper supportive care, becomes more hypoxic and requires intubation. His postintubation chest x-ray reveals multilobar infiltrates. The next treatment for this patient should be:

a. exchange transfusion
b. plasma exchange
c. acyclovir
d. heparin
e. 1 L normal saline bolus

12. A 22-year-old African American woman presents to the ED after her friend noted that her eyes looked yellow. She was recently treated for a UTI with nitrofurantoin and phenazopyridine. She has icteric sclera, and mild jaundice, but an otherwise normal physical examination. She has felt slightly fatigued but denies any other complaints. Her hemoglobin is 9.5 g/dL, with a normal WBC and platelet count. A liver profile reveals a total bilirubin of 5 mg/dL with an indirect bilirubin of 4 mg/dL. The transaminases and alkaline phosphatase are normal. Her urine is positive for blood, but no red blood cells are observed under the microscope. Which of the following is her most likely diagnosis?

a. DIC (disseminated intravascular coagulation)
b. acute hemolysis from underlying G-6-PD deficiency
c. iron deficiency anemia
d. folate deficiency
e. TTP (thrombotic thrombocytopenic purpura)

13. Which of the following laboratory findings would make the diagnosis of iron deficiency in a patient with anemia?

a. low mean corpuscular volume (MCV), low iron levels, high total iron-binding capacity (TIBC), low ferritin
b. low MCV, low iron levels, low TIBC, high ferritin
c. low MCV, low iron levels, low TIBC, normal ferritin
d. high MCV, low iron levels, high TIBC, high ferritin
e. normal MCV, low iron levels, low TIBC, normal ferritin

14. A 65-year-old man with polycythemia vera presents to the ED after experiencing transient left-sided weakness that resolved spontaneously after an hour. He no longer has any focal neurologic symptoms, but has a headache and feels weak. His neurologic examination and head CT are normal. He has a hematocrit of 65%. Which of the following treatments would be the most appropriate?

a. methotrexate
b. fibrinolytic therapy
c. phlebotomy
d. heparin
e. plasmapheresis

15. In a patient with cyanosis and normal oxygen saturation by pulse oximetry, you should suspect:

a. cyanide poisoning
b. chronic obstructive pulmonary disease
c. microcytic anemia from lead toxicity
d. methemoglobinemia
e. polycythemia vera

16. A 70-year-old man with chronic myelogenous leukemia (CML) presents to the ED with a gradual-onset severe headache that has gotten progressively worse. His wife reports that he has become more somnolent and is not responding to her questions. His head CT is negative. The laboratory calls you to tell you that the patient's peripheral blood smear is abnormal. What is the most likely finding?

a. ovalocytes
b. blasts
c. schistocytes
d. Reed–Sternberg cells
e. bands

17. Giving packed red blood cells that have been irradiated can prevent:

a. ABO incompatibility
b. pulmonary edema due to volume overload
c. transfusion-related graft-vs.-host disease in immunocompromised recipient patients
d. all of the above

18. Protamine can be used to help control bleeding in:

a. warfarin excess
b. heparin excess
c. low-molecular-weight heparin excess
d. aspirin overdose
e. both b and c

19. Hemolytic uremic syndrome is associated with:

a. methicillin-resistant *Staphylococcus aureus*
b. methicillin-sensitive *S. aureus*
c. *Escherichia coli* O157:H7
d. *Corynebacterium hemolyticum*

20. Laboratory features of hemolytic anemia include:

a. elevated haptoglobin
b. elevated mean cell corpuscular volume (MCV)
c. elevated lactate dehydrogenase (LDH)
d. decreased reticulocyte count

---

1. Answer: d

This patient had an acute hemolytic transfusion reaction as evidenced by the clinical history, positive direct Coomb test, and hemoglobinuria. **The most common cause of acute hemolytic transfusion reaction is clerical error** resulting in the **transfusion of ABO-incompatible blood.** Bacterial contamination would also be a concern based on the clinical history, but will not result in a positive direct Coomb test or other laboratory findings consistent with hemolysis.

2. Answer: a

In a patient taking warfarin that is not bleeding, acceptable options for management for an **INR between 5 and 9 include omitting the next one to two doses, or omitting one dose and administering oral vitamin K (1 to 2.5 mg).** Subcutaneous vitamin K should be avoided. A discussion with the doctor managing the patients INR should be a part of any patient encounter such as this.

3. Answer: e

A patient on **warfarin with serious bleeding requires immediate reversal of his or her coagulopathy** regardless of the degree of elevation of the INR. The most appropriate response to this question is **e**, although prothrombin complex concentrate (factor IX complex), or recombinant factor VIIa, will provide a more rapid reversal than FFP, and could be used instead of FFP if available.

4. Answer: c

Most patients with **hemophilia** that come to the ED have a known diagnosis, and present with **hemarthrosis** or **intramuscular bleeding** that is spontaneous or follows minor trauma.

5. Answer: d

Hemophiliacs with even minor head trauma require factor replacement to 50% activity level, evaluation with a head CT and admission for observation. Adequate factor replacement effectively prevents intracranial hemorrhage in hemophiliacs with normal head CTs following minor trauma, and it is extremely unlikely that this patient would require neurosurgical intervention.

6. Answer: a

DDAVP is effective in patients with mild-moderate (but not severe) hemophilia A. It does not carry the viral infection risk of FFP or cryoprecipitate, and is less expensive than recombinant or highly purified plasma-derived factor VIII. Factor IX concentrate would be appropriate for a patient with hemophilia B.

7. Answer: b

A patient with **DIC** would be expected to have some or all of the following laboratory abnormalities: **thrombocytopenia, anemia, schistocytes, on peripheral blood smear, prolonged PT/PTT, elevated D-dimer, and *decreased* fibrinogen levels.** Haptoglobin levels are decreased during hemolysis (which typically occurs in DIC).

8. Answer: d

This patient **most likely has thrombotic thrombocytopenic purpura (TTP)**—which classically features fever, hemolytic anemia, thrombocytopenia,

neurologic symptoms, and renal insufficiency. The most appropriate treatment is **plasma exchange** in consultation with a hematologist. **Platelet transfusion is contraindicated in the absence of life-threatening bleeding,** as it can cause sudden clinical deterioration or death from increased thrombus formation. Splenectomy and/or steroids are treatment options for patients that do not respond to plasma exchange. Lumbar puncture would be contraindicated in a patient with a platelet count of 20,000.

9. Answer: e

Once a patient has had HIT, they should never receive either form of heparin ever again. A faster-acting anticoagulant should be used until the patient's INR becomes therapeutic on warfarin. **Lepirudin** is one of a number of parenteral anticoagulants that could be used in place of heparin. It is **a direct thrombin antagonist.** In a patient with a deep vein thrombosis and active HIT, warfarin can cause skin necrosis by decreasing protein C levels. For this situation, heparin should be discontinued, and warfarin started only after the platelet count has returned to normal. During this time, the patient should be anticoagulated with a direct thrombin antagonist like lepirudin.

10. Answer: b

ITP is a diagnosis of exclusion, but in this well-appearing patient with no hepatosplenomegaly, and otherwise normal labs, it is the most likely diagnosis. ITP typically resolves spontaneously and does not require treatment. Admission should be considered for further evaluation to rule out other causes of thrombocytopenia.

11. Answer: a

Exchange transfusion is indicated for sickle cell patients with severe acute chest syndrome. It is thought to work by reducing the number of sickled cells without adding volume or increasing blood viscosity. Patients with acute chest syndrome may have rapid clinical improvement following exchange transfusion. Pulmonary embolus from fibrin clot is one of a number of etiologies of acute chest syndrome, but is not a common cause, and not suggested by the scenario above. Heparin, therefore, is not an appropriate choice. An IV fluid bolus would likely not be beneficial and may lead to or exacerbate pulmonary edema, which can cause acute chest syndrome.

12. Answer: b

Patients with **G-6-PD deficiency can develop acute hemolytic reactions to certain drugs (including nitrofurantoin and phenazopyridine).** The resulting anemia is usually not severe enough to require a blood transfusion, and the episodes are usually self-limited. Although **b** is the correct answer to this question, the patient would require further hematologic workup to determine if G-6-PD deficiency was truly the underlying cause of this acute hemolytic reaction.

13. Answer: a

Iron deficiency anemia causes a microcytic anemia. Low serum ferritin indicates diminished levels of stored iron. TIBC rises as iron stores diminish. Choices **b, c,** and **d** are consistent with anemia of chronic disease.

14. Answer: c

Polycythemia vera (PV) can cause both thrombotic and bleeding events. Transient ischemic attack (TIA) and stroke are two thrombotic complications associated with PV. In addition to his TIA symptoms, this patient also has a headache, weakness, and a hematocrit of 65%, which are consistent with hyperviscosity syndrome. A neurologist and hematologist should be consulted to help manage this patient. The most appropriate treatment would be phlebotomy and aspirin.

15. Answer: d

Methemoglobinemia can be congenital or acquired. Patients with congenital methemoglobinemia are generally asymptomatic (except for the cyanotic appearance) and do not typically require treatment. Acute toxic methemoglobinemia can be treated with methylene blue.

16. Answer: b

This patient has **leukostasis due to blast crisis.** With elevated blasts on his peripheral blood smear, he would require a hematology consult for emergent leukapheresis.

17. Answer: c

Giving irradiated blood to immunocompromised patients prevents transfusion-related graft-vs.-host disease. It will not affect ABO incompatibility or volume overload issues.

18. Answer: e

Protamine sulfate is used to reverse heparin and low-molecular-weight heparin excess (although it is less effective in the latter), but has no activity in warfarin excess or aspirin overdose.

19. Answer: c

The classic case is a child, usually less than 5 years of age, who has **bloody diarrhea** (due to *Escherichia coli* O157:H7) and is treated with antibiotics, but develops purpura—although this can be seen in older children and adults.

20. Answer: c

Hemolysis leads to increased red cell production in compensation; thus **reticulocyte counts should be increased.** There is **no effect on the MCV. Haptoglobin levels are decreased,** because haptoglobin binds free hemoglobin, so levels will be low. **LDH is high** as it is released from the lysed cells, but is not specific for hemolysis (i.e., can be elevated in myocardial infarction and liver disease, among other processes).

Immunologic

9

Edward A. Stettner | Bisan Salhi

9

Sarcoidosis

- Usually affects adults 20 to 40 years old
- Women affected slightly more than men
- Characterized by noncaseating epithelioid granulomas
- The etiology of sarcoidosis is unknown

SIGNS AND SYMPTOMS

- Pulmonary involvement is most common
  - Cough, dyspnea, chest tightness
  - Chest radiograph may demonstrate hilar adenopathy and/or parenchymal disease (Fig. 9-1)
  - Pulmonary fibrosis may occur late in the disease course (Fig. 9-2)
- Malaise and low-grade fevers are common
- Dermatologic involvement
  - Erythema nodosum, plaques
- Hypercalcuria and hypercalcemia
  - Decreased intestinal absorption of vitamin D
  - Increased conversion of vitamin D to active form in sarcoid granulomas
- Cardiac involvement
  - Congestive heart failure, dysrhythmias
- Neurologic involvement
  - Headaches, focal neurologic deficits, seizures, meningitis, encephalitis

DIAGNOSIS

- Clinical symptoms
- Biopsy showing noncaseating granulomas

TREATMENT

- Systemic corticosteroids
- Topical steroids may be considered for skin lesions
- Supportive care

Organ transplantation

- The treatment of patients with organ transplantation poses a unique challenge to the emergency physician
- They may suffer from problems related to their specific surgery, rejection of the transplanted organ, immunosuppression, and susceptibility to infection
- Because of denervation of the transplanted organ, as well as surgical anastomoses and altered anatomy, the transplanted patient may have vague or atypical signs of underlying disease

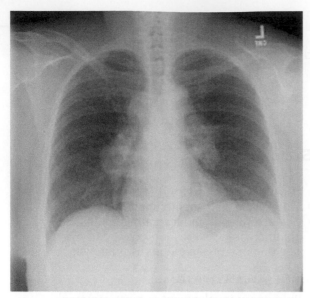

Figure 9-1. Typical chest radiographs in sarcoidosis. Stage I sarcoidosis is characterized by bilateral hilar and often mediastinal adenopathy without visible parenchymal lung disease. (From Goldman L: *Cecil medicine,* ed 23, Philadelphia, 2007, Saunders.)

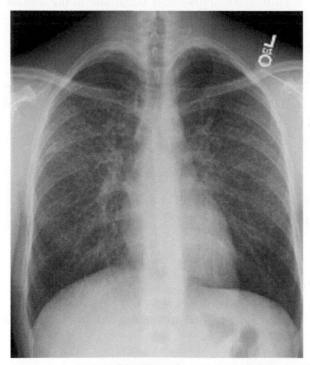

Figure 9-2. In stage III sarcoidosis, the radiograph shows parenchymal lung involvement without hilar adenopathy. (From Goldman L: *Cecil medicine,* ed 23, Philadelphia, 2007, Saunders.)

REJECTION

Liver transplant

SIGNS AND SYMPTOMS

- Symptoms may be subtle and nonspecific
- Fever
- Tenderness of the right upper quadrant

- Elevation in liver enzymes and/or prothrombin time (PT)
- Eosinophilia or lymphocytosis
- Diagnosis can be made by liver transplant ultrasound and/or liver biopsy
- Differential diagnosis includes infection, hepatic artery thrombosis, or postoperative complications

Renal transplant

SIGNS AND SYMPTOMS

- Tenderness over the transplanted kidney
- Decreased urine output
- Fever
- Malaise
- Volume overload
- Elevated creatinine (decline in glomerular filtration rate [GFR])
- Ultrasonography of the transplanted kidney is required

Lung transplant

SIGNS AND SYMPTOMS

- Cough
- Fever
- Dyspnea
- Chest tightness
- Decline in FEV-1
- Abnormal chest radiograph

Heart transplant

SIGNS AND SYMPTOMS

- Malaise
- Dysrhythmias (atrial fibrillation, ventricular tachycardia, etc.)
- Symptoms may be subtle and nonspecific
- Many patients are asymptomatic

TREATMENT

- Includes high-dose intravenous glucocorticoids once the diagnosis has been made

INFECTIONS

- There is a broad range of infections that can affect the transplant patient, which may be a serious cause of morbidity and mortality in this patient population (Fig. 9-3)

Cytomegalovirus (CMV)

- Most common infection in solid organ transplant
- Broad range of symptoms
  - Malaise, fever, hepatic infection, enteric involvement (diarrhea), pneumonitis
- Treat with ganciclovir

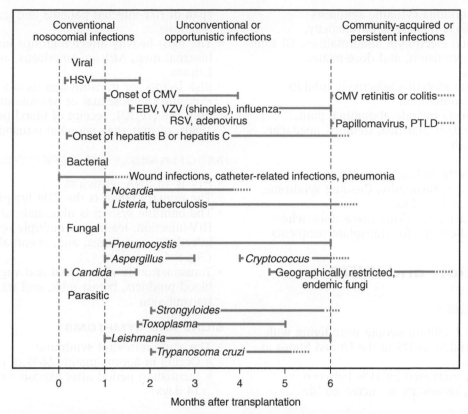

Figure 9-3. Usual sequence of infections after organ transplantation. Exceptions to the usual sequence of infections after transplantation suggest the presence of unusual epidemiologic exposure or excessive immunosuppression. *CMV*, Cytomegalovirus; *EBV*, Epstein-Barr virus; *HSV*, herpes simplex virus; *PTLD*, posttransplant lymphoproliferative disorder; *RSV*, respiratory syncytial virus; *VZV*, varicella-zoster virus. *Zero* indicates the time of transplantation, *solid lines* indicate the most common period for the onset of infection, and *dotted lines* indicate periods of continued risk at reduced levels. (Reprinted from Rubin RH, Wolfson JS, Cosimi AB, Tolkoff-Rubin NE: Infection in the renal transplant patient, *Am J Med* 70:405–411, 1981. Copyright 1981, with permission from Excerpta Medica, Inc.)

Intra-abdominal infections

- Common within the first postoperative month
- Broad-spectrum antibiotic coverage for Gram-negative organisms, enterococci, anaerobes

Pneumonia

- Common within the first 3 months after lung transplantation
- Can be community-acquired or nosocomial
- Broad-spectrum coverage is indicated
- Consider the possibility of opportunistic infections
  - CMV pneumonitis
  - PCP pneumonia

Mediastinitis

- Can be a complication in the first month after cardiac transplantation

ED EVALUATION AND TREATMENT

- Blood cultures
- Urinalysis and urine cultures
- CBC, renal, and liver function tests
- Chest radiograph

- Computed tomography (CT) and lumbar puncture in patients with neurologic complaints or headache
- Treatment is directed at the patient's infection and clinical presentation
  - Urinary tract infections and pneumonia can be treated with the usual antimicrobial agents
  - Broad-spectrum coverage should be initiated early in patients who exhibit signs of sepsis, severe illness, and/or hemodynamic compromise
- Patients should be managed in close consultation with a transplant coordinator at a transplant center

Complications of immunosuppression

- Symptoms are specific to the antirejection medications
  - Cyclosporine—a calcineurin inhibitor, inhibits lymphocyte signal transduction
    - Adverse effects include nephrotoxicity, neurotoxicity, electrolyte abnormalities, elevated bilirubin, and cholestasis
  - Azathioprine inhibits DNA and RNA synthesis, suppressing lymphocyte proliferation
    - Adverse effects include hepatotoxicity, gastrointestinal (GI) side effects, and dose-related neutropenia

- Tacrolimus—inhibits cytokine synthesis
  - Adverse effects include nephrotoxicity, neurotoxicity, electrolyte abnormalities, GI side effects, hypertension, and dose-related neutropenia
- Mycophenolate mofetil—selectively inhibits lymphocyte proliferation
  - Adverse effects include abdominal pain, vomiting and/or diarrhea, tremors, headache, flushing, rash
  - Prednisone
    - Adverse effects include hypertension, hyperglycemia, myopathy, Cushing syndrome, delayed wound healing
- Carefully consider drug–drug interactions when prescribing medications for transplant recipients

HIV infection and AIDS

EPIDEMIOLOGY

- An estimated 1.1 million people were living with HIV infection and/or AIDS in the United States at the end of 2006
- HIV prevalence increased by 11% between 2003 and 2006, secondary to increased life span of HIV-infected patients and increased diagnosis
- The most heavily affected groups include gay and bisexual men, African Americans, and Hispanics/Latinos
- Risk factors for transmission include sexual exposure (homosexual or heterosexual), intravenous drug use (IVDU), receipt of blood products in the 1980s, or maternal–neonatal transmission

MECHANISM OF INFECTION

- HIV is an RNA retrovirus
- The primary target is the CD4 lymphocyte
- The immune system is ultimately unable to control HIV-infection, leading to multiple opportunistic infections, neoplasms, and, eventually, death (Fig. 9-4)
- Transmission is via seminal and vaginal fluid, blood products, breast milk, and transplacental transmission

SIGNS AND SYMPTOMS

- The acute retroviral syndrome
  - Occurs in approximately 66% of patients
  - Incubation period after exposure is usually 10 to 14 days

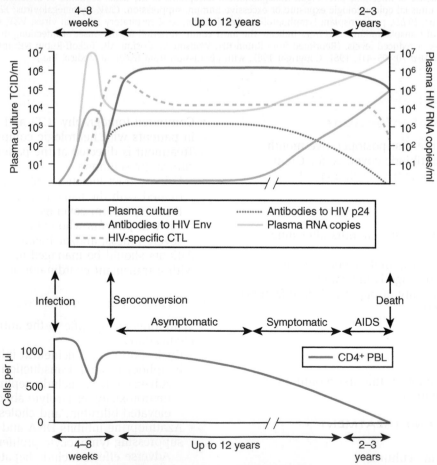

Figure 9-4. HIV-1 natural history. (Modified from Staprans SI, Feinberg MB: Natural history and immunopathogenesis of HIV-1 disease. In Sande MA, Volberding PA [eds]: *The medical management of AIDS,* ed 5, Philadelphia, 1997, Saunders, pp. 29–55.)

- Most common manifestations
  - Fever (80% to 90% of symptomatic patients)
  - Malaise (>70%)
  - Anorexia or weight loss (15% to 70%)
  - Myalgias and arthralgias (40% to 70%)
  - Headache (30% to 40%)
  - Pharyngitis (>50%)
  - Rash (20% to 70%)
- Seroconversion (a detectable HIV antibody response) occurs within 4 to 8 weeks after infection
- Following the acute retroviral syndrome, patients can be asymptomatic for years
- Early symptomatic infection is defined by an increase in community-acquired infections (not necessarily AIDS-defining illnesses)
- AIDS is defined by a CD4 <200 and/or the appearance of an AIDS-defining illness, including:
  - Cryptococcosis
  - Cryptosporidiosis
  - CMV retinitis
  - Esophageal candidiasis
  - Kaposi sarcoma
  - *Pneumocystis carinii* pneumonia (PCP)
  - Toxoplasmosis
  - Mycobacterium avium complex
  - Disseminated histoplasmosis

PULMONARY MANIFESTATIONS

- Respiratory symptoms are a common presenting complaint in the ED
- Symptoms include cough, hemoptysis, dyspnea, chest pain, or fever
- Nonopportunistic infections are most common, especially early in the course of disease
  - *Streptococcus pneumoniae*
  - *Haemophilus influenzae*
  - *Staphylococcus aureus*
  - *Mycoplasma pneumoniae*
  - *Viral pneumonia*

Pneumocystis pneumonia (PCP)

- Caused by the organism *Pneumocystis jiroveci* (formerly referred to as *Pneumocystis carinii*)

SIGNS AND SYMPTOMS

- Fever
- Nonproductive cough
- Dyspnea, especially with exertion

DIAGNOSIS

- Hypoxemia
- Increased alveolar-arterial gradient
- LDH may be elevated
- Chest radiograph
  - Diffuse interstitial infiltrate
  - May be normal early in disease (Fig. 9-5)

TREATMENT

- Prednisone in patients with a PaO$_2$ <70 mmHg

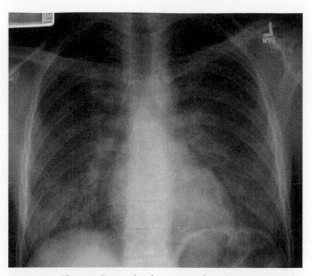

Figure 9-5. Chest radiograph of an HIV-infected person, CD4$^+$ cell count less than 200 cells/μL, demonstrating the characteristic bilateral, reticular-granular opacities of *Pneumocystis* pneumonia. Bronchoscopy with examination of bronchoalveolar lavage fluid revealed *Pneumocystis jirovecii*. (From Goldman E: *Cecil medicine*, ed 23, Philadelphia, 2007, Saunders.)

- Trimethoprim–sulfamethoxazole (TMP/SMX; Bactrim DS), 2 tabs PO thrice daily for 3 weeks, or IV TMP/SMX if severely ill
- Pentamidine (in sulfa-allergic patients)

Mycobacterium tuberculosis

- Increased incidence in HIV-infected patients
- Extrapulmonary symptoms are more common in HIV-infected patients

SIGNS AND SYMPTOMS

- Fever, night sweats, cough, hemoptysis, anorexia, weight loss

DIAGNOSIS

- Sputum cultures required for definitive diagnosis
- Purified protein derivative (PPD) may be falsely negative in anergic patients
- Chest radiograph
  - Classic findings
    - Upper lobe cavitation
    - Adenopathy
  - Atypical features
    - Lobar infiltration
    - Negative or nonspecific chest radiograph

TREATMENT

- Four-drug treatment with isoniazid, rifampin, pyrazinamide, and ethambutol for 6 months
- Some patients may have multidrug-resistant tuberculosis
- Close contacts should be evaluated and treated

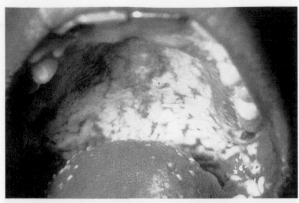

Figure 9-6. Oral candidiasis (thrush). (Courtesy of Stephen Raffanti, MD, MPH) (From Mandell GL, Bennett JE, Dolin R: *Principles and practice of infectious diseases,* ed 6, Philadelphia, 2005, Churchill Livingstone.)

Other pulmonary complications

- Cryptococcal pneumonia
- Histoplasmosis
- CMV
- Kaposi sarcoma
- Lymphoma

GASTROINTESTINAL MANIFESTATIONS

- Oral lesions
  - Oral candidiasis (thrush) (Fig. 9-6)
  - >80% of AIDS patients affected
  - Plaques from an erythematous base that can be easily scraped off
  - Tongue and buccal mucosa are most commonly involved
  - Treatment is with fluconazole 150 mg PO once daily for 7 to 14 days
- Esophageal lesions
  - Characterized by dysphagia or odynophagia
  - Can be secondary to candida, CMV, or HSV
- Enteric disease
  - Diarrhea is the most common GI symptom
    - Occurs in up to 90% of patients
  - Causes
    - Viral, bacterial, fungal, drug-related
    - Treat the underlying cause

NEUROLOGIC MANIFESTATIONS

- Infectious processes
  - Bacterial meningitis
  - Cryptococcus neoformans
  - CMV
  - Progressive multifocal leukoencephalopathy
  - Herpes simplex virus (HSV)
  - Neurosyphilis
  - Tuberculosis
- Noninfectious processes
  - CNS lymphoma
  - Stroke

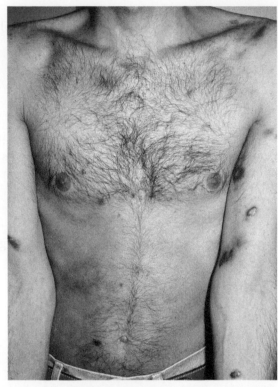

Figure 9-7. Kaposi sarcoma. (Courtesy of Benjamin K. Fisher, MD) (From Habif TP: *Clinical dermatology: a color guide to diagnosis and therapy,* ed 4, Philadelphia, 2003, Mosby.)

- Encephalopathy
- Neuropathy
- Evaluation and diagnosis includes CT of the brain and lumbar puncture (LP)

CUTANEOUS MANIFESTATIONS

- Kaposi sarcoma (Fig. 9-7)
  - Can range from isolated cutaneous lesions to disseminated disease
  - Cutaneous appearance is violaceous, pink, or red papules, plaques, nodules, and tumors
  - Treatment includes cryotherapy, radiotherapy, and intralesional or systemic chemotherapy
- Varicella zoster
  - May involve multiple dermatomes
  - Treatment
    - Single dermatomal zoster infection
      - Outpatient management with oral famciclovir (500 mg PO TID), acyclovir (500 mg PO QID), or valaciclovir (1 g PO BID)
    - Admission criteria
      - Systemic involvement
      - Ophthalmic zoster
      - Severe, multidermatomal involvement

DRUG REACTIONS

- Common in HIV-infected patients secondary to increasing use of antiretroviral drugs

- Common reactions
  - Dermatological reactions
  - Nausea and vomiting
  - Diarrhea
- Treatment is aimed at the specific symptoms and identifying and removing the offending drug

DIAGNOSIS OF HIV INFECTION

- In the acute phase
  - HIV nucleic acid amplification *or*
  - HIVp24 antigen *or*
  - A combined HIV p24 antigen–antibody test *and* a negative or indeterminate HIV-antibody (suggests incomplete seroconversion)
- After seroconversion
  - Enzyme-linked immunoassay (EIA) (99% specific, 98.5% sensitive)
  - Confirmatory Western blot (WB) assay (99.9% sensitive and specific)
  - A CD4 count can be used to differentiate between HIV infection and AIDS

TREATMENT OF HIV-RELATED INFECTIONS

- Patients with bacterial infections and/or signs of sepsis should be treated aggressively with antibiotics
- Diagnostic tests should be tailored to the patient's symptoms and clinical presentation
- Admission criteria
  - Patients with severe illness (hypotension, hypoxemia, inability to tolerate PO, etc.)
  - Patients with pneumonia, especially those with suspected tuberculosis
  - Patients with CNS symptoms
  - Patients with unreliable follow-up
- Patients may be discharged if they appear well, can be treated as an outpatient, and have adequate reliable follow up

Rheumatic fever

- A multisystem inflammatory complication resulting from infection with group A streptococcus, usually from pharyngitis
- Although the exact mechanism is unknown, it is thought to occur from an abnormal humoral response to a bacterial antigen leading to inflammation
- Typically occurs 2 to 3 weeks following an episode of acute pharyngitis, but the initial infection is not always recognized
- Typically affects those between 5 and 20 years of age, though it is occasionally seen in adults
- Leading cause of acquired heart disease in children worldwide
  - Incidence is decreasing with increased antibiotic usage
  - Rare in the United States, but isolated outbreaks still occur, especially following epidemic streptococcal pharyngitis occurrences

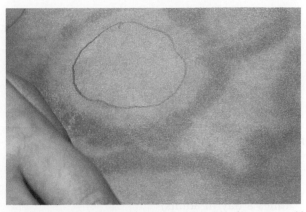

Figure 9-8. Erythema marginatum on the trunk of an 8-year-old Caucasian boy. The *pen mark* shows the location of the rash approximately 60 minutes previously. (Photograph provided by Associate Professor Mike South, Royal Children's Hospital, Melbourne, Australia) (From Cohen J, Powderly WG: *Infectious diseases,* ed 2, Philadelphia, 2004, Mosby.)

SIGNS AND SYMPTOMS

- Arthritis and arthralgias
  - Patients typically have migratory polyarthralgia
  - Usually affects the large joints
- Cardiac—30% to 50% of patients with acute rheumatic fever develop rheumatic heart disease
- 40% develop pericarditis
- Heart valves can become inflamed and develop scarring, leading to regurgitation and congestive heart failure (CHF)
  - Mitral valve most common
- Myocardial involvement can lead to cardiac conduction delays that manifest as PR prolongation on the ECG
- Dermatologic—these lesions are rare, occurring in less than 10% of cases
  - Erythema marginatum (Fig. 9-8)
    - Expanding erythematous ring that typically appears early in the disease course
  - Subcutaneous nodules
    - Firm lumps located over extensor surfaces that occur 2 to 3 weeks after disease onset
    - Associated with severe carditis
- Neurologic
  - Sydenham chorea (St. Vitus dance)
    - Nonpurposeful movements of the arms and face
    - Typically resolves by 6 weeks to 6 months

DIAGNOSIS

- Diagnosis made through the Jones Criteria. The presence of either two major criteria *or* one major and two minor criteria with a recent streptococcal infection is diagnostic
- Major criteria
  - Polyarthritis
  - Carditis
  - Chorea
  - Erythema marginatum
  - Subcutaneous nodules
- Minor criteria
  - Arthralgia

- Fever
- Elevated erythrocyte sedimentation rate (ESR) or C-reactive protein (CRP) level
- Prolonged PR interval on ECG
- Throat culture is typically negative at the time rheumatic fever is diagnosed
    - Antistreptococcal antibody titers remain positive for 4 to 6 weeks

TREATMENT

- Treat for group A streptococcus
    - 10 days oral penicillin V (250 mg three or four times a day in children; 500 mg three or four times a day in adults)
    or
    - Erythromycin (20 mg/kg two times a day, up to 250 mg)
    or
    - Intramuscular benzathine penicillin (adults: 1.2 million units; children: 0.6 million units)
- Antimicrobial prophylaxis
    - Patients with diagnosed rheumatic fever must receive prophylaxis against recurrent infection with either oral or intramuscular penicillin for at least 5 years
- Salicylates
    - High-dose aspirin very effective for fever and arthralgias
    - 80 to 100 mg/kg/day initially
- Corticosteroids
    - Used for severe carditis, although their efficacy is controversial

CARDIAC MANIFESTATIONS

- Standard treatment for CHF
- Valve replacement for severe disease
- Chorea
    - Usually self-limited, but can improve with some antipsychotic and anticonvulsant medications

Hypersensitivity reactions

- Allergic reactions represent a spectrum of diseases, ranging from minor skin irritation to life-threatening anaphylactic shock

ALLERGIC REACTIONS

Definition (allergic vs. anaphylactic)

- The Second Symposium on the Definition and Management of Anaphylaxis in 2005 developed a deliberately broad definition of anaphylaxis:
    - "Anaphylaxis is a serious allergic reaction that is rapid in onset and may cause death."
- Diagnosis of anaphylaxis should be suspected with one of the following
    - Acute onset of an illness involving skin and/or mucosal membranes *and* either respiratory symptoms or hypotension
    - At least two of the following after antigen exposure
        - Cutaneous or mucosal symptoms
        - Respiratory symptoms
        - Hypotension
        - Gastrointestinal symptoms
    - Hypotension after antigen exposure definition:
        - Pediatrics: age dependent
        - Adults: systolic BP <90 mmHg or 30% below patient's baseline

Epidemiology

- Exact incidence is unknown, but estimates are about 21/100,000 person-years
- Etiologic agents
    - Unknown in one third of cases
    - Food in one third of cases
        - Typically peanuts and seafood
        - Many other foods have been implicated
    - Hymenoptera
        - Responsible for 25 to 50 deaths annually in the United States
    - Other important causes include medications (see "Drug Allergies"), latex, and radiocontrast dye
        - Consider detergents, soaps, or other cutaneous exposure
    - Exercise can induce anaphylaxis without another cause

Pathophysiology

- Most allergic reactions occur in a two-step fashion
    - Initial *sensitization* from exposure to an antigen
        - Develops IgE antibodies
    - On *reexposure,* IgE antibodies cause a cascade of chemomediators to be released from mast cells, which cause a variety of physiologic changes
    - Most commonly affected systems include the skin, eye, nasal, respiratory, cardiovascular, and GI
    - Other reactions (such as transfusion reactions) are caused by IgM- or IgG-mediated complement activation
- Chemical mediators
    - Histamine is the primary mediator
    - H_1 receptor
        - Bronchial, intestinal, and uterine smooth muscle contraction
        - Increased vascular permeability
    - H_2 receptor
        - Increased cardiac contraction, gastric secretions, airway mucous production, and vascular permeability

Differential diagnosis

- Different manifestations of allergic reactions warrant various differential consideration
    - Dermatologic reactions may mimic other rashes, such as zoster or autoimmune conditions
        - Conditions including carcinoid and scombroid poisoning can cause flushing similar to allergic symptoms

- Patients with respiratory complaints may mimic respiratory infection, asthma, pneumonia, or pulmonary embolism
- In patients with hypotension or shock, cardiac ischemia and arrhythmias as well as infectious, toxicologic, and metabolic causes must be considered

Clinical presentation

- Allergic symptoms range from mild skin irritation to life-threatening respiratory and cardiovascular collapse
- More rapid symptom onset typically heralds more severe reaction
- The most mild allergic reactions involve primarily cutaneous symptoms
  - Contact or atopic dermatitis
- More severe reactions can involve any or all of the above organ systems (see "Anaphylaxis")
  - Patients usually have skin symptoms first, which then progress to involve respiratory and cardiac systems
  - Anaphylaxis can sometimes present precipitously, without preceding skin findings
- Some patients may have symptom recurrence between 24 to 48 hours after exposure

SIGNS AND SYMPTOMS

- Allergic reactions can affect virtually any organ system
- Skin—involved in >80% to 90% of cases
  - Urticaria
    - Pruritic, raised welts resulting from increased vascular permeability
  - Flushing
    - Results from vasodilatation
  - Angioedema (see "Angioedema")
    - Marked subcutaneous edema from increased vascular permeability
- Eye
  - Pruritic conjunctivitis with increased lacrimation
- Respiratory
  - Increased secretions in the upper airway
    - Resulting from increased vascular permeability
  - Laryngeal edema and sensation of throat closing
    - Increased vascular permeability and vasodilatation
    - May cause stridor and airway narrowing
  - Bronchospasm, causing cough and wheezing
    - Bronchial smooth muscle contraction and increased vascular permeability
- Cardiovascular
  - Hypotension and tachycardia
    - Increased vascular permeability and vasodilatation
  - Ischemic chest pain
    - Coronary smooth muscle contraction
- Gastrointestinal
  - Abdominal cramping, nausea, and vomiting
    - Gastric smooth muscle contraction and increased secretions

- Hematologic
  - Fibrinolysis and disseminated intravascular coagulation
    - Manifests with bleeding and increased bruising
    - Caused by various chemomediators

TREATMENT

- Treatment modalities depend on the severity of the reaction
- Mild cutaneous reactions, including contact dermatitis
  - Oral antihistamines for symptomatic relief
  - Consider treatment with topical steroid preparations
- More severe, multisystem reactions require more aggressive treatment regimens (see "Anaphylaxis")
  - Inhaled beta-agonists for wheezing or cough
  - Oral or intravenous H_1- and H_2-blocking antihistamines should be provided
  - Systemic corticosteroids for any angioedema or other systemic signs
    - Onset of action 4 to 6 hours
  - Subcutaneous or intravenous epinephrine for severe anaphylactic reactions with multi-system involvement
  - Anaphylactic shock requires administration of intravenous epinephrine

Disposition

- Mild to moderate allergic reactions can be discharged after a brief observation period, generally 2 to 6 hours
  - Patients should be discharged on oral antihistamines for 48 hours
  - May reduce symptom recurrence
    - Diphenhydramine hydrochloride 25 to 50 mg every 6 hours
  - Patients given steroids should be prescribed oral prednisone for 7 to 10 days
    - May reduce rebound or delayed symptoms
  - Patients with wheezing should be discharged with inhaled beta-agonists
- Patients with severe, multisystem reactions should be considered for 24- to 48-hour hospitalization for observation
- Patients with significant reactions should receive counseling on antigen avoidance
- Prescribe an epinephrine auto-injector for any patient with a moderate to severe allergic reaction
  - Consider providing multiple injectors for ease of access

ANAPHYLAXIS

- Moderate to severe allergic symptoms affecting multiple systems, which may be life-threatening
- Symptoms typically progress rapidly after antigen exposure
  - Often between 5 and 30 minutes
  - More rapid symptom onset correlates with more severe reactions

SIGNS AND SYMPTOMS

- Virtually any organ system can be affected
  - Rash and pruritis in >80% to 90%
  - Respiratory
    - Wheezing, dyspnea, and stridor
  - Cardiovascular
    - Hypotension and tachycardia
  - Gastrointestinal
    - Abdominal pain, nausea, vomiting, and diarrhea

TREATMENT

- Always remember to remove any triggering antigen if present
- **Airway**
  - Administer adequate supplemental oxygen
  - Assess airway patency; consider airway adjuncts as needed
  - Consider early intubation for airway edema
  - Consider nebulized racemic epinephrine
    - 0.5 mL of 2.25% in 2.5 mL of saline
  - Standard RSI medications may be used
    - Caution with agents that can worsen hypotension
- **Breathing**
  - Administer inhaled or nebulized beta-agonists for wheezing
- **Circulation**
  - Anaphylactic shock is multifactorial; distributive shock from vasodilatation; hypovolemic shock from extravascular extravasation due to increased blood vessel permeability
    - Obtain 2 large bore peripheral IVs
    - Administer intravenous crystalloid or colloid for hypotension (10 to 20 mL/kg boluses)
- **Specific medications**—medication choice depends largely on clinical symptoms and severity of anaphylaxis
  - Epinephrine—give immediately for any severe reaction
    - Vasopressor of choice for anaphylaxis
    - Should be given intramuscularly into anterior thigh every 5 minutes for any severe reaction
      - Adult: 0.3 to 0.5 mL of 1:1000 (1 mg/mL)
      - Pediatric: 0.01 mL/kg of 1:1000 (1 mg/mL)
    - Titrate to symptom improvement
    - IM provides more rapid absorption than subcutaneous in experiments with healthy volunteers
    - Patients in anaphylactic shock should be given intravenous epinephrine
      - 5 to 10 mcg IV of 1:10,000 (0.1 mg/mL) for hypotension
      - 0.1 to 0.5 mg IV of 1:10,000 (0.1 mg/mL) for cardiovascular collapse
      - Can start drip at 1 to 4 mcg/min IV for shock
      - Ensure continuous hemodynamic monitoring
  - Antihistamines—give immediately in any systemic allergic reaction to antagonize histamine effect and improve symptoms
    - Can be administered via intravenous or oral route
    - Both H1 and H2 blockers should be given
    - H1 blockers
      - Adult: 50 mg diphenhydramine or equivalent every 4 to 6 hours
      - Pediatric: 1 mg/kg diphenhydramine or equivalent every 4 to 6 hours
    - H2 blockers
      - Adult: ranitidine 50 mg (or equivalent)
      - Pediatric: ranitidine 1 mg/kg (or equivalent)
  - Beta-agonists—inhaled beta-agonists should be provided for any patient with wheezing, cough, or other respiratory symptoms
    - Albuterol: 2.5 to 5 mg via nebulizer
    - Levalbuterol can be used
    - Consider addition of ipratropium 0.25 to 0.5 mg via nebulizer
  - Corticosteroids are a mainstay of therapy for their anti-inflammatory properties
    - Can be given via oral or intravenous route
    - Onset of action typically 4 to 6 hours
      - IV: 1 to 2 mg/kg methylprednisolone (or equivalent) every 6 hours
      - PO: 1 mg/kg prednisone (or equivalent)
- **Additional medications**
  - Glucagon
    - Consider in patients with refractory hypotension, especially if taking beta-blocker medications
    - 1 to 5 mg IV over 5 minutes, followed by 5 to 15 mcg/min continuous infusion
    - Can causes emesis
  - Other vasopressors
    - Consider norepinepherine, dopamine, or vasopressin for refractory shock at standard doses
  - Atropine and isoproterenol occasionally needed for patients on beta-blockers

ANGIOEDEMA

- Rapid-onset swelling of skin and mucosal membranes
- Caused by increased vascular permeability, leading to plasma extravasation
- Can occur anywhere, but oral and oropharyngeal pose immediate life threat because of airway compromise

Etiology

- Multiple causes, but all are treated essentially the same
  - Allergic
    - IgE related as with anaphylaxis
    - Foods, drugs (especially antibiotics), envenomations, contrast dye
  - Hereditary
    - Compliment mediated
    - Includes C1-esterase deficiency
  - ACE inhibitor related
    - Related to bradykinin and substance P
  - Other causes exist as well

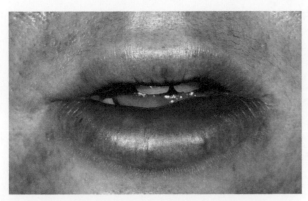

Figure 9-9. Angioedema. Swelling of the lips may be the only manifestation of angioedema. (From Habif TP: *Clinical dermatology: a color guide to diagnosis and therapy*, ed 4, Philadelphia, 2003, Mosby.)

Differential diagnosis

- Consider other causes of tissue swelling
  - Systemic allergic reactions
  - SVC syndrome can cause facial swelling
  - Erythema multiforme
  - Bullous pemphigoid

SIGNS AND SYMPTOMS

- Commonly involves the face, tongue, and lips; may extend to the oropharynx, including epiglottis (Fig. 9-9)
- Other areas include extremities and genitals
- Patients may have concomitant allergic symptoms, but this is not universal

TREATMENT

- Airway management is the most important step in treating angioedema
- Early evaluation of the posterior oropharynx and upper airway
  - Consider specialty consultation with otolaryngologist or anesthetist if a difficult airway is anticipated, as patients may require advanced or surgical airway techniques
- Early intubation is strongly advised for progressive symptoms to avoid airway obstruction
- Medications
  - Treatment for angioedema is similar to that for anaphylaxis
  - Antihistamines to block both H_1 and H_2 receptors
  - Systemic corticosteroids are typically given though there is little evidence to support their use
  - Intramuscular epinephrine may be given as well
  - For patients with hereditary angioedema with C1-esterse deficiency, fresh frozen plasma should be given
    - Contains C1 inhibitor
- Any medication suspected of causing the symptoms should be immediately discontinued

Disposition

- Patients with mild angioedema whose symptoms improve in the emergency department may be discharged on antihistamines and possibly oral corticosteroids
- Patients with significant oral or facial edema should be admitted to a monitored setting (usually the intensive care unit) where they can be closely watched for symptom progression and need for intubation

DRUG ALLERGIES

- Adverse drug reactions (ADRs) are very common in the hospital setting
- Incidence may be greater than 15% in hospitalized patients
- Incidence of fatal ADRs as much as 0.32%
- 6% to 10% of ADRs are thought to be related to allergy
- Increase in frequency because of polypharmacy

Etiologic agents

- Multiple classes of drugs are responsible for allergic reactions
- Many patient-reported allergies are not true allergic reactions. Important to have patient describe their allergic reaction (stomach upset vs rash and shortness of breath)

PENICILLIN AND DERIVATIVES

- Most common cause of drug allergies
  - 1 to 5 reactions/10,000 administrations
- Fatality rate <0.002%
- More common with parenteral rather than oral
- 10% of patients report a penicillin allergy
  - Many of these are not true allergies
  - Skin testing can identify real allergies
  - Some patients can lose, and occasionally later regain, their penicillin sensitivity
- Occurs via IgE-mediated sensitivity

CEPHALOSPORINS

- Patients can have true allergy to this class
- Share some structural similarity with penicillin
  - Historical concern over cross-reactivity in patients with penicillin allergy
  - Recent data suggest that these medications may be safe in patients with penicillin allergy
  - Administer with caution in patients with true anaphylactic penicillin allergy, but they are likely safe

CARBAPENEMS

- A newer class of antibiotic which shares some similarity to penicillin
- May be 6% to 8% incidence of allergic reaction in penicillin allergic patients

SULFONAMIDES

- Can cause any type of drug hypersensitivity reaction
- Associated with Toxic Epidermal Necrolysis and Stevens Johnson Syndrome

NSAIDS AND ASPIRIN

- Patients can be allergic to one or both
- Reactions include bronchospasm in patients with underlying reactive airway disease, angioedema, and anaphylactic shock
- True life-threatening reactions preclude administration of aspirin, even for acute coronary syndrome

LOCAL ANESTHETICS

- True allergic reactions to these medications are rare
- Most occur from the ester family, and patients can usually be safely given amides
- Multidose vials contain the preservative methylparaben, which can cause reactions

Treatment

- Therapy for allergic drug reactions consists of removing the antigen and standard treatment based on symptoms severity
- Other reactions, including toxic epidermal necrolysis, are discussed elsewhere

Disposition

- Disposition depends on the severity of the reaction, as described previously
- Patients should be advised to avoid the class of medications they reacted to, and referred for allergy testing and potential desensitization as an outpatient

Collagen vascular diseases

- Patients may present to the ED with a wide variety of symptoms and complaints ranging from the mild to life-threatening

RAYNAUD PHENOMENON

- Recurrent, episodic vasospasm of the fingers and/or toes which often occurs after exposure to cold (Fig. 9-10)

Primary (formerly Raynaud disease)

- Occurs in the absence of underlying systemic disease
- Usually milder without eventual ulceration
- Female predominance
- Onset in the 2nd or 3rd decade of life

Secondary (formerly Raynaud syndrome)

- Occurs in association with underlying disease or medication
  - Frequent association with scleroderma, rheumatoid arthritis, dermatomyositis, and systemic lupus erythematosus
- Digital ulceration and gangrene can be seen

SIGNS AND SYMPTOMS

- Typically bilateral
- Classic triphasic Raynaud attack: Digits become white (initial vasospasm) then blue (vessels relax slightly leading to diminished blood return) then red (reactive hyperemia after return of complete blood flow)
- Persistent ischemia or cyanosis may indicate acute arterial thrombosis and mandates further workup

TREATMENT

- Address any coexistent ulceration or gangrene
  - Antibiotics and surgical consultation as needed
- Rewarming should resolve symptoms

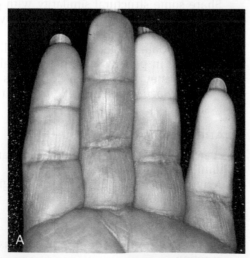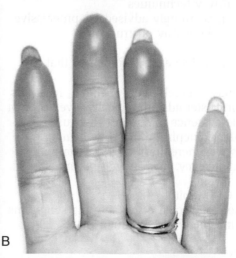

Figure 9-10. Active Raynaud phenomenon. **A,** Sharply demarcated pallor resulting from the closure of digital arteries. **B,** Digital cyanosis of the fingertips in a patient with primary Raynaud phenomenon. (From Wigley FM: Raynaud's syndrome, *New Engl J Med* 347:1001–1008, 2002. Copyright © 2002 Massachusetts Medical Society. All rights reserved.)

- Supportive therapy
  - Cold avoidance with gloves or mittens
  - Avoidance of tobacco or systemic stimulants (can cause vasoconstriction)
  - Some patients benefit from long-term vasodilators
- Referral for outpatient rheumatologic workup if discharged

REITER SYNDROME

- Reactive arthritis
- Typically occurs 2 to 6 weeks following acute dysentery (*Salmonella, Shigella, Yersinia,* or *Campylobacter*) or genitourinary infection (*Chlamydia trachomatis*)
- Male predominance during ages 15 to 35 years
- May be recurrent, with up to 20% developing severe disabling symptoms

SIGNS AND SYMPTOMS

- Classic triad (present in one third of patients):
  - Conjunctivitis (30% to 60%)
    - Usually bilateral and sterile
    - Can also see keratitis and uveitis
  - Urethritis/cervicitis (90%)
  - Arthritis (nearly universal)
    - Often polyarticular and asymmetric
    - Typically involves lower extremities
    - 50% have back pain
- Other symptoms may include enthesitis (inflammation of ligament and tendon insertion into bone), dermatologic findings (including keratoderma, balanitis, oral lesions, and nail changes)
- Neurologic and cardiac sequelae (including conduction abnormalities and aortic insufficiency) are extremely rare

DIAGNOSIS

- Based primarily on history and physical findings
- Synovial fluid with PMN predominance is usually sterile
- Serologic testing is nonspecific
  - ESR, CRP, and white blood cell counts may be elevated
  - Antinuclear antibody (ANA) and rheumatoid factor are negative

TREATMENT

- NSAIDs are first-line therapy
- Severe skin lesions treated with topical steroids and salicylic acid
- Methotrexate and etretinate may be used in refractory cases
- Antibiotic use controversial
  - May benefit *Chlamydia*-related cases

RHEUMATOID ARTHRITIS

- Chronic inflammatory autoimmune disorder causing symmetrical polyarthritis of large and small joints

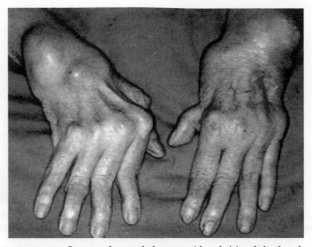

Figure 9-11. Severe advanced rheumatoid arthritis of the hands. There is massive tendon swelling over the dorsal surface of both wrists, severe muscle wasting, ulnar deviation of the metacarpophalangeal joints and swan-neck deformity of the fingers. (From Forbes CD, Jackson WF: *Color atlas and text of clinical medicine,* ed 3, London, 2003, Mosby.)

- Most common inflammatory arthritis
  - 25 per 100,000 men and 54 per 100,000 women
- Typically presents between 30 and 50 years of age

SIGNS AND SYMPTOMS

- Most patients present with symmetrical polyarticular pain, swelling, and stiffness
- Typically involves wrists, proximal interphalangeal, metacarpophalangeal, and metatarsophalangeal joints (Fig. 9-11)

DIAGNOSIS

- American College of Rheumatology criteria. Must have at least four of the following:
  - Morning stiffness >1 hour for more than 6 weeks
  - Arthritis of three or more joint areas for more than 6 weeks
  - Arthritis of hand joints for more than 6 weeks
  - Symmetric arthritis for more than 6 weeks
  - Subcutaneous rheumatoid nodules
  - Positive rheumatoid factor
  - Radiographic changes with erosion or demineralization of joints
- Serologic testing—largely nonspecific
  - Elevated ESR, CRP, and rheumatoid factor
  - Renal and liver function should be checked to help guide medication choice

TREATMENT

- NSAIDs and low-dose oral corticosteroids are first-line
- A variety of immunosuppressive agents can be used to suppress disease symptoms and progression
  - These agents should only be started once the diagnosis is confirmed and only by a rheumatologist

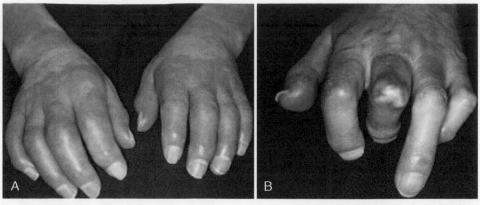

Figure 9-12. Scleroderma involving the hands. **A,** Edematous phase with diffuse swelling of fingers. **B,** Atrophic phase with contracture and thickening sclerodactyly (thick skin over the fingers). (From Goldman L: *Cecil medicine,* ed 23, Philadelphia, 2007, Saunders.)

- Patients on these medications need to be watched for complications, including infection, malignancy, and tuberculosis
- When intubating a patient with a history of rheumatoid arthritis, avoid hyperextension of the neck. Changes in the cervical spine can lead to cord injury and paralysis

SCLERODERMA

- Connective tissue disorder characterized by thickening of the skin and varying involvement of multiple organ systems
- Unknown etiology

SIGNS AND SYMPTOMS

- Scleroderma can involve any of the following systems:
  - Skin
    - Findings occur first in hands then extend to face (Fig. 9-12)
    - Thickened, taut skin with loss of creases
  - Musculoskeletal
    - Inflammatory arthritis with myopathy
    - Raynaud phenomenon seen in up to 70% at presentation
  - Gastrointestinal
    - Dysmotility in any part of the intestinal tract
    - Can develop liver cirrhosis
  - Pulmonary fibrosis and hypertension
  - Renal failure and severe hypertension
  - Other findings include hypothyroidism, erectile dysfunction, and Sjögren syndrome

CREST syndrome

- Calcinosis, Raynaud phenomenon, esophageal dysfunction, sclerodactyly, and telangiectasias

DIAGNOSIS

- Primarily clinical, based on organ system involvement
- No diagnostic lab test

TREATMENT

- No specific antiscleroderma therapy

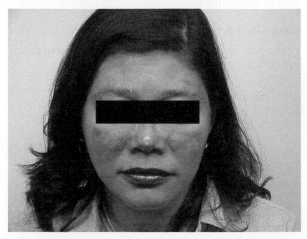

Figure 9-13. Localized acute cutaneous lupus erythematosus (malar rash). These lesions are abrupt in onset, frequently appear after exposure to the sun, and are characterized by erythema and edema. The sparing of the nasolabial folds and the absence of discrete papules and pustules help to differentiate this condition from acne rosacea (including glucocorticoid-induced rosacea). (From Firestein GS: *Kelley's textbook of rheumatology,* ed 8, Philadelphia, 2008, Saunders.)

- Treatment plans target specific organ involvement, including gastrointestinal motility agents, anti-hypertensives, and treatment for pulmonary hypertension
- 10 year survival 40% to 60%
  - Prognosis worse with pulmonary involvement

SYSTEMIC LUPUS ERYTHEMATOSUS (SLE)

- Multisystem autoimmune disorder
- 7:1 female-to-male ratio
- Classic triad of fever, joint pain, and rash in a woman of childbearing age

SIGNS AND SYMPTOMS

- Lupus is characterized by multisystem involvement
- Dermatologic
  - Malar (butterfly) facial rash seen in 40% (Fig. 9-13)

- Discoid lesions (more common in blacks) are erythematous or hypopigmented, scaly raised plaques seen in about 25% of lupus patients
- Patients often exhibit photosensitivity
- Rheumatologic
  - Polyarthralgia and myalgia almost universal
- Renal
  - Nephritis with proteinuria seen in 50%
  - Can progress to nephritic syndrome and/or renal failure
  - Hypertension common
- Neurologic
  - CNS involvement seen in up to 50% of cases
    - Seizures most common
    - Other signs include peripheral neuropathy, stroke, and lupus cerebritis (see "Complications")
- Pulmonary
  - Pleurisy and/or effusions seen in approximately 12%
  - Can develop pulmonary embolism and/or pneumonitis
- Cardiac
  - Pericarditis seen in up to 30% of patients
  - Other cardiac manifestations include myocarditis (10%) and noninfectious endocarditis with valvular vegetations
  - Now considered an independent risk factor for coronary artery disease
- Gastrointestinal—symptoms common
  - Range from oral ulcers to dysmotility to severe intestinal vasculitis
- Hematologic
  - Anemia is seen in 40% of patients, and thrombocytopenia in up to 25%
  - Thrombotic thrombocytopenic purpura and immune idiopathic thrombocytopenic purpura are seen, but are rare

DIAGNOSIS

- American College of Rheumatology developed revised criteria for diagnosis (must have at least four)
  - Includes presence of characteristic dermatologic, rheumatologic, renal, neurologic or hematologic symptoms
  - Also includes serologic findings:
    - Anti-DNA antibody
    - Anti-Sm antibody
    - Positive finding of antiphospholipid antibody
- IgG or IgM anticardiolipin antibody
- Lupus anticoagulant
  - Antinuclear antibody

TREATMENT

- NSAIDs may be used for arthritis, myalgias, and mild pericarditis or pleurisy
  - Avoid NSAIDs in patients with GI symptoms, thrombocytopenia, or renal insufficiency
- Corticosteroids often used for symptom control
  - Low dose for minor symptoms
  - High doses may be necessary for serious disease, including severe anemia or thrombocytopenia, as well as cerebritis and progressive nephritis

- Antimalarial agents can be used for cutaneous or musculoskeletal symptoms
  - Can cause reversible corneal deposits or permanent retinopathy
- Immunosuppressive agents used for severe or refractory disease

Complications

- Antiphospholipid antibody syndrome
  - Both lupus anticoagulant and anticardiolipin antibody bind to the prothrombin activator complex, increasing the risk of clotting
  - Patients can develop arterial or venous thromboemboli, including:
    - Pulmonary embolism
    - Stroke and/or myocardial infarction
    - Peripheral arterial occlusion and gangrene
    - Renal or portal arterial or venous thrombosis
  - Other complications include hemolytic anemia, thrombocytopenia, and neurologic symptoms
- Lupus cerebritis
  - Presents as mental status changes
  - Need to rule out other causes of altered mental status first (e.g., infection, cerebrovascular accident [CVA])
  - Treated with high-dose steroids
- Vasculitis—can see in any vascular bed
  - GI vascular inflammation can lead to intestinal ischemia, gangrene, and perforation
  - Coronary vasculitis can cause myocardial infarction

Special cases

- Drug-induced lupus
  - Seen in a variety of agents, including antimicrobials, anticonvulsants, antihypertensives (especially hydralazine), and antidysrhythmics (especially procainamide)
  - Usually resolves after cessation of causative agent, though may require a short steroid taper
- Pregnancy
  - Pregnancy can exacerbate SLE symptoms
  - Fetus at risk of decreased blood flow, poor development, and spontaneous miscarriage
    - Pregnant patients typically treated with aspirin and subcutaneous heparin

VASCULITIS

- The vasculitides represent a variety of multisystem diseases characterized by inflammation and destruction of blood vessels, often leading to organ system dysfunction. The conditions can best be characterized by the types of blood vessels they affect.

Large-vessel vasculitis

TAKAYASU ARTERITIS

- Chronic, recurrent inflammation of the aorta, its branches, and the pulmonary arteries

- Most common in women 20 to 30 years of age, especially Japanese
- Nonspecific symptoms including fever and weakness predominate early, but the disease can progress causing ischemia of limbs or virtually any organ system

TREATMENT

- Corticosteroids 1 mg/kg/day
- Cytotoxic agents can be used for treatment failure

TEMPORAL ARTERITIS (GIANT CELL ARTERITIS)

- Granulomatous inflammation of large arteries that most commonly affects branches of the carotid artery
- Most common in women older than 60 years of age
- Symptoms include headache, vision loss (usually unilateral), temporal artery tenderness, and jaw claudication
- Diagnosed by temporal artery biopsy, but elevated ESR and CRP are seen
  - Normal ESR increases with age

TREATMENT

- Corticosteroids 1 mg/kg/day

Medium-vessel vasculitides

BEHÇET DISEASE

- Chronic, recurrent ulcerations of oral mucosa and genitals with uveitis
- More common in men, and seen in young adult patients

DIAGNOSIS

- Based largely on history of recurrent oral and genital aphthous ulcers
- Confirmed by biopsy of affected tissue

TREATMENT

- Glucocorticoids 1 mg/kg/day
- Uveitis, optic neuritis, or CNS involvement mandates admission for chemotherapeutic agents

POLYARTERITIS NODOSA (PAN) AND MICROSCOPIC POLYANGIITIS (MPA)

- Inflammation of small and medium vessels
  - PAN affects peripheral nerves and the gastrointestinal system
  - MPA characterized by progressive glomerulonephritis and pulmonary alveolar hemorrhage

TREATMENT

- Corticosteroids ± additional immunosuppressant agents

WEGENER GRANULOMATOSIS

- Necrotizing vasculitis which primarily affects the respiratory tract and kidneys

- Slightly more common in men, with onset between 40 and 50 years of age
- Initial symptoms involve the upper respiratory tract but progresses to the lungs with cough, hemoptysis and pulmonary infiltrates
- Aggressive glomerulonephritis is a common late finding

DIAGNOSIS

- Elevated cytoplasmic anti-neutrophil cytoplasmic antibody (c-ANCA) is sensitive and specific
- Lung biopsy is definitive

TREATMENT

- Combination therapy with cyclophosphamide and corticosteroids

Small-vessel vasculitis

CHURG–STRAUSS SYNDROME

- Eosinophilic granulomatous disease associated with asthma and allergic rhinitis

SIGNS AND SYMPTOMS

- Pulmonary symptoms predominate, and precede other symptoms
- Can develop pericarditis and myocarditis
- Renal disease is uncommon

DIAGNOSIS

- Markedly elevated eosinophil counts
- Confirmed by biopsy

TREATMENT

- Responds well to corticosteroid therapy

ERYTHEMA NODOSUM (Fig. 9-14)

- Inflammation of subcutaneous venules
- More common in women
- Red nodules typically located on the anterior shin

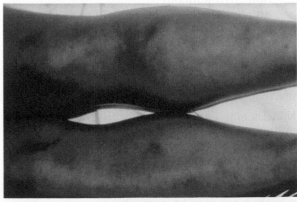

Figure 9-14. Erythema nodosum. (Courtesy of David Effron, MD) (From Marx JA: *Rosen's emergency medicine: concepts and clinical practice*, ed 6, Philadelphia, 2006, Mosby.)

- Thought to develop from hypersensitivity to an infection, drug, or systemic disease

TREATMENT

- Identify and treat underlying cause
- NSAIDs can control associated arthralgias

GOODPASTURE SYNDROME

- Results from antibodies to glomerular basement membrane
- More common in young men

SIGNS AND SYMPTOMS

- Cough with pulmonary hemorrhage, which can be severe
- Glomerulonephritis that can progress to renal failure
- Additional symptoms include fever, arthralgias, and palpable purpura
  - Diagnosis made by renal biopsy

TREATMENT

- Severe disease requires high-dose intravenous methylprednisolone (10 to 15 mg/kg)

HENOCH–SCHÖNLEIN PURPURA (HSP)
(Fig. 9-15)

- Primarily effect arterioles and capillaries

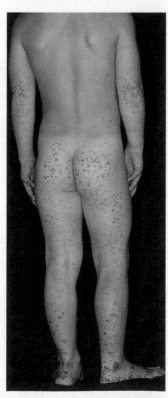

Figure 9-15. Henoch–Schönlein purpura. Palpable purpuric lesions are most common on the lower extremities and buttocks but can appear on the arms, face, and ears; the trunk is usually spared. (From Habif TP: *Clinical dermatology: a color guide to diagnosis and therapy*, ed 4, Philadelphia, 2003, Mosby.)

- Peaks between 4 and 11 years of age, but can be seen in adults, and often follows a viral illness and can be drug related

SIGNS AND SYMPTOMS

- Vasculitic rash with lower-extremity arthralgias
- GI symptoms occur in 70%
- Hematuria and red cell casts occur in 50%, but rarely lead to fulminant renal failure

TREATMENT

- Identify and treat any underlying illness or medication causing symptoms
- Corticosteroids 1 mg/kg/day

HYPERSENSITIVITY VASCULITIS

- Small-vessel vasculitis limited to the cutaneous system
- Occurs in response to a variety of medications
- Typical lesions include flat, coalescent papules or palpable purpura occurring on the lower extremities
- Withdrawal of the causative agent is usually sufficient therapy, though various chemotherapeutic agents are used in severe cases

PEARLS

- Sarcoidosis is defined by the presence of noncaseating granulomas, and any organ system may be involved.

- Patients with organ transplantation are susceptible to multiple infections, drug reactions, and postoperative complications.

- Rejection symptoms can often be vague and nonspecific, sometimes with only malaise and/or fever as indicators.

- Careful workup is indicated to differentiate rejection from infection and to identify an underlying infection, if present.

- Transplant patients should have detailed ED evaluations in close consultation with a transplant coordinator.

- When an infection is identified or suspected, appropriate antibiotics should be initiated promptly.

- The acute retroviral syndrome often presents with vague symptoms, often mistaken for the flu.

- AIDS is defined as a CD4 count < 200 and/or presence of an AIDS-defining illness.

- AIDS patients are highly susceptible to common community-acquired infections and opportunistic infections.

- In AIDS patients with neurologic complaints, it is important to obtain a CT and perform a lumbar puncture (LP).

- When diagnosing rheumatic fever, ensure that the patient has received complete treatment for group A streptococcal pharyngitis.

- Patients with severe valvular disease from rheumatic fever often require valve replacement.

- Salicylates are very effective in relieving arthralgias due to rheumatic fever.

- Any patient with a multisystem allergic reaction should be thought of as having anaphylaxis.

- Antihistamine therapy should be continued for 48 hours following an allergic reaction.

- In patients with refractory anaphylactic shock, especially those on beta-blocker, intravenous glucagon bolus followed by a drip may be effective.

- Patients with angioedema represent true airway emergencies and the emergency physician must be prepared to intervene early with a potentially very difficult airway.

- Raynaud symptoms that do not resolve should prompt evaluation for arterial insufficiency.

- The classic triad of Reiter syndrome is only present in one third of cases.

- Patients with SLE are at increased risk for all vascular occlusions, including myocardial infarction.

- Many vasculitides are associated with nonspecific symptoms, including fever, malaise, and arthralgias and can be mistaken for a viral syndrome.

- Do not delay corticosteroid therapy in any patient suspected of having temporal arteritis in order to obtain a biopsy.

BIBLIOGRAPHY

Aufderheide TP: Peripheral arteriovascular disease. In Marx JA, Hockberger RS, Walls RM (eds): *Rosen's emergency medicine: concepts and clinical practice*, ed 6, Philadelphia, 2006, Mosby.

Block JA, Sequeira W: Raynaud's phenomenon, *Lancet* 357:2042–2048, 2001.

Cannon GW: Immunosuppressive drugs including corticosteroids. In Goldman L, Ausiello DA (eds): *Cecil medicine*, ed 23, Philadelphia, 2008, Saunders. Online edition 978-0-8089-2377-0.

Carapetis JR: Rheumatic fever. In Cohen J, Powderly WG (eds): *Infectious diseases*, ed 2, Philadelphia, 2004, Mosby.

Centers for Disease Control and Prevention: New estimates of U.S. prevalence, 2006. Available at http://www.cdc.gov/hiv/topics/surveillance/resources/factsheets/prevalence.htm.

Dunmire SM: Infective endocarditis and valvular heart disease—Rheumatic fever. In Marx JA, Hockberger RS, Walls RM (eds): *Rosen's emergency medicine: concepts and clinical practice*, ed 6, Philadelphia, 2006, Mosby.

Ferri F, Wachtel T: Scleroderma (progressive systemic sclerosis). In Ferri FF: *Ferri's clinical advisor*, ed 1, Philadelphia, 2008, Mosby.

Fischer SA: Infections complicating solid organ transplantation, *Surg Clin North Am* 86:1127–1145, 2006.

Joint United Nations Programme on HIV/AIDS: AIDS epidemic update: 2006. Available at http://data.unaids.org/pub/EpiReport/2006/2006_EpiUpdate_en.pdf.

Judson MA: The management of sarcoidosis by the primary care physician, *Am J Med* 120:403–407, 2007.

Keadey MT, Lowery DW: The solid-organ transplant patient. In Marx JA, Hockberger RS, Walls RM (eds): *Rosen's emergency medicine: concepts and clinical practice*, ed 6, Philadelphia, 2006, Mosby. Online Edition 0-323-03686-4.

Lowery DW: Arthritis—acute rheumatic fever. In Marx JA, Hockberger RS, Walls RM (eds): *Rosen's emergency medicine: concepts and clinical practice*, ed 6, Philadelphia, 2006, Mosby.

Lowery DW: Arthritis. In Marx JA, Hockberger RS, Walls RM (eds): *Rosen's emergency medicine: concepts and clinical practice*, ed 6, Philadelphia, 2006, Mosby.

Majithia V, Geraci, SA: Rheumatoid arthritis: diagnosis and management, *Am J Med* 120(11):936–939, 2007.

Marco CA, Rothman RE: HIV infection and complications in emergency medicine, *Emerg Med Clin North Am* 26:367–387, 2008.

Martin JM, Barbadora KA: Continued high caseload of rheumatic fever in Western Pennsylvania: possible rheumatogenic EMM types of streptococcus pyogenes, *J Pediatr* 149(1):58–63, 2006.

McDonald M, Currie BJ, Carapetis UR: Acute rheumatic fever: a chink in the chain that links the heart to the throat? *Lancet Infect Dis* 4:240–245, 2004.

Mihailovic-Vucinic V, Jovanovic D: Pulmonary sarcoidosis, *Clin Chest Med* 29:459–473, 2008.

Rothman RE, Marco G, Yang S: AIDS and HIV. In Marx JA, Hockberger RS, Walls RM (eds): *Rosen's emergency medicine: concepts and clinical practice*, ed 6, Philadelphia, 2006, Mosby. Online edition 0-323-03686-4.

Sampson HA, Munoz-Furlong A, Campbell RL, Adkinson NF: Second Symposium on the Definition and Management of Anaphylaxis: Summary Report—Second National Institute of Allergy and Infectious Disease/Food Allergy and Anaphylaxis Network Symposium, *Ann Emerg Med* 47(4):373–380, 2006.

Sercombe CT: Systemic lupus erythematosus and the vasculitides. In Marx JA, Hockberger RS, Walls RM (eds): *Rosen's emergency medicine: concepts and clinical practice*, ed 6, Philadelphia, 2006, Mosby.

Simmons F: Anaphylaxis, *J Allergy Clin Immunol* 21:2, 2008.

Solensky R: Drug hypersensitivity, *Med Clin North Am* 90(1):23–60, 2006.

Temiño VM, Peebles RS: The spectrum and treatment of angioedema, *Am J Med* 121(4):282–286, 2008.

Tran TP, Muellman, RL: Allergy, hypersensitivity, and anaphylaxis. In Marx JA, Hockberger RS, Walls RM (eds): *Rosen's emergency medicine: concepts and clinical practice*, ed 6, Philadelphia, 2006, Mosby.

Weinberger SE: Sarcoidosis. In Goldman L, Ausiello DA (eds): *Cecil medicine*, ed 23, Philadelphia, 2008, Saunders. Online edition 978-0-8089-2377-0.

Wigley FM: Scleroderma (systemic sclerosis). In Goldman L, Ausiello DA (eds): *Cecil medicine*, ed 23, Philadelphia, 2008, Saunders.

Wu IB, Schwartz RA: Reiter's syndrome: the classic triad and more, *J Am Acad Dermatol* 59:113–121, 2008.

Zetola NM, Pilcher CD: Diagnosis and management of acute HIV infection, *Emerg Med Clin North Am* 21:19–48, 2007.

Questions and Answers

1. Chest radiograph abnormalities that can be seen in sarcoidosis include:
   a. focal consolidation
   b. parenchymal disease
   c. cavitary lesions
   d. pulmonary nodules
   e. pleural effusions

2. Treatment of CMV infection in the transplant patient includes:
   a. acyclovir
   b. ceftriaxone
   c. valacyclovir
   d. ganciclovir
   e. IV glucocorticoids

3. A 34-year-old woman with a renal transplant presents to the emergency department with 2 days of a vague right-lower quadrant pain over her transplanted kidney. Appropriate workup includes:
   a. ultrasonography
   b. computed tomography
   c. CBC, chemistry, and urinalysis
   d. MRI
   e. both **a** and **c**

4. A 24-year-old, HIV-infected man presents to the emergency department with dyspnea. He is diagnosed with PCP pneumonia. He has a sulfa allergy. The next appropriate treatment for this patient is:
   a. prednisone
   b. azithromycin
   c. doxycycline
   d. pentamidine
   e. fluconazole

5. A 34-year-old HIV-infected patient presents to the emergency department with a complaint of white plaques to his tongue. You notice that you can easily scrape off the plaques on his buccal mucosa. Appropriate treatment is:
   a. fluconazole
   b. amphotericin
   c. acyclovir
   d. doxycycline
   e. none of the above

6. Which of the following is considered a major Jones criterion for the diagnosis of rheumatic fever?
   a. fever
   b. elevated ESR
   c. arthralgia
   d. PR prolongation on ECG
   e. erythema marginatum

7. An otherwise healthy 10-year-old male patient presents complaining of low-grade fever, joint pain, and a rash for 4 to 5 days. His parents report that he had a "sore throat" 2 weeks earlier but did not seek medical attention. He has a temperature of 38.1° C, but otherwise has normal vital signs. His exam is notable for a well-appearing young male with scattered irregular, circular, erythematous lesions on his legs. He has generalized joint tenderness with a full range of motion, and has no clinical meningismus. The rest of his physical exam is normal. Which of the following choices of antibiotics would be appropriate first-line therapy for the diagnosis of rheumatic fever?
   a. penicillin V 250 mg TID for 10 days
   b. gentamicin 2.5 mg/kg IV every 8 hours
   c. azithromycin 12 mg/kg/day orally for 5 days
   d. vancomycin 1 gram IV twice a day
   e. all are appropriate

8. Which of the following is true concerning allergic reactions and anaphylaxis?
   a. patients with normal blood pressure cannot have anaphylaxis
   b. epinephrine should be administered early in patients suspected of having moderate to severe anaphylaxis
   c. the absence of cutaneous symptoms excludes patients from having anaphylaxis
   d. very few allergic reactions are mediated by IgE
   e. in patients with systemic allergic reactions whose symptoms completely resolve in the emergency department, no further treatment is needed

9. A 19-year-old male patient presents to the emergency department severely hypotensive. He has a known history of anaphylaxis to peanuts. EMS reports he was at a party where peanuts were being eaten, and he began to complain about feeling itchy, and having difficulty breathing. He tried using his epinephrine autoinjector, but within 5 minutes had collapsed. His vital signs on arrival to the ED are heart rate (HR) = 160 bpm, BP = 65/30 mmHg, RR = 4/minute, O_2 saturation 98% on a non-rebreather. He is poorly responsive, has audible stridor and wheezing, and his skin is diffusely erythematous with multiple areas of urticaria. Which of the following is most correct regarding his management?
   a. administer epinephrine 1 : 1000 0.3 mL IV
   b. there is no role for intravenous fluids in treating his hypotension
   c. oral prednisone 60 mg should be given immediately
   d. prompt airway assessment, including early intubation, should be performed

e. prior to attempting intubation, it is mandatory to administer inhaled albuterol 5 mg over 15 to 20 minutes

10. Which of the following presentations of SLE represents an indication for admission for intravenous corticosteroids?

   a. a 24-year-old woman with mild pleuritic chest pain, normal vital signs, and no evidence of pulmonary embolism or infectious complication
   b. a 24-year-old woman with isolated diffuse arthralgias
   c. a 24-year-old woman with altered depressed consciousness, normal labs, and a negative head CT and lumbar puncture
   d. a 24-year-old woma with a low-grade fever, evidence of hemolysis, and a hemoglobin of 4 mg/dL
   e. both **c** and **d**

11. A 9-year-old boy presents to the ED complaining of abdominal pain, a rash on his legs, and a low-grade fever. He is nontoxic appearing, and his parents report he has recently recovered from a viral illness. His labs show hematuria but are otherwise normal. The most likely diagnosis is:

   a. Henoch–Schönlein purpura
   b. Goodpasture syndrome
   c. giant-cell arteritis
   d. Wegener granulomatosis
   e. Churg–Strauss Syndrome

12. Goodpasture syndrome typically affects which two organ systems?

   a. lungs and GI tract
   b. kidney and GI tract
   c. CNS and lung
   d. kidney and lungs
   e. cardiac and kidney

13. Definitive diagnosis of temporal arteritis is made by:

   a. ESR
   b. CRP
   c. biopsy
   d. history of unilateral vision loss
   e. CBC

14. Typical findings of rheumatoid arthritis include:

   a. monoarticular swelling
   b. symmetrical polyarticular swelling
   c. large erythematous plaques
   d. headache and visual changes
   e. pallor of the distal extremities

15. Reiter syndrome is associated with:

   a. gonorrhea
   b. syphilis
   c. chlamydia

d. HIV/AIDS
e. group B Strep

16. Incidence of adverse drug reactions in hospitalized patients is:

   a. 5%
   b. 10%
   c. 15%
   d. 30%

17. A 63-year-old woman presents to the ED with a complaint of tongue and lip swelling. She was recently started on an ACE inhibitor for hypertension. On exam, her lips are markedly swollen and her tongue is starting to protrude. Mild stridor is present. The most important first action is to:

   a. administer IM epinephrine
   b. nebulized beta-agonists
   c. secure the airway with the help of ENT and/or anesthesia
   d. fluid resuscitation

18. A 23-year-old woman presents in extreme distress after being stung by a bee. She is altered and stridulous on arrival with a diffuse urticarial rash. Her vital signs are BP = 80/30 mmHg, HR = 130 bpm, RR = 33/minute, SaO_2 = 87% on 15 LPM of O_2 and a temp of 98.7° F. All of the following may be helpful in her care except:

   a. glucagon
   b. epinephrine
   c. ranitidine
   d. bicarbonate
   e. intubation

19. Which of the following is considered an AIDS-defining illness?

   a. CMV retinitis
   b. PCP pneumonia
   c. cryptococcosis, toxoplasmosis
   d. all of the above

20. A 68-year-old woman with a history of diabetes, hypertension, and rheumatoid arthritis presents in extreme distress due to acute pulmonary edema. On arrival, her vital signs are a BP = 210/140 mmHg, HR = 118 bpm, RR = 38/minute, SaO_2 = 89% on 15 LPM O_2 and temp 99.1° F. After maximal medical therapy and a trial of BiPAP, the patient is obtunded with no gag reflex and her vital signs are BP = 168/90 mmHg, HR = 110 bpm, RR = 30/minute, SaO_2 = 78% on 10 LPM O_2 on BiPAP. A decision is made to intubate the patient. What precaution should be taken?

   a. pretreatment with lidocaine
   b. intubation with inline cervical spine immobilization
   c. use of ketamine for induction
   d. IV fluid bolus prior to intubation
   e. no special precaution needed

1. Answer: b

Radiographic findings associated with sarcoidosis include hilar adenopathy, **parenchymal disease,** and pulmonary fibrosis.

2. Answer: d

Infection with CMV is treated with **ganciclovir.** Immunosuppression is maintained at the lowest possible dose. Immunoglobulin may be added for treatment.

3. Answer: e

This patient may be suffering from *rejection* or *infection* of her transplanted organ. Appropriate evaluation includes **ultrasonography, CBC, chemistry,** and **urinalysis** to evaluate for possible infection and renal function.

4. Answer: d

Pentamidine is an appropriate second-line agent for the treatment of PCP in sulfa allergic patients. The other antibiotic choices listed do not provide adequate coverage.

5. Answer: a

This patient is suffering from *oral candidiasis* (thrush). Appropriate treatment is with **fluconazole** or clotrimazole. Patients with suspected esophagitis are treated with fluconazole for a longer course.

6. Answer: e

The major criteria include polyarthritis, carditis, chorea, **erythema marginatum,** and subcutaneous nodules. The minor criteria include fever, arthralgia, elevated ESR and CRP, and PR prolongation.

7. Answer: a

Penicillin is still considered first-line therapy for *group A streptococcal pharyngitis* (and therefore rheumatic fever) because of its low cost, narrow spectrum, and clinical efficacy. It can be given either as a single IM injection of benzathine penicillin (adults: 1.2 million units, children: 0.6 million units) or as 10 days of oral therapy (250 mg three to four times a day in children, 500 mg three to four times a day for adults). **Gentamicin** is ineffective against group A streptococcus and is not indicated. While **azithromycin** may well be effective, it is more expensive than penicillin, has an unnecessarily broad spectrum, and faces increasing antimicrobial resistance. **Vancomycin,** while likely effective, is far stronger than what would be necessary in this case, and is usually reserved for cases of methicillin-resistant staphylococcal infections.

8. Answer: b

Epinephrine is first-line therapy for any moderate to severe allergic reaction, especially when multiple systems are involved **(b).** It should be given early once the diagnosis is suspected. Patients do not need to be hypotensive to have severe anaphylaxis, but hypotension does indicate anaphylactic shock **(a).** While most patients have cutaneous symptoms, roughly 10% to 20% of allergic reactions occur without obvious skin findings **(c).** Most allergic reactions are IgE mediated **(d).** Finally, patients treated in the emergency department for allergic reactions should be discharged on antihistamines, and often on systemic corticosteroids **(e).**

9. Answer: d

This patient is critically ill, and in profound *anaphylactic shock* with respiratory failure. He will almost certainly require immediate **intubation (d).** Although **epinephrine** should be administered immediately, the dose provided is incorrect **(a).** This patient has cardiovascular collapse and should receive intravenous epinephrine dosed at 0.1 to 0.5 mg slow IV of 1:10,000 (0.1 mg/mL), followed by a drip at 1 to 4 µg/min IV. For stable patients without profound hypotension, IM epinephrine 1:1000 (1 mg/mL) can be given in 0.3 to 0.5 mL doses every 5 to 15 minutes. Although **oral prednisone** is as efficacious as IV corticosteroids **(c),** oral medications should not be given to critically ill patients who are unable to tolerate PO. Finally, although **albuterol** may help with bronchospasm and respiratory symptoms, airway concerns override any benefit from bronchodilators, and clinical need for intubation should be the priority **(e).**

10. Answer: e

Both **c** and **d** represent severe manifestations of lupus and require admission for intravenous steroid therapy. The patient in **a** has **pleurisy** without evidence of severe complication and can be treated as an outpatient. Patients with isolated **arthralgias (b)** who are otherwise stable do not need to be admitted. Answer **c** describes *lupus cerebritis,* a severe neurologic complication requiring intensive therapy. The patient in **d** has severe *hemolytic anemia,* which requires intravenous steroid therapy.

11. Answer: a

The case described represents **HSP,** most often seen in young children. **Goodpasture syndrome** is typically accompanied by pulmonary hemorrhage and glomerulonephritis. **Giant-cell arteritis,** also known as temporal arteritis, occurs in patients older than 50 years and is associated with headache, jaw claudication, and development of vision loss. **Wegener granulomatosis** is accompanied by pulmonary symptoms, including hemorrhage, and occurs in patients who are 40 to 50 years of age. **Churg–Strauss syndrome** is associated with asthma and allergic symptoms, and is accompanied by elevated eosinophil levels.

12. Answer: d

Goodpasture syndrome results from destruction of the glomerular basement membrane as a result of immune-mediated antibody response. The **renal** and **pulmonary** systems are typically affected. Clinical presentation may include hemoptysis, cough, and glomerulonephritis progressing to renal failure

13. Answer: c

Biopsy of the temporal artery makes the definitive diagnosis. Elevated **ESR** is a common lab finding in this condition. Remember that as a patient ages, his or her normal ESR may increase. Because of the potential risk of vision loss, treatment is started prior to obtaining biopsy results

14. Answer: b

15. Answer: c

16. Answer: c

Adverse drug reactions are common and may have an incidence of **15%** or more in hospitalized patients. These reactions are common in the elderly where polypharmacy is more common. Be sure to check for potential interactions before prescribing new medications to an at-risk population.

17. Answer: c

This patient has angioedema with impending airway loss. **Airway management** is a priority in these

patients with an emphasis on early intubation. Speciality consultation may be required if available for fiberoptic guided nasal intubation.

18. Answer: d

This patient presents with *anaphylactic shock.* Treatment focuses on removal of the offending agent, airway and hemodynamic support, beta- and alpha-agonists, steroids and H_1 and H_2 blockers, and glucagon (in some cases). **Bicarbonate** does not factor into the acute management.

19. Answer: d

AIDS is defined as a CD4 count <200 or the presence of an AIDS-defining illness, which includes all of the above as well as cryptosporidiosis, esophageal candidiasis, Kaposi sarcoma, *Mycobacterium avium* complex, and disseminated histoplasmosis.

20. Answer: b

Because of changes in the cervical spine, patients with a history of rheumatoid arthritis are prone to cervical injury with hyperextension as can happen during intubation. Use of **inline cervical spine immobilization** is recommended.

Infectious Disorders 10

Jeffrey Green | Alison E. Suarez

BACTERIAL INFECTIONS

Bacterial food poisoning/diarrheal illness

Enterocolitis

Botulism

Chlamydia

Gonorrhea

Meningococcal disease

Tuberculosis (TB)

Atypical mycobacteria

Diphtheria

Gas gangrene

Bacteremia

SEPSIS

Systemic inflammatory response syndrome (SIRS)

SEVERE SEPSIS AND SEPTIC SHOCK

TOXIC SHOCK SYNDROME (TSS)

SYPHILIS

TETANUS

FUNGAL INFECTIONS

Aspergillus fumigates

Blastomyces dermatitidis

Coccidioides immitis

Histoplasma capsulatum

Mucormycosis

Sporotrichosis—*Sporothrix schenckii*

PROTOZOAN INFECTIONS

Malaria

Toxoplasmosis

TICK-BORNE ILLNESS

Ehrlichiosis

Lyme disease

Rocky Mountain spotted fever

VIRAL INFECTIONS

Hantavirus

Herpes simplex virus

Varicella zoster virus (VZV)

Infectious mononucleosis (Epstein–Barr virus [EBV])

Influenza

Parainfluenza

Rabies

Rubella

Rubeola (measles)

EMERGING INFECTIONS/PANDEMICS

Plague

SARS

Community-acquired/associated methicillin-resistant *S. aureus* (CA-MRSA)

West Nile virus

Dengue fever

Bacterial infections

BACTERIAL FOOD POISONING/ DIARRHEAL ILLNESS

- Duration of antibiotic therapy varies per author; bacterial diarrheal illness may be treated for 3 to 5 days in some instances

Campylobacter

- *Campylobacter jejuni, Campylobacter coli, Campylobacter fetus,* small Gram-negative bacteria
- Fecal–oral transmission
- Most common bacterial cause of diarrhea, most cases in young children
- Opportunistic infection in homosexual men and AIDS patients

SIGNS AND SYMPTOMS

- 2- to 5-day incubation, rapid onset of symptoms; resolves in 5 to 7 days
- Fever, crampy abdominal pain, diarrhea, anorexia, malaise, myalgias, headache
- Stool loose, bile colored, 60% to 90% have gross or occult blood, fecal leukocytes

DIAGNOSIS

- Clinical diagnosis
- Stool culture
- Sigmoidoscopy—inflammatory colitis, similar to inflammatory bowel disease (IBD)

TREATMENT

- Antibiotics not indicated when symptoms improving
- Ciprofloxacin 500 mg PO two times a day for 7 days
- Erythromycin 500 mg PO four times a day for 7 days

Salmonellosis

- *Salmonella enteritidis, Salmonella choleraesuis, Salmonella typhimurium,* Gram-negative bacilli
- Ingestion of contaminated food (poultry and eggs), excretions of household pets
- Risk factors
  - Decreased gastric acidity, alteration of intestinal flora, sickle cell, immunocompromise
  - Penetrate intestinal mucosa, lodge in lamina propria

SIGNS AND SYMPTOMS

- 8- to 48-hour incubation; resolves in 2 to 5 days
- Fever, colicky abdominal pain/tenderness, vomiting
- Loose watery diarrhea (occasionally with mucus and blood), fecal leukocytes

DIAGNOSIS

- Stool culture

TREATMENT

- Clinically improving do not require treatment
- Ciprofloxacin 500 mg two times a day for 7 days

Typhoid fever

- *Salmonella typhi*
- Invasive, bacteria replicate in Peyer's patches, mesenteric lymph nodes, spleen

SIGNS AND SYMPTOMS

- 5- to 21-day incubation period
- Sustained fever (103° to 104° F), malaise (diarrhea uncommon), apathy, confusion
- Relative bradycardia, splenomegaly, abdominal tenderness
- Rose spots on chest or abdomen (30% of patients)
- Hepatosplenomegaly, leukopenia, neutropenia
- Complications
  - Pancreatitis, cholecystitis, infective endocarditis, pneumonia
  - Liver abscess, orchitis, or focal infection

DIAGNOSIS

- Initial clinical diagnosis
- Confirmed by isolation of *S. typhi* from blood, stool, or bone marrow

TREATMENT

- Ciprofloxacin 500 mg PO two times a day for 7 to 14 days (IV if not tolerating POs)
- Ceftriaxone 1 to 2 g every 12 to 24 hours for 10 to 14 days

Shigellosis

- *Shigella sonnei, Shigella flexneri, Shigella dysenteriae*
- Fecal–oral spread, common in nursing homes, prisons, countries with poor sanitation
- Small inoculum may cause disease
- Noninvasive inflammation of bowel epithelium, bleeding from superficial mucosa

SIGNS AND SYMPTOMS

- 24- to 48-hour incubation
- Watery diarrhea with no constitutional symptoms (may progress to dysentery)
- **Dysentery:** grossly bloody diarrhea, tenesmus, fever, headache, and myalgias
- Profound dehydration and circulatory collapse

DIAGNOSIS

- Clinical diagnosis
- Stool cultures

TREATMENT

- Correction of fluid and electrolytes
- Ciprofloxacin 500 mg PO two times a day for 7 days

Yersinia

- *Yersinia enterocolitica,* Gram-negative, aerobic bacteria
- Increasing incidence worldwide, more common in children
- Invasive intestinal infection, fecal–oral transmission
- Large outbreaks because of contaminated milk

SIGNS AND SYMPTOMS

- Initially fever, colicky abdominal pain, diarrhea, anorexia, vomiting and malaise
- Symptoms persist 10 to 14 days or longer
- Ileocecitis, lower abdominal pain with minimal diarrhea, **mimics appendicitis**

DIAGNOSIS

- Stool culture, fecal leukocytes
- Ileocecitis on ultrasound, may differentiate from appendicitis

TREATMENT

- No antibiotics if symptoms improving
- trimethoprim–sulfamethoxazole (TMP/SMX) 160 mg/800 mg PO two times a day for 7 days

Vibrio

VIBRIO PARAHAEMOLYTICUS, VIBRIO VULNIFICUS

- Gram-negative bacilli, coastal seawater organism
- Ingestion of raw or undercooked seafood
- Inflammatory response in intestine

SIGNS AND SYMPTOMS

- 4- to 48-hour incubation; resolves in 24 to 48 hours
- Diarrhea, abdominal cramps, fever, nausea, headache

DIAGNOSIS

- Thiosulfate citrate bile sucrose (TCBS) agar culture

TREATMENT

- Usually self-limited
- Doxycycline 100 mg PO two times a day for 7 days for severe disease

VIBRIO CHOLERA

- Noninvasive enterotoxin production

SIGNS AND SYMPTOMS

- 24- to 48-hour incubation, resolves in 7 days
- Copious watery diarrhea, abdominal cramps, vomiting, low-grade fever, severe dehydration

DIAGNOSIS

- Fecal leukocytes and guaiac-negative stool (noninvasive)
- TCBS stool culture

TREATMENT

- WHO oral rehydration formula successful worldwide
- Doxycycline 100 mg PO two times a day for 10 days

Hemorrhagic *Escherichia coli*

- *E. coli* O157:H7
- Most common in children and elderly, outbreaks due to undercooked hamburger, raw milk, contaminated water supplies
- Produces *Shigella*-like toxin, noninvasive

SIGNS AND SYMPTOMS

- 4- to 9-day incubation; resolves in 7 to 10 days
- Bloody diarrhea (may be large quantity of blood), abdominal cramps, vomiting

DIAGNOSIS

- Sorbitol–MacConkey stool culture, latex agglutination antibody testing

TREATMENT

- Supportive care, no antibiotics (increase incidence of hemolytic-uremic syndrome)

Aeromonas

- *Aeromonas hydrophila*, Gram-negative facultative anaerobe
- Ubiquitous in fresh and brackish water
- Account for 10% to 15% of diarrhea in children, also immunocompromised adults

SIGNS AND SYMPTOMS

- Watery (nonbloody) diarrhea, vomiting, fever (2 to 10 *weeks* of symptoms)

DIAGNOSIS

- Stool culture

TREATMENT

- TMP/SMX 160 mg/800 mg PO two times a day for 7 to 14 days

Staphylococcal food poisoning

- Enterotoxin forming strain of *Staphylococcus aureus*, heat-stable toxin, direct CNS effects
- Contaminated ham, eggs, pastries, potato salad

SIGNS AND SYMPTOMS

- 1 to 6 hours post-ingestion; resolves in 8 to 24 hours
- Cramping, abdominal pain, **violent vomiting**
- Variable diarrhea (nonbloody), occasional fever

DIAGNOSIS

- Clinical diagnosis (stool cultures noncontributory)
- Food-related outbreaks after short incubation period highly suggestive

TREATMENT

- Supportive care, antibiotics of no value

Clostridium

- *Clostridium perfringens*, enterotoxin-mediated infection
- **Most common cause of acute food poisoning in the United States**
- Cooked meat or poultry dishes, ingested >24 hours later

SIGNS AND SYMPTOMS

- 6 to 24 hours post ingestion, watery diarrhea, abdominal cramps
- Outbreaks due to contaminated food
- **Enteritis necroticans**—hemorrhagic, necrotizing enterocolitis of bowel
  - Abdominal pain, diarrhea, shock, rapidly fatal

DIAGNOSIS

- Fecal leukocytes and guaiac-negative, stool cultures noncontributory

TREATMENT

- Supportive care, antibiotics not indicated

Bacillus cereus

- *B. cereus*, spore forming, Gram-positive rod, enterotoxin-mediated infection
- Poorly processed food (boiled rice), unrefrigerated, rewarmed before serving

SIGNS AND SYMPTOMS

- Vomiting, abdominal cramping, diarrhea
- Vomiting predominate: onset 2 to 3 hours; resolves in <10 hours
- Diarrhea predominate: onset 6 to 14 hours; resolves in 20 to 36 hours

DIAGNOSIS

- Isolation in suspected food source, stool cultures

TREATMENT

- Supportive care, antibiotics not indicated

Scombroid fish poisoning

- History of dark-fleshed fish ingestion (tuna, mackerel, mahi-mahi, bluefish)
- Poor refrigeration, normal marine flora produce histamine-like substances

SIGNS AND SYMPTOMS

- 20 to 30 minutes postingestion; resolves in 6 hours
- Metallic, bitter-tasting fish
- Facial flushing, injected conjunctivae, diarrhea, severe headache, palpitations, and abdominal cramps
- **Not an allergic reaction,** should not prevent future fish ingestion

DIAGNOSIS

- Clinical

TREATMENT

- Diphenhydramine 50 mg IV

Ciguatera fish poisoning

- *Gambierdiscus toxicus,* marine dinoflagellate, unicellular plankton
- Toxin accumulates in coral fish (red snapper, grouper, barracuda, sea bass, mackerel)
- Ciguatoxin, heat-stable neurotoxin, not deactivated by cooking or freezing
- Causes >50% of fish poisoning in the United States, undetectable in fish

SIGNS AND SYMPTOMS

- 2- to 6-hour incubation; usually resolves in 2 to 8 weeks
- GI symptoms (vomiting, watery diarrhea, abdominal cramps)
- Later neurologic symptoms (paresthesias, loose painful teeth, ataxia, confusion)
- **Dysesthesias (heat and cold sensory reversal) virtually pathognomonic**

DIAGNOSIS

- Clinical

TREATMENT

- Atropine for severe bradycardia and hypotension
- Alcohol abstention
- Mannitol 1 g/kg IV use is controversial for severe neurologic manifestations

ENTEROCOLITIS

- *Clostridium difficile,* toxin-producing bacteria
- Following use of oral or parenteral antibiotics (usually nosocomial)
- Clindamycin, ampicillin, cephalosporins, tetracycline, TMP-SMX, others
- Antidiarrheal medications or narcotics increase likelihood
- Proliferate when normal flora reduced by antibiotics, cytopathic toxin destroys colonic mucosa, causing pseudomembranous enterocolitis

SIGNS AND SYMPTOMS

- Up to 3 to 4 weeks after discontinuing antibiotics
- Fever, crampy abdominal pain, watery, possible bloody diarrhea

DIAGNOSIS

- *C. difficile* toxin assays best test; sensitivity increases with repeat samples
- Stool cultures not diagnostic (may grow *C. difficile* in the absence of disease)
- Sigmoidoscopy for pseudomembranous lesions

TREATMENT

- Stop causative antibiotic
- Metronidazole 250 mg PO four times a day for 10 to 14 days
- Vancomycin 125 mg PO four times a day for 10 to 14 days (500 mg four times a day if critically ill)
- Colonic resection for severe cases with bowel perforation or toxic megacolon

BOTULISM

- *Clostridium botulinum,* anaerobic, Gram-positive rod, spore forming
- Releases a potent exotoxin (most potent biologic compound known)
- Inhibits release of acetylcholine at neuromuscular junction
- Transmission
    - Undercooked or poorly preserved food
    - Contaminated "black tar" heroin
    - Honey, corn syrup, soil ingestion in infants
    - Iatrogenic from medical use of toxin

SIGNS AND SYMPTOMS

- Food born, adult
    - Onset 2 hours to 14 days postingestion
    - Dry mouth, painful tongue, lightheadedness, vomiting, constipation
    - Diplopia, dysphonia, dysphagia, dysarthria, vertigo

- Ptosis, extraocular palsies, dilated and fixed pupils, depressed or absent gag
- Extremity weakness, more pronounced in upper extremities
- Severe disease—distended bladder, tachypneic, shallow breathing
- Infantile botulism
  - Children <1 year old, peaks at 3 months
  - Constipation, poor feeding, weak cry, poor head control, hypotonia
  - Decreased muscle tone, diminished DTRs, altered facial expressions
  - Respiratory failure in 50% of cases

DIAGNOSIS

- Clinical: **GI, autonomic, and cranial nerve symptoms**
- Toxin or organism isolated in blood, GI tract, wound, or ingested food product

TREATMENT

- Supportive care, ICU admission
- Early intubation for potential respiratory compromise
- Serial vital capacities (<12 mL/kg requires ventilator support)
- Foley catheterization for urinary retention, nasogastric tube for ileus
- Antitoxin (administer as early as possible)
  - Equine trivalent compound, effective against toxin A, B and E
  - Equine heptavalent effective against all known strains—military availability
  - Skin test for hypersensitivity, then one 10-mL IV dose
  - No effect on bound toxin
  - Not indicated for infantile botulism
- Infant botulism—botulinum immune globulin (BIG)-orphan drug available through California Department of Health Services
- Alert CDC and area emergency departments of possible outbreak

CHLAMYDIA

- Obligate intracellular bacterium

Chlamydia pneumonia

- 2% to 10% of pneumonia, higher proportion in young adults, can affect all ages

SIGNS AND SYMPTOMS

- URI symptoms, cough, malaise, prolonged symptoms (fever less common)

DIAGNOSIS

- Chest x-ray (CXR)—single, subsegmental patchy infiltrate classic
  - CXR pattern cannot differentiate from other pneumonias
- Cultures of little diagnostic utility

TREATMENT

- Azithromycin 500 mg PO one time, then 250 mg PO daily for 4 days *or*
- Doxycycline 100 mg PO two times a day for 10 days

Chlamydia psittaci

- Birds (parakeets, parrots, macaws, pigeons, turkeys) major reservoir

SIGNS AND SYMPTOMS

- **Bird handlers at risk**
- 5- to 14-day incubation
- Acute febrile illness, nonproductive cough, headache, malaise
- Extensive interstitial pneumonia
- Complications: pericarditis, myocarditis, endocarditis, hepatitis

DIAGNOSIS

- Clinical diagnosis
- Fourfold antibody titer increase confirms diagnosis (titer >1 : 32 diagnostic)

TREATMENT

- Tetracycline 500 mg PO every 6 hours *or*
- Erythromycin 500 mg PO every 6 hours for 14 to 21 days

Chlamydia trachomatis

- Most common bacterial STD, transmitted via direct contact
- Linked to **Reiter syndrome** (reactive arthritis)
  - 15- to 35-year-old males
  - 2 to 6 weeks after urethritis or dysentery
  - Urethritis (non-gonococcal)
  - Arthritis (asymmetric, inflammatory polyarthritis)
  - Conjunctivitis (may progress to iritis, or corneal ulceration)
    - *S. flexneri* and *S. typhi* also implicated

SIGNS AND SYMPTOMS

- 2% to 20% asymptomatic carriers
- Cervicitis
  - Vaginal discharge, dysuria, abnormal vaginal bleeding
  - Friable, erythematous, congested cervix with purulent discharge
- Pelvic inflammatory disease
  - Lower abdominal pain, tenderness, fever, peritonitis, ascites
  - Leukocytosis, elevated ESR, C-reactive protein
- Fitz–Hugh–Curtis syndrome
  - Perihepatitis, direct extension of PID from fallopian tubes
  - Right upper quadrant abdominal pain, fever
  - "Violin string" adhesions on laparoscopy
- Urethritis
  - 10% of males asymptomatic carriers

- 6- to 12-day incubation, milder course than gonorrhea
- Urethral discharge and dysuria
- Epididymitis
  - **More common** than gonococcal epididymitis
  - Normal testicle, warm, swollen, erythematous scrotum, tenderness posterior and lateral to testicle
- Trachoma
  - Common in developing countries
  - Unilateral conjunctivitis with palpebral edema
    - Pannus over cornea
      - Lid scarring by **entrichiasis** (eyelashes turn inwards, abrade cornea)
- Lymphogranuloma venereum
  - L_1, L_2, L_3 *C. trachomatis* strains
  - Inguinal lymphadenopathy, pelvic vascular strictures
    - **Groove sign**—adenopathy above and below inguinal ligament

DIAGNOSIS

- Culture, technically difficult
- PCR (retains sensitivity with urine sampling or self-collected vaginal swabs)

TREATMENT

- Uncomplicated (cervicitis, urethritis)
  - Azithromycin 1 g PO for 1 day *or* doxycycline 100 mg PO two times a day for 7 days
- Complicated (pelvic inflammatory disease)
  - Doxycycline 100 mg IV or PO two times a day for 14 days
  - Treat for presumed gonorrhea coinfection

GONORRHEA

- *Neisseria gonorrhoeae*, encapsulated, Gram-negative diplococcus
- Consider coinfection with *C. trachomatis* (15% to 25% males, 35% to 50% females)

SIGNS AND SYMPTOMS

- Urethritis
  - 2- to 7-day incubation, urethral discharge and dysuria
- Epididymitis
  - Normal testicle, warm, swollen, erythematous scrotum, tenderness posterior and lateral to testicle
  - More commonly due to *C. trachomatis*
- Rectal gonococcal infection
  - Transmitted by receptive anal intercourse and cervicovaginal secretions
  - Anal pruritis, tenesmus, purulent discharge, rectal bleeding
- Cervicitis
  - Vaginal discharge, dysuria, abnormal vaginal bleeding
  - Friable, erythematous, congested cervix with purulent discharge
  - Bartholin cyst/abscess

- Pelvic inflammatory disease
  - Develops in 10% to 20% of cervicitis
  - Lower abdominal pain, fever, cervical motion tenderness, painful intercourse
- Fitz–Hugh–Curtis syndrome
- Pharyngitis
  - Primarily via oral sexual exposure, usually asymptomatic
  - Sore throat, tonsillar edema, exudates
- Conjunctivitis
  - Autoinoculation, photophobia, purulent exudates, corneal ulcers, blindness
  - Symptoms greatly exaggerated compared to common causes of conjunctivitis
- Gonorrhea in pregnancy
  - PID and perihepatitis uncommon
  - Spontaneous abortion, premature labor, early rupture of membranes
- Disseminated gonococcal infection (0.5% to 3% of GC infections)
  - Fever, malaise, leukocytosis
- Arthritis–dermatitis syndrome (most common presentation)
  - Arthritis—asymmetric polyarthralgias of knees, elbows, distal joints
  - Typically at least two joints
  - Dermatitis—discrete papules and hemorrhagic pustules on extremities, 5 to 40 lesions (Fig. 10-1)

DIAGNOSIS

- Obtain specimens from all potentially infected sites
- Gram stain, 95% sensitive for male urethritis, not sensitive for other sites
- Culture, Thayer–Martin agar, PCR (can use voided urine/self-collected vaginal swabs)
- Test for chlamydia coinfection
- Suspected **disseminated gonococcus**
  - Sample urethra, cervix, pharynx, rectum, affected joints (increase sensitivity)
  - Skin lesions, unroofed lesions yield purulent fluid, organisms on Gram stain

TREATMENT

- Treat for presumed *C. trachomatis* coinfection
- Urethritis, cervicitis, proctitis:
  - Cefixime 400 mg PO once *or* ceftriaxone 125 mg IM once and treatment for chlamydia (single 1-g oral dose azithromycin in urethritis/cervicitis)
- Epididymitis
  - Ceftriaxone 250 mg IM once *and* doxycycline 100 mg PO two times a day for 10 days
- Bacteremia
  - Cefotaxime 1 g IV every 8 hours *and* doxycycline 100 mg IV every 8 hours
- Pelvic inflammatory disease, disseminated gonococcus
  - Hospitalization (some cases of PID)
  - Ceftriaxone 1 g IV everyday *and* doxycycline 100 mg PO or IV two times a day for 10 days

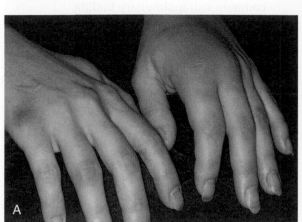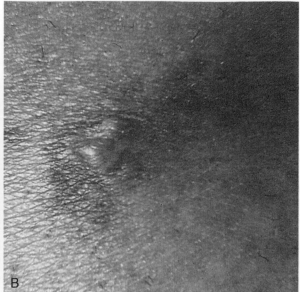

Figure 10-1. Gonococcal septicemia. **A,** There is erythema and swelling of joints on the left hand. A single vesicle is present on the right hand. **B,** More advanced lesion than that shown in **A.** Base has become hemorrhagic and necrotic. (From Habif TP: *Clinical dermatology: a color guide to diagnosis and therapy,* ed 4, Philadelphia, 2003, Mosby.)

MENINGOCOCCAL DISEASE

- *Neisseria meningitidis,* aerobic, Gram-negative diplococcus
- 2,400 to 3,000 annual cases in the United States
- Epidemic outbreaks among military recruits and college freshmen

SIGNS AND SYMPTOMS

- Variable presentation from mild febrile illness to fulminant disease and death
- Symptoms include fever, rhinorrhea, lethargy, myalgia, emesis, diarrhea, cough
- Occult bacteremia: (<1% mortality)
  - Vague symptoms with positive blood cultures, usually resolve spontaneously or with oral antibiotics, infrequently progresses to meningococcemia
- **Meningococcal meningitis:** (2% to 5% mortality)
  - Headache, fever, seizures, petechial or purpuric rash in 50% of cases
- **Meningococcemia:** (20% to 60% mortality) rapidly progressive illness, progresses from vague symptoms to multisystem organ failure and death <12 hours
  - Lethargy, cyanosis, hypo- or hyperventilation
  - Petechiae and purpura present in 50% to 60% of cases, on ankles, wrist, pressure points in contact with clothing
  - Myocarditis, vasculitis, pulmonary edema, DIC, acute tubular necrosis
- **Waterhouse–Friderichsen syndrome:** 10% to 20% of meningococcemia,
  - Rapid deterioration, diffuse petechiae/purpura, vasomotor collapse and *bilateral adrenal hemorrhage*

- Poor prognostic signs: seizures, hypothermia, hyperpyrexia, WBC <5000, platelets <100,000, petechiae, purpura, absence of meningitic signs

DIAGNOSIS

- Clinical, do not delay therapy for diagnostic tests
- Confirmed by positive culture (blood, CSF, pleura, synovium) <50% positive
- Cerebrospinal fluid analysis: elevated opening pressure, protein, WBC count, segmented neutrophils, bandemia, positive Gram stain, and low glucose

TREATMENT

- Cefotaxime 200 mg/kg/day divided every 6 hours *or*
- Ceftriaxone 100 mg/kg initial bolus, then 100 mg/kg/day divided every 12 hours *or*
- Chloramphenicol 75 to 100 mg/kg every 6 hours
- Respiratory isolation for suspected cases
- Occult bacteremia: treatment based on clinical presentation, repeat cultures, lumbar puncture for signs of meningitis, admit for observation
- Meningococcemia:
  - Prompt airway management if necessary, aggressive IV fluid hydration, vasopressor support, central venous pressure monitoring, hemodialysis for acute renal failure, fresh frozen plasma for bleeding complications
  - Dexamethasone 10 mg IV every 6 hours for 4 days if vasopressors required
  - Prophylaxis: close contacts, household, nursery school, day care center, health care workers (if mouth-to-mouth resuscitation, intubation, suctioning performed)
    - Rifampin 10 mg/kg every 12 hours × 4 doses *or*
    - Ciprofloxacin 500 mg every 12 hours × 4 doses

TUBERCULOSIS (TB)

- *Mycobacterium tuberculosis,* acid-fast bacillus, slow growing
- Transmission—respiratory droplets 1- to 5-µm diameter
- Pathogenesis
  - Stage 1: alveolar macrophage phagocytosis of inhaled bacilli
  - Stage 2: replication within macrophage, cell lysis, macrophage activation, logarithmic replication within macrophages
  - Stage 3: Cell-mediated immune response, destruction of infected macrophages (primary TB), dormant bacilli survive for years
  - Stage 4: months to years later, decreased resistance and reactivation, tubercle formation, production of large numbers of extracellular bacilli, overwhelms cell-mediated response (postprimary TB)

SIGNS AND SYMPTOMS

- *Primary*
  - Usually asymptomatic, mild fever and malaise, convert to PPD+
  - 8% to 10% convert to active TB (37% with untreated HIV)
- *Postprimary*
  - Constitutional symptoms—anorexia, weight loss, fatigue, malaise, fever
  - Cough—nonproductive to mucopurulent with hemoptysis, pleuritic chest pain
  - Pallor, fever and cachexia, posttussive rales
  - Amphoric breath sounds (hollow breath sounds heard over cavities)
  - Suspect with risk factors and vague symptoms or fever of unknown origin
  - Initially subtle presentation with HIV coinfection
- Risk factors
  - HIV infection
  - Close contact with known TB
  - Foreign born from Asia, Africa, or Latin America
  - Low-income, homeless, migrant farm workers, health care workers
  - Elderly
  - Nursing home, correctional facility residents
  - IV drug abuse
- Complications
  - Pneumothorax
  - Empyema
  - Pleural effusion
    - WBC 100 to 5000, pleural protein >50% of serum protein, glucose normal to low, few bacilli
  - Bronchopleural fistula
  - Endobronchial spread—dependent pulmonary nodules, coalesce into infiltrate
  - Airway tuberculosis—bronchiectasis, bronchial stenosis (segmental or lobar collapse), tracheal and laryngeal TB
  - Superinfection—*Aspergillus fumigatus* (fungus ball)
  - Massive hemoptysis—destroyed lung parenchyma, neovascularity
  - Pericarditis—direct extension from mediastinal lymph nodes
  - Lymphadenitis (scrofula) of the neck—most common extrapulmonary finding
  - Gastrointestinal TB—pain, diarrhea, anorexia, obstruction, hemorrhage
    - Most commonly ileocecal, may mimic appendicitis
    - Peritonitis—pain, abdominal swelling, fever, anorexia
      - Ascites with 500 to 2000 WBCs, lymphocyte predominate, elevated protein
  - Meningitis

DIAGNOSIS

- Chest x-ray
  - Primary—1% false-negative rate (7% to 15% with HIV)
    - Pneumonic infiltrate with enlarged hilar/mediastinal lymph nodes, pleural effusion, miliary TB (diffuse 1- to 3-mm nodules), Ghon focus (healed primary lesion)
  - Postprimary
    - Classically upper lobe infiltrate, with or without cavitation, can occur in any lung field
    - May progress to lobar or lung opacification
- Microbiology
  - Tuberculin skin test (antigen reaction)
    - =5 mm induration: positive with HIV or HIV risk factors, close contacts, fibrotic changes on chest x-ray
    - =10 mm induration: positive with other TB risk factors (e.g., long-term care resident)
    - =15 mm induration, positive with no risk factors
  - Spontaneous or induced sputum for acid-fast bacilli
    - Insensitive (10,000 bacilli/mL required), three specimens over 3 days improve sensitivity
  - Culture
    - Slow growing, 14 to 28 day incubation
    - BACTEC system shortens time to diagnosis to 7 to 14 days

TREATMENT

- Preventive therapy
  - INH 300 mg/day, 9 to 10 months minimum
- Suspected or confirmed pulmonary TB
  - Admit, respiratory isolation, PPD placement, serial induced sputum
- Confirmed case, multidrug therapy, minimum of 6 months
  - Isoniazid 3 to 5 mg/kg (1% to 2% hepatitis)
  - Rifampin 10 mg/kg (orange discoloration of body fluids)
  - Pyrazinamide 15 to 30 mg/kg
  - Ethambutol 15 to 25 mg/kg
  - Recommend PPD placement for all close contacts

- HIV-positive
  - INH, rifabutin, pyrazinamide, ethambutol
  - Extrapulmonary TB—may require 12-month therapy
  - Add prednisone 20 to 60 mg/kg/day for tuberculous pericarditis and meningitis
- Massive hemoptysis (= 600 mL blood in 24 hours)
  - Secure airway (8-0 endotracheal [ET] tube or larger for bronchoscopy)
  - Place bleeding lung in dependent position
- Prevention of transmission
  - Early identification, respiratory isolation for hemoptysis or TB risk factors and pulmonary symptoms
  - Respiratory isolation, negative pressure, 6 to 12 air changes per hour
  - Personal respiratory protection devices
  - PPD placement after potential exposure, annually for health care workers
  - BCG vaccine not recommended

ATYPICAL MYCOBACTERIA

- *Mycobacterium avium complex, Mycobacterium kansasii*
- Opportunistic infection, disseminated disease in up to 50% of AIDS patients

SIGNS AND SYMPTOMS

- Severe weight loss, diarrhea, fever, malaise and anorexia
- Rarely causes pulmonary disease

DIAGNOSIS

- Ziehl Neelson (acid-fast) stain of stool or other bodily fluids
- Blood culture

TREATMENT

- Azithromycin 500 mg PO daily for 14 days *and* ethambutol 15 mg/kg daily for 14 days
  - CD4 count <50 cells/mm^3, prophylaxis with clarithromycin or azithromycin

DIPHTHERIA

- *Corynebacterium diphtheriae,* encapsulated, Gram-positive bacillus
- Person-to-person spread via nasopharyngeal secretions
- Minimal incidence with adequate immunization
- Produces exotoxin, contributes to membrane formation due to localized pharyngeal necrosis, surrounding edema

SIGNS AND SYMPTOMS

- 2- to 4-day incubation
- Pharyngeal diphtheria
  - Fever, sore throat, weakness, dysphagia, headache, loss of appetite
  - Shortness of breath and cervical adenopathy
  - Neck edema (correlates with increased mortality), "bull neck" appearance
  - Pharyngeal membrane
  - Size correlates with morbidity, if limited to tonsils low morbidity, when involving entire pharynx, rapid illness onset and increased mortality
- Laryngeal diphtheria
  - Begins in larynx and spreads downward, upper airway obstruction
- Cutaneous diphtheria
  - Tropics, skin ulcer with grayish membrane
- Complications
  - 2% to 3% overall mortality
  - Airway obstruction, muscle paralysis
  - Myocarditis, congestive heart failure, cardiac conduction abnormalities

DIAGNOSIS

- Throat cultures on tellurite media, (notify laboratory of suspicion)
- 30% coinfection with group A streptococcus

TREATMENT

- Early intubation for potential airway compromise
- Equine serum diphtheria antitoxin (from Centers for Disease Control and Prevention)
  - 20,000 to 40,000 units IV after sensitivity testing
- Erythromycin 40 to 50 mg/kg/day *or*
- Aqueous crystalline penicillin 100,000 to 150,000 U/kg/day divided every 6 hours
- Cultures, immunization update and observation of close contacts

GAS GANGRENE

- Clostridial myonecrosis
  - *C. perfringens* (and other clostridial species)
  - Spore-forming bacilli, anaerobic, Gram-positive cocci
  - Found in soil and human intestinal tract
  - Rapidly progressive, muscle-necrosing infection
  - Usually due to trauma or recent surgical wounds
  - Exotoxin elaboration by clostridial bacilli
- Nonclostridial myonecrosis
  - *Bacillus fragilis* or *Peptostreptococcus*
  - Similar pathogenesis, presentation and treatment, better prognosis

SIGNS AND SYMPTOMS

- 1- to 4-day incubation
- Pale, anxious appearance, rapid progression to toxemia and shock
- Wound painful, swollen, brownish, thin exudates, soft tissue crepitus
- Brownish skin discoloration, progressing to purplish blebs
- Sickly sweet odor, muscle "cooked" appearing, does not bleed with incision

DIAGNOSIS

- Gram stain, large Gram-positive rods
- Radiographs show soft-tissue gas

TREATMENT

- Wide surgical debridement and excision
- Antibiotics—assume polymicrobial infection, aerobic and anaerobic
  - Penicillin, 2 million units IV every 3 hours *and*
  - Clindamycin 900 mg IV every 8 hours
- Monotherapy
  - Zosyn (piperacillin/tazobactam) 4.5 g every 8 hours *or*
  - Imipenem 1 g every 8 hours *or*
  - Meropenem 1 g every 8 hours
- Hyperbaric oxygen very early in disease (following debridement)

BACTEREMIA

SIGNS AND SYMPTOMS

- Asymptomatic bloodstream infection

DIAGNOSIS

- Presence of viable bacteria in blood based on positive blood cultures
- Blood cultures and cultures of all suspected infectious sites recommended for suspected sepsis (no proven impact on morbidity or mortality)
- 30% to 60% of clinically proven sepsis cases have negative blood and body fluid cultures
- False-positive result because of contaminated cultures common

TREATMENT

- Based on clinical condition and bacteriology of isolate
- Treatment generally not indicated for healthy, asymptomatic adults

Sepsis

- Systemic inflammatory response, usually due to a bloodstream infection

SIGNS AND SYMPTOMS

- Suspicion for infection
- Pneumonia, abdominal–pelvic, urinary tract, most common sources *AND*

SYSTEMIC INFLAMMATORY RESPONSE SYNDROME (SIRS)

- Systemic response to a clinical insult (can occur in the absence of infection)
- Defined as presence of at least *two* of the following:
  - Oral temperature >38° C or <35° C
  - Respiratory rate >20/minute or $PaCO_2$ of <32 mmHg
  - Heart rate >90 beats per minute (bpm)

- Total blood leukocyte count of >12,000 cells/µL or <4000 cells/µL or >10% bands

DIAGNOSIS

- Clinical, laboratory

TREATMENT

- Supportive care directed at restoring oxygenation and perfusion
- Cardiac monitor
- Supplemental oxygen
- Large-bore peripheral IV access or central line, 20 mL/kg NS fluid bolus
- Consider Foley catheter to monitor urine output (maintain 1 to 2 mL/kg/hour)
- Source identification and control (drainage, antibiotics)
- Screen for severe sepsis and septic shock

Severe sepsis and septic shock

SIGNS AND SYMPTOMS

SEVERE SEPSIS

- Sepsis with one or more signs of organ dysfunction, including:
  - Hypoperfusion
  - Clinical findings—altered mental status, cyanosis, mottled skin
  - Elevated serum lactate = 4.0 mmol/L (increased short-term mortality)
- Neurologic (10% to 70% incidence)
  - Altered mental status and lethargy "septic encephalopathy"
  - Glasgow Coma Scale score <13 correlates with 20% to 50% increased mortality
- Cardiovascular
  - Early—increased cardiac output, decreased systemic vascular resistance (distributive shock)
  - Late—direct myocardial depression, ventricular dilatation, decreased cardiac index
  - Typically recovers with treatment of infection
- Pulmonary
  - Respiratory failure, common cause of mortality
  - Catabolic state, increased respiratory demand and increased respiratory resistance

ADULT RESPIRATORY DISTRESS SYNDROME (ARDS)

- Impaired oxygenation (PaO_2/FiO_2 ≤200 irrespective of PEEP)
- Bilateral pulmonary infiltrates
- No clinical evidence of congestive heart failure
- Gastrointestinal
  - Ileus
  - Elevated AST, ALT, total bilirubin (two times normal or greater)
- Endocrine
  - Adrenal insufficiency

- Hematologic
  - Coagulopathy
  - Platelet count <100,000 cells/μL
  - Disseminated intravascular coagulation

SEPTIC SHOCK

- Severe sepsis with hypotension unresponsive to fluid resuscitation (20 to 30 mL/kg crystalloid bolus)
- Differentiate from other shock states (e.g., cardiogenic, neurogenic)
- Initially warm, flushed skin, flat neck veins, rapid, thready pulse
- Progress to hypotension, altered mental status, mottled skin, cyanosis

DIAGNOSIS

- Clinical

TREATMENT

- Source identification and control
- Early, appropriate antibiotics may reduce mortality by 30%
  - Broad-spectrum antibiotics for unidentified source
- Airway management, early intubation for potential respiratory failure
  - Decreases work of breathing
  - Low tidal volume (plateau pressure <35 cmH$_2$O) strategy, shown to decrease incidence of ARDS
- IV fluid hydration, 20 to 30 mL/kg crystalloid (normal saline or Ringer lactate) bolus for hypotension or serum lactate = 4.0 mmol/L
  - May require a large amount of crystalloid in first 24 hours
  - No evidence of improved outcome with colloids, some recommend initial colloid bolus for severe hypovolemia (CVP <4 mmHg)
  - Maintain urine output (1 to 2 mL/kg/hour) with crystalloid infusion
- Steroids
  - Theoretical benefit for persistent hypotension due to adrenal insufficiency following fluid bolus
  - No proven mortality benefit
  - Hydrocortisone 100 mg IV every 8 hours

EARLY GOAL-DIRECTED THERAPY (EGDT)

- 16% absolute mortality reduction in randomized controlled trial (>10% mortality reduction in subsequent before/after cohort studies)
- Indicated for sepsis with either:
  - Persistent hypotension (systolic blood pressure < 90 mmHg after 20 to 30 mL/kg crystalloid bolus) *or*
  - Systemic hypoperfusion (serum lactate = 4.0 mmol/L)
- Three hemodynamic outcomes independently optimized within 6 hours of ED arrival:
  - *Central venous pressure* >8 mmHg, optimized with NS bolus, 500 mL every 30 minutes (CVP >12 mmHg for intubated patients)

- *Mean arterial pressure* >65 mmHg, after initial fluid bolus, maintained with vasopressors (norepinephrine preferred)
- *Central venous oxygen saturation* >70%, maintained by PRBC transfusion to maintain hematocrit >30%, followed by dobutamine infusion to increase cardiac index if needed

Toxic shock syndrome (TSS)

- *S. aureus* or *Streptococcus pyogenes*
- Associated with high-absorbency tampons
- Nonmenstrual TSS now more common
  - Surgical procedures, focal infections, burns, heroin injection, childbirth, nasal packing, HIV coinfection
- Women 15 to 34 years most common (can affect any age)
- Case fatality rate 10%—1980, 1%—1989 and beyond
  - 30% to 50% mortality for streptococcal TSS
- Toxic shock syndrome toxin (TSS-1): Streptococcal pyrogenic exotoxin, absorbed from infection site, systemically distributed

SIGNS AND SYMPTOMS

- Fever, tachycardia, hypotension
- Rash—nonpruritic, diffuse, macular, blanching erythroderma, flaking desquamation

DIAGNOSIS

STAPHYLOCOCCAL TSS

- Temperature >102° F, characteristic rash
- Hypotension: SBP ≤90 mmHg, orthostatic DBP drop ≥15 mmHg, orthostatic syncope
- Involvement of three or more systems:
  - Gastrointestinal—vomiting or diarrhea
  - Muscular—severe myalgia or CPK at least two times normal
  - Mucous membrane—vaginal, oral, or conjunctival hyperemia
  - Renal—BUN / creatinine at least two times normal or urinary sediment with pyuria
  - Hepatic—total bilirubin, AST or ALT at least two times normal
  - Hematologic—platelets ≤100,000/mm^3
  - CNS—disorientation without focal neurologic findings
- Negative blood, throat, or CSF cultures
- Negative titers for Rocky Mountain spotted fever, leptospirosis or rubeola

STAPHYLOCOCCAL TSS

- Isolation of group A strep from body site (sterile or nonsterile) *and*
- Clinical signs
  - Hypotension *and* at least two of the following:
    - Renal impairment
    - Coagulopathy
    - Liver abnormalities

■ Acute respiratory distress syndrome
■ Extensive tissue necrosis
■ Erythematous rash

TREATMENT

■ Removal of foreign bodies, drainage of infection, debridement of infected wounds
■ Supportive care
  ■ 20 to 30 mL/kg crystalloid bolus
  ■ Hemodynamic monitoring, vasopressors for persistent hypotension
■ Clindamycin 600 to 900 mg every 8 hours
■ Intravenous immunoglobulin (IVIG) 400 mg/kg over several hours, if no response to fluids and vasopressors

Syphilis

■ *Treponema pallidum,* spirochete
■ Sexually transmitted
■ Strong correlation with HIV coinfection and men who have sex with men

SIGNS AND SYMPTOMS

PRIMARY SYPHILIS

■ Small papule at inoculation site (10 to 90 days postexposure)
■ Progresses to painless, indurated ulcer (chancre) 1 to 2 cm at transmission site
■ Nontender inguinal adenopathy

SECONDARY SYPHILIS (25% OF UNTREATED)

■ 6 to 20 weeks postexposure
■ Fever, chills, sore throat, malaise, weight loss, generalized lymphadenopathy
■ Rash—"great masquerader," variable appearance
  ■ Typical—macular or papular, symmetric, involves trunk, extremities, *palms and soles,* 0.5- to 2-cm reddish-brown lesions, can be pustular
  ■ **Condyloma lata**—large, raised gray/white lesions, involving moist areas and mucous membranes, usually proximal to primary lesion (Fig. 10-2)
■ Alopecia, hepatitis (high alkaline phosphatase), synovitis, nephrotic syndrome
■ Anterior uveitis, chorioretinitis (can lead to syphilitic meningitis)

TERTIARY SYPHILIS (25% TO 40% OF UNTREATED)

■ Gummatous syphilis
  ■ Large skin ulcers or heaped up granulomatous tissue
■ Cardiovascular syphilis
  ■ Dilated aorta, aortic regurgitation, with murmur or CHF
  ■ Coronary artery narrowing, thrombosis
■ Neurosyphilis
  ■ Meningitis—within 1 year of primary infection

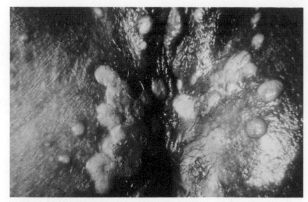

Figure 10-2. Condyloma lata of secondary syphilis. (From Marx JA, Hockberger RS, Walls RM (eds): *Rosen's emergency medicine: concepts and clinical practice,* ed 6, Philadelphia, 2006, Mosby.)

■ Headache, stiff neck, altered mental status, uveitis with vision impairment
■ Meningovascular—infectious arteritis, ischemic stroke, spinal cord infarct
  ■ Suspect in young person with ischemic stroke
■ General paresis—10 to 25 years post infection
  ■ Progressive memory and judgment deficits, dementia
  ■ Psychosis, dysarthria, facial and limb hypotonia, tremors
■ Tabes dorsalis—20-year latency, posterior columns of the spinal cord
  ■ Ataxia, lancinating pain (sudden brief stabs of pain), paresthesias, epigastric pain, nausea and vomiting
  ■ Argyll–Robertson pupil—small, accommodates, nonreactive

DIAGNOSIS

■ Dark-field microscopy—from scrapings of moist lesions
■ Serologic studies
  ■ Nontreponemal test—RPR or VDRL, sensitive, nonspecific, inexpensive
  ■ Treponemal specific test—FTA-ABS or TPPA, confirmatory study, high specificity for treponemal infection, expensive
■ Cerebrospinal fluid analysis—For clinical symptoms of meningitis, focal neurologic findings, ophthalmic involvement, tertiary syphilis, or HIV with low CD4 count
  ■ Elevated WBC 10 to 400 cells/μL, elevated protein 45 to 200 mg/dL, CSF VDRL (which is highly specific, but not sensitive); CSF FTA-ABS is less specific but is highly sensitive
■ Primary syphilis—serologic tests may be negative, scrapings from chancre or inguinal nodes show treponemes under dark-field microscopy
■ Secondary syphilis—serologic studies or rash scrapings under dark-field microscopy
■ Tertiary syphilis—clinical suspicion, confirmed by serologic studies

- HIV coinfection—may have false-negative treponemal serologic test

TREATMENT

- Primary, secondary or early latent (latent is seroreactivity without evidence of disease; early latent means acquired within past year)
  - Benzathine penicillin G 2.4 million Units IM once (highly preferred) *or*
  - Doxycycline 100 mg PO two times a day for 14 days
  - Reexamine in 6 months (clinically and repeat VDRL/RPR)
  - Refer for HIV testing (treated/followed differently)
- Late latent, unknown duration
  - Benzathine penicillin G 2 to 4 million units IM weekly for 3 weeks (highly preferred) *or*
  - Doxycycline 100 mg PO for 30 days
- Neurosyphilis
  - Aqueous crystalline penicillin G IV 3 to 4 million units every 4 hours for 10 to 14 days *or*
  - Procaine penicillin 2.4 million units IM daily *plus* probenecid 500 mg PO four times a day for 10 to 14 days (alternative regimen)
  - Jarisch–Herxheimer reaction—fever, headache, myalgias within 24 hours of treatment for syphilis. Treat with antipyretics

Tetanus

- *Clostridium tetani*—spore-forming, Gram-negative anaerobic bacilli
- Ubiquitous in soil and dust, animal feces (10% of human GI tracts)
- Noninvasive, requires portal of entry, retrograde axonal transport to CNS
- Release tetanospasmin toxin
- Blocks inhibitory neurotransmitter release, irreversible
- Causes severe muscle spasm and autonomic dysfunction

SIGNS AND SYMPTOMS

- 70% recall a history of injury
- Incubation of 1 day to several months
- Symptoms gradually progress over 10 days, then diminish, full recovery 4 weeks
- Early findings
  - Irritability, muscle weakness, myalgia, muscle cramps, dysphagia, drooling
- Delayed findings
  - Masseter spasm, risus sardonicus (characteristic facial muscle spasm)
  - Spontaneous or stimulated muscle spasm, can lead to long-bone fractures, tendon rupture and major joint dislocation
  - Laryngeal/respiratory muscle spasm leading to respiratory failure
  - Autonomic symptoms (leading cause of death)
    - Tachycardia, hyperthermia, dysrhythmia, myocarditis, pulmonary edema

DIAGNOSIS

- Clinical diagnosis
- Wound cultures insensitive, no confirmatory lab tests available

TREATMENT

- Supportive care
- Muscle spasm control
- Remove all external stimulation
- Benzodiazepine or propofol infusion, titrate to muscle spasm control
- Dantrolene may decrease need for mechanical ventilation
- Magnesium sulfate infusion, decreases autonomic instability
- Mechanical ventilation and neuromuscular blockade
  - For airway compromise or failure to control spasm
  - Avoid succinylcholine due to hyperkalemia risk
    - Contraindicated after 4 days of symptoms
- Adjunctive sedation mandatory
- Treatment of autonomic instability
  - Combined alpha/beta-antagonists (labetalol or propranolol) for hypertension
  - Pure beta-blockade could lead to uncontrolled hypertension
  - Morphine or magnesium sulfate infusions for labile blood pressure
  - Temporary pacemaker for bradydysrhythmias (avoid atropine)
- Human tetanus immunoglobulin (TIG)
  - Eliminates circulating toxin, no effect on bound toxin
  - 3,000 to 6,000 Units IM, administer at separate site from tetanus toxoid
  - Passive immunity, half life 25 days, one-time administration
- Prevention of tetanospasmin production
  - Wound debridement, only *after* TIG given
  - Metronidazole 500 mg IV every 6 hours
- Vaccination
  - Inactivated tetanospasmin toxoid
  - Nearly 100% effective after three divided doses, immunity wanes after 5 to 10 years (faster in elderly, IVDAs, and immunosuppressed)
  - Give to all suspected acute tetanus infections and as prophylaxis for routine wounds (Table 10-1)
  - Adults with uncertain history, give primary series, dose at time zero, 4 to 8 weeks and 6 to 12 months, with booster every 10 years

Fungal infections

ASPERGILLUS FUMIGATES

- *Aspergillus fumigates*, ubiquitous fungus, grows in moist soil
- Infection occurs via inhalation

SIGNS AND SYMPTOMS

- Invasive pulmonary disease
- Angioinvasion with resulting thrombosis, dissemination to other organs, and occasionally, erosion of the blood vessel wall with catastrophic hemorrhage
- Risk factors for invasive disease
  - Neutropenia, HIV, poorly controlled DM
  - Cough, pleuritic chest pain, hemoptysis, hypoxemia
- Aspergilloma
  - Fungus ball—colonization of previously existing cavitary lesion (in patients with chronic lung disease (e.g., cystic fibrosis, bronchogenic cysts)
  - Presents with hemoptysis
- Allergic **aspergillosis**
  - Hypersensitivity lung disease—episodic wheezing, expectoration of brown mucus plugs, low-grade fever, eosinophilia, transient pulmonary infiltrates
  - Most commonly in children with asthma or cystic fibrosis
  - Occurs secondary to persistent exposure to fungus

TABLE 10-1   **Guide to Tetanus Prophylaxis in Routine Wound Management in Adults**

	Clean, Minor Wounds	All Other Wounds*
History of Prior Td (doses)	*Unknown or less than 3*	*Unknown or less than 3*
Td	Yes	Yes
TIG	No	Yes
History of Prior Td (doses)	*3 or more*	*3 or more*
Td	No†	No‡
TIG	No	No

Modified from Diphtheria, tetanus, and pertussis: recommendations for vaccine use and other preventive measures. Recommendations of the Immunization Practices Advisory Committee (ACIP), *MMWR Morbid Mortal Wkly Rep* 55(RR17);1-33, 2006.
* Such as, but not limited to, wounds contaminated with dirt, feces, soil, and saliva; puncture wounds; avulsions; and wounds resulting from missiles, crushing, burns, and frostbite
† Yes if >10 years since last dose
‡ Yes if >5 years since last dose

- Eosinophilic pneumonia
- Farmer's lung
- Extrinsic allergic alveolitis

DIAGNOSIS

- Invasive pulmonary/disseminated disease
  - Bronchoscopy/lung biopsy—tissue demonstrates organism
- Aspergilloma
  - CXR—cavitary lesion with an air crescent sign (Fig. 10-3)
  - MRI/CT reveal fungus ball
  - Sputum culture
- Allergic
  - History of bronchial asthma
  - Peripheral eosinophilia, elevated serum IgE level
  - Immediate reaction to *Aspergillus fumigatus* antigen, serum precipitants to *A. fumigatus*
  - Pulmonary infiltrates on CXR, central bronchiectasis on CT imaging
- Farmer's lung
  - Clinical

TREATMENT

- Invasive pulmonary
  - Treatment failure common
  - Amphotericin B, itraconazole
- Aspergilloma
  - Surgical resection/lobectomy
- Allergic
  - Corticosteroids (recent movement towards antifungal treatment alone)
- Farmer's lung
  - Remove source

BLASTOMYCES DERMATITIDIS

- Round, thick-walled, dimorphic yeast
- Endemic to Ohio and Mississippi Valleys

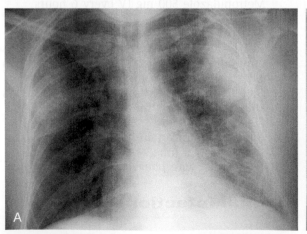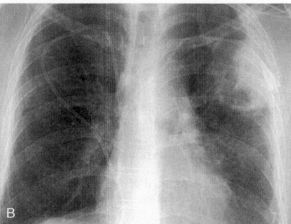

Figure 10-3. Invasive aspergillosis. A 46-year-old man on steroids and methotrexate for asthma. The patient developed cough and fever. (A) Initial chest radiograph demonstrates peripheral homogeneous opacities in both upper lobes and heterogeneous opacities in the left lower lobe. (B) A subsequent posteroanterior (PA) chest radiograph demonstrates cavitation within the peripheral left opacity following appropriate antifungal therapy and reconstitution of neutrophils 6 days into course. (From Adam A, Dixon A: *Grainger and Allison's diagnostic radiology,* ed 5, Philadelphia, 2007, Churchill-Livingstone.)

- Associated with **construction activities near waterways**
- Portal of entry—inhalation via lungs, hematogenous and lymphatic spread

SIGNS AND SYMPTOMS

- Clinical syndromes
- Pulmonary
  - Acute or chronic progressions
    - Fever, chills, cough, night sweats, hemoptysis, chest pain
    - Respiratory failure, extrapulmonary disease, ARDS
- Extrapulmonary (listed in order of decreasing frequency)
  - Skin (may occur with or without pulmonary involvement)
    - Verrucous or ulcerative lesions
  - Skeletal
  - Genitourinary

DIAGNOSIS

- Direct examination, isolation of organism in tissue

TREATMENT

- Amphotericin B
- Other options include itraconazole, ketoconazole, fluconazole
- Itraconazole/ketoconazole not used to treat genitourinary disease
- Surgical debridement may be indicated

COCCIDIOIDES IMMITIS

- Southwestern United States, persons exposed to dust in summer and fall when dust is dry
- Archeology digs, earthquakes, dust storms
- Infected individuals cannot transmit disease
- Causes **San Joaquin Valley Fever**
- Immune response T-cell mediated

SIGNS AND SYMPTOMS

- Pneumonia (most common manifestation)
  - Chest pain, pleurisy, cough, cyanosis, dyspnea, pleural friction rub
  - Constitutional—anorexia, arthralgias, chills, fatigue, fever, headache, malaise, night sweats, sore throat, tachycardia, weight loss
- Rash
  - Erythema multiforme, erythema nodosum
  - Rash signifies intense immunological response and a good prognosis
- Complications
  - Persistent pulmonary cavitary lesions
  - Disseminated disease with increased fatality
  - Immunocompromised people, elderly, neonates, pregnant women, African Americans, Filipinos
  - Meningitis (treatment is very difficult)—most common in young white males

DIAGNOSIS

- Ask about travel history
- Serology and/or biopsy
- Bronchoscopy, fine-needle biopsy, tissue biopsy, CSF stain, serology, or culture

TREATMENT

- Disease usually self-limited
- Ketoconazole for
  - Symptoms lasting >8 weeks
  - IgG >1:16
  - Bilateral pneumonia or extensive unilateral pneumonia
  - Extreme fatigue, work disability, weight loss >10%
- Treat high-risk patients even with mild disease
- Severe/rapidly progressive disease, late pregnancy—amphotericin B (nephrotoxic)
- May be lifelong treatment, relapse common in extrapulmonary/disseminated disease

HISTOPLASMA CAPSULATUM

- Thin-walled dimorphic yeast, endemic to Ohio and Mississippi Valleys
- Lives in soil enriched with bat, chicken, and bird excrement
- Spelunking, excavation—activities that disrupt soil
- Inhaled yeast deposited in alveoli, hematogenous/lymphatic spread
- Granulomas form secondary to T-cell–mediated response

SIGNS AND SYMPTOMS

- Symptoms in fewer than 5% of infected people
- Pulmonary infection
  - Fever, malaise, nonproductive cough, chest pain, fatigue
- Severe disease (exposure to high inoculum, immunocompromised)
  - Severe dyspnea and hypoxemia
- Complications (secondary to intense inflammatory reaction)
  - Acute pericarditis
  - Arthritis
  - Erythema nodosum
- Chronic infection
  - Cavitary lesions with predilection for lung apices, form over time (differential diagnosis includes TB)
  - Progressive restrictive or obstructive lung disease
  - Respiratory failure, death
- Mediastinal
  - Progressive fibrosis of mediastinum, secondary to aggressive antigenic reaction stimulated by yeast that persist in granulomas
  - **Fibrosing mediastinitis**—second-leading cause of superior vena cava syndrome

DIAGNOSIS

- Serology
- Complement fixation—titers >1:32 indicate active infection

- Immunodiffusion
- Histopathology, culture

TREATMENT

- Itraconazole
- Amphotericin B (for severe disease, immunocompromised, CNS infection)

MUCORMYCOSIS

- Risk factors
  - Immunocompromised
  - Diabetes mellitus
  - Trauma
- *Rhizopus* most common genera
- Inhalation of fungus with deposition on nasal passage
- Very aggressive, invasive, leading to hemorrhagic necrosis

SIGNS AND SYMPTOMS

- Rhinocerebral
- Initially headache, nasal stuffiness, facial pain
- Progression to orbital and intracranial invasion
- **Black eschar** on hard palate is hallmark of disease

DIAGNOSIS

- Biopsy

TREATMENT

- Correct underlying predisposing factors
- Amphotericin B
- Aggressive nasal debridement

SPOROTRICHOSIS—*SPOROTHRIX SCHENCKII*

- Schenck disease, **Rose gardener disease**
- Fungus in moist soil, sphagnum moss, decaying vegetation
- Gardeners, foresters, animal handlers (animal-to-human transmission reported)
- Forms—cutaneous, pulmonary, osteoarticular, disseminated

SIGNS AND SYMPTOMS

- Cutaneous form is most common
- Initial red raised lesions, erythematous and warm; advance proximally via **lymphatic channels,** causes lymphangitic streaking

DIAGNOSIS

- Culture or tissue biopsy with demonstration of organism

TREATMENT

- Cutaneous, lymphocutaneous, or osteoarticular disease
  - Itraconazole *or* fluconazole
  - Potassium iodide saturated solution (SSKI) is an alternative treatment

- Pulmonary
  - Surgical therapy may be needed in addition to antifungals
  - Amphotericin B for severe or life-threatening disease
- Disseminated
  - Amphotericin B

Protozoan infections

MALARIA

- Protozoan disease (four species)
  - *Plasmodium vivax; Plasmodium ovale; Plasmodium malariae; Plasmodium falciparum* (highest mortality rate)
- Species vary in morphology, degree of RBC tropism
- Vector: female *Anopheles* mosquito
- Recent incidence increase due to increased international travel; *Anopheles* resistance to insecticides; increased resistance of *plasmodium* to antimalarial medication
- Endemic regions
  - Central/South America, Caribbean, sub-Saharan Africa, Middle East, Oceania (predominant *Plasmodium* form varies among geographic regions)
- Risk of contracting disease depends on:
  - Intensity of transmission—sub-Saharan Africa has highest exposure intensity
  - Time and type of travel
  - Mode of transmission
- Exoerythrocytic
  - Mosquito feeds on human; releases sporozoites into bloodstream; travel directly to liver
- Erythrocytic
  - Direct transfusion of infected cells (e.g., needle-stick injuries)
- Transplacental

SIGNS AND SYMPTOMS

- Occur during the erythrocytic stage
- Non-falciparum malaria: symptoms cyclic every 48 to 72 hours
- Nonspecific symptoms: weakness, malaise, headache, and myalgias
- Progresses to anemia
- Intermittent fever; marked diaphoresis, profound exhaustion between fevers
- *Vivax* and *ovale*—latent disease, relapses months after initial infection
- *P. malariae* may be regular 72-hour intervals of symptoms
- Benign quartan malaria—subclinical, persists for years
- Falciparum malaria: noncyclic, rapidly progressive systemic symptoms
- Fatigue and malaise, fevers continual, some with spiking fever
- Cerebral malaria—prostration, convulsions, impaired consciousness
- Respiratory distress

Blackwater fever

- Abnormal bleeding, circulatory collapse, hypoglycemia, anemia, jaundice (excessive hemolysis and liver involvement)
- Physical examination (nonspecific)
  - Hepatosplenomegaly
- Laboratory features
  - Hemolysis resulting in normochromic, normocytic anemia
  - Also demonstrates leukopenia, thrombocytopenia, elevated ESR, LDH, bilirubin, LFTs
- Complications (very young, elderly, immunocompromised, pregnant patient, delay in care, poor compliance with chemoprophylaxis regimens, misdiagnosis)
  - Splenic rupture
  - Capillary sludging due to high parasite load
  - Immune-mediated glomerulonephritis
  - Cerebral malaria
  - Noncardiogenic pulmonary edema, ARDS

DIAGNOSIS

- Consider in patient returning from endemic region with unexplained febrile illness
- Definitive diagnosis
  - Visualization of parasite on Giemsa-stained thick and thin blood smears (most cost-effective method)
  - ELISA and PCR
- Two major considerations
  - Degree of parasitemia
  - *Plasmodium falciparum* as causative species

TREATMENT

- Decision based on presence of severe malaria, defined as
  - Parasitemia greater than 5% of red blood cells
  - Signs of central nervous system or other end-organ involvement
  - Shock, acidosis, and/or hypoglycemia
  - Agent
  - Resistance
- Hospitalization recommended
  - *P. falciparum* infection
  - Significant hemolysis
  - Significant comorbidities
  - Infants, pregnant patient, very elderly
- Agents
  - *P. malariae, P. vivax, P. ovale*
    - Chloroquine *or*
    - Primaquine (avoid in G6PD)
  - Terminal prophylaxis in *P. vivax* or *P. ovale* to prevent relapses
  - *P. falciparum* (always assume resistance)
    - Chloroquine
- If from regions with known resistance
  - Quinine
    - IV in severe cases, cardiac monitoring necessary
    - Cinchonism (headache, nausea, blurred vision, tinnitus)
    - Hypoglycemia

- *and* doxycycline *or* clindamycin
- *or* atovaquone-proguanil
- *or* mefloquine (avoid if used for chemoprophylaxis)
- Exchange transfusion for:
  - Parasitemia of >10% combined with severe disease
  - Therapeutic failure
  - Poor prognostic factors
  - Parasitemia of >30%, even in the absence of clinical complications
- Glucocorticoids are of no benefit

TOXOPLASMOSIS

- *Toxoplasma gondii,* zoonosis
- Host: cats
- Mode of transmission
  - Ingestion of uncooked, raw meat (cysts); cat or wild animal feces (oocytes)
  - Transplacental, or through transfusion or transplantation of infected blood/tissue
- Severe disease in the immunocompromised host
- Congenital toxoplasmosis
- Incidence correlates with prevalence of infection; gestational age at which pregnant woman acquires infection (increased gestational age–increased incidence); public health programs available for prevention

SIGNS AND SYMPTOMS

- Immunocompetent individuals: self-limited, nonspecific illness
  - Fatigue with/without fever
  - Lymphadenopathy—single enlarged nontender posterior cervical node
  - Chorioretinitis—4th to 6th decades, unilateral involvement, macula spared
- Myocarditis and polymyositis
  - Resembles infectious mononucleosis or cytomegalovirus (CMV)
  - Reinfection occurs, but without clinically apparent disease
- Congenital toxoplasmosis
  - Mothers acquire the infection for the **first** time during gestation
  - 85% appear normal at birth, later disease in most infected children
- **Classic triad (seen rarely)**
  - **Hydrocephalus, chorioretinitis, cerebral calcifications**
  - Disease more severe when acquired early in gestation
  - Chorioretinitis
    - Reactivation of intrauterine or postnatally acquired infection
    - Occur in second and third decades of life (it is rare after age 40); bilateral disease, retinal scars, and involvement of the macula are hallmarks of retinal disease

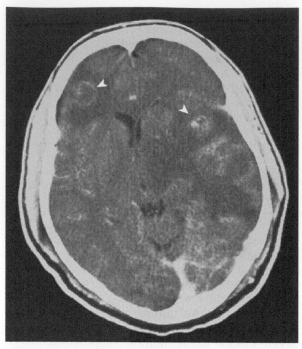

Figure 10-4. Toxoplasmic encephalitis in person who has AIDS. A cranial CT scan shows bilateral contrast-enhanced ring lesions with peripheral edema and mass effect. (From Cohen J, Powderly WG: *Infectious diseases,* ed 2, Philadelphia, 2004, Mosby.)

- Hydrocephalus, seizure disorder, developmental delay, hearing loss
- Jaundice, hepatosplenomegaly
- Pneumonitis
- Thrombocytopenia
- Immunocompromised patients
  - More severe, life threatening
  - Reactivation of previously acquired infection
  - Brain is the **most commonly** affected organ (Fig. 10-4)
  - Most common findings—hemiparesis, speech abnormalities
- Other clinical manifestations
  - Pneumonitis
  - Chorioretinitis
  - Acute respiratory failure, hemodynamic abnormalities similar to septic shock

DIAGNOSIS

- Serology, histology, mouse/tissue culture inoculation, PCR, radiologic studies

TREATMENT

- Immunocompetent adults and children
  - Do not require treatment unless symptoms are severe
  - Pyrimethamine, sulfadiazine, and folinic acid for 4 to 6 weeks is the most commonly used and recommended drug regimen
- Toxoplasmic chorioretinitis (consult ophthalmologist)
  - Pyrimethamine, sulfadiazine, and folinic acid

- Clindamycin
- Systemic corticosteroids may be required in addition to the anti-*Toxoplasma* drugs
- Infection in pregnant women
  - Spiramycin loading
  - Decreases incidence of fetal infection, continue throughout pregnancy
- Congenital toxoplasmosis
  - Sulfadiazine, pyrimethamine, and folinic acid for 12 months
- Infection in immunocompromised patients
  - Same regimen, higher doses
- Pregnant women should avoid contact with cat feces (cleaning litter boxes)

Tick-borne illness

EHRLICHIOSIS

- *Ehrlichia chaffeensis* (other species cause clinically similar disease)
  - Gram-negative pleomorphic coccobacilli
  - Infect circulating leukocytes
  - Vector: tick of the *Ixodes, Amblyomma* spp.
- Human granulocytic ehrlichiosis (HGE)
  - Predominant in NE, Midwest United States
  - Vector: *Ixodes* tick; reservoir: white-tailed deer
- Human monocytic ehrlichiosis (HME)—more common
  - Predominant in South/Southeast
  - Vector: *Amblyomma* tick, reservoir: white-tailed deer
- Acute, febrile illness similar to RMSF with exception of the following
  - Anemia, leukopenia, absolute lymphopenia (HME)
  - Lack of vasculitis
  - Rash less common
  - Age of those infected typically >40 years

SIGNS AND SYMPTOMS

- Fever, headache, malaise, vomiting, abdominal pain, anorexia, myalgias, rigors
- Rash
  - Occurs in 20% of cases, early in illness (more common with HME form)
  - Maculopapular, petechial—infrequently involves soles, palms
- Rare complications
  - Renal failure, respiratory failure, encephalitis
  - Leukocytopenia, thrombocytopenia, liver dysfunction (elevated AST/ALT)

DIAGNOSIS

- Indirect immunofluorescent antibody test
- Fourfold rise in antibody titers

TREATMENT

- Doxycycline 100 mg PO two times a day for 7 to 14 days
- Usually good prognosis unless delay in treatment

LYME DISEASE

- Most common vector-borne zoonotic infection
- Organism—*Borrelia burgdorferi,* spirochete; vector—deer tick (*Ixodes* species)
- Most prevalent in Northeast United States (3% prevalence in highly endemic areas)
- Risk of disease increases with duration of tick exposure
- <72 hours attachment almost no risk; 25% if attached >72 hours

SIGNS AND SYMPTOMS

- Primary
  - Erythema migrans (erythema chronicum migrans or ECM)—most common sign (Fig. 10-5)
    - Erythematous plaque, central clearing, vasculitis, painless, not pruritic
    - Occurs at site of bite, develops 2 to 20 days after bite
    - Incidence 60% to 80%
  - Fever, malaise, headache, mild neck stiffness, myalgia, and arthralgia
- Secondary (dissemination stage)
  - A few days to 6 months after bite
  - Rash (reflects spirochetemia with dissemination)
    - Multiple erythema migrans rashes
    - **Most characteristic component** of second stage
  - Other symptoms
    - Fever, adenopathy, arthritis
    - Neurological disturbances
      - Headache, stiff neck, photophobia, peripheral nerve, paresthesias/palsies—CN VII—can be bilateral
    - Cardiac abnormalities—first-, second-, or third-degree atrioventricular (AV) block
- Tertiary
  - **Chronic arthritis,** myocarditis, encephalopathy, polyneuropathy, leukoencephalopathy

DIAGNOSIS

- Clinical findings, epidemiologic features

- Elevated antibody response to *B. burgdorferi*
  - Lacks standardization, accuracy unsubstantiated, false-positive results common, undertake only when diagnosis strongly suspected
- Confirmatory tests
  - PCR, polyvalent fluorescence immunoassay, Western blot
  - Fourfold rise in antibody titer suggests recent infection

TREATMENT

- Doxycycline
- Children under age 12 years, pregnant
  - Amoxicillin *or* penicillin VK
- PCN allergic
  - Cefuroxime *or* erythromycin 15 to 30 days (less effective)
- Treatment during primary phase—excellent prognosis
- Duration of treatment depends on phase:
  - Primary phase: 14 to 21 days PO
  - Secondary phase: 30 days PO
  - Tertiary phase: IV treatment
- High-degree atrioventricular block may require temporary pacing
- Jarisch–Herxheimer reaction
  - Acute febrile reaction accompanied by headache, myalgia, and an aggravated clinical picture lasting less than 24 hours that can occur when therapy is initiated
  - Treat with NSAIDS, **antimicrobial agent should be continued**
- Prophylaxis
  - Not recommended routinely, consider in the following cases
    - Bitten by deer tick in highly endemic areas
    - Deer tick is partially engorged with blood while biting patient
    - Deer tick has been feeding >72 hours
  - Doxycycline 200 mg once within 72 hours of tick bite

ROCKY MOUNTAIN SPOTTED FEVER

- *Rickettsia rickettsii;* vector: *Dermacentor* tick
- Hosts: deer, rodents, horses, cattle, cats, and dogs
- Common in pet owners, animal handlers, and persons engaged in outdoor activities
- Found only in the Western Hemisphere, 50% of cases occur in the mid-Atlantic states
- 90% occur from April through September
- Highest incidence of infection—5 to 9 years old and males >60 years of age
- History of tick exposure (approximately 1/2 of patients recall tick bite)

SIGNS AND SYMPTOMS

- Systemic, small-vessel vasculitis
- Classic triad: rare, 3%
  - Fever, headache and rash

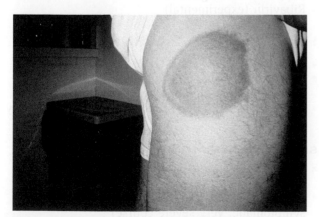

Figure 10-5. Erythema migrans. A typical annular, flat, erythematous lesion with a sharply demarcated border and partial central healing. (Courtesy of Dr. Steven Luger, Old Lyme-Connecticut, USA.) (From Cohen J, Powderly WG: *Infectious diseases,* ed 2, Philadelphia, 2004, Mosby.)

- Rash
  - Occurs day 1 to 15, absent in 20% of patients
  - Begins on hands, feet, **palms and soles,** wrists and ankles **and spreads centripetally**
  - Usually present at day 3
- Gastrointestinal
  - Nausea, vomiting, diarrhea, and abdominal pain (40% to 60% of patients)
  - Mild to moderate elevations of transaminases
- Pulmonary—most worrisome
- Neurologic (if present, indicates more severe prognosis)
  - Encephalitis
  - Headache, confusion, lethargy, delirium, ataxia, coma, convulsions
  - Lymphocytic meningitis (occurs in 30%)
- The course of untreated disease
  - Advancing severity of illness, high fevers, hemorrhage
  - Neurologic complications—paraparesis, hearing loss, peripheral neuropathy, bladder and bowel incontinence, cerebellar, vestibular, or motor dysfunction
  - Mortality is highest in males >50 years of age
- People with no recognized tick bite or attachment
  - Delay to treatment
  - Absence of rash
  - Initial presentation before the fourth day of illness (classic triad not likely to be present)
  - Usually occur in months April through September

DIAGNOSIS

- High index of suspicion based on clinical findings
- Laboratory analysis (nonspecific)
  - Neutropenia, thrombocytopenia, elevated LFTs, hyponatremia
- Confirmatory tests
  - PCR assay
  - Indirect fluorescent antibody assay, elevated titer >1:64
    - Most sensitive and specific
  - Skin biopsy with immunofluorescent staining—70% sensitivity, 100% specificity, best rapid diagnostic test if available
  - Weil–Felix test less sensitive

TREATMENT

- Indications for admission
  - Neurologic symptoms, vomiting, renal failure
- Medical therapy
  - Treatment must be administered on clinical suspicion, most effective when given in the first 3 to 5 days of illness
  - Doxycycline 100 mg PO two times a day for 7 days
    - Delayed treatment results in severe disease
    - Drug of choice in children
    - Less likely than other tetracyclines to stain developing teeth
    - More efficacious

- Chloramphenicol not recommended
  - Serious adverse effects, less effective
  - Need to monitor serum concentrations
  - No oral form in the United States

Viral infections

HANTAVIRUS

- Member of Bunyaviridae family, vector: deer mouse
- Far western United States ("four corner" states)
- Spreads by exposure to aerosolized urine and feces of infected rodents

SIGNS AND SYMPTOMS

- Pulmonary—most severe and significant form in United States
- Severe noncardiogenic pulmonary edema
- Prodrome: fever, chills, myalgias, headache, GI distress, **no cough**
- Bilateral pulmonary infiltrates, ARDS, myocardial depression
- Consider diagnosis in patients with:
  - Febrile illness temp >101° F
  - Bilateral pulmonary edema (ARDS), respiratory failure <72 hours
  - Respiratory illness in healthy persons with rodent exposure
- Hantavirus pulmonary syndrome, 50% to 70% mortality rate
- Associated thrombocytopenia
- Other forms:
  - Hemorrhagic fever, renal involvement (most common worldwide)

DIAGNOSIS

- PCR or serology (IgM-specific assay or fourfold increase in IgG antibody)

TREATMENT

- Supportive management
- Ribavirin (experimental)

HERPES SIMPLEX VIRUS

- Two types: HSV1, HSV2
- Direct contact with infected secretions on abraded skin or mucous membrane
- Remains latent in dorsal root ganglia, humans only reservoir

SIGNS AND SYMPTOMS

- Forms of infection—primary, latent, reactivation/recurrence
- Initial infection—primarily asymptomatic (if symptomatic, very severe course)
- Vesicular rash on erythematous base
- Greatest concentration of virus shed during symptomatic primary infections
- Virus can be shed when asymptomatic

- Recurrence—common, triggered by fever, ultraviolet light, friction, sexual intercourse, menstruation, stress, or fatigue

HERPES LABIALIS

- HSV 1 most common etiological agent
- Gingivostomatitis (most common form in children), fever, lymphadenopathy, multiple vesicular lesions
- Recurrence 60% to 90%, mild symptoms, vesicles on vermillion border

OPHTHALMIC HSV

- Follicular conjunctivitis, blepharitis, corneal opacities
- Common cause of blindness in developed world
- Recurrence—keratitis and deeper involvement of cornea
- Fluorescein stain—branching dendritic ulcers (Fig. 10-6)

HERPETIC WHITLOW

- Painful vesicular lesions of the finger often mistaken for bacterial infection (do not incise and drain); health care workers at risk

GENITAL HERPES

- Most common manifestation in young adults and adolescents
- HSV2 70% to 95% cases (occasionally HSV1)
- Men—lesions on glans penis, shaft; female—vulva, vagina, cervix, buttocks
- Incubation period 8 to 16 days
- Primary infection
  - Painful vesicle clusters on a red base
  - Fever, inguinal adenopathy, vaginal discharge, urinary incontinence
  - Aseptic meningitis (especially women)
- Secondary/recurrence
  - Prodrome of pain and paresthesias
  - Shorter, milder course

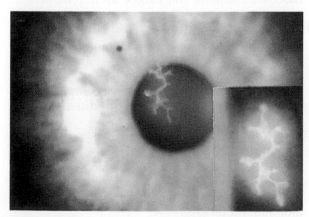

Figure 10-6. Herpes simplex corneal epithelial keratitis in diffuse light and in light passed through a cobalt blue filter after fluorescein staining (inset). Note the dendritic staining pattern characteristic of herpes simplex. (From Goldman L: *Cecil medicine,* ed 23, Philadelphia, 2007, Saunders.)

HSV ENCEPHALITIS

- Most common acute, nonepidemic encephalitis
- Fever, focal neurological signs (most commonly temporal lobe), headache, meningismus, lethargy, confusion, stupor
- Prompt treatment decreases morbidity and mortality

DIAGNOSIS—HSV

- Clinical picture
- Tzanck smear, multinucleated giant cells
- Viral culture (definitive diagnosis)
- Encephalitis—definitive diagnosis challenging
  - CSF shows nonspecific mononuclear pleocytosis
  - Culture usually negative; PCR amplification is best assay for encephalitis
  - MR imaging—usually abnormal (80% temporal lobe findings)
  - Biopsy of lesion with culture

TREATMENT—HSV

- Acyclovir 400 mg PO three times a day for 7 to 10 days, heals sooner if <72 hours from onset
- Acyclovir 400 mg two times a day suppressive—decreased incidence and severity of recurrence
- Famciclovir and valacyclovir regimens for acute, recurrent, and suppressive as well
- Indications for admission
  - Severe pain or dehydration (herpes labialis, gingivostomatosis)
  - Systemic symptoms
  - Complications (e.g., meningitis, neuropathic bladder)
  - Large or rapidly progressive lesions
- Ophthalmic keratitis
  - Consult ophthalmology
  - Topical steroids contraindicated—increase depth of injury, blindness
- Encephalitis
  - Acyclovir IV 10 mg/kg every 8 hours

VARICELLA ZOSTER VIRUS (VZV)

- Transmission via direct contact, airborne droplets, transplacental passage
- VZV latent in dorsal root ganglia
- Reactivation occurs many years after initial infection

SIGNS AND SYMPTOMS

CHICKEN POX

- Late winter to early spring, commonly children <10 years (rate decreased secondary to immunization); lifelong immunity after infection
- Fever, malaise
- Rash
  - Initially maculopapular, then vesicular
  - "Dew drop on rose petal" appearance
  - 3 days, scab forms
  - Several stages of healing present at same time

- Infectious 48 hours before rash until **all** lesions have crusted
- Risk factors for severe/disseminated disease
  - Adult onset
  - Children with leukemia/immunocompromised state
  - Neonate <10 days
  - Mothers in perinatal period, congenital varicella syndrome
- Complications
  - Sepsis, encephalitis, pneumonia

HERPES ZOSTER/SHINGLES

- Reactivation infection, lifetime incidence 20%
- Majority with no underlying illness
- Risk factors
  - Increasing age, immunosuppression, spinal surgery
- 1 to 3 day prodrome of tingling paresthesias, pain, fever, malaise
- Rash
  - Dermatomal, unilateral, up to three consecutive dermatomes, vesicular
  - Thoracic/lumbar dermatomes most common
  - Lasts for 2 weeks
- Can transmit virus to susceptible persons
- Cranial nerve involvement/cervical dermatome
  - Ophthalmic branch of trigeminal nerve
    - **Hutchinson sign**—vesicles on tip of nose indicate nasociliary nerve and inevitable ocular involvement
    - Keratitis, dendritic lesions on fluorescein examination
  - Ramsay–Hunt syndrome
    - Bell palsy, vesicular lesions in external auditory meatus or on TM
  - Post-herpetic neuralgia
    - Incidence increases with age, common, difficult to treat

DIAGNOSIS

- Clinical characteristics
- Confirmed if necessary by Tzanck smear or culture

TREATMENT

- Do not give aspirin to children—Reye syndrome
- Chicken pox
  - Acyclovir: treat adults
    - 800 mg five times a day (IV in severe cases, immunocompromised)
  - Vaccine
    - Live attenuated—children <12 months (avoid in immunocompromised)
    - >12 years, two doses recommended 4 to 8 weeks apart
    - Recommended for postexposure prophylaxis in nonimmune host
- Herpes zoster
  - Acyclovir, 800 mg five times a day *or* valacyclovir, 1 g three times a day
  - Decreases severity and duration of long-term pain syndromes

- Indications for IV acyclovir in herpes zoster
  - Disseminated, complicated course
  - Involvement of multiple dermatomes or disseminated disease
  - Involvement of ophthalmic branch trigeminal nerve
- Prompt analgesic control of pain
- Corticosteroids not recommended except in age >50 years (taper over 21 days)
- Isolate hospitalized patients
- Immunization/vaccination
- Post exposure: prevents infection/reduces severity if <72 hours
  - Exposed are at risk and infectious for 21 days
  - Exposure criteria: continued household contact, prolonged face-to-face contact (same room), or indoor playmate >1 hour

INFECTIOUS MONONUCLEOSIS (EPSTEIN–BARR VIRUS [EBV])

- Adolescents, young adults, incubation 4 to 6 weeks
- Secretion of virus in saliva up to 1 year, personal contact required for transmission
- EBV also associated with lymphoproliferative diseases—African Burkitt lymphoma, nasopharyngeal carcinoma

SIGNS AND SYMPTOMS

- Severe exudative pharyngitis, fever, posterior lymphadenopathy, fatigue, jaundice, hepatosplenomegaly
- Rash more common in patients treated with ampicillin
- Complications
  - Severe tonsillar swelling resulting in airway compromise
  - Splenic rupture
  - Neurologic—encephalitis, aseptic meningitis, transverse myelitis, Guillain–Barré syndrome
- Symptoms may persist 1 to 3 weeks
- Associated malaise and fatigue up to 3 months

DIAGNOSIS

- Clinical picture coupled with laboratory testing
- Atypical lymphocytes >10%
- Heterophile antibody test (Monospot) is highly sensitive/specific, positive early in disease

TREATMENT

- Supportive
- Avoid contact sports until spleen no longer palpable
- Avoid ampicillin or amoxicillin (nonallergic morbilliform rash)
- Steroids
  - Impending airway obstruction from severe pharyngitis
  - Hemolytic anemia or thrombocytopenia

INFLUENZA

- Groups A, B, C (ability to undergo rapid antigenic change results in epidemics of febrile respiratory disease affecting all age groups)
- Types A and B associated with most widespread epidemics/pandemics and most mortality
- Transmission person to person by respiratory droplets, contaminated surfaces
- Most common cause of viral pneumonia in adults
- Usually occurs November–April

SIGNS AND SYMPTOMS

- Symptoms begin 1 to 4 days after exposure
- Fevers, myalgias, coryza, conjunctivitis, headache, nonproductive cough
- Complications
  - Influenza pneumonia (may progress to ARDS)
  - Elderly, pregnant, cardiac disease at risk
  - Secondary bacterial pneumonia (staphylococcal, streptococcal)

DIAGNOSIS

- Clinical presentation
- Viral culture criterion standard
- Rapid direct antigen assay

TREATMENT

- Antivirals, when administered within 48 hours of illness onset, reduce severity and duration (by 1 day) of influenza A (**not** B) in young, healthy adults
  - Neuraminidase inhibitors (administer within 2 days of symptoms)
    - Zanamivir (10 mg two times a day), oseltamivir (75 mg two times a day)
  - Amantadine 100 mg PO two times a day (effective against Type A **not** B), resistance increasing
- Vaccination (administer yearly based on viral epidemiology)
  - Age >65, immunocompromised, chronic disease, second and third trimester of pregnancy, health care workers
  - Most severe side effect—Guillain–Barré syndrome
- Avoid aspirin in children—associated with Reye syndrome

PARAINFLUENZA

- Parainfluenza types 1 and 2—predominant cause of acute laryngotracheobronchitis (croup; inflammation of the subglottic trachea)
- Second most common cause of pneumonia in children
- Most common in fall and winter months in children 6 months to 3 years
- Transmission person to person by direct contact, respiratory tract droplets
- Most common viral cause of respiratory tract infection requiring hospitalization

SIGNS AND SYMPTOMS

- Barking, "seal-like" cough, worse at night
- Inspiratory stridor (subglottic swelling)
- Febrile illness lasting 4 days, associated rhinorrhea
- Complications
  - Bacterial superinfection, laryngotracheitis
  - Respiratory compromise—higher risk in children with medical history, narrowing of the upper airway (subglottic stenosis and tracheomalacia)

DIAGNOSIS

- Clinical picture
- X-ray not necessary for the diagnosis of croup
  - AP neck shows subglottic narrowing—"steeple sign"
  - Lateral neck films help to rule out other processes such as epiglottitis ("thumb sign")

TREATMENT

- Goal: reduce upper airway edema and inflammation
- Mist inhalation, heliox
- Racemic epinephrine for
  - Stridor at rest
  - Severe respiratory distress (nasal flaring, suprasternal/intercostal retractions, tachypnea, hypoxia)
  - Failure to respond to humidified air
- Reevaluate at 2 to 4 hours—risk of "rebound" swelling
- Dexamethasone associated with decreased hospitalization and severity of disease
- Intubation for severe distress or airway collapse—anticipate difficult airway

RABIES

- Caused by neurotropic rhabdovirus—*Lyssavirus*
- Public health problem in the Third World
- Human rabies virus
  - United States: bats most important reservoir/transmitter (88% of human rabies)
  - Also raccoon, skunks, foxes, coyotes, and woodchucks
  - Worldwide: dogs, cats more common
  - No human rabies from rodent or lagomorph (rabbits, hares) except woodchucks and beavers
- Rabid animals may display aggressive behavior, ataxia, excessive salivation
- Behavior *not* a reliable sign of the rabid state
- 50 times greater risk of transmission via bite
- Pathophysiology
  - Multiplication of virus within local monocytes
  - Virus spreads across motor end plate, replicates along peripheral nerve axoplasm, enters CNS thru dorsal root ganglia
  - Replication of virus in CNS gray matter, spreads via peripheral nerves

SIGNS AND SYMPTOMS

- Prodrome
  - General, nonspecific symptoms (may last several days to weeks)
  - Headache, fever, rhinorrhea, myalgias, gastrointestinal disturbance
  - Back pain, muscle spasms
  - Paresthesias, pain at site of bite
- Full-blown rabies
  - Encephalitic "frenzy" form
  - Agitation, hydrophobia, aerophobia, irritability
  - Hemodynamic lability (tachycardia, tachypnea, fever)
  - Hydrophobia (even the site of water can elicit choking fit)
- "Dumb" form
  - Limb weakness with spared consciousness initially
- Forms overlap
- Coma within 1 week, death 3 to 20 days

DIAGNOSIS

- Ante mortem, diagnosis helpful in limiting contacts
- Isolation of virus, detection of antigen from peripheral nerves
- CSF analysis: nonspecific pleocytosis, rabies virus RNA detection via PCR
- Postmortem: Negri bodies (eosinophilic cytoplasmic viral inclusion distributed throughout the brain—pathognomonic) or rabies antigen in brain tissue

TREATMENT

- No specific treatment exists, primarily supportive; case reports of survival
- Human rabies immune globin (HRIG) and human diploid cell vaccine (HDCV) no effect once symptoms have developed
- Postexposure prophylaxis, administration depends on
  - Local rabies epidemiology—discuss with public health officials
  - Type of exposure
  - Bite or exposure to open wound, mucous membrane
  - Oddly behaving animal that bites without being provoked
  - Location of incident, endemic area
  - Species of biting animal
- High-risk animals in areas where rabies endemic
  - Treat immediately
  - Quarantine animal, euthanize, send brain to lab for testing
- Domestic animals in endemic area
  - Observe animal for 10 days (dog, cat, ferret)
  - Withhold PEP unless animal becomes ill
- Low threshold for prophylaxis with bat *exposure* (infection has occurred when no report of bite but mere presence of bat in vicinity)
- If decision made to administer PEP (failure to adhere to all steps listed below may result in treatment failure)

- Wound care: **most crucial step, decreases viral inoculum**
  - Scrub/clean/irrigate wound with soap and water
  - Do not suture or close would if rabies transmission is suspected
- Immunoprophylaxis
  - Passive immunization
    - HRIG 20 IU/kg, as much as possible at site of wound intradermally, remainder IM at site away from vaccine
  - Active immunization
    - HDCV 1 mL IM deltoid, away from site of HRIG administration
      - Administer days 0, 3, 7, 14 (day 28 if immunocompromised)
      - If previously vaccinated: no HRIG, HDCV 1 mL IM days 0 and 3
      - Safe in pregnancy (as is HRIG)

RUBELLA

- German measles, "third disease"
- Transmission via respiratory droplets
- Incubation 12 to 23 days
- Highly contagious 1 week before and 4 days after onset of rash

SIGNS AND SYMPTOMS

- Prodromal symptoms of eye pain, sore throat, headache, fever, cough, myalgia, nausea, URI symptoms
- Fine maculopapular rash, from face to extremities within 24 hours, lasts 3 days
- Posterior auricular, occipital and posterior cervical lymphadenopathy
- Complications in children: encephalitis, thrombocytopenia, arthritis
- Complications in adults: myocarditis, orchitis, neuritis, erythema multiforme
- Congenital rubella syndrome
  - Hearing loss, cataracts, retinopathy, mental retardation, cardiac abnormalities
- **Highest risk** if infected before 12 weeks' gestation

DIAGNOSIS

- Clinical

TREATMENT

- Supportive care
- Vaccination—should occur before 15 months
- No evidence of decreased immunity with age

RUBEOLA (MEASLES)

- Epidemic systemic viral illness of children and young adults
- Transmission via respiratory droplets
- Communicable 3 to 5 days prior to rash and up to 4 days after rash appearance
- Reportable disease

SIGNS AND SYMPTOMS

- Prodromal phase
  - Cough, coryza, conjunctivitis, fever >101° F
  - **Koplik spots**—white papules on an erythematous base, "grains of sand" pathognomonic, located on buccal mucosa, present before the rash
- Exanthem phase
  - Rash—maculopapular, confluent, spreads caudally from head to extremities
  - Lasts >3 days
- Complications
  - Otitis media, pneumonia, laryngotracheitis
  - Meningoencephalitis, **subacute sclerosing panencephalitis**
  - Myocarditis/pericarditis
  - Thrombocytopenia purpura

DIAGNOSIS

- Clinical
- Positive serological test for measles IgM, rise in measles antibody level

TREATMENT

- Isolation
- Supportive care
- Indications for hospitalization
  - Respiratory distress, encephalopathic
- Vitamin A
- Vaccine for postexposure prophylaxis

Emerging infections/ pandemics

PLAGUE

- *Yersinia pestis,* Gram-negative bacillus; reservoir: rodents
- Responsible for numerous epidemics, three pandemics
- Asia, Africa, South America, North America and Europe
- Spread by contact with infected tissues, bodily fluids, or respiratory droplets
- Flea bite deposits inoculum just under skin, spreads to regional lymph nodes

SIGNS AND SYMPTOMS

- Fever, chills, headache, malaise, prostration, leukocytosis
- Bubonic (most common form)
  - 2 to 8 days after flea bites
  - Regional lymphadenitis, enlargement and necrosis of lymph nodes (bubo), eschar
  - Pneumonia, sepsis
  - Septicemic
- Primary or secondary form (complication of bubonic form)
  - DIC, necrosis of small vessels, gangrene fingers and nose (**"Black Death"**)

- Pneumonic
  - Most likely form in bioterrorism-related event
  - Spread by inhalation of droplets or hematogenous spread
  - Productive cough, chills, body aches
  - Fatality rate high within 48 hours
  - Chest x-ray may show patchy or confluent infiltrate

DIAGNOSIS

- Gram, Wright, Giemsa, and Wayson stains
- PCR
- Serum antibody titers four times normal, antigen detection by fluorescent assay
- Confirmatory
  - Culture of blood or lymph node, isolation of *Y. pestis*

TREATMENT

- Place in isolation with droplet precaution (especially pneumonic form)
- Streptomycin, 15 to 22.5 mg/kg IM two times a day for 10 days *or*
- Gentamicin 2 mg/kg IV three times a day for 10 days
- Alternatives: doxycycline, ciprofloxacin, chloramphenicol

SARS

- Coronavirus (SARS-CoV)
- Pandemic 2002-2003
- Spread by inhalation of respiratory droplets, direct person-to-person contact, contact with fomites followed by autoinoculation

SIGNS AND SYMPTOMS

- 2 to 10 days after exposure, most contagious during second week
- Variable, nonspecific symptoms
- Flu-like symptoms (no initial respiratory symptoms in some reported cases)
- Fever, diarrhea, respiratory compromise
- Severe sepsis, respiratory failure requiring mechanical ventilation
- Poor prognostic indicators
  - Male
  - Hyponatremia
  - Left shift
  - Elevated LDH
  - Age >60

DIAGNOSIS

- High suspicion—from endemic areas (Hong Kong, mainland China, Taiwan) with symptoms consistent for SARS
- WHO definition
  - Fever >38° C
  - Evidence of lower respiratory tract infection
  - Chest x-ray—evidence of pneumonia (78% one side consolidation or ARDS)
  - No other diagnosis attributable to symptoms

- Lab studies (nonspecific)
  - Leukopenia, lymphocytopenia, thrombocytopenia
  - Elevated PTT, AST, CK, LDH
  - Reverse transcriptase PCR or isolation of SARS-CoV

TREATMENT

- Isolation precautions and strict adherence to hygiene is of utmost importance
- Often require ICU supportive care
- No effective definitive treatment

COMMUNITY-ACQUIRED/ASSOCIATED METHICILLIN-RESISTANT *S. AUREUS* (CA-MRSA)

- Emerged in 1990s, genetically distinct from hospital variant—HA-MRSA
- Predominantly minor skin/soft tissue infection
- CA-MRSA is commonly resistant **only** to beta-lactams
- Virulent, only susceptible to narrow-spectrum antibiotics
- Causes infection in healthy, predominantly young hosts with no co-morbidities
- Risk factors (different from HA-MSRA)
  - Infection has appearance of furuncle
  - Household contacts of infected individuals
  - People living/spending long periods of time together with close quarters
    - Jail detainees, military recruits, sports teams, homeless
  - Men who have sex with men
  - Pregnant, post-partum, neonates
  - African Americans, Pacific islanders, Native Americans
  - Panton–Valentine leukocidin (PVL) toxin, associated with soft tissue infections, severe necrotizing pneumonia

SIGNS AND SYMPTOMS

- Skin and soft tissue infection
  - Predominant form of disease
- Furuncle most common, may be cellulitis, erysipelas, impetigo
- Infections typically described as occurring spontaneously
- Necrotizing fasciitis
- Deep infections
- Septic arthritis, osteomyelitis, pyomyositis
- Necrotizing pneumonia
  - May follow influenza
  - Presentation identical to other forms of bacterial pneumonia

DIAGNOSIS

- Culture
- Deep infection
  - MRI (most sensitive)
- Septic arthritis
  - Joint fluid aspiration/analysis consistent with bacterial infection, culture

- Osteomyelitis
  - MRI has replaced bone scan as preferred modality
- Pneumonia
  - Prodrome of influenza-like symptoms
  - Prior CA-MRSA or contact with infected individual
  - Hemoptysis, hypotension, leukopenia
  - Chest x-ray demonstrating ARDS-like pattern

TREATMENT

- Skin/soft tissue infection
  - Cellulitis/impetigo
    - TMP/SMX ± cephalexin (to cover group A streptococcus)
  - Uncomplicated abscess
    - I&D
  - Complicated abscess (surrounding cellulitis + fever + lymphadenopathy)
    - I&D plus antibiotics
  - PO therapy
    - TMP/SMX
    - Clindamycin (beware of inducible clindamycin resistance)
  - IV therapy
    - Vancomycin *or*
    - Linezolid
- Deep infection/osteomyelitis/pneumonias
  - Parenteral vancomycin *or* linezolid
  - Discuss with Infectious Disease consultants

WEST NILE VIRUS

- This arbovirus emerged in the late 1990s, likely due to migration of infected birds
- Vector: *Culex* mosquito; reservoir: infected birds, primarily crows
- Endemic to Middle East, Africa, Europe

SIGNS AND SYMPTOMS

- 20% develop symptoms, 10% actually seek medical attention
- West Nile Fever—80%
  - Sudden onset: fever, malaise, myalgias, eye pain, anorexia, headaches, nausea, vomiting, lymphadenopathy, morbilliform rash
- "West Nile Encephalitis"
  - Most common neurological form
  - Neck stiffness, headache, seizures
  - Mental status changes, indicating encephalitis
  - Movement disorders such as tremor or Parkinsonism
  - Acute flaccid paralysis with or without meningitis or encephalitis
- Guillain–Barré syndrome
- Risk for life-threatening neuroinvasive disease
  - Immunosuppression, DM, age >50
- Poor prognostic factors include profound weakness, coma, immunosuppression, advanced age, and severe comorbidity

DIAGNOSIS

- CSF
  - Viral profile with pleocytosis and increased protein
- Definitive
  - Isolation of virus-specific IgM (may persist for up to 1 year)
  - >4 times increase in virus-specific serum antibody
  - Isolation of virus from tissue/body fluid
- Will not be diagnosed in ED
- High index of suspicion
  - Febrile or acute neurologic illness
  - Recent exposure to mosquitoes, blood transfusion, or organ transplantation
  - Child born to an infected mother

TREATMENT

- Primarily supportive
- Pay close attention to epidemiological alerts
- Intravenous IgG and plasmapheresis for Guillain–Barré syndrome
- Prevention is focus
- Health education regarding insect repellant
- Insecticide dissemination with elimination of vector

DENGUE FEVER

- Arbovirus transmitted by mosquito *Aedes aegypti, Aedes albopictus*
- South America, Southeast Asia, endemic to Hawaii
- 16% of febrile illness in travelers from endemic regions

SIGNS AND SYMPTOMS

- 2 to 8 days after mosquito bite
- Fever, headache, retro-orbital pain, chills, photophobia, nausea, vomiting, severe muscle and back pain ("**breakbone fever**")
- Maculopapular rash, lymphadenopathy, hemorrhage (nosebleed, GI bleed)
- Dengue hemorrhagic fever (mostly children <15 years old)
  - Fever, epistaxis, gum bleeding
  - Thrombocytopenia
  - Increased capillary fragility and permeability

DIAGNOSIS

- Viral culture
- Serological testing

TREATMENT

- Primarily supportive

PEARLS

- *Yersinia enterocolitica* infection may mimic appendicitis.

- Infection due to poorly preserved raw seafood is likely *Vibrio parahaemolyticus*. Treatment is supportive care; doxycycline is reserved for severe cases.

- Outbreaks of vomiting and abdominal pain related to food left at room temperature (church picnic) are likely *Staphylococcus aureus*. Treatment is supportive.

- Scombroid fish poisoning (facial flushing, headache) is not an allergic reaction to fish.

- Dysesthesias (heat and cold sensory reversal) are pathognomonic for ciguatera fish poisoning.

- *Botulism* causes a combination of GI, autonomic, and cranial nerve symptoms.

- Bird handlers are at risk of developing *Chlamydia psittaci* infection. Treatment is tetracycline.

- Disseminated gonococcal infection presents with asymmetric polyarthralgias and a discrete papular rash (5 to 40 lesions) on the extremities.

- An absence of meningeal signs is a *poor* prognostic indicator in meningococcemia.

- Streptococcal toxic shock syndrome has a higher mortality than the staphylococcal version.

- Serologic tests may be negative during primary syphilis.

- Herpetic whitlow presents as vesicular lesions on fingertips and is commonly seen in health care workers.

- Negri bodies are eosinophilic intracellular lesions found within cerebral neurons, and are pathognomonic for rabies.

- Administration of postexposure prophylaxis for rabies should be discussed with a local public health official or done with knowledge of local disease epidemiology.

- The most common tick-borne illness is Lyme disease.

- The rash associated with RMSF begins on the wrists and ankles, involves palms and soles, then spreads centripetally to involve the rest of the body.

- *Plasmodium falciparum*, the deadliest form of malaria, is spread by the female *Anopheles* mosquito.

- The vesicular lesions of *Varicella* are classically "dew drops on a rose petal" and are in different stages of healing.

- Hutchinson sign—presence of a vesicular lesion on tip of nose, indicating zoster involving the nasociliary nerve and possible ocular involvement.

- Influenza A is the most common form of virus, associated with epidemics/pandemics.

- Patients with infectious mononucleosis treated with ampicillin classically develop a morbilliform rash.

- Dexamethasone in the treatment of croup secondary to the *Parainfluenza* virus is associated with a decreased rate of hospitalization.

- Koplik spots are pathognomonic for rubeola (measles). They are present before the skin rash.

- CA-MRSA causes infection in healthy, predominantly young hosts with no predisposing comorbidities.

BIBLIOGRAPHY

Adedipe A, Lowenstein R: Infectious emergencies in the elderly, *Emerg Med Clin North Am* 24:443–448, 2006.

Band J: Malaria. In Tintinalli JE, Kelen GD, Stapczynski JS (eds): *Emergency medicine: a comprehensive study guide*, ed 6, New York, 2004, McGraw-Hill, pp. 953–958.

Becker BM, Cahill JD: Parasites. In Marx JA, Hockberger RS, Walls RM (eds): *Rosen's emergency medicine: concepts and clinical practice*, ed 6, Philadelphia, 2006, Mosby, p. 2096.

Birnbaumer DM, Anderegg C: Sexually transmitted diseases. In Marx JA, Hockberger RS, Walls RM (eds): *Rosen's emergency medicine: concepts and clinical practice*, ed 6, Philadelphia, 2006, Mosby, p. 1556.

Bolgiano EB, Sexton J: Tick-borne illnesses. In Marx JA, Hockberger RS, Walls RM (eds): *Rosen's emergency medicine: concepts and clinical practice*, ed 6, Philadelphia, 2006, Mosby, p. 2116.

Brice JH, Myers JB: Reportable infectious diseases. In Tintinalli JE, Kelen GD, Stapczynski JS (eds): *Emergency medicine: a comprehensive study guide*, ed 6, New York, 2004, McGraw-Hill, pp. 987–993.

Browstein RA: Common viral infections: influenzaviruses and herpesviruses. In Tintinalli JE, Kelen GD, Stapczynski JS (eds): *Emergency medicine: a comprehensive study guide*, ed 6, New York, 2004, McGraw-Hill, pp. 919–924.

Center for Disease Control and Prevention (website). Available at www.cdc.gov/malaria/.

Center for Disease Control and Prevention (website). Available at www.cdc.gov/tetanus/.

Chlapek BH: Dermatologic emergencies. In Stone CK, Humphries R (eds): *Current diagnosis and treatment emergency medicine*, ed 6, Norwalk, 2008, Connecticut.

Drew LW: Miscellaneous systemic viral syndromes. In Wilson WR, Sande MA (eds): *Current diagnosis in infectious disease*. New York, 2001, McGraw-Hill, pp. 463–470.

Drew LW: Herpesvirus. In Wilson WR, Sande MA (eds): *Current diagnosis in infectious disease*. New York, 2001, McGraw-Hill, pp. 400–412.

Fernandez MF: Bacteria. In Marx JA, Hockberger RS, Walls RM (eds): *Rosen's emergency medicine: concepts and clinical practice*, ed 6, Philadelphia, 2006, Mosby, p. 2001.

Folstad SG: Soft tissue infections. In Tintinalli JE, Kelen GD, Stapczynski JS (eds): *Emergency medicine: a comprehensive study guide*, ed 6, New York, 2004, McGraw-Hill, pp. 979–987.

Freer L: North American wild mammalian injuries, *Emerg Med Clin North Am* 22:445–473, 2004.

Klig JE: Ophthalmologic complications of systemic disease, *Emerg Med Clin North Am* 26:217–231, 2008.

Kman NE, Nelson RN: Infectious agents of bioterrorism: a review for emergency physicians, *Emerg Med Clin North Am* 26:517–547, 2008.

Lawrence DT, Dobmeier SG, Bechtel LK, Holstege CP: Food poisoning, *Emerg Med Clin North Am* 25:357–373, 2007.

McKinzie J: Sexually transmitted diseases, *Emerg Med Clin North Am* 19:723–744, 2001.

Meislin HW, Guisto JA: Soft tissue infections. In Marx JA, Hockberger RS, Walls RM (eds): *Rosen's emergency medicine: concepts and clinical practice*, ed 6, Philadelphia, 2006, Mosby, p. 2195.

Mell HK: Management of oral and genital herpes in the emergency department, *Emerg Med Clin North Am* 26:457–473, 2008.

Meredith JT: Zoonotic infections. In Tintinalli JE, Kelen GD, Stapczynski JS (eds): *Emergency medicine: a comprehensive study guide*, ed 6, New York, 2004, McGraw-Hill, pp. 969–978.

Moran GJ, Talan DA: Pneumonia. In Marx JA, Hockberger RS, Walls RM (eds): *Rosen's emergency medicine: concepts and clinical practice*, ed 6, Philadelphia, 2006, Mosby, p. 1131.

Moran GJ, Talan DA, Abrahamian FA: Antimicrobial prophylaxis for wounds and procedures in the emergency department, *Infect Dis Clin North Am* 22:117–143, 2008.

Perry SJ, Booth AE: Toxic shock syndrome and streptococcal toxic shock syndrome. In Tintinalli JE, Kelen GD, Stapczynski JS (eds): *Emergency medicine: a comprehensive study guide*, ed 6, New York, 2004, McGraw-Hill, pp. 913–918.

Pickering L (ed): *Red book®: 2006 report of the committee on infectious disease*, ed 27, Elk Grove Village, Ill, 2006, American Academy of Pediatrics.

Polis MA, Haile-Mariam T: Viruses. In Marx JA, Hockberger RS, Walls RM (eds): *Rosen's emergency medicine: concepts and clinical practice*, ed 6, Philadelphia, 2006, Mosby, p. 2033.

Rothman RE, Hsieh YH, Yang S: Communicable respiratory threats in the ED: Tuberculosis, influenza, SARS and other aerosolized infections, *Emerg Med Clin North Am* 24:989–1017, 2006.

Saks MA, Karras D: Emergency medicine and the public's health: emerging infectious diseases, *Emerg Med Clin North Am* 24:1019–1033, 2006.

Shah S, Sharieff GQ: Pediatric respiratory infections, *Emerg Med Clin North Am* 25(4):961–979, 2007.

Shapiro NI, Zimmer GD, Barkin AZ: Sepsis syndromes. In Marx JA, Hockberger RS, Walls RM (eds): *Rosen's emergency medicine: concepts and clinical practice*, ed 6, Philadelphia, 2006, Mosby, p. 2211.

Sokolove PE, Chan D: Tuberculosis. In Marx JA, Hockberger RS, Walls RM (eds): *Rosen's emergency medicine: concepts and clinical practice*, ed 6, Philadelphia, 2006, Mosby, p. 2145.

Stanley J: Malaria, *Emerg Med Clin North Am* 15:113–155, 1997.

Talan DA, Moran GJ, Abrahamian FA: Severe sepsis and septic shock in the emergency department, *Infect Dis Clin North Am* 22:1–31, 2008.

Weber DJ, Wohl DA, Rutalla WA: Rabies. In Tintinalli JE, Kelen GD, Stapczynski (eds): *Emergency medicine: a comprehensive study guide*, ed 6, New York, 2004, McGraw-Hill, pp. 946–953.

Weber EJ: Rabies. In Marx JA, Hockberger RS, Walls RM (eds): *Rosen's emergency medicine: concepts and clinical practice*, ed 6, Philadelphia, 2006, Mosby, p. 2061.

Questions and Answers

1. A 37-year-old man presents with 2 days of nausea, constipation, and a dry, painful mouth. He recalls eating homemade pickles the day before his symptoms started. On physical examination, he demonstrates dry mucous membranes, drooping eyelids, and bilateral upper extremity weakness. The most appropriate treatment for this patient would be:
   a. admission for neurologic workup
   b. doxycycline 100 mg PO three times a day for 21 days for possible Lyme disease
   c. ICU admission with serial vital capacity measurement for possible respiratory compromise
   d. edrophonium stimulation test for possible new-onset myasthenia gravis

2. A 43-year-old-male migrant farmer sustains a forearm laceration from a soiled plow blade. He is uncertain of his prior tetanus status. In addition to careful wound debridement and repair, appropriate tetanus prophylaxis would include:
   a. inactivated tetanus toxoid (Td), first dose, with planned follow-up for vaccination series completion
   b. Td first dose with follow-up for vaccination series completion and TIG 3000 Units IM at separate site
   c. TIG 3000 Units IM with close follow-up for tetanus titer testing and vaccination if indicated
   d. Td first dose with follow-up for vaccination series completion and TIG 1500 Units IM at separate site

3. Of the following species of tick, which one is well known to transmit the organism *Borrellia burgdorferi*?
   a. *Ixodes scapularis*
   b. *Amblyomma americanum*
   c. *Dermacentor variabilis*
   d. *Dermacentor andersoni*

4. The most common clinical manifestation associated with Lyme disease is a rash that is commonly referred to as:
   a. erythema nodosum
   b. erythema marginatum
   c. erythema migrans
   d. erythema multiforme

5. Approximately what percentage of patients with Rocky Mountain spotted fever present with classic triad of fever, headache and rash?
   a. 50%
   b. 25%
   c. 10%
   d. 3%

6. A 27-year-old man presents to the Emergency Department complaining of a sore throat, malaise and chills. He denies past medical history. On physical examination he has a temperature of 101.4° F, heart rate = 113 beats per minute (bpm), blood pressure = 118/73 mmHg, respiratory rate = 20/minute. He appears comfortable. He has lymphadenopathy of the anterior and posterior cervical chain, axillary, and inguinal lymph nodes. He has a symmetric maculopapular rash of the trunk and extremities involving the palms and soles. He is sexually active but has never had an HIV test. What is the most appropriate treatment for this patient?
   a. aqueous crystalline penicillin G 3 to 4 million units every 4 hours for 10 to 14 days
   b. benzathine penicillin G 2.4 million Units IM weekly for 3 weeks
   c. probenecid 500 mg PO two times a day for 10 to 14 days
   d. benzathine penicillin G 2.4 million units IM for 1 dose
   e. ceftriaxone 1 g IV everyday for 10 days

7. A 67-year-old man with a history of diabetes mellitus, hypertension, and benign prostatic hypertrophy presents complaining of a fever and generalized weakness. Vital signs are temperature = 102.8° F, heart rate = 128 bpm, blood pressure = 84/53 mmHg, and respiratory rate = 24/minute. Urinalysis shows positive leukocyte esterase and nitrite test and large WBCs and Gram-negative bacteria on microscopic examination. The patient is placed on a monitor and given broad-spectrum antibiotics and an IV fluid bolus (20 mL/kg NS), after which his blood pressure is 89/55 mmHg. The patient's serum lactate is 4.2 mmol/L. What is the next step in this patient's management?
   a. continued crystalloid IV fluids, ICU admission and vasopressors
   b. central line placement; optimization of central venous pressure (CVP) >12 mmHg with fluids; systolic blood pressure (SBP) >70 mmHg with vasopressors; and central venous oxygen saturation ($S_{cv}O_2$) >65% with blood products and inotropes
   c. central line placement, optimization of CVP >8 mmHg with fluids, SBP >90 mmHg with vasopressors, and $S_{cv}O_2$ >70% with blood products and inotropes
   d. central line placement, optimization of CVP >4 mmHg with fluids, SBP >90 mmHg with vasopressors, and $S_{cv}O_2$ >65% with blood products and inotropes
   e. supportive care, the patient has a poor prognosis

8. A 37-year-old man had an episode of epistaxis 3 days ago. Hemostasis was achieved in the ED with an adsorbent packing placed in the right nare. He presents to the ED complaining of fever, fatigue, diffuse myalgias, dizziness, and diarrhea. He also complains of a diffuse macular rash to the trunk and extremities. Past medical history includes untreated hypertension. On examination, the vital signs are temperature 103° F, blood pressure = 103/57 mmHg, heart rate = 118 bpm, respiratory rate = 24/minute. He appears to be in moderate distress, with rapid shallow breathing. His mucous membranes are hyperemic and he has a diffuse, blanching macular rash. In addition to removal of nasal packing, which of the following should be part of this patient's initial treatment?

   a. admission to a general medical floor
   b. Intravenous immunoglobulin (IVIG) 400 mg/kg intravenous piggyback (IVPB) over several hours
   c. cardiac monitoring, vasopressors and an IV fluid bolus (10 mL/kg crystalloid)
   d. clindamycin 600 mg IV every 6 hours
   e. ampicillin 1 g IV every 8 hours

9. A 23-year-old woman presents to your ED with a history of fever, headache, retro-orbital pain, photophobia, nausea, vomiting, and severe muscle and back pain. She also has an associated maculopapular rash, lymphadenopathy, and a nosebleed. She tells you she recently returned from a trip to Southeast Asia. Which of the following is the next best step in management of this patient?

   a. immediately place the patient in isolation
   b. administer chloroquine and primaquine
   c. supportive care
   d. doxycycline or chloramphenicol

10. An archeologist who was recently working at an excavation site in New Mexico presents to your emergency department with fever, weight loss, and a dry cough associated with pleuritic chest pain. You note multiple erythematous, tender nodules on the anterior aspect of the patient's lower extremities. Which diagnosis is most likely?

   a. Q fever due to *Blastomyces dermatitidis*
   b. San Joaquin Valley fever due to *Coccidioides immitis*
   c. atypical pneumonia due to *Histoplasma capsulatum*
   d. Q fever due to *Coxiella brunetti*

11. A patient who recently returned from a hiking trip in North Carolina presents to the ED with fever, headache, nausea, and vomiting. A petechial rash that started 5 days ago on the wrists and ankles now covers most of her body. Which of the following factors regarding this particular patient would contribute to increased mortality?

   a. the patient is 40 years old
   b. the patient is female
   c. increased time between onset of symptoms and commencement of treatment
   d. the history of a confirmed tick bite.

12. Which of the following signs or symptoms is typical of disseminated gonococcal infection?

   a. generalized maculopapular rash involving mucous membranes
   b. symmetric bilateral arthralgia of the major joints
   c. discrete papules and hemorrhagic pustules on hands and feet
   d. rapidly progressive illness leading to multisystem organ failure

13. Scombroid fish poisoning is caused by which of the following mechanisms?

   a. normal marine flora produce histamine-like compounds that accumulate in fish
   b. IgE = mediated allergic reaction leading to histamine release by mast cells
   c. *Gambierdiscus toxicus*, a unicellular plankton, releases a heat-stable neurotoxin
   d. mediated by a bacterium that produces heat-stable spores and releases enterotoxin

14. A 53-year-old woman presents with 4 hours of violent vomiting. She also complains of generalized abdominal cramps, fever, and diarrhea. She was at a work party a few hours before her symptoms started and two of her colleagues have similar symptoms. What is the most likely cause of her symptoms?

   a. *Staphylococcus aureus*
   b. *Clostridium perfringens*
   c. *Shigella sonnei*
   d. *Campylobacter jejuni*
   e. *Yersinia enterocolitica*

15. A 74-year-old male presents to the ED with a rash located on his face. The rash is vesicular, extremely painful, extends over the right side of his forehead, and involves the tip of his nose. Which of the following statements regarding this patient's condition is accurate?

   a. an eye is examination, including slit-lamp, is mandatory in this patient
   b. rarely seen in the elderly
   c. the described condition is not contagious
   d. the patient can be safely discharged on oral acyclovir with no further workup.

16. A 17-year-old female presents to ED with a sore throat, fever, malaise, fatigue, and abdominal pain. Physical examination reveals exudative pharyngitis with tender posterior cervical

lymphadenopathy and hepatomegaly. Which is the most sensitive and specific test available to diagnose this patient's condition?

a. peripheral blood smear
b. throat culture
c. monospot test
d. increased antibody titer

17. A 37-year-old HIV+ male presents complaining of a cough with blood-tinged sputum for 3 weeks. He has lost 20 pounds in the past month and is having frequent night sweats. Which of the following would confirm an active tuberculosis infection?

a. chest x-ray showing a right upper lobe infiltrate with hilar adenopathy
b. tuberculin skin test with 10 mm of induration
c. induced sputum showing acid-fast bacilli
d. none of the above

18. The animals most commonly associated with transmission of rabies worldwide are:

a. rats
b. bats
c. dogs
d. raccoons

19. Which of the following statements regarding herpes simplex virus (HSV) is true?

a. HSV-1 is responsible for up to 30% of urogenital infections
b. administration of acyclovir decreases viral shedding but does affect duration of symptoms and does not cure herpes
c. lesions typically follow a dermatomal distribution
d. during asymptomatic periods, infected individuals are not capable of transmitting virus

20. Which of the following statements is true regarding influenza?

a. early administration of amantadine decreases the duration of symptoms for patients with influenza A and B
b. the most severe side effect of influenza vaccine is rash
c. influenza A and B subtypes are associated with most epidemics
d. influenza vaccine is not safe in pregnancy

21. A diffuse, fine, maculopapular rash spreading from the face to the extremities within 24 hours and lasting 3 days accompanied by fever, malaise, posterior auricular, occipital, and posterior cervical lymphadenopathy best describes which if the following viruses?

a. rubeola
b. rubella
c. parvovirus
d. roseola

1. Answer: c

The patient is likely suffering from food-borne *botulism*. Poorly preserved canned food is a risk factor for botulism. **ICU admission** is mandated for presumed botulism infection **with serial vital capacity monitoring** for possible respiratory compromise. **Floor admission (a)** is not an appropriate disposition as this patient could rapidly develop respiratory failure. **Lyme disease (b)** does not typically present with weakness or autonomic symptoms. **Myasthenia gravis (d)** does not include autonomic symptoms.

2. Answer: b

For this patient with a *high-risk tetanus-prone wound* and unknown prior vaccination status, **Td should be given on presentation with repeat vaccinations planned at 4 to 8 weeks and 6 to 12 months postexposure.** This schedule provides nearly 100% active immunization to adults. In addition, the patient should be provided passive immunity via **TIG 3000 Units IM at a site separate from the Td vaccination.** TIG provides adequate passive immunity to prevent tetanus infection from the acute injury. Providing only the Td vaccine **(a)** would be inadequate prophylaxis for this high-risk wound. Patients with unknown or incomplete tetanus vaccination history should receive the first dose of Td as soon as possible after an injury **(c)**. The correct dose for TIG is 3,000 to 6,000 Units IM at a site separate from the Td vaccination **(d)**.

3. Answer: a

The deer tick of the *Ixodes* species **(a)** is responsible for the transmission of the organism responsible for causing *Lyme disease, B. burgdorferi.* The *Amblyomma* species **(b)** is associated with transmission of organism that causes ehrlichiosis. RMSF is caused by *Rickettsia rickettsii,* which is transmitted by the tick of the *Dermacentor* sp. **(c, d)**.

4. Answer: c

Erythema migrans (c) is an erythematous plaque with central clearing that enlarges (or migrates). It is a vasculitis that is warm to touch, painless, and is not pruritic. It occurs at the tick bite site and is the *most common* clinical manifestation associated with *Lyme disease,* present in 60% to 80% of patients in the first stage of Lyme disease. It can develop within 2 to 20 days of the tick bite and it may last for up to 1 month. **Erythema nodosum (a)** appears as painful red nodules, most commonly on the shins. It is related to a nonspecific inflammatory response. **Erythema marginatum (b)** presents as pink rings on the trunk and inner arms. It is associated with rheumatic fever. **Erythema multiforme (d)** typically presents as multiple, symmetric, "target" lesions on the extremities. It is mediated by an autoimmune process. It can progress to Stevens–Johnson syndrome.

5. Answer: d

The classic triad of fever, headache, and rash associated with *Rocky Mountain spotted fever* is rare and seen in **only approximately 3% of patients** with disease **(d)**. This fact makes it imperative for patients to be treated for disease when clinical suspicion is high. It has been found that the prognosis of the disease improves with early treatment. The classic petechial rash that begins on the wrists and ankles and spreads centripetally is absent in 20% of patients.

6. Answer: d

This patient has a rash characteristic of *secondary syphilis*. Although secondary syphilis can present with a variety of skin rashes, a symmetric maculopapular rash involving the palms and soles with generalized adenopathy is the most likely presentation. The appropriate treatment is **benzathine penicillin G 2.4 million units IM once (d)**. Choices **(a)** and **(c)** would be appropriate treatment options for neurosyphilis. Latent, late, or unknown-duration syphilis is treated with benzathine **penicillin G 2.4 million units IM weekly for 3 weeks (b)**. **Third-generation cephalosporins** are not considered to be first-line treatment for syphilis **(e)**.

7. Answer: c

This patient is in *septic shock* based on the evidence of systemic infection and persistent hypotension after a fluid bolus. Patients in septic shock benefit from Early Goal-Directed Therapy (EGDT). The patient should have a **central line placed** (subclavian or internal jugular). **Three therapeutic outcomes (CVP >8 mmHg with fluids, SBP >90 mmHg with vasopressors, and $S_{cv}O_2$ >70% with blood products and inotropes)** should be optimized within 6 hours of ED arrival **(b, c, d)**. If this is accomplished, the patient's short-term mortality could be reduced by as much as 16% from the previous standard care **(a)**. With early aggressive care, the patient's prognosis may improve significantly **(e)**.

8. Answer: d

The patient's fever, rash, and relative hypotension (patient has a history of untreated hypertension) are consistent with **toxic shock syndrome (TSS)**. There is also evidence of multisystem organ involvement (diarrhea, myalgia, mucous membrane hyperemia). Clindamycin 600 mg IV every 6 hours **(d)** is a first-line treatment for presumed TSS. Admission to an intensive care unit, not a general medical floor, would be appropriate **(a)**. IVIG **(b)** is recommended for patients that do not respond initially to fluids and vasopressors. Cardiac monitoring, vasopressors, and an IV fluid bolus of 20 to 30 mL/kg of crystalloid **(c)** would represent appropriate hemodynamic support for this patient. Ampicillin **(e)** is not recommended for treatment of presumed TSS.

9. Answer: c

The patient in the above clinical scenario most likely has *Dengue fever*, which is caused by an Arbovirus transmitted by the *Aedes* mosquito. It is common in

South America and Southeast Asia, is endemic to Hawaii, and has recently been reported in Key West, Florida. It accounts for 16% of febrile illness in travelers from the stated endemic regions. Patients present typically 2 to 8 days after being bitten by mosquito. Symptoms include fever, headache, retro-orbital pain, photophobia, nausea, vomiting, severe muscle/back pain *("breakbone fever")*, maculopapular rash, lymphadenopathy, and hemorrhage secondary to thrombocytopenia and capillary fragility. **Supportive therapy** is the mainstay of treatment **(c)**. Patients with Dengue fever do not need to be placed in **isolation (a)**. Malaria is a febrile illness caused by *Plasmodium* species. Endemic regions include Central/South America, Caribbean, sub-Saharan Africa, Middle East, and Oceania. The clinical presentation depends on which species of plasmodium is responsible for disease, with *P. falciparum* causing the most morbidity and mortality. Fever, jaundice, and hemolytic anemia are among the signs and symptoms present in those afflicted with malaria. **Chloroquine, primaquine, and mefloquine** are among agents used to treat malaria **(b)**. RMSF is often described as illness in adolescents following camping trips to the Carolinas that develop fever, headache, and rash. **Doxycycline** and **chloramphenicol** are agents used to treat this tick-borne disease **(d)**.

10. Answer: b

Coccidioides immitis causes fungal pneumonia in persons who live or travel to the southwestern U.S. and inhale dust, especially in summer and fall months when the dust is dry **(b)** (archaeologic digs, earthquakes, dust storms). Infected individuals cannot transmit disease. Most of those infected are asymptomatic; however, only a small inoculum is needed to cause disease. Immune response is T-cell mediated, and the development of *erythema nodosum* signifies a good immune response and portends a good diagnosis. *B. dermatitidis* **(a)** is largely found in the Mississippi Valley of the United States. *H. capsulatum* **(c)** is caused by ingestion of contaminated soil and cave exploration. *C. brunetti* **(d)** causes **Q-fever**. Infection is usually related to occupational exposure to cattle or sheep.

11. Answer: c

Rocky Mountain spotted fever (RMSF) is a tick-borne illness caused by *R. rickettsii*, transmitted by the female *Dermacentor* tick. It causes a febrile illness that is associated with a headache and rash, although this classic triad is only present in 3% of those infected. Early antibiotic therapy significantly reduces the mortality rate. Initiation of treatment relies on strong clinical suspicion. Mortality is higher in patients **more than 50 years old (a)**, **males (b)**, patients with a **delay in treatment (c)**, and patients with **no confirmed history of a tick bite (d)**.

12. Answer: c

Disseminated gonococcal infection is characterized by a dermatitis made up of **discrete papules** and

hemorrhagic pustules, mostly found on the extremities **(c)**. There are typically 5 to 40 lesions in disseminated infection. The rash is typically not generalized and **does not involve mucous membranes (a)**. The associated arthritis is typically an **asymmetric polyarthralgia** of the knees, elbows, and distal joints (knees > wrists > ankles > elbows) **(b)**. Disseminated gonococcal infection, unlike meningococcemia, **does not typically cause a rapidly progressive illness leading to multisystem organ failure (d)**.

13. Answer: a

Scombroid fish poisoning is caused by normal marine flora that produce **histamine and histamine-like compounds (a)**. These compounds accumulate mostly in dark skinned fish (tuna, mackerel, bluefish). Ingestion of contaminated, undercooked fish leads to a histamine-mediated reaction, including facial flushing, diarrhea, severe headache, palpitations, and abdominal cramps. The reaction is **not an IgE-mediated allergic reaction to fish (b)**. Affected patients should be informed that they are not allergic to the involved fish. *G. toxicus* **is a unicellular plankton that releases a heat-stable neurotoxin called ciguatoxin,** leading to ciguatera fish poisoning **(c)**. *Bacillus cereus* food poisoning is mediated by bacteria that produce **a heat-stable spore that release an enterotoxin (d)**.

14. Answer: a

This patient most likely has **staphylococcal food poisoning (a)**. Epidemic outbreaks of food-related gastroenteritis are most commonly caused by *S. aureus*. Undercooked or poorly preserved food is the most common cause. Patients typically present with violent, repetitive vomiting, and abdominal cramps. They sometimes also present with fevers and diarrhea. *C. perfringens* **(b)** infection is commonly food-mediated, but typically has a more delayed presentation and diarrhea is the predominant symptom. *Shigella* **(c)** has a 24- to 48-hour incubation period and causes bloody diarrhea. *C. jejuni* **(d)** is typically spread by fecal–oral transmission, has a 2- to 5-day incubation and presents predominantly with diarrhea. *Y. enterocolitica* **(e)** also features diarrhea, and typically is transmitted via contaminated water or milk, not by poorly preserved food.

15. Answer: a

The patient described in the scenario has *herpes zoster,* caused by reactivation of varicella virus that lies dormant in dorsal root ganglia after initial infection. *Herpes zoster ophthalmicus* results specifically from reactivation of the latent virus in the trigeminal ganglion. Patients present with pain, paresthesias, tearing, and unilateral vesicular eruption in the distribution of the ophthalmic branch of the trigeminal nerve. Lesions present on the tip of the nose *(Hutchinson sign)* signal involvement of the nasociliary nerve. Ocular lesions are likely. A careful eye examination is required to measure visual acuity and **slit-lamp examination (a)** for dendritic lesions. If visual acuity is diminished or dendritic lesions are visualized on slit-lamp examination, immediate ophthalmology consultation is warranted. Herpes zoster occurs predominantly in the **elderly (b)** and is **highly contagious (c)**. Patients with herpes zoster ophthalmicus should be admitted and started on **IV acyclovir (e)**.

16. Answer: c

Diagnosis of *infectious mononucleosis is* based on clinical characteristics in conjunction with laboratory testing. Heterophile antibody testing **(monospot test)** is the most sensitive and specific single test for infectious mononucleosis **(c)**. Atypical lymphocytes on the **peripheral blood smear** are consistent with infectious mono, but do not have as useful test characteristics as the monospot test **(a)**. **Throat culture (b)** and **antibody titers** are not useful for diagnosing infectious mono.

17. Answer: d

A **right upper lobe infiltrate with hilar adenopathy** also could be caused by community-acquired pneumonia **(a)**. **10 mm of induration after tuberculin skin testing** is consistent with prior exposure to *Mycobacterium tuberculosis,* but does not confirm active infection **(b)**. **Induced sputum showing acid-fast bacilli** is most likely due to *M. tuberculosis,* but infection with atypical mycobacterium is possible **(c)**. Only sputum culture positive for *M. tuberculosis* confirms active infection. The culture can take 7 to 14 days to grow, so suspected cases of tuberculosis should be treated presumptively.

18. Answer: c

Worldwide, **dogs (c)** are most responsible for transmission of rabies. *Rabies* has never been transmitted to a human from **rats (a)**, rabbits or hares (lagomorphs) (they are capable of being infected but are not known to infect humans). In the United States, **bat species (b)** are considered the most important reservoir for maintenance and transmission of rabies. In the United States, the animals most commonly infected are **raccoons (d)**, skunks, foxes, and coyotes.

19. Answer: a

Herpes simplex virus has two variants: type 1 and type 2. HSV, while predominantly responsible for nongenital lesions, is also found to be responsible for anywhere from **10% to 30% of urogenital lesions (a)**. Acyclovir remains the drug of choice of herpes simplex infections, primarily urogenital. It has been found to **decrease shedding** and to **shorten duration of symptoms (b)**. It does not cure herpes. Patients who suffer from frequent recurrences have found that daily prophylaxis decreases the recurrence rate by close to 80%. Lesions associated with HSV infections **do not follow dermatomal distribution** as do lesions associated with herpes zoster **(c)**. Patients should be informed that **transmission of virus can occur during asymptomatic periods** because of continuous viral shedding **(d)**.

20. Answer: c

The three most common types of influenza virus include type A, B, and C. Types **A and B are responsible for most epidemics** due to rapid antigenic change **(c)**. When amantadine is administered within 48 hours of illness onset, there is a **reduction in the severity and duration (by 1 day) of influenza A, but not influenza B (a)**. Neither amantadine nor rimantadine is effective against influenza B infections. **Guillain–Barré syndrome is the most severe side effect** of the vaccine **(b)**. Patients >65 years of age, those who are immunocompromised, **pregnant patients** in the second and third trimester, and health care workers should receive the vaccine **(d)**.

21. Answer: b

The signs and symptoms of *rubella, also known as German measles* **(b)**, include a fine maculopapular rash that lasts 3 days ("3-day measles") accompanied by generalized malaise and fever. Posterior cervical lymphadenopathy may also be present. **Rubeola**, also known as measles **(a)**, is characterized by cough, coryza, and conjunctivitis. In addition, the presence of Koplik spots on the buccal mucosa are pathognomonic findings in patients infected with rubeola virus. The rash associated with rubeola is a generalized, maculopapular, confluent rash that centrifugally spreads from the head to the extremities and usually lasts greater than 3 days. **Fifth disease,** caused by **parvovirus B19 (c)**, is a mild illness that occurs most commonly in children. The child develops a "slapped-cheek" rash on the face and a lacy red rash on the trunk and limbs. The rash may be accompanied by fever, malaise, and "flu-like" symptoms for a few days prior to rash development. The rash resolves in 7 to 10 days. **Roseola (d)** is typically characterized by a history of high fever followed by rapid defervescence and a characteristic rash that fades within a few hours to 2 days. The rash is maculopapular or erythematous, typically begins on the trunk, and may spread to involve the neck and extremities. The rash is nonpruritic and blanches on pressure.

Musculoskeletal Disorders (Nontraumatic)

Sanjey Gupta | Steven S. Wright

BONY ABNORMALITIES
Aseptic necrosis of hip (avascular necrosis [AVN])
Osteomyelitis (CM)

MUSCULOSKELETAL TUMORS
Benign bone tumors
Malignant bone tumors
Soft-tissue sarcomas
Pathologic fractures

DISORDERS OF THE SPINE
Disk herniation
Diskitis
Inflammatory spondylopathies

LOW BACK PAIN
Cauda equina syndrome
Sacroiliitis (SI)
Low back pain: sprains and strains

JOINT ABNORMALITIES
Arthritis

PEDIATRIC JOINT ABNORMALITIES
Congenital dislocation of hip
Slipped capital femoral epiphysis (SCFE)
Osgood Schlatter disease

MUSCLE ABNORMALITIES
Myositis/myonecrosis
Rhabdomyolysis

OVERUSE SYNDROMES
Bursitis
Tendinitis
Muscle strains
Peripheral nerve syndromes/ entrapment neuropathies

SOFT-TISSUE INFECTIONS
Paronychia
Felon
Tenosynovitis
Fasciitis
Myositis/myonecrosis
Gangrene

Bony abnormalities

ASEPTIC NECROSIS OF HIP (AVASCULAR NECROSIS [AVN])

- Interruption of blood flow to bone leads to cellular death, then collapse of bone. Most often affects bones with limited collateral circulation, or single terminal blood supply—femoral head, talus, carpal bones

Causes

- Trauma, systemic steroids, systemic lupus erythematosus (SLE), alcohol abuse, slipped capital femoral epiphysis (SCFE), Legg–Calve–Perthes, renal failure/transplant, sickle cell disease, hemoglobinopathies

Epidemiology

- More common in males (except with SLE), middle age; bilateral in 50%

SIGNS AND SYMPTOMS

- Pain in joint, often complain of groin pain with standing, gradually worsens
- Joint function becomes limited; tenderness to palpation; limping

DIAGNOSIS

- MRI most sensitive (procedure of choice); reactive zone is diagnostic for AVN, showing low intensity on T1, high intensity on T2, after initial nonspecific water signal suggesting edema
- Plain films not as sensitive, but show diffuse porosis and sclerosis in the precollapse phase

TREATMENT

- Medical care: limited effect, does not slow progression, pain control
- Surgical care: core decompression, bone graft, total hip arthroplasty

OSTEOMYELITIS (OM)

- Acute or chronic inflammation of bones and surrounding structures due to infection

Hematogenous OM: Seeding of bacteria from distant site

- Acute: children, usually no preceding illness
- Subacute/chronic: adults
- *Staphylococcus* most common in all ages
- Illicit drug user—*Staphylococcus, Candida, Serratia, Pseudomonas*
- Intravenous drug users (IVDU): joints affected include sternoclavicular, sacroiliac, or pubic symphysis
- Sickle cell disease: *Salmonella* common

SIGNS AND SYMPTOMS

- Hematogenous OM: high fever, often abrupt
- Malaise, irritability, fatigue
- Restriction of movement
- Local edema, erythema, tenderness

Hematogenous vertebral OM: Seeding of bacteria from distant site

- Adults >45 years old
- Uncommon
- Lumbar vertebrae most common, then thoracic, next cervical
- Risk factors include diabetes mellitus (DM), hemodialysis, IVDU, cancer, long-term catheter placement

SIGNS AND SYMPTOMS

- Insidious onset
- Acute bacteremic episode history
- Local edema, erythema, tenderness
- Extension leading to abscesses, meningitis

Direct/contiguous OM

- Seeded directly from trauma, or spread from adjacent site of infection or surgery
- Most common in adults/teens
- Normal vasculature: *Staphylococcus aureus, Staphylococcus epidermidis*
- Vascular insufficiency/DM: polymicrobial, anaerobes too
- Puncture wound through tennis shoe: *S. aureus, Pseudomonas*
- Sickle cell disease—*S. aureus, Salmonella*

SIGNS AND SYMPTOMS

- Local pain, redness, warmth, edema
- Fever

Chronic OM

- Necrotic bone is characteristic
- *S. epidermidis, S. aureus, Pseudomonas, Serratia, Escherichia coli*

SIGNS AND SYMPTOMS

- Chronic fatigue, malaise
- Sinus tract drainage
- Nonhealing ulcers

Diagnosis of osteomyelitis

LABORATORY

- WBC may be elevated, but frequently normal; increased polymorphonuclear leukocytes (PMNs), left shift
- Erythrocyte sedimentation rate (ESR)/C-reactive protein (CRP) elevated but nonspecific
- Blood cultures positive in >50% children
- Culture and bone biopsy are standard of care

RADIOLOGY

- X-rays initially normal 7 to 10 days after symptom onset
  - Periosteal elevation is earliest finding
  - Cortical erosions
  - New bone formation
  - Need 40% to 50% bone loss to visualize lucency
- Bone scan: Technetium-99 initial imaging of choice
  - Measures increase in bony activity
  - Abnormal after 1 to 2 days
  - 95% sensitive, less specific than MRI
- MRI: effective in early detection
  - Detects bone edema, periosteal reaction, cortical destruction, soft-tissue involvement earlier than x-rays
  - Test of choice for vertebral OM
- CT: may detect abnormal ossification, calcification, intracortical abnormalities, foreign bodies, gas
- Ultrasound (US): may detect changes as early as 1 to 2 days
  - Allows for US-guided aspiration
  - Detects soft-tissue abscess, periosteal elevation, fluid collections
- **Diagnosis** requires 2 of 4 of the following:
  - Purulent aspiration
  - Positive blood or bone culture
  - Classic physical findings of erythema, edema, tenderness
  - Positive radiological result

TREATMENT

- ED—empiric antibiotics—nafcillin vs. vancomycin *plus* ceftriaxone or cefotaxime
- Orthopedic and infectious disease consult
- Sickle cell anemia: ciprofloxacin or levofloxacin
  - Alternative—third generation cephalosporin
- Postnail puncture through tennis shoe: ceftazidime or ciprofloxacin

DISPOSITION

- Admit those with acute OM
- Discharge subacute or chronic if outpatient IV antibiotics and appropriate follow-up can be arranged

Musculoskeletal tumors

- Musculoskeletal tumors can arise in the bone, muscle, or nerve; can be benign or malignant, primary, or secondary

BENIGN BONE TUMORS

- Occur first 3 decades of life; can arise from bone, cartilage or other cells; generally do not extend beyond cortex of bone, but can be aggressive leading to bone destruction
  - Often surrounded by radiodense bony margin
  - Pain may or may not be present
  - Most common site: metaphysis
  - Treatment includes surgical excision

MALIGNANT BONE TUMORS

- Associated with deep, aching, constant pain that persists at rest
  - Metastases are common, especially to the lung
  - Most common: osteosarcoma (mainly adolescents, knee joint)
  - Treatment: surgical, including orthopedics; radiation

SOFT-TISSUE SARCOMAS

- Malignant tumors arising in the muscles and the soft tissues
  - Can arise anywhere, but most common in the extremities
  - Present as a musculoskeletal lump, usually painless
  - Found on physical examination, usually supplemented with imaging studies (MRI)
  - Biopsy will confirm whether mass is malignant
  - Treatment-wide surgical resection, often radiation therapy

PATHOLOGIC FRACTURES

- Tumors gradually erode bone, weakening it to point that the bone cannot withstand normal stress
  - Often associated with minimal trauma
  - Benign tumors are often asymptomatic before fracture
  - Examples include solitary bone cyst, fibrous dysphasia, nonossifying fibroma, endochondroma
  - Dull, aching pain may precede fractures associated with malignant bone tumors or metastatic tumors

Disorders of the spine

DISK HERNIATION

- Disk is composed of gelatinous nucleus pulposus surrounded by a fibrous annulus fibrosus
- "Slipped disk" is usually a posterior herniation of the nucleus pulposus with nerve root or spinal cord impingement
- May cause **anterior cord syndrome**—paralysis (corticospinal tracts) and loss of pain/temperature sensation (spinothalamic tracts) occur below level of injury, with preservation of posterior column function (vibration, position sense, crude touch—light touch is in the spinothalamic tracts and dorsal columns)

Types of disk herniation

CERVICAL

- Cervical spine involvement
- C5-C6 (C6 root): 20% of cases
- C6-C7 (C7 root): 70% of cases

SIGNS AND SYMPTOMS

- Sharp, intense pain with burning sensation
- Radicular symptoms radiate to trapezius, periscapular area, down arm
- Numbness and motor weakness in myotomal distribution
- Myelopathy may include hyperreflexia, gait disturbance, sexual or bladder dysfunction, reduced fine-hand motor coordination, upper or lower extremity weakness or spasticity

DIAGNOSIS

- Physical examination
- MRI for patients with evidence of myelopathy

TREATMENT

- Pain management
- Evidence of myelopathy: treatment decisions made in conjunction with neurosurgical consultation

THORACIC/LUMBAR

- Uncommon thoracic
- Mostly in mid-to-lower thoracic spine
- **Lumbar** L4-L5 (L5 nerve root) or L5-S1 (S1 nerve root): 95% cases

SIGNS AND SYMPTOMS

- Sharp, intense pain with burning sensation
- Radicular symptoms: 90% along L5-S1 nerve root radiating below knee to foot
  - L5: sensory—great toe webspace; motor—foot dorsiflexion
  - S1: sensory—lateral foot; motor—foot plantar flexion
- Numbness and motor weakness in myotomal distribution
- Monitor for signs of epidural compression syndrome, for example, cauda equina syndrome, conus medullaris syndrome (urinary retention, perineal anesthesia, fecal incontinence, bilateral leg pain)

DIAGNOSIS

- Lumbar x-ray—not helpful for diagnosis of disk herniation
- Emergent MRI if epidural compression considered

TREATMENT

- Pain management
- Epidural compression: treatment decisions made in conjunction with stat neurosurgical consultation
  - Dexamethasone 10 mg IV

DISKITIS

- Infection of nucleus pulposus
- Increased incidence in immunocompromised, postsurgical, and patients with systemic infections, IVDU
- Lumbar spine most common site

SIGNS AND SYMPTOMS

- Fever
- Pain at level of involvement often with radicular symptoms
- No neurological deficits

DIAGNOSIS

- X-ray
  - Plain films positive after 2 to 4 weeks of disease
  - Disk space narrowing
  - Irregular destruction of end plates of vertebral body
- MRI
- Elevated ESR and CRP, but WBC count usually normal

TREATMENT

- Intravenous antibiotics

INFLAMMATORY SPONDYLOPATHIES

- Inflammation of axial joints (sacroiliac most common), asymmetric oligoarthritis (lower extremities), enthesitis, genital/skin lesions, eye and bowel inflammation, flexor tenosynovitis. Often associated with HLA B27

Undifferentiated spondyloarthritis

SIGNS AND SYMPTOMS

- Musculoskeletal features
- Inflammatory back pain 70%
- Peripheral asymmetric arthritis usually of knees and ankles
- Enthesitis (inflammation at site of ligament or tendon insertion): most commonly at heels with insertion of Achilles tendon or plantar fascia ligament
- Dactylitis (sausage fingers)
- Eye disease (conjunctivitis or uveitis)
- Bowel inflammation: two thirds of patients; symptoms usually silent

DIAGNOSIS

- HLA-B27 positive (70%)
- Testing for bacterial or HIV infection
- ESR/CRP
- X-ray may show sacroiliitis with symmetric syndesmophytes
- MRI

TREATMENT

- Pain management

- Anti-tumor necrosis factor (TNF)-alpha agents: etanercept, infliximab, adalimumab
- Sulfasalazine
- Methotrexate
- Glucocorticoids (ocular glucocorticoids with uveitis)

Ankylosing spondylitis

- Disease of axial skeleton with back pain and progressive stiffness of spine
- Young adult peak age 20 to 30, predominately male
- Prevalence 5% to 6% those who are HLA-B27 positive

SIGNS AND SYMPTOMS

- Reduced range of motion of low back
  - *Schober test:* 5th lumbar spinous process marked by pen, additional marks made 10 cm above and 5 cm below pen mark in midline
  - Normal spine mobility: increase measured distance in lumbar full flexion (between upper and lower marks) of 5 cm
- Sacroiliac or hip joint pain or tenderness

DIAGNOSIS

- X-ray
  - Abnormal-appearing sacroiliac joint (widening, erosions, sclerosis, ankylosis)
  - *Bamboo spine:* ossification of annulus fibrosis with development of continuous (bridging) syndesmophytes
- Laboratory
  - HLA-B27 positive >90% cases
  - ESR/CRP elevated

TREATMENT

- Pain management/anti-inflammatory

Psoriatic arthritis

- Distal interphalangeal joints and spine are affected in 40% to 50% of cases

SIGNS AND SYMPTOMS

- DIP joint involvement
- Asymmetric oligoarthritis (<5 joints) or symmetric polyarthritis
- Destructive arthritis (arthritis mutilans) in 20%
- Sacroiliitis and spondylitis
- Soft-tissue inflammation and ocular involvement as seen in other arthritides
- Nail lesions—nail pitting (Fig. 11-1) and onycholysis (separation of nail from its bed)

DIAGNOSIS

- Arthritis in presence of psoriasis
- X-ray-presence of erosive changes and new bone formation in distal joints, gross destruction isolated joints, boney changes at enthesitis
- MRI: sacroiliitis 1/3 patients
- Laboratory: ESR and CRP elevated, HLA-B27 positive

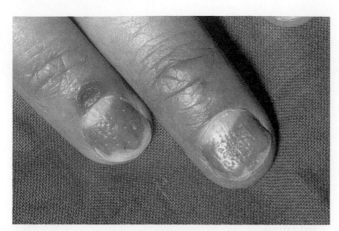

Figure 11-1. Nail pitting in psoriasis. The pits are more discrete and regular compared with pits affecting the nail plate in dermatitis. (From Goldman L: *Cecil textbook of medicine,* ed 23, Philadelphia, 2007, Elsevier.)

TREATMENT

- Pain management/anti-inflammatory agents
- Disease modifying drugs (e.g., methotrexate, cyclosporine A, sulfasalazine, TNF-alpha)

Low back pain

CAUDA EQUINA SYNDROME

- Cauda equina formed by nerve roots distal to spinal cord termination (usually L2)
- May result from any lesion that compresses these nerve roots
- Uncommon disease
- Usually from lumbar disk herniation, tumor, infection (epidural abscess), or trauma

SIGNS AND SYMPTOMS

- Low back pain often with radiation to legs
- Variable lower extremity sensory and motor abnormality with diminished reflexes
- Saddle anesthesia
- Urinary (overflow) and fecal incontinence
- Poor anal sphincter tone

DIAGNOSIS

- X-ray to evaluate for bony lesions
- MRI

TREATMENT

- Steroids if noninfectious
- Antibiotics if infectious
- Immediate neurosurgical or orthopedic consultation

SACROILIITIS (SI)

- See discussion from "Inflammatory Spondylopathies"
- Often related to seronegative spondyloarthritides—ankylosing spondylitis, reactive arthritis (e.g.,

Reiter syndrome), psoriatic arthritis, arthropathy related to inflammatory bowel disease
- SI joint involvement
- Related to HLA-B27 marker
- Inflammation around entheses
- Rheumatoid factor negative
- Dactylitis
- Conjunctivitis or uveitis

SIGNS AND SYMPTOMS

- Inflammatory back pain: presence of 4/5 of the following has 75% sensitivity
  - Onset before age of 40
  - Insidious onset
  - Persistence of minimum 3 months
  - Morning stiffness
  - Improvement with exercise
- SI joint tenderness and alternating buttock pain
- Decreased range of motion of back

DIAGNOSIS

- X-ray—takes many years for radiographic SI to appear
  - Typically symmetric
  - Early sign is indistinctness of joint
  - Progresses to widening, erosions, sclerosis, or ankylosis
  - Late stage—joint is thin line or not present at all
- MRI: subchondral bone marrow edema adjacent to the SI joint or rarely SI joint effusion

TREATMENT

- Pain management: NSAIDS to reduce inflammation, opiates for severe pain

LOW BACK PAIN: SPRAINS AND STRAINS

- Presumed pain from muscles and ligaments
- Usually no specific preceding event causing pain
- 75% to 90% have complete resolution of symptoms within 6 weeks

SIGNS AND SYMPTOMS

- Usually unilateral
- May extend to buttock or posterior thigh, but not past the knee
- Pain exacerbated with movement, patients can usually find a position of comfort
- Should not present with any lower extremity numbness, weakness, or urinary or sphincter abnormalities

DIAGNOSIS

- X-ray—indications for radiographs
  - Extremes of age: <18 or >50 years old
  - History of malignancy
  - Recent trauma with significant mechanism of injury
  - Duration longer than 4 to 6 weeks

- History of fever, immunocompromise, or IVDU
- Possibly prior to specialty referral

TREATMENT

- NSAIDs or opioids for short course
- Muscle relaxants generally offer no additional benefit
- Advocate continuation of normal activities, no "bed rest"
- Advocate exercise program

Joint abnormalities

ARTHRITIS

Septic arthritis

- Typically single joint
- A patient with monoarticular arthritis with unexplained inflammatory fluid is considered to have septic arthritis until proven otherwise by appropriate culture
- Bacteria reach joint by hematogenous spread, by direct inoculation, and by direct spread from bony or soft-tissue infection
- In children, hematogenous spread is the most common source
- Increased risk in elderly, those with prosthetic joints, IVDU, or immunocompromised patients; those with underlying chronic arthritis; joint instrumentation
- *S. aureus* is the most common cause of monoarthritis
- *Neisseria gonorrhoeae* accounts for 20% of monoarticular septic arthritis
    - Most commonly presents as migratory polyarthritis, asymmetric
- Children <6 months at risk for *S. aureus, E. coli/Enterobacteriaceae,* and group B streptococcal species
- Children 6 to 24 months: *S. aureus, Kingella kingae* (gram-negative rod), and *H. influenzae* (significantly reduced incidence due to vaccination)
- IVDU: *S. aureus* or gram-negative organisms
- Iatrogenic: *S. aureus* (most likely), *S. epidermidis,* gram-negative rods, anaerobes

SIGNS AND SYMPTOMS

- Painful, swollen, hot joint with tenderness to movement
- Most common is knee (40% to 50%), hip (20%), shoulder, wrist/ankle, elbow, hand and foot joints in this order
- Fever or chills

DIAGNOSIS

- CBC with possible leukocytosis, ESR elevation, blood culture (will be positive 50% of time)
- Acutely no bony changes in radiographs of joints
- Definitive diagnostic test is arthrocentesis with synovial fluid analysis

- Typically have leukocyte counts 50,000 to 150,000 cells/mm^3 (50% to 70%)
- "Left shift" of polymorphonuclear leukocytes (>75% to 85%)
- Cell count may be low in immunocompromised patients
- Gram stain positive in 50% to 70%
- Culture should be sent in all cases
- Viscosity: decreased
- Clarity: cloudy fluid

TREATMENT

- Pain control/immobilization
- Immediate orthopedic consultation for joint irrigation
- Intravenous antibiotic

Gouty arthritis

- Deposition of uric acid crystals into joints with resulting inflammatory response
- All patients with gout have hyperuricemia at some point during disease
- Patients with an acute gouty attack may have a normal or elevated uric acid level

SIGNS AND SYMPTOMS

- 80% of attacks involve single joint
- Typically lower extremity, most often first metatarsal phalangeal joint (podagra), ankle, or knee
- Up to 40% may experience polyarticular involvement, especially in repeat attacks
- Red, warm, painful, inflamed joint with exquisite tenderness at onset of attack
- May be indistinguishable from acute septic arthritis
- Attacks are self-limiting with intercritical periods
- Long-term disease: presence of tophi or renal stones

DIAGNOSIS

- Arthrocentesis with synovial fluid analysis
    - Leukocytosis generally up to 50,000 WBC/mm^3 with >75% PMNs
    - Presence of needle-shaped, negatively birefringent crystals
    - Gram stain and culture are negative
- CBC with leukocytosis and elevated ESR
- Uric acid is not helpful in acute gouty attack as it may be normal
- Acute radiographs may be normal
    - Long-standing disease produces asymmetric bone erosions

TREATMENT

- Colchicine: inhibits microtubule formation
    - Inhibits inflammatory response to crystals in the joint
    - Oral dose 0.6 mg orally every 1 to 2 hours until pain control or maximum of 4 to 6 mg (8 to 10

tablets), or until the presence of gastrointestinal side effects; lower dose maximum (3 mg) in elderly, renal/hepatic impairment; smaller body mass
  - Narrow therapeutic window; dosing maximum is controversial; not usually first-line therapy; wait at least 3 days between accelerated dosing
- NSAIDs
- Oral steroids (e.g., prednisone)
  - 40 mg/day for 3 to 5 days ± taper depending on duration of inflammation
- Joint injection with steroids
- Other analgesics (e.g., acetaminophen, opiates)
- Long-term therapy
  - Allopurinol: decreases uric acid production
  - Probenecid: increases uric acid excretion

Pseudogout (calcium pyrophosphate dihydrate crystal deposition disease)

- Self-limited attacks of arthritis involving one or several joints
- Knee most commonly involved (>50%), then wrist, ankle, elbow

SIGNS AND SYMPTOMS

- Red, hot, painful, swollen joint
- Symptoms not as severe as gouty attack

DIAGNOSIS

- X-ray: chondrocalcinosis in articular hyaline or fibrocartilaginous tissue
- CBC with leukocytosis and elevated ESR
- Arthrocentesis with synovial fluid analysis
  - Leukocytosis generally up to 50,000 WBC/mm³ with >75% polymorphonuclear leukocytes
  - Presence of rhomboid-shaped positively birefringent crystals
  - Gram stain and culture are negative

TREATMENT

- Similar to that of gout
- Colchicine: inhibits microtubule formation and inflammatory response in joint; not usually first-line therapy; see "Gouty Arthritis" for dosing
- NSAIDs

Osteoarthritis

- Most common form of arthritis in adults
- Loss of articular cartilage, micro-fractures of subchondral bone, and formation of osteophytes to repair damage

SIGNS AND SYMPTOMS

- Pain and lack of systemic symptoms
- General clinical characteristics (especially for knee)
  - >50 years old
  - Morning stiffness
  - Crepitus on active or passive motion of joint

- Bony tenderness and enlargement
- No palpable warmth
- Hand—Bouchard's nodes at PIP, Heberden's nodes DIP

DIAGNOSIS

- Laboratory tests are generally normal
- X-rays: joint space narrowing with osteophyte formation near joint margins
- Synovial fluid analysis not necessary, if obtained, appears noninflammatory

TREATMENT

- Pain management
- Specialty referral

Pediatric joint abnormalities (see also Chapter 24, Pediatrics)

CONGENITAL DISLOCATION OF HIP (ALSO KNOWN AS DEVELOPMENTAL DYSPLASIA OF THE HIP)

- Abnormal formation of hip joint, which ranges from subluxation to full hip dislocation
- More common in Native American and Caucasian populations
- More common in females and more commonly unilateral

SIGNS AND SYMPTOMS

- Variable presentation depending on severity of hip dislocation
- 4 to 6 months: examination of leg lengths, skin fold, asymmetry in the range of motion of hips, *Ortolani sign* (palpable gliding of the femoral head in and out of the acetabulum), *Barlow test* (provoked dislocation of the hip with adduction of the flexed hip with pressure posteriorly in line with the shaft of the femur)
- >4 to 6 months: *Galeazzi sign* (asymmetry in the levels of the patient's knees when supine, knees/hips flexed, and feet flat on the table) and skinfold asymmetry
- Walking age: *Trendelenburg sign:* while standing, the patient lifts a leg, and the body tilts toward that (normal) side—away from the weight-bearing side (affected) side—as a result of weakened pelvic girdle musculature

DIAGNOSIS

- 4 to 6 weeks of age—ultrasound
- >6 weeks—radiographs

MANAGEMENT

- <6 months old—Pavlik harness
- >6 months—hip spica cast or possibly surgery
- >2- to 3-year-old—femoral or pelvic osteotomy

SLIPPED CAPITAL FEMORAL EPIPHYSIS (SCFE) (Fig. 11-2)

- Posterior and inferior slippage of the proximal femoral epiphysis on the metaphysis
- Boys affected twice as often as girls, African Americans more than Caucasians
- Peak incidence during adolescent growth spurt
- Bilateral in up to 80% of cases
- Most cases idiopathic and related to obesity

SIGNS AND SYMPTOMS

- Limp
- Pain to hip, thigh, groin, or knee
- Present often after sports injury or fall

DIAGNOSIS

- Differential diagnosis: Legg–Calve–Perthes disease (AVN of femoral head with subchondral stress fracture—usually ages 4 to 9 years with chronic pain and limp); septic arthritis; toxic tenosynovitis; and fractures
- Anteroposterior (AP) pelvis and frog-leg view lateral pelvis x-rays (see Fig. 11-2)

TREATMENT

- Non–weight-bearing status
- Immediate orthopedic consultation
  - Internal fixation with a solo central screw

OSGOOD SCHLATTER DISEASE

- Adolescent orthopedic knee disorder; 3 : 1 male predominance
- Quadriceps contraction stress over time cause inflammatory changes at patellar tendon insertion on the tibial tuberosity
- Pain and tenderness over anterior knee, especially over tibial tuberosity, which appears enlarged

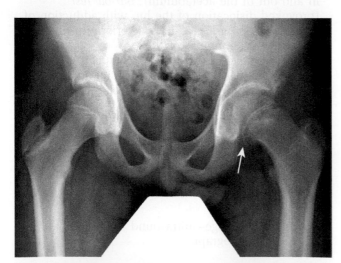

Figure 11-2. Anteroposterior pelvis radiograph demonstrating a left mild stable slipped capital femoral epiphysis. (From Frontera WR, Micheli LJ, Silver JK, Herring SA (eds): *Clinical sports medicine: medical management and rehabilitation*, Philadelphia, 2006, Saunders.)

- No knee effusion
- Conservative treatment

Muscle abnormalities

MYOSITIS/MYONECROSIS (SEE "SOFT-TISSUE INFECTIONS")

RHABDOMYOLYSIS

- Pathophysiology: release of intracellular contents (including myoglobin, creatine phosphokinase [CPK], aldolase, lactate dehydrogenase [LDH], potassium) due to musculoskeletal injury—most commonly disrupting Na–K–ATPase pump and calcium transport, leading to increased intracellular calcium and cell necrosis
- Most common causes: alcohol/drug abuse, trauma, systemic infection, heat-related illness, strenuous activity (athletes and military recruits), toxins, seizures

SIGNS AND SYMPTOMS

- Include myalgias, stiffness, weakness, nausea, vomiting, low-grade fever, dark urine, and tenderness of affected muscles
  - Absence of the above symptoms does not rule out rhabdomyolysis

DIAGNOSIS

- Myoglobin: unreliable marker for rhabdomyolysis, half-life of 1 to 3 hours, may clear within 6 hours
- Urinalysis: brown urine with large amount of blood on urine dipstick but few RBCs on microscopy
- CPK: more sensitive than myoglobin in detecting rhabdomyolysis, peak levels occur 24 to 36 hours after muscle injury
  - CK levels correlate well with severity of disease
- Electrolytes
  - Hypocalcemia—most common abnormality
  - Hyperkalemia, hyperphosphatemia, hyperuricemia, hypoalbuminemia

COMPLICATIONS

- Acute renal failure
- Disseminated intravascular coagulopathy: thrombocytopenia, hypofibrinogenemia, increased fibrin split products, elevated coagulation studies, abnormal liver panel
- Compartment syndrome
- Peripheral neuropathy

TREATMENT

- Mainstay is aggressive early hydration with intravenous fluids to maintain urine output at 200 to 300 mL/hour, which decreases incidence of acute renal failure
- Urine alkalinization: maintain urine pH >6.5; commonly done, but not proven to change outcomes compared with aggressive hydration

- Mannitol: osmotic diuretic expands intravascular volume, increases renal blood flow, free radical scavenger; works to prevent obstruction from renal casts, decreases tubular obstruction
- Avoid loop diuretics (furosemide), which can acidify urine
- Electrolyte abnormalities
  - Hyperkalemia: treat as other patients with hyperkalemia
  - Hypocalcemia: avoid intravenous calcium; ineffective if phosphate is elevated; may cause precipitates
  - Dialysis may be necessary
  - Compartment syndromes: suggestive symptoms or CPK levels that fail to decline after 48 hours may suggest compartment syndrome and necessitate fasciotomy

Overuse syndromes

BURSITIS

- Bursae are closed flat sacs lined with synovial membranes, approximately 150 bursae are located at sites of friction between bones, ligaments, muscles, tendons, and skin, providing lubrication for movement
- Etiology
  - Trauma is most common cause
  - Crystal deposition of urate, calcium pyrophosphate
  - Infection: risk increases with DM, uremia, gout, immunosuppressants
    - *S. aureus*, *S. epidermidis* >90%; streptococcal species
  - Systemic disease: rheumatoid arthritis, gout, SLE, psoriatic arthritis, ankylosing spondylitis
- Affected joints (most common)
  - Shoulder: **subacromial bursitis** is synonymous with supraspinatus tendinitis; pain, tenderness to lateral aspect of shoulder, painful arc with abduction from 70 to 100 degrees
  - Elbow: **olecranon bursitis** features tense edematous bursa, tender to palpation, frequently warm, erythematous, high incidence of infection
  - Hip: **trochanteric bursitis** is more common among older females, acute or chronic pain overlying greater trochanter and lateral thigh, increased with lying on hip/walking
  - Knee: **prepatellar bursitis** (housemaid's knee)— may affect any of four extensor bursae, results from chronic irritation, overuse, trauma
    - Pyogenic less common than olecranon, more common in children
  - Ankle/foot: **calcaneal bursitis** may result from improper shoes/high heels

SIGNS AND SYMPTOMS

- Localized pain
- Decreased active range of motion (passive maintained)
- Localized swelling
- Overlying warmth, erythema; low grade fever if infectious

DIAGNOSIS

- Suspicion of infection mandates aspiration; hip/deep bursae referred to orthopedics
  - Laboratory: CBC; glucose; evaluation for systemic disease
  - Bursal fluid analysis: cell count and differential; glucose, total protein, crystals, Gram stain, culture
- Normal fluid: WBC 0 to 200/hpf, clear yellow, low protein/glucose
- Traumatic bursitis: WBC <1200, bloody, xanthochromatic, many RBCs, low protein, normal glucose
- Septic bursitis: purulent; WBC generally much lower than in septic arthritis; may be between 5,000 and 20,000; predominantly polymorphonuclear leukocytes, increased protein, decreased glucose, positive Gram stain 70%
- Radiology
  - X-rays if indicated to rule out fracture or foreign body
  - MRI/US—may aid in ascertaining extent of infection

TREATMENT

- Immobilization if pain is severe
- Immobilize shoulders for less than 2 to 3 days to prevent adhesive capsulitis
- Ice
- NSAIDs
- Steroid injections
- Septic bursitis—orthopedic consult for I&D of bursa, antibiotics based on Gram stain result
- Management of systemic diseases causing bursitis

TENDINITIS

- Refers to inflammation of the tendon only. *Tenosynovitis* includes tendon and sheath, poor distinction between two entities

SIGNS AND SYMPTOMS

- Classically presents with pain, swelling, warmth, tenderness, decreased range of motion
- Pain often resolves quickly after initial movement only to return as throbbing after exercise
- Increased pain with active contraction against resistance or passive stretching

Pathophysiology

- Mechanical overload or repetitive/overuse
- Release of vasoactive and chemotactic mediators, causing vasodilation, edema, and increased inflammation
- Continued irritation leads to fibrosis
- Association with fluoroquinolone use

Most common

- **Supraspinatus tendinitis:** tendon sits between humerus and acromion as part of rotator cuff, causing compression and impingement with motion; *Neer classification of impingement syndrome*
  - Stage I: <25 years old, repetitive overhead motions such as swimming and pitching cause edema and hemorrhage within tendon
    - Dull ache, tenderness over greater tuberosity with abduction/flexion, no weakness, loss of strength
  - Stage II: 25 to 40 years old, constant pain, worse at night, limited active but retained passive range of motion, diffuse pain, fibrosis, edema, tendon thickening
  - Stage III: >40 years old, partial to complete tears
  - Classic test: Impingement by raising humerus in forced forward flexion while preventing scapular rotation reproduces pain
- **Calcific tendinitis:** may affect any tendon of rotator cuff, most commonly supraspinatus in patients >40 year of age
  - Asymptomatic; x-rays show calcium deposition
  - Spontaneous resorption causes discomfort
  - Trauma may cause crystal release causing acute attacks
- **Bicipital tendinitis:** pain in anterior shoulder radiating to radius, worse when sleeping/rolling on shoulder, trying to reach back pocket
  - Tenderness in bicipital groove, worse with flexing shoulder/supinating forearm
  - *Yergason test:* elbow is flexed to 90° using thorax to stabilize the upper arm as the forearm is held pronated. The examiner resists supination while the patient also laterally rotates the arm against resistance. The test is positive if the patient experiences discomfort or pain in the bicipital groove or if the tendon pops out of the bicipital groove
- **De Quervain tendinitis:** abductor pollicis longus and extensor pollicis brevis inflammation from thumb overuse, with tenderness along radial aspect of wrist and distal forearm
  - *Finkelstein test:* with thumb held inside clenched fist, forced ulnar deviation of wrist causes pain to radial styloid, also can occur with OA, and gonococcal tenosynovitis
- **Trigger finger:** pain and popping on extension, locking in flexion when proximal portion of flexor tendon sheath stenoses and "catches" on metacarpal head. Most common in middle age or pregnant females
- **Achilles (calcaneal) tendinitis:** strongest, longest tendon in body, overuse causes inflammation, eventual scar formation, and degeneration of tendon. Most common in young male athletes, and those with trauma or systemic disease

DIAGNOSIS

- Made by history and physical examination
- US is the criterion standard for evaluating tendon injury with trauma/rheumatologic disease, limited use in ED
- X-ray to rule out acute fracture if necessary

TREATMENT

- Immobilization, rest, decrease activity
- Ice first 24 to 48 hours, NSAIDs, steroid injection, range-of-motion exercises, physical therapy

MUSCLE STRAINS

- Common overuse injury, occurs with muscle contraction, stretch with active use, or excessive stretch, mainly at muscle–tendon junction
- Most susceptible muscles are the ones that have complex arrangement or cross multiple joints
- Candidates for poor healing and possible surgery include those who have injuries that involve the rectus femoris, the biceps femoris origin, and the abdominal wall

SYMPTOMS

- Include pain, muscle weakness, stiffness, ecchymoses, swelling, and decreased mobility

TREATMENT

- Ice during the first 24 to 48 hours, rest, immobilization, elevation, NSAIDs, possible referral if severe

PERIPHERAL NERVE SYNDROMES/ ENTRAPMENT NEUROPATHIES

- Feature pain or loss of function due to chronic compression, resulting in focal segmental demyelination of the nerve as it passes between bony surface and ligamentous canal

Most common

- Median nerve entrapment: carpal tunnel syndrome (see below)
- Ulnar nerve entrapment

CUBITAL TUNNEL SYNDROME (ELBOW)

- Numbness/weakness in the fourth and fifth digits; exacerbated by holding elbow in full flexion; thumb adduction may be weak (adductor pollicis) with a *positive Froment sign* (need to flex proximal phalanx to hold paper tightly between thumb and proximal index finger)

GUYON CANAL SYNDROME (WRIST)

- Numbness in fourth and fifth digits (hand is spared) and Froment sign is absent

RISK FACTORS

- Trauma, repetitive motion, pregnancy, diabetes, and other systemic diseases

SYMPTOMS

- Weakness, paralysis, paresthesias, pain, hypersensitivity

CARPAL TUNNEL SYNDROME

- Median nerve compression at wrist
- Dull aching pain from wrist through forearm to elbow, worse at night
- Wake-up with paresthesias to index finger and thumb
- *Phalen sign:* forced maximal flexion at wrist causes increased pain/paresthesia
- *Tinel sign:* tapping over volar aspect of wrist overlying median nerve reproduces symptoms (poor sensitivity)

TREATMENT

- Conservative at first: avoid repetitive motions, wrist splint, treat underlying conditions, NSAIDs
- Progress to bupivacaine/dexamethasone injection, surgical/orthopedic referral

Soft-tissue infections

PARONYCHIA

- Acute or chronic inflammation of nail folds caused by disruption to cuticle or nail fold, allowing entry of bacteria or yeast to eponychial space
  - Occurs with frequent hand wetting, water exposure, nail biting, thumb sucking, aggressive manicures, and is more common in diabetics
  - *S. aureus,* streptococcal species
  - *Candida,* other fungi, coexist with *S. aureus*
  - Chronic nail biting, thumb sucking can lead to anaerobic mouth flora in pediatric patients

SIGNS AND SYMPTOMS

- Acute: pain, erythema, swelling, tenderness of nail fold, abscess formation
- Chronic: slower onset, symptoms intermittent, cuticle can become retracted, nail plate examination reveals horizontal ridges

TREATMENT

- Acute: early without purulence—oral antibiotics such as cephalexin or clindamycin (trimethoprim–sulfamethoxazole if community-acquired methicillin-resistant *S. aureus* is a concern), warm soaks
- Purulent: incision and drainage between nail plate and cuticle, gentle pressure to express pus, consider digital block if warranted, warm soaks
- Chronic: keep hands dry, avoid prolonged water exposure, stop manicures, wear gloves at work
  - 2% to 4% thymol, drying agent
  - Topical antifungal
  - Acute flares are treated with antibiotics
  - Dermatology referral

FELON

- Infection of the pulp space to the distal digit
- Septa of the finger pad produce separate compartments, confining infection under pressure

- Gradually spread forming multiple abscesses
- *S. aureus* is most common pathogen

Mechanism

- Minor trauma, mainly penetrating, to the dermis of the finger pad, with secondary bacterial infection

Clinical features

- Severe throbbing pain, swelling, pressure to pulp space

TREATMENT

- Early and complete incision and drainage, irrigation, culture
  - Approach is controversial
- Unilateral longitudinal—spares sensate volar pad, allows adequate drainage, do not extend to distal interphalanx (DIP)
- Central longitudinal incision—recommended when felon points towards volar fat pad, fewer long-term complications
  - Packing, splint, oral antibiotic covering *S. aureus*

COMPLICATIONS

- Flexor tenosynovitis, osteomyelitis, cellulitis, and septic arthritis of adjacent joint

TENOSYNOVITIS

- Inflammation/infection of tendon/tendon sheath and synovial spaces

Flexor tenosynovitis

- Acute synovial space infections involving flexor tendon sheaths, with tendency to spread along midpalmar, thenar, lumbrical areas
- Mechanism—penetrating trauma, less commonly hematogenous spread
- *S. aureus* is most common; streptococcal species; anaerobes

SIGNS AND SYMPTOMS

- **Kanavel's four cardinal signs**
  - Flexed posture of digit at rest
  - Symmetric swelling ("sausage digit")
  - Tenderness of flexor sheath
  - Pain elicited with passive extension (most important sign)

MANAGEMENT

- Surgical emergency: hand/orthopedic admission for open drainage or closed-sheath irrigation
- Intravenous antibiotics: anti-staphylococcal, consider disseminated gonorrhea coverage with ceftriaxone
- If early, may consider oral antibiotics with hand surgeon consultation

FASCIITIS

- Infection of skin, subcutaneous tissue, and fascia, does not include but can spread to muscle leading to myositis/myonecrosis

SIGNS AND SYMPTOMS

- Erythema, edema (which can be massive, may lead to blebs, bullae, crepitus, frank necrosis)
- Moderate to severe systemic toxicity (fever, tachycardia, altered mental status, shock)
- Systemic signs often out of proportion to skin findings
- Severe types (below)

Necrotizing fasciitis

- Uncommon, potentially lethal, more common in men, lower extremities, anaerobic, mixed aerobic gram-negative organisms, can progress to wet gangrene

Clostridial cellulitis

- Anaerobic, local gas gangrene; spreads through fascial planes, but not in muscle
- Pain is variable as cutaneous nerves may be destroyed, leading to worsening condition without normal pain response

TREATMENT

- Intravenous fluid resuscitation
- Surgical consult for operative debridement
- Broad-spectrum antibiotics initially, then follow Gram stain and culture
- Intravenous calcium to reverse hypocalcemia from subcutaneous fat necrosis
- Transfusion or treatment of disseminated intravascular coagulopathy if needed

MYOSITIS/MYONECROSIS

- Deep soft-tissue infection involving surrounding tissues, causing muscular compromise

SIGNS AND SYMPTOMS

- Skin changes range from minimal redness to gangrene, massive edema may be present

Types

CLOSTRIDIAL MYONECROSIS ("GAS GANGRENE")

- Rapidly progressive necrotizing infection of the muscle, usually secondary to trauma, recent surgery
- Spore-forming gram-positive, anaerobic bacilli found in soil, GI tract, incubation 1 to 4 days
- Skin/wound is very painful
- Marked edema turns to brownish exudate, crepitus within hours
- Blebs/bullae

- "Sweet odor"
- Pain out of proportion to examination
- Shock may be present
- Muscle does not bleed when cut at time of surgery

NONCLOSTRIDIAL MYONECROSIS

- *B. fragilis*, *Peptostreptococcus*, *Staphylococcus*
  - Better prognosis
  - Synergistic necrotizing cellulitis—rapidly progressive, involving legs, perineum
  - More common in the immunocompromised and diabetics and patients with peripheral vascular disease
  - Skin appears murky
  - Discharge: blebs, crepitus, necrosis, multiple flora present
  - Hemolysis occurs; high mortality

TREATMENT

- Broad-spectrum intravenous antibiotics
- Surgical admission for wide excision and debridement
- Intravenous fluid resuscitation
- Consider hyperbaric oxygen therapy

GANGRENE

- Decay or death of tissue or organ due to lack of blood supply; can be complicated by injury, infection, inflammatory processes, or chronic diseases

Risk factors

- Immunocompromise, DM, alcoholism, peripheral vascular disease, IVDU
- Malignancy (especially gastrointestinal and hematologic)

SIGNS AND SYMPTOMS

- Fever, tachycardia, tachypnea
- Pain out of proportion to examination findings
- Diarrhea, vomiting
- Altered mental status
- Shock

Types

- "Dry gangrene"
  - Blood supply to tissue becomes obstructed
  - Tissue slowly dies, turns cold, numb, pale, then black
  - No infection occurs
  - Area may be marked by red line indicating affected tissue
  - Most commonly due to arteriosclerosis
  - Patients generally present without systemic signs of toxicity, unless superinfected
- "Wet gangrene"—blood flow suddenly stops, usually traumatic
- Sensation of heaviness followed by severe pain (also gas gangrene)

- Usually affects lower extremities, toes, feet
- Bacterial invasion as blood flow ceases, allowing multiplication without immune response
- Foul smelling
- *Streptococcus, Staphylococcus*
- Group A streptococcal disease is a serious, rare form, can progress to synergistic gangrene, more commonly called necrotizing fasciitis

DIAGNOSIS

- Clinical picture
- Laboratory evaluation
  - Metabolic acidosis
  - Leukocytosis
  - Coagulopathy, anemia, thrombocytopenia
  - Myoglobinemia, myoglobinuria
  - Liver/renal insufficiency
  - Gram stain of bullae: few WBC, positive bacilli with or without spores, RBCs
  - Radiography: may show gas within soft-tissue fascial planes (Fig. 11-3)

TREATMENT

- Dry gangrene
  - If no acute infection present, consult vascular surgeon
- Wet gangrene or gas gangrene
  - Broad-spectrum intravenous antibiotics
  - Surgical admission for wide excision and debridement
  - Intravenous fluid resuscitation
  - Consider hyperbaric oxygen therapy
  - Tetanus booster, if needed

PEARLS

- MRI is the most sensitive test for OM.

- In adolescents (especially male) with a limp and pain in the thigh, groin, or knee, consider SCFE and x-ray the affected hips and knee(s).

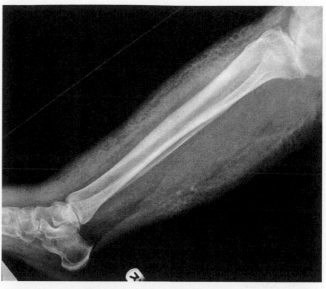

Figure 11-3. Radiologic image of leg. Note the appearance of gas in the soft tissues. (From Anesti E, Brooks P, Majumder S: Images in emergency medicine, *Ann Emerg Med* 50:14, 2007.)

BIBLIOGRAPHY

http://www.emedicine.com/emerg
http://www.utdol.com
Campana B: Soft tissue spine injuries and back pain. In Marx JA, Hockberger RS, Walls RM (eds): *Rosen's emergency medicine: concepts and clinical practice*, ed 5, St. Louis, 2002, Mosby, pp. 606–625.
Lowery DW: Arthritis. In Marx JA, Hockberger RS, Walls RM (eds): *Rosen's emergency medicine: concepts and clinical practice*, ed 5, St. Louis, 2002, Mosby, pp. 1583–1599.
McQuillen KK. Musculoskeletal disorders. In Marx JA, Hockberger RS, Walls RM (eds): *Rosen's emergency medicine: concepts and clinical practice*, ed 5, St. Louis, 2002, Mosby, pp. 2370–2392.
Rodgers KG, Jones JB: Back pain. In Marx JA, Hockberger RS, Walls RM (eds): *Rosen's emergency medicine: concepts and clinical practice*, ed 5, St. Louis, 2002, Mosby, pp. 233–240.
Uehara DE, Chin HW: Injuries to the elbow and forearm. In Tintinalli JE, Kelen GD, Stapczynski JS (eds): *Emergency medicine: a comprehensive study guide*, ed 5, New York, 2000, McGraw Hill, pp. 1763–1772.

Questions and Answers

1. What is the earliest x-ray finding of osteomyelitis?

   a. periosteal elevation
   b. new bone formation
   c. bony lucency
   d. cortical erosion

2. What is the most common cause of osteomyelitis in a sickle cell patient?

   a. *Salmonella* species
   b. *Staphylococcus aureus*

   c. *Pseudomonas aeruginosa*
   d. anaerobes

3. What is the most common location for lumbar disk herniation?

   a. T12-L1
   b. L1-L2 or L3-L4
   c. L4-L5 or L5-S1
   d. L3-L4 or L4-L5

4. A 46-year-old runner with no past medical history stepped on a nail while out running 4

weeks ago. The patient has had progressive pain to the ball of his right foot since the injury and now complains of low-grade fever and difficulty walking. In the ED, the patient's WBC count and ESR are elevated. A plain radiograph of the right foot reveals cortical erosions of the second metatarsal. The best choice of antibiotics should cover the following pathogens:

  a. *S. aureus* and *Pseudomonas*
  b. *Salmonella* and *S. aureus*
  c. *Staphylococcus epidermidis* and *Serratia* spp.
  d. anaerobes

5. What is the most common location for cervical disk herniation?

  a. C4-C5
  b. C5-C6
  c. C3-C4
  d. C6-C7

6. A 26-year-old male presents to the ED with 2 weeks of atraumatic lumbar back pain. The patient denies radicular symptoms, denies fecal incontinence or urinary retension, denies fever, and is able to perform the activities of daily living as well as those at work. The patient's physical examination is normal except for muscular lumbar tenderness. The next best is action is:

  a. lumbar x-ray
  b. analgesics and discharge
  c. MRI
  d. neurosurgical consultation

7. A 65-year-old woman with a history of osteoarthritis presents to the ED with increasing pain, redness, and swelling to her right knee. She normally has knee pain, but this pain is worse and she has increased difficulty walking. The next best course of action is:

  a. MRI of the knee
  b. knee immobilizer and discharge
  c. arthrocentesis
  d. physical therapy referral

8. A 47-year-old, overweight, sedentary patient presents to the ED the morning after the Super Bowl. The patient complains of pain in the large toe of the left foot and difficulty walking. Physical examination reveals redness, swelling, and tenderness at the first metatarsal-phalangeal joint. Which of the following has the *least* utility in establishing a diagnosis?

  a. x-ray of foot
  b. serum uric acid level
  c. synovial fluid analysis

9. Which is the following is **not** an HLA-B27-associated arthritis syndrome?

  a. ankylosing spondylitis
  b. psoriatic arthritis

  c. reactive arthritis (Reiter's syndrome)
  d. gouty arthritis

10. Which of the following is an indication for lumbar x-ray in low back pain?

  a. age of 35 to 40 years
  b. history of remote trauma
  c. duration of 2 weeks
  d. history of lung cancer

11. Which bacterium is most responsible for septic mono-arthritis in adult patients?

  a. *S. aureus*
  b. *Neisseria gonorrhoeae*
  c. *S. epidermidis*
  d. *Escherichia coli*

12. Which of the following is **true** in the diagnosis of gouty arthritis?

  a. the majority of attacks involve multiple joints
  b. presence of needle-shaped, positively birefringent crystals on synovial fluid analysis
  c. uric acid levels may be normal during an acute attack
  d. tenderness usually develops 24 to 48 hours after onset of attack

13. What is the most common laboratory abnormality in acute rhabdomyolysis?

  a. hypocalcemia
  b. hyperuricemia
  c. hyperphosphatemia
  d. hypoalbuminemia

14. A 13-year-old boy presents with knee pain and limp for 2 weeks. The patient is obese and stated that the pain began after playing soccer at school. On physical exam, the knee has no deformity or tenderness, and has full range of motion. The next best course of action would be:

  a. knee immobilization
  b. anteroposterior (AP) pelvis and frog-leg view pelvis x-ray only
  c. knee x-ray only
  d. AP pelvis and frog-leg view pelvis x-ray/knee x-ray
  e. analgesics and discharge

15. A 21-year-old man has had back pain for 8 weeks. The patient has also complained of eye redness and pain to his ankle and knees. He has also experienced increased pain to his heels when walking. His condition is most likely to be related to:

  a. gonorrhea infection
  b. parvovirus B19
  c. HLA-B27
  d. endocarditis

16. Which of the following is *not* a sign of flexor tenosynovitis?
    a. flexed posture of digit at rest
    b. symmetric swelling of the digit
    c. tenderness of flexor sheath
    d. pain elicited with passive flexion

17. A 57-year-old diabetic patient had a puncture wound to the right ankle. A small area of cellulitis formed around the puncture. The cellulitis rapidly expanded with intense pain and bullae formation. The patient spiked a temperature of 39° C with a blood pressure of 90/60 mmHg and heart rate of 110 beats per minute. The next most important action is:
    a. intravenous calcium
    b. acetaminophen for fever control
    c. immediate surgical consultation
    d. arterial Doppler ultrasound

18. A 34-year-old woman who ran a marathon the previous day presents to the ED with global muscle pain, muscle weakness, and nausea. The patient reports her urine being tea-colored. Laboratory studies reveal a total serum CPK of 25,000 U/L. The best initial treatment option is:
    a. intravenous fluids to maintain urine output at 200 to 300 mL/hour
    b. urine alkalinization to maintain pH above 7.5
    c. intravenous furosemide
    d. intravenous calcium

19. A 24-year-old woman presents with a progressively painful right wrist for 1 week. She admits to frequent use of her cellular phone to send text messages. She has no history of arthritis or other systemic disease. On physical examination, she is afebrile. Examination of her right upper extremity reveals tenderness and mild edema overlying the radial aspect of her wrist extending proximally into her forearm. On examination, one would expect a positive
    a. Phalen test
    b. Froment test
    c. Finkelstein test
    d. Tinel test

20. A 67-year-old man with a history of prostatic enlargement presents with a painful right ankle for 5 days. He denies trauma or overuse. He recently finished a course of unknown antibiotics for an unspecified condition; he denies diarrhea or fever. On physical examination, he appears well and his vital signs are within normal limits. Examination of his right ankle reveals no bony tenderness, no deformity, normal color, and normal neurovascular findings. There is appreciable tenderness over the calcaneal tendon without evidence of rupture (Thompson test is negative). This patient most likely finished a recent course of

    a. ciprofloxacin
    b. trimethoprim–sulfamethoxazole
    c. amoxicillin clavulanate
    d. doxycycline

---

1. Answer: a

Periosteal elevation is the first radiographic finding in osteomyelitis, appearing 7 to 10 days after onset of symptoms (a). **New bone formation** and **cortical erosion** occur after long-standing disease. **Lucencies** become apparent after 40% to 50% bony loss from the infection.

2. Answer: b

The most common cause of osteomyelitis of patients with sickle cell disease is *S. aureus*. *Salmonella* infection is also common for sickle cell patients. *Pseudomonas* is a recognized cause of osteomyelitis resulting from puncture wound through a "tennis" shoe. Patients with diabetes mellitus often suffer from osteomyelitis caused by a polymicrobial/**anaerobic** infection.

3. Answer: c

About 95% of cases of lumbar disk herniation occur at **L4-L5 (L5 nerve root)** or **L5-S1 (S1 nerve root)**.

4. Answer: a

Puncture wounds through a tennis shoe most often will cause an osteomyelitis from *S. aureus* or *Pseudomonas*. Patients with sickle cell disease may have osteomyelitis caused by *Salmonella* or *S. aureus*. Chronic osteomyelitis may be caused by *S. epidermidis, Serratia, Pseudomonas,* or *E. coli*. Diabetics often have osteomyelitis caused by multiple pathogens or **anaerobes.**

5. Answer: d

About 70% of cases of cervical disc herniation occur at **C6-C7** disk level, affecting the C7 nerve root. About 20% of cases of cervical disc herniation occur at the **C5-C6** disk level, affecting the C6 nerve root.

6. Answer: b

A **lumbar x-ray** is indicated after 4 to 6 weeks of back pain symptoms. The patient displays no symptoms of acute cord compression (pain, hyperreflexia, gait disturbance, sexual or bladder dysfunction, reduced fine motor coordination, lower extremity weakness or spasticity) or epidural compression syndrome (urinary retention, perineal anesthesia, fecal incontinence, bilateral leg pain) that would necessitate **MRI** and **neurosurgical consultation.** Thus, **analgesics** and **discharge** are most appropriate.

7. Answer: c

New redness, swelling, and pain to a joint is considered septic arthritis until proven otherwise. **Arthrocentesis** with Gram stain, cell count, and culture will help to support or refute the diagnosis of septic arthritis.

8. Answer: b

In gout, **serum uric acid levels** may be normal in an acute attack. **Radiographs** may reveal tophi or bony erosions in long-standing gouty disease. **Synovial fluid analysis** may reveal negatively birefringent crystals or uric acid deposition.

9. Answer: d

Psoriatic arthritis, reactive arthritis (formerly Reiter syndrome), and **ankylosing spondylitis** are all considered inflammatory spondylopathies. These all share in common sacroiliac involvement, HLA-B27 marker association, inflammation around entheses, rheumatoid factor negativity, dactylitis, and conjunctivitis/uveitis. **Gouty arthritis** is as a consequence of deposition of uric acid crystals into joints with a subsequent inflammatory response.

10. Answer: d

Indications for performing a lumbosacral x-ray include extremes of age <18 years or >50 years; history of **malignancy;** recent trauma; duration longer than 4 to 6 weeks; history of fever, immunocompromise, IV drug use, or possibly prior to specialty referral.

11. Answer: a

S. aureus is the most common cause of mono-arthritis in an adult patient. **N. gonorrhoeae** accounts for about 20% of septic monarthritis. **S. epidermidis** is often responsible for septic arthritis is cases with an iatrogenic cause (e.g., joint aspiration, arthroscopy). Children less than 6 months old are at risk for **E. coli** infection.

12. Answer: c

In gout, 80% of attacks involve a single joint (a), classically the first metatarsal–phalangeal joint (podagra). Synovial fluid analysis reveals needle-shaped, negatively birefringent crystals. **Uric acid levels** may be normal during an acute attack, limiting the usefulness of obtaining a uric acid level for diagnostic testing in a suspected gouty attack. Tenderness develops at onset of attack.

13. Answer: a

Hypocalcemia is the most common laboratory abnormality in acute rhabdomyolysis. All of the other above electrolyte derangements may also occur in acute rhabdomyolysis.

14. Answer d

The patient is at risk for osteosarcoma (mostly affects adolescents and often affects knee joint) and SCFE in light of his age and presentation; thus, it is appropriate to **x-ray both the knee and the hip.**

15. Answer: c

The spondyloarthrides are related to **HLA-B27** positivity state and include ankylosing spondylitis, reactive arthritis (e.g., Reiter syndrome), psoriatic arthritis, arthropathy related to inflammatory bowel disease. The signs and symptoms include sacroiliac involvement, inflammation around entheses, rheumatoid factor negativity, dactylitis, and conjunctivitis or uveitis.

16. Answer: d

Flexor tenosynovitis is a hand surgery emergency often occurring as a consequence of penetrating trauma. The most important sign is the elicitation of **pain with passive extension, not flexion.** All of the other answers are among Kanavel's signs of flexor tenosynovitis.

17. Answer: c

Necrotizing fasciitis is a **surgical emergency** for debridement of infected and necrotic tissue. **Intravenous calcium** may be needed in the course of management to treat hypocalcemia secondary to myonecrosis. **Acetaminophen** may be administered for fever control, but is not critical. **Doppler ultrasound** is not necessary.

18. Answer: a

Aggressive hydration is the mainstay of treatment of *rhabdomyolysis.* **Urine can be alkalinized** to maintain a **pH above 6.5,** but whether this is of significant benefit over appropriate intravenous fluid hydration is controversial. **Loop diuretics** should be avoided as they acidify the urine. **Calcium** may need to be administered if the patient experiences hypocalcemia from the disease process.

19. Answer: c

Clinically, this patient has *De Quervain tendinitis* or *tenosynovitis* from overuse of her thumb. Forced ulnar deviation of the wrist while the thumb is held within the clenched fist should result in increased pain (positive **Finkelstein test**). **Froment test** is the inability to hold a piece of paper between adducted thumb and index finger without flexion of the interphalangeal joint, and suggests cubital tunnel syndrome. **Phalen** and **Tinel tests** are tests for carpal tunnel syndrome, and involve eliciting pain/paresthesias in a median nerve distribution by either maximal wrist flexion (Phalen's) or tapping over the nerve at the volar wrist crease (Tinel's).

20. Answer: a

The fluoroquinolones have been associated with tendinitis and tendon rupture, so **ciprofloxacin** (perhaps for a urinary tract infection) is a possible contributing factor to the development of this apparent case of *calcaneal tendinitis.*

Nervous System Disorders 12

Jeffrey Barrett

Cranial nerve disorders

IDIOPATHIC FACIAL NERVE PARALYSIS

- The facial nerve (CN VII) supplies:
  - Motor innervations to the muscles of facial expression,
  - Parasympathetic fibers to the lacrimal and salivary glands, and
  - Sensory innervations to the anterior portion of the tongue and the auditory canal
- Peripheral facial nerve palsies can be secondary to trauma, infection, or neoplasm. A large proportion of cases, however, are idiopathic
- *Bell palsy* is a term commonly used to describe idiopathic facial nerve paralysis
  - Some recent data have suggested that these cases may actually be precipitated by viral infections, and clinical trials using antivirals and corticosteroids have shown some efficacy in the treatment of this disorder

SIGNS AND SYMPTOMS

- Weakness or paralysis of the muscles of facial expression, including the forehead on the affected side. If the forehead is spared, the deficit should be assumed to be central in origin
- Sensation intact
- Decreased tear production, otalgia, disturbances of taste, and hyperacusis
- Onset over 1 to 3 days
- Absence of other neurologic findings

DIAGNOSIS

- History and physical examination
- Check the ear on the affected side for vesicular lesions indicating *Ramsay–Hunt syndrome* (zoster infection involving the facial nerve)
- Consider testing for Lyme disease in endemic areas

TREATMENT

- 10-day steroid taper starting at 60 mg of prednisone in adults
- 7-day course of antiviral agent (acyclovir, valacyclovir, etc.)
- Ophthalmic lubricant, and taping the eye shut at bedtime
- 80% will have satisfactory recovery within weeks

TRIGEMINAL NEURALGIA

- Characterized by paroxysms of pain in one or more divisions of the trigeminal nerve (CN V)
- It tends to occur in the 6th and 7th decade of life, more commonly in women than in men
- It is thought to be caused by vascular compression of the nerve root by tortuous vessels

SIGNS AND SYMPTOMS

- Sharp, severe, transient paroxysms of pain in the trigeminal nerve distribution
- Pain is often triggered by movement or temperature changes
- Pain is transient, lasting less than 2 minutes
- It tends not to occur during sleep

DIAGNOSIS

- The diagnosis is clinical, primarily based on the history
- Any abnormal physical findings or neurologic deficits should lead one to reconsider the diagnosis
- In older patients, always consider and exclude temporal arteritis

TREATMENT

- Carbamazepine has been shown to be efficacious
- Open surgical or minimally invasive techniques are also options
- Referral for neurologic follow-up is recommended to exclude secondary causes such as tumor, aneurysm, or demyelinating process

Demyelinating disorders

MULTIPLE SCLEROSIS (MS)

- MS is an inflammatory disease of the nervous system that causes focal areas of demyelination
- It is generally considered an autoimmune disease and tends to occur with a higher frequency in women and individuals of western European descent

SIGNS AND SYMPTOMS

- Clinical manifestations are varied depending on the neurologic territory affected
  - May present with cognitive impairment, cranial nerve deficits, motor, sensory, or cerebellar deficits
  - Optic neuritis in a young, otherwise healthy patient is strongly suggestive of MS
  - Afferent pupillary defect or internuclear ophthalmoplegia may be seen
- The relapsing remitting clinical subtype is most common at onset
- A minority of patients contract primary progressive MS, which is characterized by a progressive worsening of symptomatology without discreet exacerbations

DIAGNOSIS

- There is no laboratory test diagnostic for MS
- Roughly 70% of patients will have an elevated CSF IgG
- Electrophoresis of the CSF will show oligoclonal bands in 85% to 95% of patients
- An MRI can demonstrate areas of focal demyelination

TREATMENT

- Medical therapy has three objectives: preventing acute exacerbations, treating acute exacerbations, and managing complications
- Interferon-B and glatiramer acetate are immune modulators used to suppress disease
- Intravenous methylprednisolone is effective in treating acute exacerbations
- Analgesics and antispasmodics such as baclofen can be used to treat painful sensory disturbances and spasticity

Headache

TENSION-TYPE HEADACHE (TTH)

- Most common type of headache, occurring in most people at some point in their lives. Despite how pervasive it is, the pathophysiology behind it has still not been uncovered

SIGNS AND SYMPTOMS

- Location is bilateral, described as "pressing" or "tightening" in quality, mild to moderate intensity, not exacerbated by routine activities, not associated with vomiting

DIAGNOSIS

- The diagnosis is based on the above clinical characteristics and the lack of any other evident cause for the headache
- There should be no neurologic findings on physical examination
- Severe pain should prompt a search for other causes
- Diagnosis of exclusion once more serious causes of headache have been investigated

TREATMENT

- NSAID drugs are the mainstay of therapy, and should be sufficient to control pain, although other drugs have shown efficacy as well

MIGRAINE HEADACHE

- Tends to present after adolescence, more often in women
- It is characterized by recurrent episodes, moderate to severe in intensity
- The etiology is thought to be abnormal serotonergic activity in the brainstem, which leads to vasoconstriction followed by vasodilatation

- This vasoconstriction is considered the cause of the neurologic symptoms sometimes experienced prior to the onset of the headache, commonly referred to as the "aura"
- Migraine headaches have historically been divided into two subtypes: common and classic
  - Classic migraines are preceded by an aura, common migraines are not
  - The aura is a reversible neurologic symptom, most commonly visual, but may manifest as other motor or sensory abnormalities

SIGNS AND SYMPTOMS

- "Pulsating" in quality, often unilateral, moderate to severe intensity, worsened by routine activity, associated with nausea, vomiting, photophobia, and/or phonophobia

DIAGNOSIS

- Primarily a clinical diagnosis
- Neuroimaging should not be routine, but can be justified when the headache is new, sudden, particularly severe, or otherwise different from the patient's typical migraine headache

TREATMENT

- Prochlorperazine and metoclopramide are effective in treating acute attacks
- Sumatriptan, a 5-HT receptor agonist, is also effective in treating the acutely painful migraine in the ED, but is contraindicated in those with coronary or peripheral vascular disease
- Narcotics are generally not as effective as neuroleptics or triptans and carry the risk of dependency

TEMPORAL ARTERITIS

- A vasculitis that tends to affect medium-sized arteries, most often the extracranial branches of the aortic arch. Not confined to the temporal artery
- It's most feared complication, blindness, is a manifestation of inflammation in the ophthalmic artery
- It tends to affect the elderly, women more than men, and is very rare before the age of 50

SIGNS AND SYMPTOMS

- Headache (not necessarily temporal), jaw claudication, myalgias, fever, malaise, amaurosis fugax (transient monocular blindness)
  - 30% of patients may present without headache

DIAGNOSIS

- Tenderness of the temporal scalp may be present but should not be relied on
- The ESR is typically very elevated
- Histologic changes in the temporal artery noted on biopsy is the gold standard

TREATMENT

- Corticosteroids are the mainstay of treatment and are usually very effective
- If the diagnosis is strongly suspected, treatment should begin as soon as possible

CERVICAL ARTERY DISSECTION

- Uncommon but devastating cause of headache
- Cervical artery dissections can occur in all age groups
- Associated with mechanical trauma to the vessel as well as genetic factors in the patient
- The **carotid** and **vertebral arteries** are thought to be more at risk for this phenomenon because of their mobility and location

SIGNS AND SYMPTOMS

- Unilateral head, neck, and/or orbital pain
  - Often gradual in onset, but may be sudden
- Partial Horner syndrome in the case of carotid dissection
- Neurologic deficit
  - May present as a stroke-like syndrome
  - Attributable to the anterior circulation in the case of carotid dissections
  - Attributable to the posterior circulation in the case of vertebral dissections
  - Neurologic symptoms may be transient in nature
- Delayed thromboembolic events may occur days to weeks after the acute dissection

DIAGNOSIS

- MR, CT, or conventional angiography
- Doppler ultrasound

TREATMENT

- As thromboembolism and ischemia are the main complications of cervical artery dissections, anticoagulation with heparin is the preferred initial treatment

Hydrocephalus

NORMAL PRESSURE HYDROCEPHALUS (NPH)

- Idiopathic, chronically developing form of hydrocephalus.
- Caused by an obstruction in the normal circulation of CSF, which slowly leads to enlargement of the ventricles
- Although less than 2% of cases of dementia are thought to be caused by idiopathic NPH, it is important to recognize because its symptoms can be reversible with proper treatment

SIGNS AND SYMPTOMS

- NPH is associated with a classic triad:
  - Gait disturbance, incontinence and dementia ("wobbly, wet, and wacky")

- The impairment in gait is often the first symptom to manifest, followed by incontinence, and only then by slow cognitive decline
- NPH causes an apraxic gait. This type of gait is characterized by broad-based stance, reduced walking speed, short stride, and difficulty making turns

DIAGNOSIS

- Neuroimaging typically demonstrates ventriculomegaly

TREATMENT

- Treatment is large-volume CSF drainage by lumbar puncture
- Clinical response to this empiric treatment is also thought to be the criterion standard for diagnosis

THE PATIENT WITH THE VP SHUNT

- Cerebrospinal fluid is produced in the ventricles by the choroid plexi and circulates through the ventricular system until it eventually passes through the arachnoid villi into the venous system
- When this circulation of fluid is somehow blocked, the volume and pressure within this system increases
- Ventricular shunts create a pressure-regulated pathway between the ventricles and, most often, the peritoneal cavity
- It is estimated that roughly one half of these shunts will fail in the first 2 years after insertion
- Shunt failures can be secondary to infection or they can be mechanical in nature (i.e., disconnection or fracture of the shunt)

SIGNS AND SYMPTOMS

- Signs of increased ICP (headache, lethargy, nausea/vomiting)
- Irritability, diplopia, papilledema, cranial nerve defects, ataxia, hyperreflexia
- The presentation of an increased intracranial pressure can be very nonspecific in infants
- CSF shunts can also malfunction by withdrawing too much fluid. This is known as "overshunting" and can also present with a headache. A useful historical clue to differentiate the two causes is that this headache should be positional and improved when recumbent

DIAGNOSIS

- An unenhanced CT of the brain is first used to determine if there is an increased ventricular size, implying shunt malfunction
- Plain films (shunt series) are examined for evidence of catheter obstruction, disruption, or migration

TREATMENT

- Surgical repair

Infectious and inflammatory disorders

EPIDURAL ABSCESS

- Infection in the potential epidural space surrounding the brain and spinal cord
- Mass effect created by the resultant fluid collection is harmful to sensitive underlying neurologic structures
- Infecting organisms gain entry to this region either by hematogenous spread through the dense venous plexus surrounding the area, or through extension from osteomyelitis in a contiguous vertebral body
- This condition is relatively rare, but should always be considered in patients with specific risk factors for recurrent bacteremia and/or an impaired immune response
  - Intravenous drug use, diabetes, chronic renal failure, alcoholism

SIGNS AND SYMPTOMS

- Back or neck pain with or without a radicular distribution
- Pain "out of proportion"
- Fever, chills, and/or rigors
- Neurologic deficits
- The classic triad of fever, back pain, and a neurologic deficit is usually *not* present on evaluation in the emergency department

DIAGNOSIS

- WBC count and ESR are often elevated, but nonspecific
- MRI is the diagnostic test of choice (Fig. 12-1)
- CT myelography is able to visualize bony destruction as well as compression of the thecal sac

TREATMENT

- Broad-spectrum intravenous antibiotic coverage
- Prompt surgical decompression is mandatory if the collection is surgically approachable
  - If decompression occurs before paralysis, there is usually a good outcome, but if decompression is delayed more than 12 hours from the time of paralysis, the deficit is usually irreversible
- Some patients may be candidates for CT-guided drain placement by an interventional radiologist

MENINGITIS

- A potentially life-threatening infection of the subarachnoid space and the fluid contained within it
- Caused by bacterial, viral, and fungal causes (Tables 12-1 and 12-2)
- The latter two etiologies are often together referred to as "Aseptic" meningitis
- In case of bacterial meningitis, the inflammatory response generated by the infection and the immune response leads to increased permeability of the blood–brain barrier, cerebral edema,

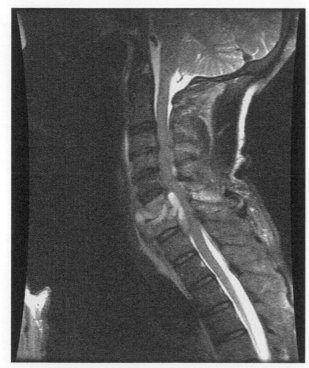

Figure 12-1. T2 weighted MRI image demonstrating an epidural abscess in the cervical region causing spinal cord compression.

TABLE 12-1 Causes of Bacterial Meningitis by Age

Age Group	Typical Organisms
Neonate	Group B strep
	Escherichia coli
	Listeria monocytogenes
Adolescent/adult	*Streptococcus pneumoniae*
	Neisseria meningitidis
Elderly/	*S. pneumoniae*
immunocompromised	*Neisseria meningitides*
	L. monocytogenes

TABLE 12-2 Causes of Aseptic Meningitis

Enteroviruses (comprise 80%)
Echoviruses
Coxsackie viruses
HSV
Mumps
HIV
Cytomegalovirus
Varicella-zoster
Noninfectious causes
Rheumatologic diseases
Drug reactions
Malignancy

decreased cerebral perfusion, and ultimately death if not treated promptly and appropriately

SIGNS AND SYMPTOMS

- Headache, fever, nausea, vomiting, photophobia, seizures, altered mental status, meningismus, neurologic deficits

TABLE 12-3 CSF Profiles in Bacterial and Viral Causes of Meningitis

	WBC Count	% Neutrophils	Protein	Glucose
Bacterial	>1000	>80%	Elevated	Decreased
Viral	<300	<20%	Normal	Normal

TABLE 12-4 Empiric Antibiotic Treatment of Meningitis by Age

Demographic	Empiric Antibiotic
Neonates	Vancomycin, cefotaxime, and ampicillin
Adolescent and adults	Vancomycin and ceftriaxone
Age >50 years or immunosuppressed	Vancomycin, ceftriaxone, and ampicillin

- Classic triad of fever, neck stiffness, and altered mental status present in less than 50% of patients
- However, one of three, most commonly fever, is present in 95% of cases
- Kernig and Brudzinski signs have been shown to have a sensitivity of 5%
- "Jolt accentuation test" has shown more promise in unveiling subtle signs of meningeal irritation
  - The patient rotates his/her head horizontally two to three times per second
    - Positive if it worsens the patient's headache
    - One series has shown this test to have a 97% sensitivity for the diagnosis of meningitis

DIAGNOSIS

- A CT or MRI is obtained to exclude mass effect or shift prior to lumbar puncture if there is any suggestion of increased ICP (neurologic deficit, altered consciousness, or papilledema)
- Lumbar puncture/CSF studies (Table 12-3)
- Treatment should *not* be delayed for diagnostic testing

TREATMENT

- Systemic corticosteroids: dexamethasone 10 mg IV is recommended in suspected acute bacterial meningitis prior to antibiotic administration, as it has been shown to improve outcomes in those cases
- Intravenous antibiotics (Table 12-4)
- Intravenous acyclovir should be added if herpes meningoencephalitis is considered

ENCEPHALITIS

- Defined as invasive infection and inflammation of the brain parenchyma itself
- As opposed to meningitis where the infection is partitioned by the pia mater and is confined to subarachnoid space and the cerebrospinal fluid within it

TABLE 12-5 **Major Causes of Encephalitis in Immunocompetent Hosts**

Herpes simplex virus type 1 (HSV)	Flaviviral infections
St. Louis encephalitis	Japanese encephalitis
West Nile virus	Rickettsial infections
Enteroviruses	HIV
Cytomegalovirus	Epstein–Barr virus
	HHV-6

TABLE 12-6 **Causes of Transverse Myelitis**

Infectious	Inflammatory
Schistosomiasis	Postinfectious (autoimmune)
Lyme disease	Vaccinations
Epstein–Barr virus (EBV)	Paraneoplastic
Cytomegalovirus (CMV)	Rheumatologic disorders
West Nile virus (encephalomyelitis)	

- In reality, the two processes are not always distinct, as parenchymal infection and brain abscesses occur in advanced bacterial meningitis, and concomitant infection of the brain parenchyma and cerebrospinal fluid occurs in some viral infections
- The term *meningoencephalitis* is the more appropriate descriptor when the process encompasses both anatomic regions
- For common causes, see Table 12-5

SIGNS AND SYMPTOMS

- Headache, hallucinations or personality changes, fever, confusion, seizures, vomiting, neurologic deficits, altered level of consciousness (most consistently present)

DIAGNOSIS

- CSF profile similar to viral meningitis
- HSV encephalitis may show increased red blood cells and/or xanthochromia
- PCR amplification of viral DNA shows great sensitivity and specificity, but is not routinely available at most institutions
- An unenhanced CT of the brain may be normal in early meningoencephalitis, but may show hypodense lesions suggestive of inflammation
- An MRI may demonstrate characteristic increased T2 signal in temporal lobes in herpes encephalitis
- The EEG in herpes meningoencephalitis shows a very distinctive pattern that may be useful in distinguishing it when other modalities are inconclusive

TREATMENT

- Supportive care
- Specific antimicrobial therapy such as acyclovir is effective for HSV encephalitis, but not flavivirus infections

MYELITIS

- Myelitis or transverse myelitis are terms used to describe inflammation of the spinal cord
- Refers to a heterogeneous group of causes that all culminate in a common clinical syndrome characterized by back pain and findings suggestive of spinal cord transection (Table 12-6)
- This rare syndrome may coexist with encephalitis when caused by certain viral pathogens. When this

is the case it is more appropriately termed encephalomyelitis

SIGNS AND SYMPTOMS

- Neck or back pain, weakness, sensory disturbances, bilateral motor and sensory deficits localized to a spinal level, autonomic dysfunction

DIAGNOSIS

- MRI: demonstrates characteristic inflammation in the involved regions of the cord
- CSF analysis: cellular pleocytosis, elevated protein level

TREATMENT

- Treat specific infections if possible (e.g., Lyme)
- Immune globulin
- Corticosteroids

Movement disorders

DYSTONIA

- Movement disorder characterized by sustained and directional muscle contractions
- Dystonias may be primary, but the type of dystonia seen in the emergency department is most often secondary, more specifically in reaction to a medication the patient has taken
- The mechanism of a dystonic reaction is thought to be blockage of the dopaminergic pathways in the nigrostriatum
- Although there is a clear association of these types of reactions with anti-dopaminergic agents, many drugs have been implicated as causing them

SIGNS AND SYMPTOMS

- Patients present with sustained, directional muscle contraction in a specific region of the body
- Most commonly in the cervical region
- Common presentations:
  - Torticollis, lateralcollis, blepharospasm, oromandibular dysphonia, oculogyric crisis, opisthotonos

DIAGNOSIS

- Clinical
- The patient may relate the reaction temporally to ingestion of an offending drug

TREATMENT

- Anticholinergic drugs, through their effect on acetylcholine pathways in the nigrostriatum, are effective in providing relief
- Diphenhydramine or benztropine are typically used

Neuromuscular disorders

GUILLAIN–BARRÉ SYNDROME (GBS)

- An acute, progressive, demyelinating polyneuropathy
- Thought to be an autoimmune response that manifests as lymphocyte- and macrophage-mediated demyelination of peripheral nerves
- An increased rate of seropositivity to *Campylobacter jejuni* suggests an antecedent infection, with that organism playing a role in provoking this immune response
- GBS is slightly more common in males, and tends to present bimodally in young adults and the elderly

SIGNS AND SYMPTOMS

- Classically, presents as ascending weakness progressing to paralysis over a period of days to weeks
- The Miller–Fischer variant, presents with descending paralysis
- Nonspecific paresthesias, decreased lower extremity DTRs
- Nausea and vomiting is sometimes present from an ileus
- Autonomic dysfunction manifesting as abnormal vital signs

DIAGNOSIS

- Lumbar puncture and CSF analysis may reveal an elevated protein (90% sensitive) with an occasional cellular pleocytosis
- MRI: should demonstrate nerve root enhancement
- Forced vital capacity (FVC) should be measured to gauge the degree of respiratory muscle involvement. Any patient with an FVC of less than 20 mL/kg should be admitted to the ICU, while any patient with an FVC of less than 15 mL/kg should be endotracheally intubated and mechanically ventilated
- Nerve conduction studies can be diagnostic, but are not practical in the ED

TREATMENT

- Intravenous immunoglobulin (IVIG)
- Steroids have been shown to hasten recovery when used with IVIG
- Plasma exchange has been shown as effective as IVIG, but is not synergistic
- Supportive care, particularly airway management

MYASTHENIA GRAVIS (MG)

- An autoimmune disease where antibodies to the nicotinic acetylcholine receptors at the neuromuscular junction are produced, causing weakness
- This predominately affects the facial muscles and causes a weakness that is exacerbated by repeated use and improved by rest
- Slightly more common in women, and is associated with thymic hyperplasia, which may be seen incidentally on a chest x-ray
- Myasthenic crisis: Acute worsening of weakness. Respiratory distress is the feared complication

SIGNS AND SYMPTOMS

- Weakness, primarily of the bulbar muscles (ptosis, ophthalmoplegia)
- Less commonly proximal muscle and limb weakness
- Typically worsens with use and improves with rest

DIAGNOSIS

- The edrophonium (Tensilon) test
  - Edrophonium is a cholinesterase inhibitor with a very short half-life. Administration of this agent should prompt a rapid but transient improvement in muscle strength in those with a myasthenic crisis. There may also be associated symptoms typical of cholinergic stimulation (salivation, lacrimation, bronchospasm, etc.)
- The ice pack test
  - This test takes advantage of the fact that cooling improves neuromuscular function in MG. Cooling the eyelid with an icepack for several minutes should lead to a noticeable improvement in the patient's ptosis if the patient is in a myasthenic crisis
- A CXR may demonstrate thymic hyperplasia

TREATMENT

- Address any respiratory insufficiency with ventilatory support. There is data suggesting that noninvasive positive pressure ventilation can reduce the rate of endotracheal intubations in patients with weakness of the respiratory muscles.
- Pyridostigmine is a cholinesterase inhibitor that can be helpful in treating the weakness resulting from a myasthenic crisis

PERIPHERAL NEUROPATHIES

- A heterogeneous group of disorders with many potential causes
- They can be broadly categorized into seven classes depending on whether they are proximal, distal, symmetric, asymmetric, motor, or sensory (Table 12-7)

SIGNS AND SYMPTOMS

- The neuropathy can be classified according to the location of the deficit:

TABLE 12-7 **Classification of Peripheral Neuropathies**

Type 1: Proximal and distal, symmetric, sensorimotor	Guillain–Barré syndrome	HIV	Hepatitis B	Malignancy
Type 2: Distal, symmetric, sensorimotor	Diabetes	Charcot–Marie–Tooth	Nutritional deficiencies	Paraproteinemias	Toxic causes
Type 3: Proximal and distal, asymmetric, sensorimotor (e.g., plexopathy)	Penetrating trauma	Sports-related (e.g. "stingers")	Neoplasm	Radiation
Type 4: Distal, asymmetric, sensorimotor, mononeuropathy	Anatomic factors	Acromegaly	Hypothyroidism	
Type 5: Distal, asymmetric, sensorimotor, mononeuropathy multiplex	Diabetes	Vasculitis	Sarcoid	Lyme	HIV
Type 6: Distal, asymmetric, motor	Motor neuron diseases (e.g., amyotrophic lateral sclerosis)			
Type 7: Distal, asymmetric, sensory (sensory ganglionopathy)	Herpes simplex I, II	Varicella zoster	Pyridoxine overdose	Cisplatin	Methyl mercury

- Proximal, distal, or both
- Motor, sensory, or both
- Symmetric or asymmetric
- This allows the patient's condition to be classified into one of the seven types of neuropathies above

DIAGNOSIS

- The diagnostic approach depends on the type of neuropathy the patient is suspected of having
- For example, a patient who sustained trauma to the proximal fibula and subsequently developed peroneal nerve palsy may need only a plain film to exclude a fracture. At the other end of the spectrum, a patient who presents with multiple distal mononeuropathies may need a workup for systemic vasculitis

TREATMENT

- Treatment is dependent on the underlying diagnosis

Other conditions of the brain

DEMENTIA

- The gradual loss of cognitive function (Table 12-8)
- There are multiple causes of dementia (Table 12-9)
- Diagnosis not frequently made in the ED
- The emergency physician must be able to distinguish acute delirium superimposed on chronic dementia, as this may represent a medical emergency
- Delirium is defined as an alteration of consciousness and cognition that begins abruptly and fluctuates in severity
- The diagnosis of dementia also influences emergency department care by affecting the

patient's ability to follow instructions after discharge

TABLE 12-8 **American Psychiatric Association Diagnostic Criteria for Dementia**

APA Criteria for Dementia
Memory impairment
Impairment in one or more of the following: aphasia, apraxia, agnosia, executive functioning
These deficits cause impairment in functioning
These deficits do not occur in the setting of delirium

TABLE 12-9 **Major Causes of Dementia**

	Cortical	Subcortical
Primary	Alzheimer Pick disease	Huntington Parkinson
Secondary		Multi-infarct Drug/toxin induced Hydrocephalus

SIGNS AND SYMPTOMS

- Memory impairment
- Difficulty remembering words, faces, objects
- Gait disturbances
- Subcortical dementias can often lead to a disheveled appearance

DIAGNOSIS

- The focus should be on identifying treatable issues

TREATMENT

- Generally speaking, treatment of dementia is not an endeavor undertaken in the emergency department

PARKINSON DISEASE (PD)

- A progressive neurodegenerative condition that is more prevalent in elderly persons
- Results from the premature demise of a cluster of neurons within the substantia nigra pars compacta of the midbrain
- Projections from these neurons comprise the striatum and use dopamine as their primary neurotransmitter
- The striatal dysfunction that results from the lack of input from these neurons influences other parts of the brain, giving rise to the constellation of findings that comprises the clinical syndrome of Parkinson disease

SIGNS AND SYMPTOMS

- Resting tremor
- Increased motor tone
- "Lead pipe" or "cogwheel" rigidity
- Impaired postural stability, difficulty initiating gait
- Difficulty with handwriting
  - Handwriting that starts with large letters and progresses to very small ones is characteristic of Parkinson disease
- Nonmotor symptoms like depression, anxiety, and insomnia

DIAGNOSIS

- Emergent neuroimaging would be necessary only to exclude other conditions being considered in the differential diagnosis

TREATMENT

- Treatment is aimed at increasing dopaminergic activity in the central nervous system (CNS) nonselectively
- The most effective and commonly used medication is a combination of levodopa and carbidopa. Carbidopa serves to inhibit the peripheral metabolism of levodopa, allowing it to enter the CNS
- Anticholinergic agents are useful because cholinergic neurons antagonize the function of dopaminergic neurons in the striatum
- Monoamine oxidase type-B (MAO-B) is an enzyme that metabolizes dopamine in the CNS. Inhibition of this enzyme allows for greater presynaptic levels of dopamine

IDIOPATHIC INTRACRANIAL HYPERTENSION (IIH)

- Also referred to as *pseudotumor cerebri*
- A poorly understood condition most common in young women characterized by an elevated intracranial pressure (ICP) without ventriculomegaly and without an apparent cause
- The pathophysiologic consequence to this increased ICP is optic nerve ischemia

- IIH has been associated with obesity, steroids, oral contraceptives, and tetracycline use, but a precise etiology has yet to be pinpointed
- This condition should be included in the differential of young women presenting to the emergency department with subacute to chronic headache syndromes, as it could eventually lead to permanent visual loss if left untreated

SIGNS AND SYMPTOMS

- Daily, throbbing headache that is often retro-ocular in location
- Visual complaints such as diplopia, obscurations, or transient visual loss
- Papilledema
- Cognitive disturbances
- Arthralgias

DIAGNOSIS

- Papilledema is a diagnostic requirement, but it may be unilateral
  - An elevated ICP without papilledema has been described in patients with *cerebral venous sinus thrombosis*. This finding should prompt the consideration of a sinus thrombosis as a diagnostic possibility
- A CT or MRI should be performed to exclude a mass or vascular lesion
- There should be NOT be any ventriculomegaly
  - The ventricles have been described as "slit-like"
- Lumbar puncture: in the lateral recumbent position, not sitting up
  - An opening pressure should be measured and be greater than 25 cm of water

TREATMENT

- Acetazolamide and loop diuretics can decrease CSF production
- CSF shunts
- Optic nerve sheath fenestration

Seizure disorders

NEONATAL SEIZURES

- The developing neonatal brain is more susceptible to seizure activity than the adult brain, due to a developmental imbalance of excitatory and inhibitory neurons
- This is thought to be a major reason why the highest incidence of seizure activity is within the first year of life
- Recognition of seizures and prompt treatment is essential
- Similar to the adult brain, prolonged neuronal firing can lead to excitotoxicity and permanent neuronal loss
- The neonatal brain also has a relative impairment of vascular autoregulation and, in the setting of seizure activity, the induced increase in blood flow

TABLE 12-10 **Causes of Seizures in Neonates**

Hypoxia
Intraventricular/intraparenchymal hemorrhage
Sepsis
Meningitis
Metabolic disorders
Hypoglycemia
Hypocalcemia
Hypomagnesemia
Hyper/hyponatremia

TABLE 12-11 **Medical Therapy for Status Epilepticus**

Benzodiazepines (e.g., lorazepam)
Phenytoin
Phenobarbital
Propofol
General anesthesia

can cause hemorrhage into vulnerable portions of the brain

- Recognition of seizures in neonates can be difficult because the relatively obvious generalized tonic–clonic variety is rare. Subtle manifestations are much more common
- When a neonate presents to the emergency department with seizures, there is often a serious underlying cause that needs to be addressed (Table 12-10)
- Hypoxia is the most common culprit, but electrolyte disturbances and infectious causes are also frequently noted
- An underlying metabolic cause for the seizures should always be considered

SIGNS AND SYMPTOMS

- Repetitive movements
- Eye movements (most common)
- Facial movement
- Bicycling movements
- Apnea

DIAGNOSIS

- Seizures in neonates do not always produce characteristic electroencephalographic abnormalities; the diagnosis is made by recognizing the movement patterns as seizure-like

TREATMENT

- Correct any hypoglycemia with IV dextrose
- Benzodiazepines
- Fosphenytoin is preferred over phenytoin in infants
- Phenobarbital

STATUS EPILEPTICUS

- Defined as continuous or serial seizure activity for 30 minutes or more without an interictal recovery
- Patients may present with continuous convulsive activity or with multiple, discreet convulsive episodes where there is no return to a normal level of consciousness in between
- More rarely, patients may present comatose without any overt convulsive activity at all (nonconvulsive status epilepticus)
- Status epilepticus is a neurological emergency, and treatment should be prompt and aggressive

- Neuronal damage and loss increases with seizure duration
- The longer a seizure continues, the more refractory to pharmacotherapy it becomes

SIGNS AND SYMPTOMS

- Partial seizures
  - Simple partial
  - Motor
  - Somatosensory
  - Autonomic
- Complex partial
  - Consciousness is impaired, not lost
  - Automatisms
  - Hallucinations
- Generalized
  - Convulsive
  - Nonconvulsive

DIAGNOSIS

- The generalized convulsive seizure is common and easily recognized in the emergency department
- An EEG can be obtained to confirm seizure activity if suspected

TREATMENT

- Airway protection
- Support hemodynamics
- Medical therapy (Table 12-11)

Spinal cord compression

- A frequent complication of advanced malignancy
- Pathophysiologically, the problem usually begins when metastases in the vertebral bodies extend into the epidural space, compressing the thecal sac
- Although much less common, there can also be direct metastasis to the epidural space
- Most likely to occur at the thoracic level, followed by the lumbar and cervical regions
- The most common culprits are breast, lung, and prostate cancers
- The tumor's encroachment, while gradual, eventually reaches a critical point where venous compression and vasogenic edema ensue
- This results in clinically apparent signs and symptoms

- Subsequently there is ischemic and hypoxic injury that causes permanent neurologic damage

SIGNS AND SYMPTOMS

- Back pain
- Weakness
- Bowel and bladder dysfunction

DIAGNOSIS

- MRI with contrast (tumors show enhancement with gadolinium)
- CT myelogram: not ideal, but acceptable when MRI is contraindicated
- Plain films alone can be negative in up to 20% of cases

TREATMENT

- Decompressive laminectomy and debulking
- Dexamethasone is used for ameliorating the associated vasogenic edema
- Local radiation therapy is sometimes helpful depending on the radiosensitivity of the underlying malignancy
- Prognosis is most dependent on neurologic function at the time treatment is initiated

Stroke

- Stroke is a syndrome with multiple etiologies where the commonality is neuronal destruction within the brain
- Most commonly, stroke is a result of atherothrombosis in the cerebral vasculature, which causes local ischemia and cell death
- It can also be a consequence of thromboembolism, hemorrhage, or venous thrombosis

ISCHEMIC STROKE

- Typically caused by one of two mechanisms
  - Atherothrombosis within the vessel
  - Embolism from another location, usually the heart

SIGNS AND SYMPTOMS

- A neurologic deficit localizable to a specific region of the CNS
- There usually is not pain unless pain is part of the stroke syndrome itself (e.g., thalamic infarction)

DIAGNOSIS

- An unenhanced CT of the brain may not show any changes in the first few hours after the event, but later may show poor differentiation of gray and white matter in the region of the brain affected
- Subtle signs may occasionally be seen on the initial unenhanced CT (Fig. 12-2)
- Although not yet the standard of care, perfusion CT may aid in distinguishing ischemic areas from infarcted ones

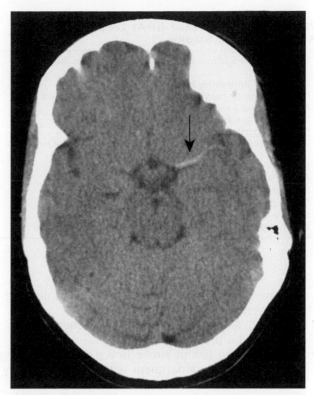

Figure 12-2. The hyperacute MCA sign. In patients with acute ischemic strokes there is sometimes dense material visible on an unenhanced CT in the proximal MCA. This is thought to be thrombus. The CT image above belonged to a patient who presented with right-sided weakness and aphasia. Note the density of the left MCA compared with the contralateral side. Subsequent perfusion CT and MRI confirmed an infarct in the left MCA distribution.

TREATMENT

- The primary treatment for ischemic stroke is supportive
- Intravenous recombinant tissue plasminogen activator (tPA), a fibrinolytic agent that dissolves thrombus nonspecifically throughout the body
- tPA treatment is advocated by the American Heart Association only when the duration of symptoms is 4.5 hours or less
- There is a significant probability of hemorrhage associated with the use of intravenous tPA for stroke, so it is important to thoroughly screen the patient for contraindication prior to administering the drug (Table 12-12)
- Many institutions have protocols for use of the drug and a checklist of contraindications

TRANSIENT ISCHEMIC ATTACK (TIA)

- Defined as a brief episode of neurologic dysfunction caused by brain or retinal ischemia without evidence of infarction
- These symptoms are usually brief, lasting less than 1 hour
- Although a TIA itself by definition causes no long-term impairment, studies have shown an

TABLE 12-12 **List of Contraindications to Tissue Plasminogen Activator (tPA) Treatment for Acute Ischemic Stroke**

Symptoms >4.5 hours in duration or unknown time of onset
A minor or improving neurologic deficit
Head trauma or previous stroke in the last 3 months
MI in the last 3 months
GI bleed in the last 3 weeks
Major surgery in the last 2 weeks
Arterial puncture at a non-compressible site in the previous 7 days
Evidence of active bleeding
INR of >1.7
Platelets <100,000/mm³
Blood glucose <50 mg/dL
History of seizure at onset
Any hypodensity visible on CT >1/3 of the hemisphere

increased rate of stroke in the short term following these events
- 15% to 20% of patients with acute ischemic strokes had a preceding TIA
- The short-term risk of stroke in a patient presenting to the emergency department with a TIA is roughly 5%
- There are several factors that raise a patient's risk for a subsequent stroke
  - Age >60 years
  - Diabetes
  - Symptoms >10 minutes in duration
  - Symptoms include weakness or impairment of speech

SIGNS AND SYMPTOMS

- Transient neurologic deficit or stroke syndrome lasting less than 1 hour
- No new neurologic deficits on examination

DIAGNOSIS

- Diagnosis is usually based on the history
- Neuroimaging should not demonstrate any evidence of infarction

TREATMENT

- Treatment revolves around identifying any areas of cerebral infarction and reducing the risk of subsequent stroke
- Duplex ultrasound, MR angiography, or CT angiography for evaluation of carotid stenosis
- Echocardiogram for identification of cardiogenic source of emboli
- Initiation of antiplatelet therapy (ASA is first-line, clopidogrel is acceptable)

SPONTANEOUS INTRACEREBRAL HEMORRHAGE

- A type of stroke caused by hemorrhage from small cerebral arteries
- Often secondary to hypertension

- Mass effect from the resultant hematoma tends to increase intracranial pressure more than in ischemic strokes
  - Makes patients with this condition more likely to have headaches, vomiting, and a depressed level of consciousness

SIGNS AND SYMPTOMS

- Neurologic deficit
- Headache
- Depressed level of consciousness
- Occasional seizures

DIAGNOSIS

- An unenhanced CT of the brain has excellent diagnostic sensitivity for hemorrhage

TREATMENT

- Treatment options are generally limited to mitigating the neuronal damage by optimizing cerebral perfusion pressure and managing the airway
- Blood pressure should be controlled to maintain a systolic of less than 180 mmHg and a mean arterial pressure of less than 130 mmHg
- Any seizure activity should be treated aggressively with the usual agents

SUBARACHNOID HEMORRHAGE (SAH)

- Most often caused by rupture of an aneurysm into the subarachnoid space
- Can also be caused by bleeding from an arteriovenous malformation 20% of the time
- The subarachnoid space is usually filled with only CSF, and hemorrhage into it acutely causes an increase in intracranial pressure, which can manifest as a sudden headache
- Important subacute complications from this bleeding is vasospasm, which may cause ischemic stroke, and hydrocephalus caused by obstruction of the normal passage of CSF into the venous system through the arachnoid villi

SIGNS AND SYMPTOMS

- Severe headache, classically sudden in onset
- Seizure or syncope at onset of the headache
- Meningismus
- Vomiting
- Altered level of consciousness

DIAGNOSIS

- An unenhanced CT of the head is very sensitive initially (97%), but that sensitivity decreases as a function of time (Fig. 12-3)
- If an unenhanced CT of the head is negative and SAH is suspected, a lumbar puncture should be performed
- CT angiography, at this point in time, has not replaced lumbar puncture but can be useful when

Subarachnoid basal cisterns
containing blood

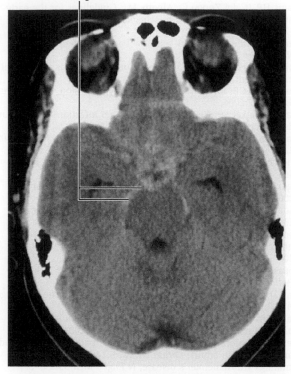

Figure 12-3. Subarachnoid hemorrhage. Axial CT scan of brain. (From Drake R, Vogl W, Mitchell AWM: *Gray's anatomy for students,* ed 2. Philadelphia, 2009, Churchill Livingstone.)

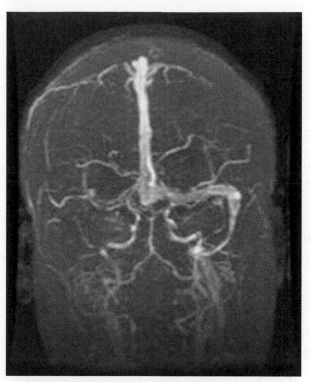

Figure 12-4. Magnetic resonance venogram demonstrating thrombosis of the sigmoid and transverse sinus

lumbar puncture is contraindicated or when the results are indeterminate
- CSF analysis may show RBCs in the thousands and xanthochromia, which is a product of the breakdown of hemoglobin in the CSF
- Xanthochromia is very specific, but takes up to 12 hours to form once there is blood within the CSF

TREATMENT

- Treatment in the emergency department is supportive
- Leaking aneurysms are sometimes amenable to surgical clipping or coiling by the interventional radiologist
- Nimodipine, a calcium-channel blocker with selectively for cerebral vessels, lessens the rate of vasospastic stroke, a complication that usually occurs 2 to 4 days later

DURAL SINUS THROMBOSIS

- A thrombotic obstruction of the venous sinuses that form the venous outflow tract from the cerebral circulation
- This process causes venous engorgement, cytotoxic as well as vasogenic edema, petechial hemorrhage, and infarction
- Dural sinus thrombosis occurs in women twice as often as in men, usually strikes younger patients, the vast majority of whom have an identifiable risk

factor such as oral contraceptive use, being in the peripartum period, or head trauma

SIGNS AND SYMPTOMS
- Neurologic deficits
- Headache
- Seizures

DIAGNOSIS
- An unenhanced CT of the head may show venous infarcts or petechial hemorrhage, but also may be normal
- An MRV is the test of choice and will reliably demonstrate the thrombus (Fig. 12-4)

TREATMENT
- Anticoagulation with unfractionated heparin

Tumors

- There are many different types of intracranial tumors
- Some are primary, while others secondarily metastasize from systemic sites
- Metastatic lesions are much more common
- The heterogeneity of causes leads to a varied clinical course and prognosis
- Although most tumors grow slowly, they can exert effects that lead to sudden changes in symptomatology

- For example, acute hemorrhage may occur into a slow-growing and asymptomatic glioma and cause a very sudden onset of headache and associated neurologic symptoms
- These are the types of events that lead to the patient presenting to the emergency department

SIGNS AND SYMPTOMS

- Headache
- Seizures
- Confusion or an altered level of consciousness
- Neurologic deficits
- Papilledema

DIAGNOSIS

- An unenhanced CT of the brain can reliably detect mass effect and shift
- MRI is more sensitive than CT and superior for detecting vasogenic edema

TREATMENT

- Consultation with a neurosurgeon is indicated to determine surgical options
- Mannitol: transient effect, but useful for acute decompensation
- Steroids: dexamethasone frequently used to help ameliorate vasogenic edema

PEARLS

- Peripheral facial nerve deficits should always involve the forehead as well as the face. If the forehead is spared, the deficit should be presumed to be central.

- Always consider Lyme disease as a potential etiology of peripheral facial nerve palsy.

- Normal pressure hydrocephalus presents with gait disturbance, incontinence, and dementia ("wobbly, wet, and wacky").

- Consider the use of steroids prior to antibiotics in patients with bacterial meningitis.

- In patients with epidural abscess, the classic triad of fever, back pain, and a neurologic deficit is usually NOT present on evaluation in the emergency department.

- In patients with suspected SAH, LP is necessary after CT to rule out the disease.

- Magnetic resonance venogram (MRV) is the test of choice for dural sinus thrombosis.

- An unenhanced CT does not definitively exclude a brain tumor when evaluating headache in the emergency department. It does, however, exclude complications from that tumor that need to be addressed emergently.

BIBLIOGRAPHY

Adams HP Jr, del Zoppo G, Alberts MJ: Guidelines for the early management of adults with ischemic stroke, *Stroke* 38:1655–1711, 2007.

Ahmed M, Modic MT: Neck and low back pain: neuroimaging, *Neurol Clin* 25:439–471, 2007.

Albin RL: Parkinson's disease: background, diagnosis, and initial management, *Clin Geriatr Med* 22:735–751, 2006.

Alex K, Ball CE: Idiopathic intracranial hypertension, *Lancet Neurol* 5:433–442:2006.

Allan R, Tunkel SP: Central nervous system infections in injection drug users, *Infect Dis Clin North Am* 16:589–605, 2000.

Allan Purdy R, Kirby S: Headaches and brain tumors, *Neurol Clin* 22:39–53, 2004.

Benecke JE: Facial paralysis, *Otolaryngol Clin North Am* 35:357–365, 2002.

Bogduk N: The neck and headaches, *Neurol Clin* 22:151–171, 2004.

Broder J, Snarski JT: Back pain in the elderly, *Clin Geriatr Med* 23:271–289, 2007.

Broderick JA: Guidelines for the management of spontaneous intracerebral hemorrhage in adults, *Stroke* 38:2001–2033, 2007.

Brousseau T: Newborn emergencies: the first 30 days of life, *Pediatr Clin North Am* 53:69–84, 2006.

Chao D, Nanda A: Spinal epidural abscess: a diagnostic challenge, *Am Fam Physician* 65(7):1341–1346, 2002.

Chaudhuri A: Adjunctive dexamethasone treatment in acute bacterial meningitis, *Lancet Neurol* 3:54–62, 2004.

Chen JW, Wasterlain CG: Status epilepticus: pathophysiology and management in adults, *Lancet Neurol* 5:246–256, 2006.

Cummings JL: Alzheimer's disease, *N Engl J Med* 351:56–67, 2004.

Dalmau J, Rosenfeld MR: Paraneoplastic syndromes of the CNS, *Lancet Neurol* 7:327–340, 2008.

Daniel J, Bonthius BK: Meningitis and encephalitis in children—an update, *Neurol Clin North Am* 20:1013–1038, 2002.

Darouiche RO: Spinal epidural abscess, *N Engl J Med* 355:2012–2020, 2006.

de Seze J, Lanctin C, Lebrun C et al: Idiopathic acute transverse myelitis: application of new diagnostic criteria, *Neurology* 65:1950–1953, 2005.

Diederik van de Beek JD: Community-acquired bacterial meningitis in adults, *N Engl J Med* 354:44–53, 2006.

Emre M: Dementia associated with Parkinson's disease, *Lancet Neurol* 2:229–237, 2003.

Factora R, Luciano M: Normal pressure hydrocephalus: diagnosis and new approaches to treatment, *Clin Geriatr Med* 22:245–267, 2006.

Fitch MT, van de Beek D: Emergency diagnosis and treatment of adult meningitis, *Lancet Infect Dis* 7:191–200, 2007.

Friedman DI: Pseudotumor cerebri, *Neurol Clin North Am* 22:99–131, 2004.

Frohman EM, Racke MK, Raine CS: Multiple sclerosis—the plaque and its pathogenesis, *N Engl J Med* 354:942–955, 2006.

Fumal A, Schoenen J: Tension-type headache: current research and clinical management, *Lancet Neurol* 7:70–83, 2008.

Giles MF, Rothwell PM: Risk of early stroke after transient ischaemic attack: a systematic review and meta-analysis, *Lancet Neurol* 6:1063–1072, 2007.

Gladstein J: Headache, *Med Clin North Am* 90:275–290, 2006.

Goetz C: *Goetz: textbook of clinical neurology*, ed 3, Philadelphia, 2007, Elsevier.

Goudreau JL: Medical management of advanced Parkinson's disease, *Clin Geriatr Med* 22:753–772, 2006.

Graff-Radford NR: Normal pressure hydrocephalus, *Neurol Clin* 25:809–832, 2007.

Greenberg BM, Thomas KP, Krishnan C et al: Idiopathic transverse myelitis: corticosteroids, plasma exchange, or cyclophosphamide, *Neurology* 68:1614–1617, 2007.

Hawker K, Frohman E: Multiple sclerosis, *Prim Care: Clin Office Pract* 31:201–226, 2004.

Heather S, Hammerstedt JA: Emergency department presentations of transverse myelitis: two case reports, *Ann Emerg Med* 46:256–259, 2005.

Howard L, Geyer SB: The diagnosis of dystonia, *Lancet Neurol* 5:780–790, 2006.

Irani DN: Aseptic meningitis and viral myelitis, *Neurol Clin* 26:635–655, 2008.

Jankovic J: Treatment of dystonia, *Lancet Neurol* 5:864–872, 2006.

Jeha LE, Sila CA, Lederman RJ et al: West Nile virus infection, a new paralytic illness, *Neurology* 61:55–59, 2003.

Joseph S: Guillain-Barré syndrome, *Adolesc Med* 13(3):487–494, 2002.

Kantarci OH, Weinshenker BG: Natural history of multiple sclerosis, *Neurol Clin* 23:17–38, 2005.

Kaushal H, Shah JA: Transient ischemic attack: review for the emergency physician, *Ann Emerg Med* 43:592–604, 2004.

Kirsten K, Calder FA: Surgical emergencies in the intravenous drug user, *Emerg Med Clin North Am* 21:1089–1116, 2003.

Krafft RM: Trigeminal neuralgia, *Am Fam Physician* 77:1291–1296, 2008.

Kulchycki LK, Edlow JA: Geriatric neurologic emergencies, *Emerg Med Clin North Am* 24:273–298, 2006.

LaMonte MP: Evaluation and management of transient ischemic attacks, *Clin Geriatr Med* 23:401–412, 2007.

Lewis R: Chronic inflammatory demyelinating polyneuropathy, *Neurol Clin* 25(1):71–87, 2007.

Leys D, Hénon H, Mackowiak-Cordoliani M-A, Pasquier F: Post-stroke dementia, *Lancet Neurol* 4:752–759, 2005.

Lonneke ML de Lau, Breteler MMB: Epidemiology of Parkinson's disease, *Lancet Neurol* 5:525–535, 2006.

Lublin FD: Clinical features and diagnosis of multiple sclerosis, *Neurol Clin* 23:1–15, 2005.

Mace SE: Acute bacterial meningitis, *Emerg Med Clin North Am* 38:281–317, 2008.

Marx JA, Hockberger RS, Walls, RM: *Rosen's Emergency Medicine*, ed 6, Philadelphia, 2006, Mosby.

Massey J: Acquired myasthenia gravis, *Neurol Clin* 15(3):577–595, 1997.

Meierkord H, Holtkamp M: Non-convulsive status epilepticus in adults: clinical forms and treatment, *Lancet Neurol* 6:329–339, 2007.

Michael E, Shy JY: Hereditary motor and sensory neuropathies: a biological perspective, *Lancet Neurol* 1:110–118, 2002.

Michael E, Winters PK: Back pain emergencies, *Med Clin North Am* 90:505–523, 2006.

Mirski MA, Varelas PN: Seizures and status epilepticus in the critically ill, *Crit Care Clin* 24:115–147, 2008.

Newswanger D: Guillain-Barré syndrome, *Am Fam Physician* 69(10):2405–2410, 2004.

Noseworthy JH, Lucchinetti C, Rodriguez M, Weinshenker BG: Multiple sclerosis, *N Engl J Med* 343(13):938–952, 2000.

Nutt JG, Wooten GF: Diagnosis and initial management of Parkinson's disease, *N Engl J Med* 353:1021–1027, 2005.

Peter M, Rothwell AB: Recent advances in management of transient ischemic attacks and minor ischemic strokes, *Lancet Neurol* 5:323–331, 2006.

Prasad D, Schiff, D: Malignant spinal-cord compression, *Lancet Oncol* 6:16–24, 2005.

Rao SS, Hoffman LA, Shakil A: Parkinson's disease: diagnosis and treatment, *Am Fam Physician* 74:2046–2054, 2006.

Roos KL: Encephalitis, *Neurol Clin* 17(4):813–834, 1999.

Rothrock JF: Headaches due to vascular disorders, *Neurol Clin* 22:21–37, 2004.

Rothrock JF: Headaches due to vascular disorders, *Neurol Clin North Am* 22:21–37, 2004.

Rozen TD: Trigeminal neuralgia and glossopharyngeal neuralgia, *Neurol Clin North Am* 22:185–206, 2004.

Ryan RE, Pearlman SH: Common headache misdiagnoses, *Prim Care: Clin Office Pract* 31:395–405, 2004.

Said G: Infectious neuropathies, *Neurol Clin* 25:115–137, 2007.

Samuel R, Browd ON: Failure of cerebrospinal fluid shunts: part II: overdrainage, loculation, and abdominal complications, *Pediatr Neurol* 34:171–176, 2006.

Samuel R, Browd ON: Failure of cerebrospinal fluid shunts: part I: obstruction and mechanical failure, *Pediatr Neurol* 25:809–832, 2007.

Scher MS: Neonatal seizures and brain damage, *Pediatr Neurol* 29:381–390, 2003.

Schievink WI: Spontaneous dissection of the carotid and vertebral arteries, *N Engl J Med* 344(12):898–906, 2001.

Schiff D: Spinal cord compression, *Neurol Clin North Am* 21:67–86, 2003.

Solomon T: Flavivirus encephalitis, *N Engl J Med* 351:370–378, 2004.

Syed A, Rizvi MA: Current approved options for treating patients with multiple sclerosis, *Neurology* 63:S8–S14, 2004.

Taylor FR: Diagnosis and classification of headache, *Prim Care: Clin Office Pract* 31:243–259, 2004.

Ted M, Burns GA: Vasculitic neuropathies, *Neurol Clin* 25:89–113, 2007.

Tiemstra JD, Khatkhate N: Bell's palsy: diagnosis and management, *Am Fam Physician* 76:997–1002, 2007.

Tolosa E, Wenning G, Poewe W: The diagnosis of Parkinson's disease, *Lancet Neurol* 5:75–86, 2006.

Wilber ST: Altered mental status in older emergency department patients, *Emerg Med Clin North Am* 24:299–316, 2006.

Wilson RK, Williams MA: Normal pressure hydrocephalus, *Clin Geriatr Med* 22:935–951, 2006.

Younger DS: Headaches and vasculitis, *Neurol Clin North Am* 22:207–228, 2004.

Zupanc ML: Neonatal seizures, *Pediatr Clin North Am* 51:961–978, 2004.

Questions and Answers

1. Which of the following is TRUE regarding acute bacterial meningitis?
   a. Kernig and Brudzinski signs are highly sensitive for the diagnosis
   b. the classic triad of fever, neck stiffness, and altered consciousness is present in 90% of cases
   c. CT should always be performed prior to lumbar puncture
   d. antibiotics should be withheld pending the results of LP analysis
   e. systemic corticosteroids administered prior to antibiotics has been shown to improve outcomes

2. What sign/symptom most strongly argues *against* the diagnosis of Bell palsy?
   a. an occipital headache
   b. arthralgias
   c. a corneal ulceration ipsilateral to the affected side of the face
   d. hyperacusis
   e. sparing of the forehead musculature

3. A 32-year-old man is brought to your emergency department after a motor vehicle accident. He was a restrained driver and did not lose consciousness. He now complains of posterior right neck and facial pain. Which of the

following findings would support the diagnosis of a vertebral artery dissection as the cause of this patient's pain?

a. ipsilateral ptosis
b. left-sided weakness
c. confusion
d. ataxia

4. A 40-year-old woman with a history of migraine headaches presents to your emergency department with a sudden-onset, unilateral, throbbing headache without an aura. She describes nausea, vomiting, and photophobia. Her level of consciousness and neurologic exam is normal. What symptom is most concerning to you?

a. vomiting
b. photophobia
c. the lack of an aura
d. the sudden onset

5. Which of the following statements is *false?*

a. tortuous vasculature compressing sensory nerves is thought to be the pathologic basis of trigeminal neuralgia
b. a typical presentation of trigeminal neuralgia in a young healthy person needs no further workup
c. any abnormal neurologic findings cast doubt on the diagnosis of trigeminal neuralgia
d. the pain of trigeminal neuralgia is often severe and sharp in quality
e. trigeminal neuralgia does not usually wake the patient from sleep

6. An 18-year-old woman with a history of hydrocephalus and ventriculoperitoneal shunt placement several years ago presents to your emergency department with a headache. It is positional, improving when she is recumbent. She is afebrile and is without any neurologic deficits. You order an unenhanced CT of the brain to exclude the possibility of a shunt malfunction and it demonstrated what the radiologist described as "slit-like" ventricles. What is the most likely diagnosis?

a. overshunting of cerebrospinal fluid
b. shunt obstruction
c. idiopathic intracranial hypertension
d. shunt-associated meningitis with resultant cerebral edema
e. fracture of the shunt

7. What physical exam finding is a common early manifestation of multiple sclerosis?

a. hemiplegia
b. ataxia
c. sensory deficits
d. cognitive deficits
e. an afferent pupillary defect

8. A 23-year-old woman presents to your emergency department with diplopia. On exam, you note that her right eye fails to deviate medially when she looks left, with concomitant nystagmus in the left eye. Anatomically, where is the lesion?

a. the 3rd nerve nucleus
b. the occipital cortex
c. the medial longitudinal fasciculus
d. the cerebellum

9. Which of the following statements is *false?*

a. blepharospasm is involuntary closing of the eyes
b. all dystonic reactions involve outwardly visible, directional movements
c. oromandibular dystonia is characterized by lip and tongue movements
d. empirically treating presumed dystonic reactions with an anticholinergic agent, like diphenhydramine, is reasonable

10. An 82-year-old man presents to your emergency department with urinary urgency and mild confusion. A urinalysis performed by the triage nurse is without evidence of infection. What test would be most useful in establishing a diagnosis for this patient's problem?

a. a urine culture
b. a complete blood count
c. an unenhanced CT of the abdomen and pelvis to exclude nephrolithiasis
d. an evaluation of the patient's gait

11. A 35-year-old male intravenous drug user presents to your emergency department with midthoracic back pain. It is described as severe, radiating to his chest, and unremitting for 2 weeks. It has not been relieved by the oxycodone/acetaminophen prescribed to him at his last visit 1 week ago. He is afebrile and does not have any neurologic deficits on your exam. What is the appropriate imaging test to order?

a. plain films
b. an unenhanced CT of the thoracic spine
c. a chest x-ray
d. an enhanced MRI of the thoracic spine

12. A 65-year-old man presents to your emergency department with symptoms suggestive of infectious meningitis. What is the appropriate medical therapy for this patient?

a. dexamethasone, ceftriaxone
b. dexamethasone, ceftriaxone, vancomycin
c. dexamethasone, ceftriaxone, vancomycin, ampicillin
d. ceftriaxone and vancomycin

13. A patient presents to your emergency department with progressive weakness and paresthesias over the last week, worse in the lower extremities. He

does not complain of any back pain. On examination, the patient is barely able to lift his legs off the stretcher, and you cannot elicit patellar or Achilles reflexes. He is only slightly weak in his upper extremities. What diagnostic test can be performed in the emergency department to rapidly clarify the diagnosis?

a. a CT of the lumbar spine
b. an MRI of the brain
c. lumbar puncture
d. nerve conduction studies
e. forced vital capacity

14. A patient presents to your emergency department with diplopia. On examination, she seems to have bilateral ptosis. You apply an ice pack to one of her eyes, and when removed, the ptosis of that eye seems improved. What does this indicate?

a. her weakness is likely the result of autoantibodies directed to the nicotinic acetylcholine receptors at the neuromuscular junction
b. she has contracted foodborne botulism
c. she has the Miller–Fisher variant of Guillain–Barré syndrome
d. she had a brainstem stroke

15. Which of the following dementias is secondary and subcortical?

a. Alzheimer
b. Huntington
c. multi-infarct dementia
d. Parkinson

16. A 23-year-old woman presents to your emergency department with a headache for 2 weeks. On examination, you note papilledema but do not detect any focal deficits. After a mass lesion is excluded by CT, you perform an LP and obtain an opening pressure, which is 30 cm of water. Which of the following plans would be appropriate?

a. you start the patient on acetazolamide
b. you start the patient on acetazolamide and dexamethasone
c. you arrange an outpatient MRI/MRV to exclude a venous sinus thrombosis or an occult mass
d. consult a neurosurgeon emergently for shunt placement

17. Why is it important to recognize status epilepticus early and treat it aggressively?

a. seizure activity can become self-propagating and more difficult to treat
b. prolonged seizure activity may lead to excitotoxicity and permanent neuronal damage
c. rhabdomyolysis may ensue and cause acute renal failure

d. prolonged seizure activity and impairment in mental status increase the risk of aspiration and respiratory compromise
e. all of the above

18. A 59-year-old man with a history of non–small cell lung cancer presents to your emergency department with midthoracic back pain for 2 weeks. Today, his legs feel weak and he is unable to walk. You attempt to order an MRI to exclude cord compression, but the patient reports he is unable to obtain an MRI because he has a pacemaker. What test will enable you to rapidly diagnose this problem?

a. plain films
b. a CT of the thoracic spine
c. a bone scan
d. an MRI without gadolinium
e. a CT myelogram of the thoracic and lumbar spine

19. A patient presents to your emergency department with headaches over the last month. On exam, there are no focal neurologic deficits, but you notice papilledema. You order an unenhanced CT, which demonstrates a right parietal extra-axial mass with compression of the lateral ventricle. There is no midline shift. What is your next move?

a. IV Mannitol to emergently decrease intracranial pressure
b. a CT of the brain with contrast
c. an MRI of the brain
d. neurosurgical consultation
e. **a** and **b**
f. **c** and **d**

20. A 55-year-old woman presents to your ED complaining of transient vision loss and jaw claudication, and her ESR is measured at 90 mm/hour. Which of the following is true regarding her diagnosis?

a. all patients present with a recent history of headache
b. steroids should be withheld until the performance of a temporal artery biopsy
c. scalp tenderness is always present
d. the most feared complication is blindness
e. it affects men more than women

---

1. Answer: e

Kernig and **Brudzinski signs** have very poor sensitivity for the diagnosis of bacterial meningitis, and the **classic clinical triad is present in less than half of cases. LP may be safely performed without CT if there are no signs of increased intracranial pressure** (papilledema, altered consciousness, neurologic deficit). **Antibiotics should not be withheld** pending the outcome of CSF analysis.

Systemic corticosteroids prior to antibiotic administration have been shown to improve outcomes in acute bacterial meningitis.

2. Answer: e

Bell palsy is a peripheral deficit of the facial nerve, CN7. Peripheral deficits should involve the entire face, inclusive of the forehead. **Central lesions characteristically spare the forehead. Arthralgias** are common in Lyme disease, which is a very common cause of Bell palsy. **Ocular findings are not unusual** as patients may be unable to blink the eye on the affected side, possibly leading to **corneal ulceration** or even globe perforation. For this reason ocular lubricants should be included in the medication regimen. **Hyperacusis** and disturbances of taste are also frequently seen in Bell palsy.

3. Answer: d

Vertebral artery dissections may be caused by trauma or may occur spontaneously. Flow through the dissected artery is turbulent and thrombogenic, which may lead to embolic ischemic events involving the posterior circulation. **Ataxia** is a symptom that could result from brain stem or cerebellar ischemia; thus, it is plausibly consistent with a vertebral artery dissection. A *carotid dissection* may cause an **ipsilateral ptosis** and **miosis** by interrupting the sympathetic innervation of that side of the face. It may also lead to embolic phenomena involving the anterior circulation, which may manifest with **contralateral weakness.**

4. Answer: d

One of the more concerning historical features of a headache is a **sudden onset.** A truly sudden headache is more likely to represent a serious underlying problem. Migraine headaches are commonly unilateral and throbbing, and nausea, **vomiting,** and **photophobia** are actually included in the diagnostic criteria for migraine headaches. Classic migraines are associated with an **aura,** whereas common migraines are not.

5. Answer: b

Pain syndromes clinically indistinguishable from trigeminal neuralgia can be caused by aneurysms or malignancy. **Imaging would at some point be indicated** for a young healthy person with symptoms suggestive of trigeminal neuralgia, although not necessarily emergently. The remaining answer choices are all true statements.

6. Answer: a

"Overshunting" is when excess cerebrospinal fluid is drained by the shunt, causing intracranial hypotension and headache. The headache is often positional, being improved when the patient is recumbent. Neuroimaging often demonstrates small or even "slit-like" ventricles, which is a term also used to describe the ventricles in idiopathic intracranial hypertension. A mechanical malfunction of the shunt will cause increased intracranial pressure and ventriculomegaly.

7. Answer: e

An **afferent papillary defect** is when the pupil dilates in response to a light that was directed into the contralateral pupil being redirected to the ipsilateral pupil (the swinging flashlight test). This finding indicates an optic nerve deficit. This is commonly seen in optic neuritis, which is a common early manifestation of MS. **Hemiplegia, ataxia, sensory deficits,** and **cognitive deficits** usually occur in advanced cases of MS.

8. Answer: c

The patient is demonstrating internuclear ophthalmoplegia. This is a consequence of a lesion in the medial longitudinal fasciculus (MLF), which connects the gaze centers of the cortex with the oculomotor nerve nuclei. A lesion in the MLF is a common early manifestation of MS, but can also be a consequence of stroke. In this particular patient, being in a demographic very unlikely to harbor cerebrovascular disease, it is highly suggestive of MS.

9. Answer: b

Dystonic reactions are defined as sustained and directional muscle contractions, but they **need not be visible. Spasmodic dysphonia** is characterized by contractions involving the vocal cords, and **no muscle contractions may be apparent on examination** of the patient.

10. Answer: d

Normal pressure hydrocephalus presents classically with the triad of a gait disturbance, incontinence, and dementia. The incontinence, however, may not be overt, and **usually begins with urinary urgency.** An evaluation of the patient's gait can be very helpful, as a somewhat characteristic "magnetic" gait may be observed with a wide stance and decreased foot clearance. There will also be difficulty initiating turns. A **urine culture** is not likely to be helpful here because a urinalysis is a fairly sensitive test for a urinary tract infection. An obstructing stone at the uterovesicular junction can cause urinary symptoms suggestive of a urinary tract infection, but this is unlikely in the absence of pain.

11. Answer: d

Epidural abscesses rarely present with the classic triad of fever, back pain, and neurologic deficit. The single biggest risk factor for their occurrence is intravenous drug use, and pain out of proportion to physical findings in a patient with risk factors should lead the clinician to consider the diagnosis. Although **plain films** may be useful if the abscess began as osteomyelitis in an adjacent vertebral body, they are not helpful for visualizing the abscess itself or for visualizing compression of the thecal sac and spinal cord. A **CT scan,** although very sensitive for detecting bony destruction, is also unable to visualize whether there is any nerve root or spinal cord compression, and this often is what determines the need for operative intervention. A **contrast-enhanced MRI** will demonstrate not only spinal osteomyelitis, but also diskitis, which can progress to epidural abscess. In addition, an MRI can demonstrate compression of nerve roots and the thecal sac, as well as the spinal cord.

12. Answer: c

Current recommendations call for the administration of **dexamethasone** 10 mg prior to the administration of antibiotics in patients suspected of having meningitis. An appropriate antibiotic regimen is **ceftriaxone** in meningitic doses (2 g, not 1 g as used in pneumonia), and **vancomycin.** Because *Listeria* is also a consideration in the immunosuppressed, neonates, and the elderly, **ampicillin** should be added to the regimen in this particular case (*listeria* is not covered by cephalosporins).

13. Answer: c

Ascending weakness and lower extremity paresthesias with areflexia on exam is a classic presentation of *Guillain–Barré syndrome* (GBS). Inability to raise the leg corresponds to weakness at the L2 level, but the lack of any back pain makes a **CT of the lumbar spine** very unlikely to yield a positive result. It would be unlikely for a central process to cause bilateral lower extremity weakness with relative sparing of the upper extremities, so an **MRI of the brain** is not likely to be useful. **Nerve conduction studies** would likely be diagnostic, but are not likely to be practical in the ED setting. A **lumbar puncture** in the setting of GBS is likely to show an elevated protein level with minimal or slight cellularity. Although a normal CSF profile cannot exclude GBS because 10% of the time it can be normal, this CSF profile can be strongly suggestive of GBS and rapidly obtained in the ED setting.

14. Answer: a

Although toxicity from **botulinum toxin** may cause ptosis and ophthalmoplegia, it should not be improved by cooling the affected body part. The **Miller–Fisher variant of GBS** may cause these symptoms as well, but similarly should not be improved by cooling of the affected body part. This patient has a positive "Ice pack test," which has been described in **myasthenia gravis,** which is a disease caused by the **production of autoantibodies to the acetylcholine receptors at the neuromuscular junction.**

15. Answer: c

Alzheimer disease is a primary cortical degenerative process, whereas **Huntington** and **Parkinson disease** are primary, subcortical degenerative processes. **Multi-infarct dementia,** the third most common cause of dementia, is not a primary degenerative process but rather secondary to multiple infarcts.

16. Answer: a

Increased intracranial pressure is defined as an opening pressure on LP of at least 25 cm of water. This procedure must be performed while the patient is recumbent for the pressure to be valid, as the pressure will be artificially increased if it is performed with the patient sitting up. It is reasonable to consider obtaining an MRI and/or MRV as both occult tumors and a venous sinus thrombosis may not be evident on CT, but the patient should still be treated with acetazolamide presumptively for idiopathic intracranial hypertension (IIH), as permanent damage to the optic nerve may ensue if treatment is withheld. Thus, it would not be appropriate to withhold treatment pending the results of an outpatient MRI. Acetazolamide is used as a treatment for IIH because it decreases the production of cerebrospinal fluid, thereby lowering ICP. The patient should still be referred for follow-up with a neurologist and an ophthalmologist, as further treatments such as CSF shunting or optic nerve fenestration may be necessary.

17. Answer: e

If generalized seizure activity is prolonged, it can lead to the loss of inhibitory pathways, become self-propagating, and become very difficult to treat. Excitotoxicity may also lead to permanent neuronal damage. Rhabdomyolysis and aspiration are potential complications of prolonged seizure activity, so their occurrence should be anticipated, or, in the case of aspiration, prevented by endotracheal intubation.

18. Answer: e

This patient has a history suggestive of *malignant spinal cord compression.* **Plain films** in this setting may be completely normal. Even if bony metastasis is noted on plain films, visualization of compression of the cord and thecal sac is not possible with plain x-rays, necessitating further studies to clarify the diagnosis before potentially risky surgery is planned. A **CT scan** has the same limitations, although it is superior to plain x-rays at visualizing the bony anatomy. An **MRI** cannot be obtained, with or without contrast, because of the presence of the patient's pacemaker. A **CT myelogram,** with contrast injected into the subarachnoid space, is invasive but allows visualization of the bony anatomy as well as the thecal sac and can make the diagnosis rapidly. Because this is an invasive test, it would be prudent to perform the scan of the lumbar region as well to avoid the patient's needing to repeat the procedure in short order.

19. Answer: f

The gradual presentation and extra-axial position of this tumor on noncontrast CT is suggestive of a meningioma. Although neurosurgical intervention is likely to be needed, this need not be emergent. A CT with contrast may be better at visualizing certain intraparenchymal tumors, but in this case an MRI is a superior test and is preferred in the nonemergency circumstance. IV Mannitol to lower intracranial pressure emergently is only necessary in the event of acute decompensation.

20. Answer: d

This woman has temporal arteritis. Approximately 30% of patients will not have a headache, and the presence of scalp tenderness is variable. It affects women more than men, and typically affects patients over 50. Treatment should not be withheld pending the biopsy. Blindness is the most feared complication of temporal arteritis.

Vagina, cervix, and sexually transmitted disease (STD)

NONSEXUALLY TRANSMITTED CAUSES OF VAGINITIS AND DISCHARGE

Bacterial vaginosis

- Polymicrobial—for example, *Gardnerella vaginalis, Mycoplasma hominis,* anaerobes
- Not an STD

SIGNS AND SYMPTOMS

- Gray-white malodorous discharge

DIAGNOSIS

- Clue cells on wet mount (cytoplasm of epithelial cells studded with coccobacilli)
- "Whiff-test"—fishy odor after adding KOH to sample
- pH >4.5

TREATMENT

- Metronidazole 500 mg PO two times a day for 7 days
- Single-dose therapy not as effective
- Do not treat the sex partner

Candida vaginitis

- Yeast
- Most common cause of vaginitis
- Not an STD

RISK FACTORS

- Antibiotic use
- Pregnancy

- Oral contraceptives
- Steroid use
- Diabetes mellitus
- Tight clothes

SIGNS AND SYMPTOMS

- Pruritic, sticky, "cottage cheese" discharge

DIAGNOSIS

- Wet mount with KOH; visualize budding spores and pseudo-hyphae
- pH <4.5

TREATMENT

- Nonpregnant—fluconazole 150 mg PO single-dose or topical antifungals
- Pregnant—topical antifungal
- Do not treat partner, unless recurrent infection or male has yeast balanitis

Miscellaneous causes of vaginitis and discharge

- Foreign bodies
- Chemical (douching)
- Atrophic vaginitis
  - Diminished levels of estrogen in menopause
  - Topical estrogen cream

SEXUALLY TRANSMITTED DISEASE: CERVICITIS AND VAGINITIS

Chlamydia

- Obligate intracellular parasite
- Most common STD
- May be asymptomatic
- Major cause of infertility
- Commonly coexists with gonorrhea
- Leading cause of "NGU" (nongonococcal urethritis)

SIGNS AND SYMPTOMS

- Mucopurulent, yellow discharge
- Dysuria
- Cervical edema and erythema
- Men and women may be asymptomatic
- May cause **Reiter syndrome** (urethritis, conjunctivitis, rash, and arthritis)

DIAGNOSIS

- ELISA and DNA probes

TREATMENT

- Azithromycin 1 g PO single dose
- Doxycycline 100 mg PO two times a day for 7 days

Gonorrhea (GC)

- Intracellular gram-negative diplococcus

SIGNS AND SYMPTOMS

- Three patterns of disease in women
  - Asymptomatic: 30% to 40%
  - Pelvic inflammatory disease (PID): 20% to 40%
  - Cervicitis: 20% to 30%
- Most common manifestations—purulent cervical discharge, dysuria, abnormal vaginal bleeding
- Men are symptomatic in 80% to 90% of cases
  - Dysuria and penile discharge
- Infections of pharynx, conjunctiva, and rectum are possible
- Disseminated GC
  - Hematogenous spread
  - 2% of untreated cases
  - **Arthritis-dermatitis syndrome**
    - Asymmetric arthralgia, septic arthritis, tenosynovitis
      - Petechial, pustular or acral skin lesions (see Fig. 10-1A and B)
    - Meningitis

DIAGNOSIS

- Culture or DNA-based tests

TREATMENT

- Cervicitis
  - Ceftriaxone 125 mg IM single dose (250 mg IM single dose for PID)
  - Cefixime 400 mg PO single dose
  - Ciprofloxacin (and all fluoroquinolones) no longer recommended for treatment of GC
- Disseminated
  - Hospitalization
  - Ceftriaxone 1 g IV every 24 hours for 1 to 2 days after clinical improvement, then oral treatment for a total of at least one week

Trichomonas vaginitis

- Protozoan

SIGNS AND SYMPTOMS

- Profuse, pruritic, white, yellow, gray-green or frothy, malodorous discharge
- Strawberry cervix

DIAGNOSIS

- Wet mount and direct visualization of motile trichomonads (Fig. 13-1)

TREATMENT

- Metronidazole 2 g PO single dose

SEXUALLY TRANSMITTED DISEASES: UPPER TRACT INFECTION

Pelvic inflammatory disease (PID)

- Spectrum of infections involving the upper female genital tract

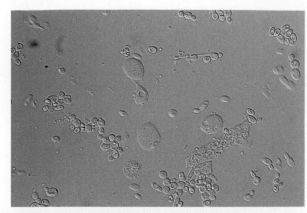

Figure 13-1. Trichomonal Infection. Saline mount of *Trichomonas vaginalis:* characteristic ovoid shape and flagella can be seen. (From Cohen J, Powderly WG: *Infectious diseases,* ed 2, Philadelphia, 2004, Mosby.)

- 10 to 20 cases per 1000 women or approximately 1 to 1.5 million cases per year
- 25% of women may experience chronic pain, infertility or ectopic pregnancy
- 12% to 15% increased risk of fatal ectopic pregnancy
- 12% to 50% increased risk of tubal factor infertility due to scarring of fallopian tubes
- Polymicrobial etiology
  - *Neisseria gonorrhoeae* and *Chlamydia trachomatis* (isolated in 80% of cases) initiate inflammatory process, which then allows for secondary infection with multiple anaerobes and gram-negative rods
  - Other organisms include *G. vaginalis, M. hominis,* and *Ureaplasma urealyticum*
- Predisposing factors
  - Multiple sexual partners, history of previous STDs, douching, recent menses or abortion, IUD use

SIGNS AND SYMPTOMS

- Multiple presentations, including acute, chronic, intermediate
- **May be asymptomatic; major cause of future infertility**
- Lower abdominal pain is the most frequent complaint
- Other presentations may include abnormal vaginal bleeding, painful sexual intercourse or postcoital bleeding, nausea, vomiting, fever, or urethritis
- Cervical motion tenderness is the hallmark on physical examination
- Adnexal fullness and tenderness and mucopurulent discharge

DIAGNOSIS

- Primarily based on history and physical. No one single diagnostic criterion. Laboratory studies and diagnostic procedures play a supporting role
- Maintain a high index of suspicion and have a low threshold to initiate treatment

- Laboratory testing
  - Pregnancy test, wet mount (looking for WBCs), Gram stain and culture or DNA probes for likely organisms
  - Consider HIV and syphilis testing
- Transvaginal pelvic ultrasound may show thickened endometrium or the presence of pelvic or tubo-ovarian abscess (TOA)
- Culdocentesis and endometrial biopsy have limited value in the ED
- Laparoscopy considered criterion standard. Still may fail to diagnose 20% of cases

TREATMENT

- Low threshold to initiate treatment given severity of possible complications
- Parenteral and oral treatment considered equally as effective
- Oral regimen
  - Ceftriaxone 250 mg IM in a single dose plus doxycycline 100 mg orally twice a day for 14 days with or without metronidazole 500 mg orally twice a day for 14 days
  - Cefoxitin 2 g IM in a single dose and probenecid, 1 g orally administered concurrently in a single dose, plus doxycycline 100 mg orally twice a day for 14 days with or without metronidazole 500 mg orally twice a day for 14 days
- Parenteral regimen
  - Cefotetan 2 g IV every 12 hours or cefoxitin 2 g IV every 6 hours plus doxycycline 100 mg orally or IV every 12 hours
  - Clindamycin 900 mg IV every 8 hours plus gentamicin loading dose IV or IM (2 mg/kg of body weight), followed by a maintenance dose (1.5 mg/kg) every 8 hours. Single daily dosing may be substituted
  - Ampicillin/sulbactam 3 g IV every 6 hours plus doxycycline 100 mg orally or IV every 12 hours
- Indications for hospitalization
  - Surgical emergency cannot be excluded
  - Pregnancy
  - Failure of outpatient regimen
  - Unable to tolerate PO medications
  - Poor compliance
  - Tubo-ovarian abscess
  - Nulliparous women
  - HIV-positive patients

Fitz–Hugh–Curtis syndrome (gonococcal perihepatitis)

- Complication of PID
- Fibrous adhesions between liver capsule and abdominal wall secondary to inflammation

SIGNS AND SYMPTOMS

- Sudden-onset severe, sharp, pleuritic right upper quadrant (RUQ) pain several weeks after acute episode of PID
- Significant tenderness to palpation in RUQ

DIAGNOSIS

- History and physical

TREATMENT

- May require laparoscopic lysis of adhesions

SEXUALLY TRANSMITTED DISEASES: GENITAL LESIONS

Genital herpes simplex

- DNA virus: HSV1 and HSV2
- HSV1—mostly causes oral lesions
- Chronic illness with acute exacerbations
- **Primary HSV illness**
  - More severe than recurrences
  - May last 3 to 4 weeks
  - May be asymptomatic but contagious

SIGNS AND SYMPTOMS

- Painful, grouped, vesicular, or ulcerated lesions on vagina, pre-labia, and labia
- Fever, abdominal pain, myalgia possible
- Aseptic meningitis, headache, photophobia possible
- **Recurrent infection**
  - Virus remains dormant in spinal root ganglia
  - Reactivation at irregular intervals as a result of unknown triggers
  - Less severe; resolves in 9 to 10 days
  - No systemic symptoms

DIAGNOSIS

- Physical examination
- Tzanck prep or ELISA

TREATMENT

- Primary
  - Acyclovir 400 mg PO three times a day for 7 to 10 days
  - Famciclovir 250 mg PO three times a day for 7 to 10 days
  - Valacyclovir 1 g PO two times a day for 7 to 10 days
- Secondary (selected regimens; there are many)
  - Acyclovir 400 mg PO three times a day for 5 days
  - Famciclovir 125 mg PO two times a day for 5 days
  - Valacyclovir 500 mg PO two times a day for 3 days
  - Suppressive daily regimens in patients with frequent attacks

Syphilis

- Spirochete *Treponema pallidum*
- Strong association with HIV co-infection

SIGNS AND SYMPTOMS

- Primary
  - Small papule that progresses to *painless* ulcer 10 to 90 days post-exposure

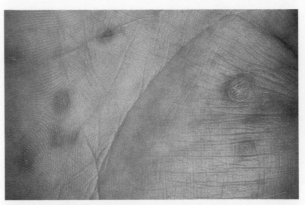

Figure 13-2. Lesions on palms and soles occur in the majority of patients with secondary syphilis. Coppery color resembling that of clean-cut ham is characteristic of secondary syphilis. (From Habif TP: *Clinical dermatology: a color guide to diagnosis and therapy,* ed 4, St. Louis, 2004, Mosby.)

- Resolves after 4 to 5 days
- May be RPR-negative
- Secondary
  - 3 to 6 weeks after resolution of primary stage
  - Nonspecific symptoms: fever, headache, sore throat, rash and lymphadenopathy are most common
  - Rash—classically dull, red, papular rash on trunk, flexor surfaces, palms of hands and soles of feet (Fig. 13-2)
  - Self-limiting
  - **Condylomata lata**—moist, verrucous lesions resembling genital warts (HPV), frequently in moist places (perianal or vulvar in women; scrotal in men) (see Fig. 10-2)
- Tertiary
  - Rarely seen in the ED
  - 3 to 20 years after initial infection
  - Cardiac and neurologic manifestations; gummas

DIAGNOSIS

- Dark-field microscopy identifies treponemes in scrapings from primary lesions
- Serology testing:
  - Nontreponemal—RPR, VRDL
  - Turn positive 14 days after appearance of primary lesion
- Specific treponemal antibody testing—FTA-ABS

TREATMENT

- Primary and secondary (early latent)
  - Benzathine PCN G 2.4 million units IM as a single dose
  - Doxycycline 100 mg PO two times a day for 2 weeks in PCN allergy
- Secondary late latent, or latent and unknown duration
  - Benzathine PCN 2.4 IM every week for 3 weeks
- Tertiary
  - Benzathine PCN 2.4 million units IM every week for 3 weeks

- Neurosyphilis or syphilitic eye disease
  - PCN G 3 to 4 million units IV Q 4 hours for 10 to 14 days

Lymphogranuloma venereum (LGV)

- *C. trachomatis*

SIGNS AND SYMPTOMS

- Painless vesicle, pustule, or ulcer on labia 7 to 21 days postexposure
- Lymphadenopathy
- Characteristic finding 2 to 12 weeks after initial lesion appears
- **Groove sign**—bulky lymphadenopathy above and below the inguinal ligament
- May ulcerate, rupture, or drain

DIAGNOSIS

- Serology testing
- Clinical diagnosis

TREATMENT

- Doxycycline 100 mg PO two times a day for 21 days

Chancroid

- Gram-negative bacillus; *Haemophilus ducreyi*
- HIV and syphilis coinfections are common

SIGNS AND SYMPTOMS

- Painful papule develops 4 to 10 days postexposure
- Becomes a very painful ulcer: single or multiple
- Painful unilateral bubo in 50% of patients; may rupture

DIAGNOSIS

- Gram stain reveals gram-negative bacilli in characteristic "school of fish" pattern

TREATMENT

- Azithromycin 1 g PO single dose *or*
- Ceftriaxone 250 mg IM single dose

Granuloma inguinale (Donovanosis)

- Gram-negative bacillus *Klebsiella* (formerly *Calymmatobacterium*) *granulomatis*
- Rare in the United States; more common in Southeast Asia, South America, Australia, and the Caribbean

SIGNS AND SYMPTOMS

- Painless genital papule(s) progress to a large ulcer or ulcers (Fig. 13-3)
- Pseudo-buboes: subcutaneous granulomas

DIAGNOSIS

- Visible Donovan bodies on smear

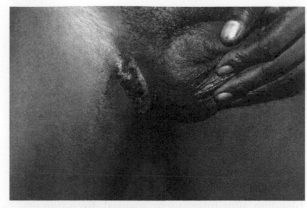

Figure 13-3. Granuloma inguinale. The chronic, granulomatous, beefy-red ulcer without suppuration is typical. (From Cohen J, Powderly WG: *Infectious diseases,* ed 2, Philadelphia, 2004, Mosby. Photo supplied by J. K. Maniar.)

TREATMENT

- Continue all regimens until lesions resolve
  - Doxycycline 100 mg PO two times a day for at least 3 weeks

Condylomata acuminata (venereal warts)

- Human papilloma viruses (HPV), DNA viruses
- Types 6 and 11 most common (virus typing not recommended at diagnosis)
- Carcinogenic
  - Types 16 and 18 frequent association
  - 90% of cervical and 50% of penile cancer

SIGNS AND SYMPTOMS

- Flesh-colored, cauliflower-like lesions on the external genitalia
- 1- to 8-month incubation

DIAGNOSIS

- Clinical

TREATMENT

- Cryotherapy, lasers, or topicals

Bartholin gland abscess

- Polymicrobial infection of Bartholin gland or duct cyst
- *N. gonorrhoeae, C. trachomatis, Escherichia coli, Proteus mirabilis*

SIGNS AND SYMPTOMS

- Unilateral pain and swelling at the lower lateral vaginal opening
- Painful sexual intercourse and painful when walking

DIAGNOSIS

- Clinical

TREATMENT

- Incision and drainage
- Word catheter placed to promote drainage
- Gynecology follow-up for definitive management

CERVICAL CANCER

- **Risk factors:** multiple sexual partners, smoking (increases the risk 3 to 5 times), HPV infection (Types 16 and 18), HIV, early first intercourse

SIGNS AND SYMPTOMS

- Postmenopausal bleeding **(most common),** bleeding after intercourse, vaginal discharge or pain, leg swelling
- Speculum examination may reveal mass or ulcerated lesion on cervix

DIAGNOSIS

- Biopsy

TREATMENT

- Surgical and radiation therapy

Ovary

CYSTS

- In the nonpregnant patient, the majority are functional cysts related to the menstrual cycle
- Pregnant patient: corpus luteum cyst
  - Corpus luteum supports the pregnancy in the first 8 weeks
- Majority resolve within two to three menstrual cycles
- They may rupture or lead to ovarian torsion

SIGNS AND SYMPTOMS

- Sudden-onset unilateral pelvic pain
- May cause vaginal bleeding
- Rupture or hemorrhage may cause peritoneal irritation
- Pelvic examination is not sensitive or specific

DIAGNOSIS

- Pelvic ultrasound primarily to rule out torsion, or ectopic in the pregnant patient
- Laparoscopy may be required to distinguish from ectopic in pregnant patients

TREATMENT

- Gynecologic follow-up
- Cystectomy if necessary

OVARIAN TORSION

- **Surgical emergency to preserve fertility**
- Results from twisting of the vascular pedicle
- Risk factors include large cysts, ovarian masses, and pelvic adhesions

SIGNS AND SYMPTOMS

- Sudden-onset unilateral pelvic pain
- Onset may be spontaneous or related to exercise, sexual intercourse, or trauma
- Pain may be intermittent if the ovary is twisting and untwisting

DIAGNOSIS

- Pelvic ultrasound

TREATMENT

- Early operative intervention

POLYCYSTIC OVARIAN SYNDROME (PCOS)

- Hyperandrogenism with associated menstrual disorder (oligo- or amenorrhea)
- Ovulatory failure
- Onset usually post-menarche
- 40% are obese; associated hyperinsulinism and insulin resistance
- Treated with hormonal therapy, metformin

OVARIAN CANCER

- 25,000 new cases per year
- 1% to 2% in women with no family history
- 50% mortality
- Risk factors: infertility, family history, low parity, high-fat diet
- Oral contraceptives thought to be protective

SIGNS AND SYMPTOMS

- 55 to 65 years old
- Abdominal pain, bloating, weight loss, pleural effusion
- New diagnosis of ascites in women 55 to 65 years old is presumed to be ovarian cancer until proven otherwise
- Many women do not present until an advanced stage

DIAGNOSIS

- Maintain a high index of suspicion
- CT scan
- DO NOT aspirate ascites as there is a risk of peritoneal seeding
- Surgical staging

TREATMENT

- Surgery, radiation, and chemotherapy

Uterus

DYSFUNCTIONAL UTERINE BLEEDING

- One of the most common presenting complaints of women in the ED

- Multiple causes, depending on the age of the patient and whether or not they are pregnant
  - Children: foreign body, trauma, severe vulvovaginitis, sexual abuse
  - Childbearing age: anovulatory bleeding, fibroids, endometriosis, STDs, threatened abortion, ectopic pregnancy, placenta previa, placental abruption, ovarian cyst rupture, or cancer
- Specific conditions addressed below

ENDOMETRIOSIS

- Ectopic growth of endometrial glands and stroma in the ovary, pelvic peritoneum, and other distant pelvic sites

SIGNS AND SYMPTOMS

- Women in their 30s
- Irregular bleeding and menstruation
- Unusually painful periods
- Physical examination and ultrasound are unreliable
- Direct visualization with laparoscopy

TREATMENT

- Hormone therapy
- Pregnancy may cause remission

LEIOMYOMA (FIBROIDS)

- Most common pelvic tumor
- More common in the 4th decade and in African Americans

SIGNS AND SYMPTOMS

- Acute or chronic pain usually due to ischemia of the tumor because of its poor blood supply
- Vaginal bleeding
- Ultrasound (US) confirms the diagnosis

TREATMENT

- Pain control
- Hormone therapy
- Spectrum of surgical interventions from selective embolization to hysterectomy

UTERINE CANCER

- Most common GYN cancer
- 32,000 cases per year
- 25% in women less than 40 years of age; most often presents in the 6th and 7th decades
- Risk factors: late menopause, nulliparity, obesity, diabetes, hypertension, and exogenous estrogen exposure

SIGNS AND SYMPTOMS

- Postmenopausal bleeding and/or abnormal vaginal discharge
- Biopsy
- Surgical staging

TREATMENT

- Surgery, radiation, and chemotherapy

Normal pregnancy

- 40 weeks
- Gestational age calculated from the first day of the last menstrual period
- Weeks 2 to 8 are the embryonic stage and account for most organogenesis
- Three trimesters: first, conception to 14 weeks; second, 14 to 28 weeks; third, 28 to 42 weeks
- Term is considered greater than 37 weeks

PHYSIOLOGIC CHANGES

- **Cardiovascular:** increases in heart rate, blood volume, and cardiac output. Decrease in blood pressure
- **Respiratory:** increase in tidal volume. Respiratory rate remains unchanged
- **Gastrointestinal:** increased risk of gastritis, reflux, and gallstones; displacement of abdominal contents creates atypical presentations (e.g., appendicitis may manifest as right upper quadrant abdominal pain)
- **Hematologic:** anemia secondary to dilution (but not below 11 g/dL hemoglobin); leukocytosis (roughly 5 to 12 thousand cells/mm^3)

Complications of pregnancy

ECTOPIC PREGNANCY

- Pregnancy implanted outside the uterus; majority in the fallopian tube; may occur in the ovary or cervix
- Increasing incidence—up to 1:100 pregnancies
- Second-leading cause of maternal death
- Heterotopic pregnancy: a normal intrauterine pregnancy and an ectopic pregnancy—1:5000 pregnancies
- Risk factors: PID, history of tubal surgery, previous ectopic, fertility treatments, intrauterine device

SIGNS AND SYMPTOMS

- Varied presentation and may be vague
- High index of suspicion
- Suspect the diagnosis in any childbearing-age women with lower abdominal pain, syncope, evidence of hypovolemia, or vaginal bleeding
- Most common presentation: missed menses, vaginal bleeding, and abdominal pain
- May present as or with: shoulder pain, peritonitis, tachycardia, bradycardia, adnexal tenderness

DIAGNOSIS

- Positive urine pregnancy test. Dilute urine may give a false negative

- US is often diagnostic
  - Transvaginal is more sensitive than transabdominal
- **Discriminatory zone:** level of beta-hCG at which an intrauterine pregnancy can be seen on US
  - Transabdominal: 6000 mIU/mL
  - Transvaginal: 1500 mIU/mL; at a beta-hCG of 3000, an IUP should absolutely be visible on transvaginal US
  - Many ectopic pregnancies can present with beta-hCG less than 1500 and US should be done in all cases regardless of the beta-hCG
  - Culdocentesis: advent of ultrasound has reduced the need for this invasive procedure
    - It is still indicated if there is no available ultrasound
    - Aspiration of any blood is considered positive
  - Laparoscopy: used in patients with nondiagnostic ultrasound and a strong clinical suspicion

TREATMENT

- Decision point: hemodynamically stable versus unstable
- Unstable: 20% of cases, requires immediate surgical intervention
- Stable patients with a confirmed ectopic
  - May consider methotrexate therapy
  - Indications include: hemodynamic stability, less than 4 cm mass, beta-hCG less than 4000, ability to follow-up
  - Pelvic pain is a common side effect of treatment. Requires reassessment to rule out acute rupture of the ectopic
- Stable patients with a beta-hCG less than 1500 and an indeterminate ultrasound
  - May be discharged with a repeat beta-hCG in 48 hours, repeat outpatient ultrasound, and GYN follow-up

SPONTANEOUS ABORTION

- Loss of a pregnancy before 20 weeks' gestation
- Affects 20% to 40% of pregnancies
- 75% occur in the first 8 weeks
- 50% of women with bleeding in the first trimester will miscarry
- Types
  - Threatened: os closed
  - Inevitable: os open
  - Incomplete: passage of partial products of conceptions (POC)
  - Missed: fetal demise before 20 weeks and no passage of tissue within 4 weeks of demise
  - Septic: infection at any stage

SIGNS AND SYMPTOMS

- Vaginal bleeding and/or cramping abdominal pain in the first trimester

TREATMENT

- Pelvic examination: assessment of the os
- Beta-hCG, type and Rh

- RhoGAM as indicated
- Ultrasound to rule out ectopic
- Other laboratory tests as indicated
- Threatened: pelvic rest and close follow-up
- Inevitable or missed: D&C
- Septic: broad-spectrum antibiotics, D&C, admission

HELLP SYNDROME: *HEMOLYSIS, ELEVATED LIVER ENZYMES, LOW PLATELETS*

- Occurs after 20 weeks' gestational age
- May develop in the postpartum period
- 1 : 1000 pregnancies
- Results from endothelial cell dysfunction, leading to microvascular thrombi and hemolysis
- End-organ damage and DIC may result. Hepatic rupture has been reported

SIGNS AND SYMPTOMS

- RUQ or epigastric pain
- Symptomatic anemia
- Lab studies including liver panel, complete blood count, fibrinogen, lactate dehydrogenase and coagulation studies

TREATMENT

- Timely delivery
- Supportive care

VAGINAL BLEEDING AFTER 20 WEEKS

- Associated with 30% fetal mortality regardless of cause

Abruptio placentae

- Premature separation of a normally implanted placenta
- 1% of pregnancies
- Risk factors: hypertension is the most common, trauma, increased maternal age, smoking, cocaine use, previous abruption
- May be partial, complete, or concealed (no vaginal bleeding)

SIGNS AND SYMPTOMS

- Sudden-onset abdominal pain with/without vaginal bleeding
- Hypertonic uterus with contractions
- Fetal distress on cardio-tocographic monitoring is a key feature
- Ultrasound to rule out placenta previa but may not (necessarily) diagnose the abruption

TREATMENT

- Delivery

Placenta previa

- Implantation of the placenta over the os

SIGNS AND SYMPTOMS

- Painless bright-red bleeding
- Ultrasound makes the diagnosis
- Speculum and digital exams are contraindicated

TREATMENT

- Cesarean section

HYPEREMESIS GRAVIDARUM

- Nausea and vomiting affect 60% to 80% of pregnancies
- Hyperemesis is severe intractable vomiting, dehydration, weight loss, hypokalemia, and ketonemia

SIGNS AND SYMPTOMS

- Abdominal pain is very unusual and should prompt a search for other causes

TREATMENT

- Anti-emetics
- Rehydration and clearance of ketonemia

PREGNANCY-INDUCED HYPERTENSION

- A common cause of maternal death
- More common after 20 weeks
- May occur in the first trimester with molar pregnancy or multiple gestations
- May precipitate abruption, preterm delivery, or low-birth-weight babies
- 140/90 mmHg or a 20-mmHg increase in systolic BP or a 10-mmHg increase in diastolic BP over the nonpregnant state
- A "normal"-appearing BP may be pathologic in the pregnant female

PRE-ECLAMPSIA

- Hypertension, proteinuria, and peripheral edema after 20 weeks
- Results from a dysfunction of the vasculature of the placenta
- 5% to 10% of pregnancies
- Risk factors: increased maternal age, pre-pregnancy hypertension, molar pregnancy, diabetes, multiple gestations, and renal disease
- May present up to 6 weeks postpartum

SIGNS AND SYMPTOMS

- Epigastric or right upper quadrant abdominal pain, headache, visual disturbances, dizziness, edema, hypertension

TREATMENT

- OB-GYN consultation
- Magnesium sulfate, hydralazine, delivery

ECLAMPSIA

- Seizures in the pre-eclamptic patient
- Treat with magnesium sulfate, 6 g over 15 minutes and then 2 g/hour, monitoring deep tendon reflexes and respiratory status
- Hydralazine is the traditional agent to lower BP
- Benzodiazepines for seizures
- Prompt OB-GYN consultation
- Prompt delivery

GESTATIONAL TROPHOBLASTIC DISEASE

- Also known as a molar pregnancy
- Disordered proliferation of the chorionic villi
- Complete hydatiform mole: no fetal tissue
- Incomplete hydatiform mole: fetal tissue is present
- May undergo malignant transformation and metastasize

SIGNS AND SYMPTOMS

- Extremely high beta-hCG for dates
- Large fundus for dates
- Evidence of hyperemesis, hypertension, or pre-eclampsia in the 1st trimester
- Ultrasound shows characteristic "snowstorm" appearance (Fig. 13-4)

TREATMENT

- D&C

RH SENSITIZATION

- Results when an Rh-negative mother is exposed to Rh-positive blood
- Sensitization occurs at delivery, with threatened abortions, ectopic pregnancy, or trauma
- Kleihauer–Betke test can detect fetal RBCs in maternal blood and quantify the amount of exposure, although this is often not practical in the ED
- Anti-D immunoglobulin (RhoGAM) should be given when sensitization may have occurred
- Dosing recommendations vary
- 300 mcg IM is the standard dose

Normal labor and delivery

- Majority of pregnancies proceed without problems and result in a smooth healthy delivery
- Labor can present as abdominal pain, back pain, nausea and vomiting, urinary or fecal urgency
- When a woman in labor presents to the ED, an assessment of that hospital's resources in terms of OB physician and nursing staff, as well as NICU availability, should inform a transfer decision
- **False labor:** also known as Braxton–Hicks contractions; uncoordinated, nonprogressive uterine contractions that subside

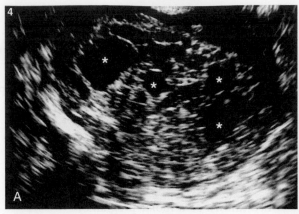
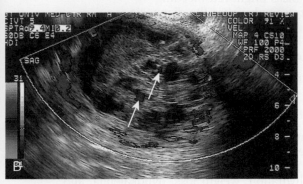

Figure 13-4. Gestational trophoblastic disease. Transverse transvaginal ultrasound (US) **(A)** shows an echogenic mass with multiple cystic spaces within the endometrial cavity (the "snowstorm" or "cluster of grapes" appearance) in a woman with a molar pregnancy. The small cystic spaces (*, **A**) are felt to represent hydropic villi. Sagittal transvaginal US with color flow (*arrows*, **B**) documents flow to the mole. (From Adam A, Dixon A: *Grainger and Allison's diagnostic radiology*, ed 5, Philadelphia, 2008, Churchill Livingstone.)

- **True labor:** cyclical uterine contractions of increasing strength and frequency

STAGES OF LABOR

- First stage: onset of contractions to complete dilation of cervix
  - Average 8 hours in the nulliparous and 5 hours in multiparous
- Second stage: cervical dilation to delivery of fetus
  - 50 minutes in the nulliparous and 20 minutes in the multiparous
  - Fetal cardio-tocographic monitoring is recommended
- Third stage: delivery of the fetus to delivery of the placenta
  - 5 to 10 minutes postdelivery of the fetus
  - Placental separation evidenced by
    - Rush of blood
    - Lengthening of the umbilical cord
    - Placental passage into the vagina
    - Firming of the uterus

DELIVERY

- If ED delivery cannot be avoided and birth is imminent, prepare a radiant warmer and neonatal resuscitation equipment
- Slow, controlled delivery of the fetus is desired
- When the child's head is crowning gentle pressure should be held on the presenting part while supporting the perineum
- Delivery of the head should prompt immediate suctioning of the oropharynx and nose and a check for a nuchal umbilical cord
- Gentle downward pressure delivers the anterior shoulder followed by upward movement to deliver the posterior shoulder
- Child then delivers spontaneously
- Keep the baby low or at the level of the perineum to maximize cord blood flow

- Clamp cord 10 cm from the abdomen and place a second clamp 5 cm from the first
- Delivery of the placenta is often spontaneous
- Massage the uterus and assess postpartum hemorrhage

Complications of labor

PREMATURE LABOR

- Cervical change and contractions before 37 weeks
- 8% to 10% of pregnancies
- Risk factors: extremes of maternal age, smoking, drug use, multiple gestations, history of first-trimester bleeding

SIGNS AND SYMPTOMS

- Fluid leak (see below)
- Vaginal bleeding, contractions

TREATMENT

- Unless delivery is imminent, transfer to OB-GYN

PREMATURE RUPTURE OF MEMBRANES

- Rupture of the amniotic sac prior to onset of labor
- 3% of pregnancies
- Increased risk of infection

SIGNS AND SYMPTOMS

- History of fluid leak or rush of fluid
- Sterile speculum exam may show pooling of fluid in the vaginal vault
- Digital exam is contraindicated
- Test the fluid pH with Nitrazine paper. Amniotic fluid is pH 7.1 to 7.3 versus vaginal pH of 3.0 to 3.5
- Microscopic exam will show a characteristic ferning pattern

TREATMENT

- Make the diagnosis
- Unless delivery is imminent, transfer to OB-GYN

UTERINE RUPTURE

- Increased risk with vaginal delivery after cesarean section (VBAC)
- 0.3% to 1.7% of VBACs
- Increased risk with a previous vertical or classic incision or more than three c-sections

SIGNS AND SYMPTOMS

- Often in the first stage of labor
- Spectrum of presentations from simple scar separation to complete expulsion of the fetus
- Fetal mortality can be as high as 20%
- May be painless
- Fetal distress

TREATMENT

- C-section within 30 minutes to maximize survival

UTERINE INVERSION

- In the third stage of labor
- Extreme pain and life-threatening hemorrhage
- 1:2500 deliveries
- Attempt to replace the uterus with counter pressure
- Operative repair

FETAL DISTRESS

- Fetal cardio-tocographic monitoring is the key
- Not usually done in the ED
- Manifest as decelerations of fetal heart rate
- Variable or early decelerations
  - Common
  - Drop in heart rate at the start of a contraction with quick recovery
  - Due to fetal head or cord compression
  - Often easily corrected with maternal positioning
- Late decelerations
  - Decrease in heart rate after the maximum uterine contraction
  - Due to hypoxia
  - Urgent delivery, often surgical, and anticipate need for neonatal resuscitation

Complications of delivery

- Only the most imminent deliveries should be done in the ED
- If it is inevitable, prepare and anticipate
- Get help—OB, Pediatrics, and Anesthesia

MALPRESENTATION OF THE FETUS

- Breech presentation is the most common malpresentation

- 4% of births
- Cervical dilation is incomplete, leading to entrapment of the head
- Cord prolapse may occur

SIGNS AND SYMPTOMS

- Mother may know the baby is breech
- Palpation of the head at the fundus
- Ultrasound

TREATMENT

- Transfer to labor and delivery unless delivery is imminent
- Consider manually displacing the presenting part from the umbilical cord and transferring to labor and delivery
- If delivery must be done in the ED
  - Fetal monitoring is essential
  - Liberal and generous episiotomy
  - Free 10 to 15 cm of cord when it presents to give more room
  - **Mauriceau maneuver:** using the fetal mouth to tuck chin to chest to allow delivery of the head and prevent dystocia

DYSTOCIA

- Shoulder dystocia is the most common form
- 0.3% of births
- Develops during labor
- Impacted anterior shoulder against the bony pelvis
- Risk factors: diabetic mother and high-birth-weight baby

SIGNS AND SYMPTOMS

- Inability to deliver the shoulders
- Turtle sign: retraction of the fetal head
- Shoulders in a vertical axis

TREATMENT

- Fetal monitoring and OB to bedside if not already present
- Episiotomy
- **McRoberts maneuver:** mother into extreme knee-chest position and suprapubic pressure
- **Rubin maneuver:** pushing most accessible shoulder toward the chest combined with fetal rotation (corkscrew movement)
- Attempt delivery of the posterior shoulder by sweeping the fetal arm across the chest up to chin and out of the vagina

MULTIPLE GESTATIONS

- 1% of deliveries
- Often known to the mother
- In those without prenatal care, bedside ultrasound
- 60% of multiple gestations have a malpresented fetus. Usually twin B
- Unless delivery is imminent, transfer to labor and delivery

UMBILICAL CORD EMERGENCIES

Cord prolapse

- Umbilical cord is the presenting part
- More common in premature rupture of membranes or malpresentation
- Cord prolapse may be the first sign of malpresentation
- 15% perinatal mortality

TREATMENT

- Immediate C-section; mortality decreases to 5% if delivery within 10 minutes
- Preservation of cord flow
  - Mother into Trendelenburg and knee-to-chest position
  - Manual displacement of the presenting part
- **Cord entanglement**
  - Nuchal cord is the most common, may be wrapped around more than once
  - Check for and reduce manually with delivery of the head
  - If it cannot be reduced, clamp and cut the cord

Postpartum complications

HEMORRHAGE

- Greater than 500 mL of blood loss
- 6% of deliveries
- Immediate: within the first 24 hours
- Delayed: 24 hours to 6 weeks

Uterine atony

- 50% of cases
- Uterine massage and oxytocin as treatment

Delivery trauma

- 20% of cases
- Tears of the vagina and surrounding tissue
  - First degree: vaginal mucosa
  - Second degree: into the perineal fascia and muscle
  - Third degree: into the anal sphincter
  - Fourth degree: into the rectal mucosa

Retained products

- 10% of cases
- Most commonly the placenta

Management principles

- Uterine exploration and removal of POC; done by OB
- Uterine packing

- Pelvic vessel embolization
- Hysterectomy

ENDOMETRITIS

- 5% of all pregnancies
- Infection of the endometrial tissue
- Risk factors: C-section, premature rupture of membranes, prolonged labor
- Polymicrobial

SIGNS AND SYMPTOMS

- Fever
- Uterine tenderness
- Foul discharge

TREATMENT

- Broad-spectrum antibiotics

PEARLS

- Chlamydia and gonorrhea are often asymptomatic in women.

- Gonorrhea may be asymptomatic in women, but is almost always symptomatic in men.

- The ulcers associated with primary syphilis and granuloma inguinale are painless.

- The ulcers associated with herpes simplex and chancroid are painful.

- The "groove sign" is associated with lymphogranuloma venereum (LGV), and is caused by bulky lymphadenopathy above and below the inguinal ligament.

- Asymptomatic pelvic inflammatory disease (PID) is a major cause of infertility.

- Consider hospitalizing nulliparous women with PID to protect future fertility.

- Many ectopic pregnancies present with a beta-hCG less than 1500.

BIBLIOGRAPHY

Centers for Disease Control and Prevention, Workowski KA, Berman SM: Sexually transmitted diseases treatment guidelines, 2006, *MMWR Recomm Rep* 55:1–94, 2006.

Centers for Disease Control and Prevention (website). Available at www.cdc.gov/std/.

Fauci AS, Braunwald E, Kasper DL et al (eds): *Harrison's principles of internal medicine*, ed 17, New York, 2008, McGraw-Hill.

Marx JA, Hockberger RS, Walls RM (eds): *Rosen's emergency medicine: concepts and clinical practice*, ed 6, Philadelphia, 2006, Mosby.

Tintinalli JE, Kelen GD, Stapczynski JS (eds): *Emergency medicine: a comprehensive study guide*, ed 6, New York, 2004, McGraw-Hill.

Questions and Answers

1. Which of the following is true regarding the HELLP syndrome?
   a. occurs in the first trimester
   b. stands for Hypertension, Elevated LDH, Low Platelets
   c. affects 1 : 10,000 pregnancies
   d. does not lead to DIC
   e. may occur in the post-partum period

2. A 20-year-old woman presents with several grouped painful ulcers on her labia that appeared yesterday. She states that she has unprotected sex with several partners. She has never had these symptoms before. The most appropriate treatment for this patient would be:
   a. acyclovir 400 mg three times a day for 7 to 10 days
   b. acyclovir 400 mg three times a day for 3 to 5 days
   c. valacyclovir 500 mg two times a day for 3 days
   d. benzathine penicillin G 2.4 million units IM as a single dose
   e. ceftriaxone 125 mg IM

3. A 34-year-old sexually active woman presents to the emergency department with bulky lymphadenopathy above and below the inguinal ligament. She reports that she had a painless labial ulcer last month. Her symptoms are most likely due to:
   a. *Klebsiella granulomatis*
   b. *Chlamydia trachomatis*
   c. Human papilloma virus (HPV)
   d. *Haemophilus ducreyi*
   e. *Treponema pallidum*

4. New onset of ascites in women between the ages of 55 to 65 years is associated with:
   a. uterine cancer
   b. fibroid tumors
   c. cervical cancer
   d. ovarian cancer
   e. menopause

5. Indications for hospitalization of women with PID include:
   a. nulliparous women
   b. tubo-ovarian abscess
   c. poor compliance
   d. failure of outpatient regimen
   e. all of the above

6. A 19-year-old woman presents to the ED requesting to be checked for STDs. She states that her partner was recently treated for a confirmed case of gonorrhea. She denies any vaginal discharge, abdominal pain, genital lesions, or fever. On examination, her vital signs are within normal limits. Her pelvic examination reveals a yellow white discharge from the cervix. What percentage of women with gonococcal cervicitis are asymptomatic?
   a. 10% to 15%
   b. 20%
   c. 30% to 40%
   d. 90%

7. Which STD is associated with an increased risk of cervical cancer?
   a. HPV
   b. chlamydia
   c. syphilis
   d. PID
   e. gonorrhea

8. A 21-year-old woman presents complaining of a frothy, malodorous, grey-green vaginal discharge for 3 days. She denies any abdominal pain, nausea, or vomiting. Her vital signs are temperature (T) = 98.7° F, heart rate (HR) = 65 beats per minute (bpm), blood pressure (BP) = 100/60 mmHg. Pelvic examination is significant for copious frothy discharge and the wet mount reveal multiple, mobile, flagellated organisms. What is the characteristic description of the cervix in this condition?
   a. friable
   b. vesicular
   c. strawberry
   d. geographic

9. Missed abortion is defined as:
   a. fetal demise before 20 weeks and no passage of tissue within 1 week of demise
   b. fetal demise before 20 weeks and no passage of tissue within 4 weeks of demise
   c. fetal demise before 20 weeks and no passage of tissue with in 2 weeks of demise
   d. fetal demise after 20 weeks and no passage of tissue within 2 weeks of demise
   e. fetal demise after 20 weeks and no passage of tissue within 4 weeks of demise

10. A 36-year-old woman presents complaining of a thick white curd-like itchy discharge for 1 week. She denies recent intercourse and has no history of STDs. She has a history of diabetes that she admits is poorly controlled. She denies abdominal pain, fevers, nausea, or vomiting. Her vital signs are T = 97.9° F, HR = 96 bpm, BP = 140/78 mmHg, respiratory rate (RR) = 12/minute. Her blood glucose level in the ED is 397 mg/dL. Her pelvic examination is significant for erythema and excoriation of the labia and a thick white discharge from the vagina. Wet

mount shows multiple budding hyphae. Which of the following is NOT a risk factor for this condition?

a. recent antibiotic use
b. diabetes
c. hypertension
d. tight clothes
e. oral contraceptives

11. Placing the mother in an extreme knee-chest position and applying suprapubic pressure in an attempt to reduce shoulder dystocia is known as the:

a. McRoberts maneuver
b. Rubin maneuver
c. Mauriceau maneuver
d. McNamara maneuver
e. McBurney corkscrew

12. A 28-year-old woman presents to the ED in acute distress from left-sided abdominal pain that she states started 20 minutes prior to arrival. Patient states that she was having sexual intercourse when she developed a severe constant LLQ pain. She reports several episodes of nonbloody, nonbilious vomiting. She has a history of ovarian cysts and had her right ovary removed due to "a problem with cysts." She has noticed brief episodes of similar pain on the left side while exercising in the past 2 weeks. In the ED, she is in acute distress and vomiting. Her vital signs are T = 99.8° F, HR = 120 bpm, BP = 140/60 mmHg, and RR = 28/minute. Her urine pregnancy test is negative. This patient's presentation is most concerning for:

a. ruptured Bartholin's cyst
b. ectopic pregnancy
c. PID
d. ovarian torsion
e. pyosalpinx

13. An 18-year-old girl has just undergone emergent delivery of a full-term baby in the ED. After delivery of the placenta, brisk painless bleeding continues. The patient denies pain and remains hemodynamically stable. The most common causes of postpartum hemorrhage include:

a. uterine atony
b. birth trauma
c. retained placenta
d. all of the above

14. Fetal malpresentation complicates what percentage of births?

a. 0.3%
b. 1%
c. 4%
d. 10%
e. 14%

15. A key component of making the diagnosis of abruptio placentae is a history of painful vaginal bleeding in the third trimester and what modality?

a. fetal cardiotocographic monitoring for fetal distress
b. ultrasound
c. speculum examination
d. digital examination
e. MRI

16. A 17-year-old girl is brought in by friends after she passed out at the mall. The patient is now awake and alert and is complaining of mild left lower pelvic pain. She says that her period has been irregular but she thinks it is starting today because she noticed some spotting this morning. Her vital signs are T = 99.9° F, HR = 75 bpm, BP = 95/40 mmHg, and RR = 18/minute and her urine pregnancy test is positive. Concerned for ectopic pregnancy, you order a pelvic ultrasound. At what serum beta-hCG should an intrauterine pregnancy (IUP), if present, **absolutely** be visible on transvaginal ultrasound?

a. 1000 mIU/mL
b. 1500 mIU/mL
c. 3000 mIU/mL
d. 4500 mIU/mL

17. A 36-year-old woman G3 P2 at 39 weeks' gestational age presents complaining of painless bright-red blood from her vagina. She has received no prenatal care for this pregnancy and reports intermittent abdominal cramping. Her vital signs are stable and a fetal heart rate is measured at 150 bpm. Her presentation is most concerning for:

a. placenta previa
b. abruptio placentae
c. preterm labor
d. preterm rupture of membranes
e. vasa previa

18. A 39-year-old woman G2P2 who is 3 weeks postpartum presents to the ED by EMS actively having a seizure. The paramedics report that the patient underwent an emergency cesarean section for an unknown complication and that she was given 2 mg of lorazepam in the field, with no cessation of her seizure activity. On arrival, the patient is actively having convulsions and her vital signs are T = 99.9° F, HR = 139 bpm, BP = 168/100 mmHg, RR = 40/minute, O_2 saturation 89% on 15 LPM O_2, with a fingerstick blood glucose level of 120 mg/dL. Which of the following medications, in addition to benzodiazepines, is likely to be most effective in treating her seizures?

a. hydralizine
b. magnesium sulfate
c. calcium gluconate

d. hypertonic saline
e. vitamin B$_6$

19. Which STD has been associated with Reiter syndrome?

    a. trichomonas
    b. gonorrhea
    c. bacterial vaginosis
    d. chlamydia
    e. lymphogranuloma venereum

20. Heterotopic pregnancy, that is, a normal IUP and a second ectopic pregnancy, affects how many pregnancies?

    a. 1:100
    b. 1:1000
    c. 1:5000
    d. 1:20,000
    e. 1:30,000

---

1. Answer: e

The HELLP syndrome stands for **hemolysis, elevated liver enzymes, low platelets**. It occurs after **20 weeks' gestational age** and results from endothelial cell dysfunction. It affects **1:1000 pregnancies,** and complications may include **DIC,** multiorgan failure, and hepatic rupture. It has been reported to occur in the **postpartum period.**

2. Answer: a

This patient is having a primary outbreak of *genital herpes simplex*. This is treated for **7 to 10 days** with **acyclovir, famciclovir,** or **valacyclovir.** Shorter durations of treatment are used for recurrent outbreaks **(b, c). Benzathine penicillin G** is used for the treatment of syphilis **(d),** and **ceftriaxone** at this dose is used for simple gonococcal cervicitis, urethritis, proctitis, pharyngitis, or chancroid **(e).**

3. Answer: b

This patient is suffering from *lymphogranuloma venereum (LGV)*, which may present with either a painless vesicle, pustule, or ulcer on labia 7 to 21 days post-exposure, or 2 to 12 weeks later with bulky lymphadenopathy on either side of the inguinal ligament (the "groove sign"). LGV is caused by *C. trachomatis* and is treated with 21 days of oral doxycycline. *Klebsiella granulomatis* causes granuloma inguinale **(a),** and **HPV** causes condyloma acuminata **(c).** *Haemophilus ducreyi* **(d)** causes chancroid, which is characterized by a painful ulcer. Syphilis, caused by *Treponema pallidum* **(e),** may present with a painless ulcer but does not cause the bulky, inguinal adenopathy characteristic of LGV.

4. Answer: d

Ovarian cancer affects 1% to 2% of women with no family history of the disease and carries a 50% mortality. The slow-growing nature of the cancer often results in delayed diagnosis. New-onset ascites

in a woman 55 to 65 years of age is considered ovarian cancer until proven otherwise.

5. Answer: e

Other considerations include pregnancy, inability to exclude a surgical emergency (e.g., appendicitis), inability to tolerate oral medications, and HIV-positive patients.

6. Answer: c

Thirty percent to 40% of women with gonococcal cervicitis may be asymptomatic as opposed to men with gonococcal urethritis, who are symptomatic in 80% to 90% of cases. A high index of suspicion is necessary, and if there is any doubt regarding the possibility of the diagnosis clinicians should err on the side of treatment.

7. Answer: a

Human papilloma virus infection (genital warts) with HPV subtypes 16 and 18 carries an increased risk of cervical cancer.

8. Answer: c

This patient has *trichomonas vaginitis*. The classic description is of a **strawberry cervix.** A copious amount of frothy, malodorous discharge is also common. The diagnosis is confirmed by the presence of mobile trichomonads seen on wet mount. Treatment is generally a single-dose 2-g oral dose of metronidazole.

9. Answer: b

10. Answer: c

This patient has *candida vaginitis*. Commonly known as a "yeast-infection," common risk factors include **recent antibiotic use, diabetes, steroid use, oral contraceptives,** and **tight clothing. Hypertension** is not a known risk factor. Not considered a sexually transmitted disease, treatment for this entity is with topical or oral antifungal agents.

11. Answer: a

Dystocia is a rare complication of delivery in which a fetal part becomes impacted on the maternal pelvis and prevents delivery. Shoulder dystocia is the most common form. It affects 0.3% of deliveries. The **McRoberts maneuver,** as described, is the most common method to attempt to relieve the dystocia. **Rubin maneuver,** also used in dystocia, involves pushing the accessible shoulder toward the chest and a corkscrew movement to facilitate delivery. **Mauriceau maneuver** is used in a breech delivery and involves placing a finger in the fetal mouth to attempt to tuck the chin and deliver the head. The last two options do not exist.

12. Answer: d

The presentation is most concerning for **ovarian torsion.** Twisting of the vascular pedicle of the ovary compromises blood flow and causes sudden onset of unilateral severe pain. Risk factors include ovarian cysts or masses that may predispose to twisting. Ovarian torsion represents a true gynecologic emergency requiring surgical intervention to preserve fertility, especially in this patient who has but one ovary. Diagnosis is confirmed by vascular ultrasound showing impaired flow to the affected ovary, and treatment is surgical.

13. Answer: d

Postpartum hemorrhage complicates approximately 6% of all deliveries and is defined as blood loss of 500 mL or more. It may be acute or delayed. Management focuses on uterine massage, the use of oxytocin to stimulate uterine contraction, laceration repair, and evacuation of retained products.

14. Answer: c

15. Answer: a

Fetal distress is one of the best indicators of abruptio placentae in the setting of painful vaginal bleeding in the third trimester. **Ultrasound** may help with the diagnosis but may miss a concealed abruption. **Speculum and digital examinations** are generally to be avoided in the setting of third-trimester bleeding because of concern for placenta previa, and **MRI** does not have a role.

16. Answer: c

The serum level of beta-hCG at which an IUP can be visualized on either transabdominal or transvaginal ultrasound is called the discriminatory zone. At a **beta-hCG of 1500 mIU/mL,** an IUP can be seen with transvaginal ultrasound. At a beta-hCG level of **6000 mIU/mL** an IUP can be visualized with transabdominal ultrasound. At a **beta-hCG of 3000 mIU/mL if an IUP is present it should absolutely be visible on transvaginal ultrasound.** If the beta-hCG is 3000 mIU/mL or greater and no IUP is seen, it is highly suspicious for an ectopic pregnancy.

17. Answer: a

Painless bright-red bleeding in the third trimester is most concerning for **placenta previa.** Placenta previa occurs when the placenta implants over the cervical os partially or completely. The diagnosis is made by ultrasound and requires delivery by cesarean section. Internal vaginal examination is contraindicated.

18. Answer: b

This patient is most likely presenting with *eclampsia.* Pre-eclampsia affects 5% to 10% of pregnancies, typically after 20 weeks' gestational age. Hypertension, proteinuria, and peripheral edema are the characteristic findings. Eclampsia is the development of seizures in the pre-eclamptic patient. Both conditions may present up to 6 weeks postpartum. Treatment of eclampsia focuses on the use of benzodiazepines and **magnesium sulfate.**

19. Answer: d

Reiter syndrome is a triad of symptoms that include arthritis, urethritis, and conjunctivitis, and has been associated with **chlamydial infections.**

20. Answer: c

Heterotopic pregnancies, although rare, have increased in frequency with the advent and increased usage of fertility treatment. They are thought to affect **1:5000 pregnancies.**

Addictive behavior

SUBSTANCE ABUSE

SIGNS AND SYMPTOMS

- Acute substance use, intoxication, or withdrawal

DIAGNOSIS

- Recurrent substance use resulting in role failure at work, school, or home
- Recurrent substance use in physically hazardous situations
- Recurrent substance-related legal problems
- Continued substance use despite persistent social or interpersonal problems

TREATMENT

- Detoxification with agent of abuse-specific medication
- Prevention of relapse with pharmacologic prevention and behavior therapy

DRUG DEPENDENCE

DIAGNOSIS

- Tolerance requiring increased drug amounts or diminished effect with same amount
- Withdrawal causing clinical syndrome or requiring similar substance to avoid withdrawal symptoms
- Substance taken in larger quantities and for a longer time than intended
- A great deal of time is spent to obtain the substances
- Loss of social, occupational, or recreational activities because of use
- Continued use despite knowledge of physical or psychological dependence

TREATMENT

- Detoxification with agent of abuse-specific medication
- Prevention of relapse with pharmacologic prevention and behavior therapy

ALCOHOL DEPENDENCE

SIGNS AND SYMPTOMS

- Intoxication symptoms such as impaired social and occupational functioning, labile mood, poor judgment, slurred speech, incoordination, unsteady

gait, nystagmus, impairment in attention or memory, or stupor or coma
- Withdrawal symptoms such as psychomotor distress; visual, auditory, and tactile hallucinations; autonomic hyperactivity (tachycardia and diaphoresis); nausea and vomiting; tremors and seizures; and mentally, emotionally, and physically unstable

DIAGNOSIS

- Recent use of alcohol
- Clinically significant maladaptive behavior or psychological changes during or after use
- Signs and symptoms of alcohol intoxication or withdrawal
- Symptoms are not the result of another medical or psychiatric condition

TREATMENT

- Detoxification with benzodiazepines as needed
- Prevention of relapse with pharmacologic prevention (e.g., naltrexone, acamprosate, disulfiram, and topiramate), and behavior or support therapy (e.g., Alcoholics Anonymous)

EATING DISORDERS

- Affect 5% to 10% of young women; 0.1% of males. Found across all racial and socioeconomic groups and in patients between the ages of 8 and 80. The onset of anorexia is usually between the ages of 12 to mid-30s; onset of bulimia is between the ages of 17 and 25

Anorexia nervosa

SIGNS AND SYMPTOMS

- Weight loss of unknown origin
- Exercise or laxative abuse
- Membership in a weight-restricted group (e.g., models, wrestlers, ballet dancers, jockeys)
- Unexplained growth retardation or primary amenorrhea
- Unexplained hypercholesterolemia or carotenemia in a thin person

DIAGNOSIS

- Refusal to maintain minimum body weight expected for age and height leading to body weight 15% below expected
- Intense fear of becoming overweight even when underweight
- Perception disturbance in body weight, shape, or size
- Absence of at least three consecutive expected menstrual cycles

TREATMENT

- Nutritional rehabilitation; may require total parenteral nutrition with hospitalization

- Psychiatric interventions: medication and counseling
- Hospitalization
  - Weight loss >30% over 3 months, severe metabolic derangements, suicide risk, psychosis, outpatient failure

Bulimia nervosa

SIGNS AND SYMPTOMS

- Weight loss or weight fluctuation of unknown origin
- Parotid or submandibular gland swelling, esophageal injuries from repeated vomiting
- Membership in a weight-restricted group (e.g., models, wrestlers, ballet dancers, jockeys)
- Unexplained hypokalemia, secondary amenorrhea
- Loss of dental enamel or scars on the knuckles of the hand

DIAGNOSIS

- A minimum average of two binge eating episodes per week for at least 3 months
- Lack of control over behavior during binge episodes
- Perception disturbance in body weight, shape, or size
- Self-induced vomiting, use of laxatives, dieting or fasting, and excessive exercising

TREATMENT

- Nutritional rehabilitation
- Medication with antidepressants (e.g., consider SSRIs such as fluoxetine)
- Psychiatric counseling

Mood disorders

- Most prevalent of the major psychiatric disorders, affecting about 10% to 15% of the general population. Depressive disorders are the major cause of completed suicide

MAJOR DEPRESSION

- More common in women or people with a family history; lifetime risk of suicide is 15%

SIGNS AND SYMPTOMS

- Thoughts and feelings (psychologic)
  - Lack of interest (anhedonia), guilt, feelings of worthlessness and hopelessness, inability to experience pleasure, recurrent thoughts of death or suicide, psychotic features may be present
- Physiologic
  - Loss (or gain in atypical variant) of appetite and weight, fatigue, sleep disturbance, insomnia, inability to concentrate, psychomotor agitation and retardation, vague weakness, or somatic pain

DIAGNOSIS

- Persistent sad mood or pervasive loss of interest in usual activities, lasting for at least 2 weeks characterized by the above symptoms and low self-esteem

TREATMENT

- Assessment of suicide risk
- Antidepressant medications
- Emergent psychotherapy referral

SUICIDAL RISK

- Men are two to three times more likely to complete suicide than women; women are two to three times more likely to attempt than men

Risk factors

- Separated, divorced, or widowed marital status
- Family history of suicide; family conflict or chaos
- Unemployed job status or socially isolated
- Recent conflict or loss of a relationship
- Disciplinary or legal trouble
- Physical health conditions such as acute or chronic illness or substance abuse
- Mental health conditions such as mood disorder (depression/bipolar), somatoform disorder, or thought disorder (schizophrenia)
- Frequent, intense, or prolonged suicidal ideation
- Suicide attempts that are repeated, realistic, high risk; or with persistent guilt or wish to die
- Religion without suicide taboo

DIAGNOSIS

- Most threatening risk factors prior to completion of suicide
  - Suicide attempt with violent or lethal means (hanging, shooting)
  - Accidental discovery of a suicide attempt
  - Elderly men with suicidal ideation or attempt
  - Suicidal ideation with a clear plan, a history of previous attempts, or possession of weapons
- Most common risk factors presenting as suicide evaluation
  - Depressive thoughts or expressions ("Life is not worth living")
  - Suicidal gestures such as nonlethal ingestions
  - Cutting/self-mutilators with multiple hesitancy marks
  - Threat of suicide for secondary gain

TREATMENT

- Assessment of lethality of suicide attempt
  - Trauma: evaluate for use of weapons (gun, knife, or blunt) or ligature marks (neck)
  - Medical: evaluate for ingestions
- Identify what substance, amount and time
- Consider drug and toxicology levels, screens, or antidotes as needed

- Closely monitored suicide precautions with physical or chemical restraints as needed
- Medications for rapid tranquilization (benzodiazepines and/or antidepressants) as needed
- Emergency involuntary commitment for psychotherapy referral

BIPOLAR DISORDER

- Previously called manic/depressive disorder; characterized by alternating mania and depression (depressive episodes more common); equal gender predilection; complications include suicide and substance abuse

SIGNS AND SYMPTOMS—MANIA

- Thoughts and feelings (psychologic)
  - Elation or irritability
  - Expansive; "on top of the world"
  - Delusions of grandeur, where patients believe they may be famous, wealthy, or blessed with special powers or abilities
  - Poor judgment, e.g., spending all of their money or risky hypersexual behaviors
  - Labile personality; become argumentative, hostile, or sarcastic if plans become undone
  - Psychotic features may be present (if mixed mood and thought disorder)
- Physiologic
  - Rapid pressured speech, racing thoughts ("flight of ideas"), decreased need for sleep or energetic, increased activity or psychomotor agitation

DIAGNOSIS

- Clinical diagnosis of one or more abnormal episodes of elevated mood termed mania (or less severe termed hypomania) in a patient who has a history of or will have future episodes of depressed mood

TREATMENT

- Assessment of suicide risk and evaluation of risky behaviors and consequences
- Bipolar medications or medications for rapid tranquilization if danger
- Emergent psychotherapy referral

DYSTHYMIC DISORDER

SIGNS AND SYMPTOMS

- Lifelong gloomy outlook/pessimistic; psychotic features not seen

DIAGNOSIS

- Chronic and less severe depressed mood present most of the day, more days than not, for 2 years

TREATMENT

- Assessment of suicide risk
- Antidepressant medications (patient's own)
- Psychotherapy referral

GRIEF REACTION

SIGNS AND SYMPTOMS

- Acute
  - Initial 5- to 15-minute "psychic pain spike," in which bereaved cannot process decisions
  - Denial, anger, bargaining, guilt, and then acceptance
- Normal grieving (can last 6 to 8 months)
  - Physical
    - Headache, irritability, fatigue, insomnia, restlessness, dyspnea, anorexia
  - Emotional
    - Guilt, denial, anger, depression, difficulty concentrating, lack of organization and preoccupation with the deceased
- Pathologic grieving (8 months and beyond or heightened intensity of symptoms)
  - Include heightened intensity of physical and emotional symptoms of normal grieving
  - Physical disability, apathy, panic attacks, overactivity, hostility with paranoia, flat affect, symptoms resembling those of the deceased

DIAGNOSIS

- Clinical

TREATMENT

- Recognize survivors at risk for pathologic grief
  - Sudden or unexpected death, death of infant or child, death related to homicide or suicide, and spousal death

Acute

- Facilitate the acute grieving steps or process (without tranquilization, which impedes the normal grieving time and process) and address survivor's guilt
- Allow an opportunity for viewing the prepared deceased
- Concluding process (autopsy, organ donation, funeral home arrangements, release of the body to the family, and release of the family from the ED to home)

Normal grieving

- Recognition, reassurance, and psychological referral

Pathologic grieving

- Tranquilization with benzodiazepines as needed, address high risks (e.g., suicide) and comprehensive psychotherapy plan

Thought disorders

- Psychotic features in thought disorders include delusions and hallucinations
  - *Delusions* are fixed false beliefs not shared by others of a similar cultural background. Delusions include several types, including those of persecution, grandeur, or bizarre type
  - *Hallucinations* are false perceptions occurring in clear consciousness; auditory are the most common in thought disorders, followed by visual, tactile, olfactory, and gustatory

SCHIZOPHRENIA

- The most prevalent psychosis. Usually begins in late adolescence or early adulthood. Schizophrenics constitute a large portion of the chronic homeless population

SIGNS AND SYMPTOMS

- Social withdrawal
- Poor insight into disease process
- Pervasive impairment in self-care, work, and social relations
- Positive symptoms
  - Delusions
  - Hallucinations
  - Disorganized thought (e.g., loose associations: unconnected illogical thoughts)
  - Disorganized speech or behavior
  - Catatonia: extreme motor immobility or purposeless hyperactivity; resistance to being moved; mutism; or repeating sounds (echolalia) or movements (echopraxia)
- Negative symptoms
  - Flat or blunted affect
  - Poverty of speech (alogia)
  - Inability to experience pleasure (anhedonia)
  - Lack of motivation (avolition)

DIAGNOSIS

- Deterioration in functioning in the presence of positive or negative symptoms for most of the time for at least 1 month continuously
- Self-care, social or occupational dysfunction during the illness much below patient's baseline
- Persistent signs of the disturbance in the duration of at least 6 months
- No mood or developmental disorder can be present; diagnosis cannot be as a result of a general medical condition or a substance
- Subtypes
  - Paranoid type: delusions of persecution and hallucinations
  - Disorganized type: disorganized thought, speech, behavior, and flat affect
  - Catatonic type: catatonic stupor and waxy flexibility
  - Undifferentiated type: psychotic symptoms present but not in previous subtypes
  - Residual type: positive symptoms present in low intensity

TREATMENT

- Ensure patient and staff safety if patient agitated or assaultive

- Antipsychotic medications usually reduce the severity of positive (not negative) symptoms
- Emergency psychiatry referral for dangerous and risky behavior or suicide risk
- Benzodiazepines for active catatonia symptoms

ACUTE PSYCHOTIC EPISODE/BRIEF PSYCHOTIC DISORDER

SIGNS AND SYMPTOMS

- Psychosis, emotional turmoil, confusion, and bizarre speech and behavior

DIAGNOSIS

- Psychotic episode for less than 4 weeks
- Psychosis occurring after exposure to an extremely traumatic life experience (family death, natural disaster, or military combat)

TREATMENT

- Ensure patient and staff safety if patient agitated or assaultive
- Antipsychotic medications usually reduce the severity of positive (not negative) symptoms
- Emergency psychiatry referral for dangerous and risky behavior or suicide risk

DELUSIONAL DISORDER

SIGNS AND SYMPTOMS

- Delusions

DIAGNOSIS

- Different from schizophrenia because of less bizarre delusions overall
- Rare impairment in daily functioning, interpersonal relationships, or occupation
- Delusional disorder subtypes
  - Delusions of persecution: patient feels conspired against, poisoned, followed, or cheated
  - Delusions of jealousy: unsubstantiated conviction of an unfaithful partner
  - Somatic delusions: unsubstantiated belief of emitting a foul odor or infested with insects

TREATMENT

- Ensure patient and staff safety if patient agitated and assaultive
- Antipsychotic medications usually reduce the severity of positive (not negative) symptoms
- Emergency psychiatry referral for dangerous and risky behavior or suicide risk

Organic psychoses

CHRONIC ORGANIC PSYCHOTIC CONDITIONS

SIGNS AND SYMPTOMS

- Global impairment in cognitive function and memory

DIAGNOSIS

- Clinical diagnosis due to a general medical condition

TREATMENT

- Identify the underlying etiology
- Symptomatic and supportive care with special attention to patient and staff safety using physical and chemical restraints as needed

DELIRIUM

SIGNS AND SYMPTOMS

- Rapid global impairment in cognitive function
- Clouding of consciousness resulting in a decreased awareness of the external environment
- Difficulty sustaining attention
- Varying degrees of alertness ranging from drowsiness, stupor, and sensory misperception
- Vivid visual hallucinations that cause the patient to react strongly
- Extreme changes in psychomotor activity ranging from restlessness and hyperactivity to stupor

DIAGNOSIS

- Acute, rapid global impairment in cognitive function with rapid deterioration in hours or days, where the severity of illness fluctuates over the course of hours

TREATMENT

- Identify the underlying etiology
- Symptomatic and supportive care, with special attention to patient and staff safety using physical and chemical restraints as needed

INTOXICATION

SIGNS AND SYMPTOMS

- Impairment of judgment, perception, attention, emotional control, or psychomotor activity
- Stigmata of substance abuse (e.g., crack pipe, heroin needles, bottles of alcohol)
- Specific intoxication of drugs of abuse
  - Sympathomimetics (e.g., cocaine/amphetamine): tachycardia, hypertension, sweating, pupillary dilation, agitation
  - Opiates (e.g., heroin): respiratory depression, coma, pupillary constriction
  - Hallucinogens (e.g., LSD, mushrooms) or dissociatives (e.g., ketamine, PCP): hallucinations or altered sense of reality
  - Ethanol: ataxia, slurred speech, fetor of ethanol, coma
  - Toxic alcohols (same as ethanol plus):
    - Methanol—blindness, abdominal pain
    - Ethylene glycol—renal failure
    - Isopropyl alcohol—profound drunken state
  - Anticholinergics (e.g., jimson weed): mental status change ("mad as a hatter"); pupillary

dilation ("blind as a bat"); hyperpyrexia ("hot as a hare"); dry skin ("dry as a bone")
  ■ Depressants (e.g., benzodiazepines, barbiturates, and GHB): respiratory depression, coma

DIAGNOSIS

■ Recent ingestion of specific substance produces maladaptive behavior and clinical symptoms
■ Patient admission of substance
■ Laboratory analysis (e.g., serum alcohol level or urine presence of drugs of abuse) as needed
■ Clinical diagnosis by toxidrome or by antidote success (e.g., naloxone treatment for opiates)

TREATMENT

■ Identify the underlying substance and use antidotes if needed
  ■ Sympathomimetics (e.g., cocaine and amphetamine): treat with benzodiazepines
  ■ Opiates (e.g., heroin): treat with naloxone
  ■ Hallucinogens (e.g., LSD, mushrooms) or dissociatives (e.g., ketamine, PCP): treat with benzodiazepines, antipsychotics, or supportive care
  ■ Ethanol: treat symptomatically; toxic alcohols: treat with ethanol or fomepizole
  ■ Anticholinergics (e.g., jimson weed): treat symptomatically, consider physostigmine if severe and life threatening
  ■ Depressants (e.g., benzodiazepines, barbiturates, and GHB): Treat supportively with attention to respiratory depression
■ Symptomatic, supportive care with special attention to patient and staff safety using physical and chemical restraints as needed

WITHDRAWAL

SIGNS AND SYMPTOMS

■ Impairment of judgment, perception, attention, emotional control, or psychomotor activity
■ Stigmata of substance abuse (e.g., crack pipe, heroin needles, bottles of alcohol)
■ Alcohol withdrawal and delirium tremens continuum
  ■ Confusion, hallucination, tachycardia, agitation, tremor, diaphoresis, seizure, coma

DIAGNOSIS

■ Acute cessation or reduction in use of a substance of abuse
■ Alcohol withdrawal and delirium tremens continuum (four stages)
  ■ Autonomic hyperactivity (sweating, tremors, tachycardia 6 to 8 hours after ETOH cessation) = withdrawal
  ■ Hallucinations (24 hours after ethanol cessation) = delirium tremens
  ■ Major motor seizures (1 to 2 days after ethanol cessation) = delirium tremens
  ■ Global confusion (3 to 5 days after ethanol cessation) = delirium tremens

TREATMENT

■ Identify the underlying substance
■ Symptomatic and supportive care with special attention to patient and staff safety using physical and chemical restraints as needed
■ Treat alcohol withdrawal with benzodiazepines (e.g., chlordiazepoxide, lorazepam) and consider in- or outpatient management depending on the patient's examination, vital signs, and response to treatment
■ Treat delirium tremens with benzodiazepines and admit to the intensive care unit

Factitious disorders

DRUG-SEEKING BEHAVIOR

SIGNS AND SYMPTOMS

■ Multiple doctor visits to obtain prescriptions for controlled substances
■ Multiple somatic complaints and vague symptom complexes
■ Overreporting of symptoms and multiple drug allergies
■ Insistence on specific medications and refusal of generic equivalents
■ Arguments about pharmacology, polypharmacy demands, and veiled threats
■ Self-asserted high tolerance
■ Flattery followed by prescription requests
■ Lost or stolen prescriptions

DIAGNOSIS

■ Clinical

TREATMENT

■ Ensure no new or worse disease process exists
■ Contact personal physician, pharmacy, or previous medical records/visits

MUNCHAUSEN SYNDROME

SIGNS AND SYMPTOMS

■ Exaggerations of symptoms of a previously diagnosed illness or those difficult to disprove
  ■ Include pain syndromes, suicidality, pseudoneurologic symptoms, intentionally misusing medications
■ Male predominance

DIAGNOSIS

■ Extreme form of feigning illness ("career medical imposter")
■ Aware of deception but helpless to control behavior (compulsion)

TREATMENT

■ Ensure no new or worse disease process exists
■ Contact personal physician, pharmacy, or previous medical records and visits

MUNCHAUSEN-BY-PROXY

SIGNS AND SYMPTOMS

- Exaggerations of symptoms of a previously diagnosed illness or those difficult to disprove
- Female predominance

DIAGNOSIS

- Feigning physical or psychiatric illness in a child by the child's guardian
- Can be active (symptom production) or passive (neglect) and represents child abuse

TREATMENT

- Ensure no new or worse disease process exists
- Contact personal physician, pharmacy, or previous medical records and visits
- Extended child abuse evaluation, including reporting to protective services and authorities

MALINGERING

SIGNS AND SYMPTOMS

- Exaggerations of symptoms of a previously diagnosed illness or those difficult to disprove

DIAGNOSIS

- Feigning illness for the purpose of avoiding something unpleasant or to gain some reward
- Aware of deception and in control of the behavior

TREATMENT

- Ensure no new or worse disease process exists
- Contact personal physician, pharmacy or previous medical records and visits

Neurotic disorders

ANXIETY

- Defined as an unpleasant emotional state consisting of psychological and physiological responses to the anticipation of real or imagined danger
- Seen more frequently in women
- Anxiety disorders account for the most common psychiatric illnesses diagnosed in children, adolescents, and older adults

SIGNS AND SYMPTOMS

- Physical signs
  - Autonomic physiologic response
- Diaphoresis, tachycardia, tachypnea, tremor
  - Fight-or-flight awareness response
- Avoidance, hypervigilance, restlessness, pressured speech, startle response
- Somatic symptoms
  - Cardiovascular system (CVS): chest pain, palpitations, dyspnea
  - Central nervous system (CNS): headache, lightheadedness, paresthesias
  - Gastrointestinal system (GI): abdominal pain, nausea, frequent stools, and flatulence
  - Genitourinary system (GU): frequent urination, erectile dysfunction, a/dysmenorrhea
  - General: dry mouth, choking sensation, muscle tightness, fatigue
- Cognitive symptoms
  - Examples include intrusive and racing thoughts, irritability, fear, emotional lability, amnesia, apprehension, depersonalization, derealization, distractibility, flashback images

DIAGNOSIS

- *Generalized anxiety disorder:* at least 6 months of persistent and excessive anxiety
- *Panic attack:* a short period of sudden onset of intense worry, fear, and terror accompanied by feelings of impending doom
- *Panic disorder:* recurrent, unexpected panic attacks with persistent concern
- *Obsessive–compulsive disorder:* characterized by anxiety-provoking obsessive thoughts requiring repetitious anxiety-calming compulsions (actions) that interferes with interpersonal relationships (e.g., being late for work because of checking the pilot light on the stove five times in a row for fear of a fire)
- *Post-traumatic stress disorder:* recurrent experiencing of an extremely traumatic event accompanied by symptoms of increased arousal and avoidance of event-associated stimuli
- *Acute stress disorder:* symptoms occur immediately after an extremely traumatic event
- *Agoraphobia:* anxiety and subsequent avoidance of situations or places from which escape or help may be difficult
- *Social phobia:* significant anxiety provoked by exposure to social or performance situations leading to avoidance behavior
- *Specific phobia:* significant anxiety provoked by exposure to a specific and identifiable fear, object, or situation leading to avoidance behavior
- Anxiety disorder related to a general medical condition or substance abuse

TREATMENT

- Calm, quiet room with the use of an empathetic tone and willingness to listen
- Ensure no medical or organic disease process exists
- Benzodiazepines are first-line agents for pharmacologic management
- Address homicidal or suicidal ideation, self-care ability, and presence of reliable follow-up

Patterns of violence, abuse, and neglect

THE VIOLENT, AGITATED, AND HOSTILE PATIENT

- 90% cases involve the patient; 10% involve the patient's family/visitors

SIGNS AND SYMPTOMS

- Risk factors
  - Evidence of agitation (e.g., pacing, yelling, pronounced hand gestures, restlessness)
  - Substance abuse
  - Escalating psychiatric illness (paranoid schizophrenia, personality disorders, or mania)
  - Prior history of violence
  - Arrival to the ED in police custody
  - Male gender

DIAGNOSIS

- Clinical

TREATMENT

- De-escalation techniques (do's)
  - Disrobe (and gown) and disarm all patients (metal detectors)
  - Set aside an examination room where objects in the room cannot be used as weapons
  - Remove all your own personal objects (e.g., stethoscope) that could be used as a weapon
  - Ensure patient comfort (e.g., food, blankets)
  - Use a calm voice, explain plan or delays, and set limits for inappropriate behavior
- De-escalation techniques (do not's)
  - Block exits or leave the patient between you and the exit
  - Shout, yell, argue or challenge the patient
  - Allow your emotions to affect your judgment and professionalism
- Ensure no underlying treatable and reversible medical condition
  - Glucose abnormalities, trauma, abnormal temperature, infection, hypoxia or hypercarbia, delirium
- Physical and chemical restraints (e.g. butyrophenones [e.g., haloperidol] or benzodiazepines [e.g., lorazepam]) when needed with a clear plan and at least one person per extremity
- Emergency psychiatric referral as indicated

HOMICIDAL RISK

SIGNS AND SYMPTOMS

- Family history of conflict or chaos
- Unemployed job status or socially isolated
- Recent conflict or loss of a relationship
- Disciplinary or legal trouble
- Physical health conditions such as acute or chronic illness or substance abuse
- Mental health conditions such as mood disorder (depression/bipolar), somatoform disorder, thought disorder (paranoid schizophrenia), or personality disorder (antisocial)
- Frequent, intense, or prolonged homicidal ideation with a plan or means

DIAGNOSIS

- Clinical

TREATMENT

- Evaluate for underlying and reversible medical condition (e.g., delirium)
- Closely monitored homicidal precautions with physical or chemical restraints as needed
- Medications for rapid tranquilization (benzodiazepines and/or antidepressants) as needed
- Emergency involuntary commitment for psychotherapy referral
- Must report the homicidal plan to the individual and the police, overriding patient confidentiality (*Tarasoff vs. Regents of the University of California 1976*)

CHILD ABUSE AND NEGLECT

SIGNS AND SYMPTOMS

- Physical abuse (e.g., shaking, twisting extremities, immersion, burning, bites)
- Sexual abuse
  - Genitourinary symptoms: discharge, bleeding, infections, dysuria
  - Behavior disturbances: masturbation or fondling, sexually oriented or provocative behavior
  - Psychological disturbances: nightmares, regression
- Emotional abuse (e.g., insulting, blaming, or yelling at the child)
- Parental substance abuse
- Physical, nutritional, and emotional neglect: inadequate food, shelter, clothing, health care, or schooling
- Failure to thrive in children (mostly under the age of 3)
  - Poor physical care and hygiene
  - Little subcutaneous tissue, with protruding ribs and loose skin in buttocks
  - Alopecia over a flattened occiput (baby lying on back all day)
  - Varying muscle tone (usually lower extremity hypertonia)
  - Child avoids contact and is irritable
  - Child spends time with hand in mouth and prefers inanimate objects
  - Child has a body mass index less than the 5th percentile for age
- Supervision neglect: burns or fractures from lack of supervision
- Munchausen syndrome by proxy: parent feigning illness in a child to secure contact with health care providers

DIAGNOSIS

- Clinical
  - Retinal hemorrhages in "shaken baby syndrome"
  - Burns: stocking glove pattern of immersion; circumferential cigarette pattern; or metal shape pattern (e.g., irons, radiators)
  - Child or parental behavior suggestive of abuse
  - Pelvic or genital examination with evidence of abuse

- Weight gain after admission is the sine qua non of failure to thrive
- Radiographs
  - Skeletal survey showing multiple fractures in varying stages of healing
  - Spiral or metaphyseal chip fractures
  - Unusual sites of fracture (e.g., ribs, lateral clavicle, sternum, or scapula)
  - Abdominal x-ray showing "double-bubble sign" of duodenal hematoma

TREATMENT

- Treat injuries and illnesses resulting from abuse or neglect and document the ED record
- Hospitalize the child as indicated
- Every case of suspected child abuse must be reported to law enforcement and protective services

INTIMATE PARTNER VIOLENCE

- Defined as a pattern of assault and coercive behaviors that may include physical injury, psychological abuse, sexual assault, progressive social isolation, stalking, deprivation, intimidation, and threats aimed at establishing control over the victimized

SIGNS AND SYMPTOMS

- Characteristic injuries: fingernail abrasions, bites, cigarette burns, strangulation bruises, or rope burns
- Defensive injuries: forearm contusions or fractures
- Central pattern of injuries (e.g., head, neck, face, thorax, or abdominal injuries)
- Inconsistent injuries: contusions or abrasions anatomically inconsistent with reported mechanism of injury
- Multiple injuries in different stages of healing reported as "accidents" or "clumsiness"
- Delayed injuries: victims wait several days before seeking care
- Minor injuries without evidence: frequent ED visits as a "cry for help"
- Suicide attempts
- Obstetric or gynecologic complaints
  - Sexual coercion or rape
  - Unwanted pregnancies; sexually transmitted diseases
  - Pregnancy complications, including abdominal trauma, substance abuse, prenatal neglect
- Inappropriate partner behavior
  - Controlling or abusive
  - Patient's fear of the partner
  - Partner will not allow for private physician communication and will give all responses

DIAGNOSIS

- Clinical history, examination or diagnostic findings suggestive (e.g., x-ray with fractures in different stages of healing)

TREATMENT

- Treat injuries and illnesses resulting from abuse or neglect and document the ED record
- Acknowledgement of violence or abuse and providing insight to the patient about the future health and safety of the patient and children
- Safety assessment of high-risk indicators of potentially lethal situation
  - Escalation of frequency and severity of violence
  - Use of weapons (e.g., firearms)
  - Victim obsession, hostage taking or stalking
  - Homicidal or suicidal threats
  - Substance abuse
- Referral to experts (e.g., social workers, community advocates, mental health care)
- Reporting to law enforcement as required by your local and state regulations

ELDER ABUSE AND NEGLECT

- Approximately 3% of the elderly experience abuse or neglect

SIGNS AND SYMPTOMS

- Physical: hitting, burning, and improper use of restraint
- Sexual: rape, sexual threats, and innuendoes
- Emotional or psychological: threats to institutionalize or withhold medication, food, or water
- Financial or material exploitation: stealing, forgery, financial coercion, or blackmail
- Neglect: withholding meds, food, water, clothing, shelter, supervision, or social support
- Abandonment: desertion by custodian or responsible caregiver
- Self-neglect: failure to provide for one's own mental health and medical care

DIAGNOSIS

- Clinical history
  - Detect presence of caretaker mental illness, drug use, incapacity, or antecedent stress
  - Look for a pattern of family violence
  - Ascertain caretaker dependence on the elder patient for housing and finances
  - Detect risk factors for patient isolation
  - Identify if patient and caregiver live together
- Clinical physical observations
  - Elderly patient fearful of caretaker
  - Conflicting accounts of injury and illness from the patient and caretaker
  - Caretaker is angry or indifferent to the patient
  - Ascertain caretaker dependence on the elder patient for housing and finances
  - Caretaker inappropriately concerned about the cost for treatment
  - Caretaker denies patient–physician private interaction
- Clinical physical examination
  - Mental status examination for medication toxicity or withholding

- Poor hygiene, dehydration, malnutrition, worsening decubiti, soiled clothing
- Unexplained trauma: contusions, fractures, dislocations, burns, lacerations
- Sexually transmitted diseases

TREATMENT

- Ensure no underlying treatable and reversible medical condition
- Treat injuries and illnesses resulting from abuse or neglect and document the ED record
- An intervention including resolution of problems brought on by the caregiver, admitting the elderly patient to the hospital, and mandatory reporting to adult protective services
- Emergency psychiatric referral as indicated

SEXUAL ASSAULT

- 1% of all violent crimes; 90% female assault, 10% male assault. "Rape" is a violent crime motivated by the need for power and control. Lack of genital injuries does not imply consensual intercourse

SIGNS AND SYMPTOMS

- Body trauma: contusions, fractures, abrasions, lacerations, bites
- Genital trauma: oral, vaginal or penile, anal penetration and injuries
- Psychological trauma (e.g., post-traumatic stress, anxiety, shame, or feelings of violation)
- Possible drug abuse, intoxication, or poisoning

DIAGNOSIS

- Assault history
  - Who, what, where, when, drug-facilitated, cleaning (e.g., shower or clothing change)
- Medical history
  - Birth control use, menstrual history, last consensual intercourse, prior sexual assault
- Physical examination
  - Vital signs and level of consciousness
  - Document body trauma in detail on a body map paying careful attention to the face, oral cavity, neck, breasts, wrists, thighs, buttocks, perineum
  - Document pelvic trauma, performing a speculum examination or anoscopy as indicated
- Chain of evidence and sexual assault kit
  - Samples (hair, saliva, urine, blood), swabs (skin, oral, vaginal or penile, anal), clothing

TREATMENT

- Physician must report sexual assault to the police
- Manage the physical injuries and psychological needs
- Pregnancy prophylaxis
  - Ascertain baseline pregnancy status
  - Hormonal therapy with medications for nausea
- Sexually transmitted disease prophylaxis
  - Ascertain baseline pregnancy status
  - Gonorrhea prophylaxis with ceftriaxone
  - Chlamydia prophylaxis with azithromycin or doxycycline
- Hepatitis B prophylaxis with vaccination series as indicated
- HIV postexposure prophylaxis as indicated
- Psychological and social support with rape counselor
- Ensure close follow-up to evaluate injuries, lab results, and psychological needs

Personality disorders

- Personality refers to an enduring pattern of perception, relation, and reaction to one's environment and interpersonal relationships. When a lifelong maladaptive pattern of behavior forms that causes significant social or occupational distress, a personality disorder is present. Patients may or may not be aware of their behavior.

SIGNS AND SYMPTOMS

- Cluster A
  - Eccentric, odd, isolated, withdrawn, suspicious, inhibited, no friends, overly sensitive
- Cluster B
  - Emotional, dramatic, angry, seductive, impulsive, erratic
- Cluster C
  - Anxious, fearful, nervous, cautious

DIAGNOSIS

- Cluster A
  - Paranoid personality: irrational suspicious, mistrust
  - Schizoid: isolated and withdrawn, no interest in social relationships
  - Schizotypal: odd behavior, isolated from social relationships out of fear
- Cluster B
  - Antisocial: maladaptive pattern of disregard for the law and rights of others
    - Disproportionately represented in emergency visits manifested by criminal behavior, lying, abuse and neglect of dependents or spouses, financial irresponsibility, recklessness, and inability to sustain enduring relationships
    - Sociopathic behavior in adolescence, but diagnosis after age of 18
    - More frequent in males, lower socioeconomic class, and families with substance abuse
    - Complications include drug abuse, imprisonment, multiple divorces, traumatic injury, accidental and violent deaths, and poor medical compliance
  - Histrionic: pervasive attention-seeking, sexual seductiveness, shallow or exaggerated emotional behavior
  - Borderline: pervasive instability in relationships, self-image, and identity; interpersonal relationships characterized by "splitting": either "best friend" or "worst enemy" exaggerated dichotomy
  - Narcissistic: pervasive grandiosity, need for admiration, and lack of empathy; self-centered behavior characterized by preoccupation with adequacy, power and prestige

- Cluster C
  - Dependent: psychological dependence on other people and their approval
  - Avoidant: social inhibition, inadequacy, extremely sensitive to negative evaluation
  - Obsessive–compulsive: rigid conformity to rules, moral codes and order; perfectionist

TREATMENT

- Recognition of the disorder and high-risk behavior
- Ensure no medical or organic disease process exists
- Set limits; provide information about medical problems; referral for substance abuse and psychotherapy

Psychosomatic disorders

SOMATIZATION

SIGNS AND SYMPTOMS

- Chronically and persistently "sick" patients with numerous vague complaints involving multiple organ systems
- Patients thrive on "sick role" despite negative evaluations or interventions (diagnostics and surgery)

DIAGNOSIS

- Pain in at least four distinct body locations or conditions
- Two or more nonpainful gastrointestinal symptoms
- One or more sexual dysfunction symptoms
- One or more neurological symptoms
- Symptoms not medically explainable and not feigned by patient

TREATMENT

- Recognition and reassurance after ensuring no serious underlying disease

CONVERSION DISORDER

SIGNS AND SYMPTOMS

- Acute, episodic onset of one sign or symptom involving limited organ systems
- Common symptoms include anesthesia or paresthesia, tremor, paralysis, ataxia, syncope, seizure, vertigo or dizziness, visual changes (diplopia or blindness), deafness, coma, and globus hystericus
- *"La belle indifference,"* characterized by incongruous disinterest in one's own illness

DIAGNOSIS

- Complaints generally sensory-motor with identifiable stressor
- Symptoms not medically explainable and not feigned by patient
- Psychogenic or somatoform pain disorder
  - Conversion limited to pain, usually brought on by stress from a traumatic injury

- Pseudocyesis
  - Conversion related to pregnancy (including amenorrhea) without positive gestation

TREATMENT

- Recognition and reassurance after ensuring no serious underlying disease

HYPOCHONDRIASIS

SIGNS AND SYMPTOMS

- Frequent physician visits and tests at significant time and cost; excessive focusing on symptoms, self-diagnosis, and disbelief in health care professionals' diagnosis

DIAGNOSIS

- Preoccupation with fear of illness despite negative testing and reassurance from a health care professional; or if medical illness is present, concerns are excessive for severity of disease

TREATMENT

- Recognition and reassurance after ensuring no serious underlying disease

BODY DYSMORPHIC DISORDER

SIGNS AND SYMPTOMS

- Typically in women in vocations dealing with body image
- Encountered by plastic surgeons and body enhancement industry

DIAGNOSIS

- Preoccupation with an imagined defect in physical appearance

TREATMENT

- Recognition and reassurance

PEARLS

- Criteria to admit anorexic patients: weight loss >30% over 3 months; severe metabolic derangements; suicide risk; psychosis; or outpatient failure.
- Patients with major depression have a lifetime risk of suicide of 15%.
- Gender and "2-3 times rule": Men are two to three times more likely to complete suicide; women are two to three times more likely to attempt than men.
- The greatest suicide risk would involve an elderly man with a history of previous attempts and a clear plan, accidentally discovered attempting suicide with violent/lethal means.

■ Schizophrenia is the most common psychosis and is characterized by positive and negative symptoms, impairment in daily functioning, and a duration of greater than 6 months of progressive symptoms; schizophreniform disorder is diagnosed when symptoms are present between 1 and 6 months.

■ Delirium is an acute, rapid global impairment in cognitive function with rapid deterioration in hours or days where the severity of illness fluctuates; it differs from dementia in its onset, duration, fluctuations in alertness and awareness of the external environment, psychomotor activity, and visual hallucinations.

■ Neurotic and anxiety disorders are the most common psychiatric illnesses diagnosed in children, adolescents, and older adults.

■ The physician has a duty to report a homicidal plan to the individual being targeted and the police (overriding patient confidentiality).

■ Every case of child or elder abuse must be reported to law enforcement and child-protective services.

■ Somatization disorder is characterized by multiple chronic, vague complaints in differing organ systems where conversion disorder is characterized by acute, episodic complaints limited to specific body parts and predominate with motor and sensory complaints.

BIBLIOGRAPHY

American Psychiatric Association: *Diagnostic and statistical manual of mental disorders*, ed 4, Washington, DC, 2000, American Psychiatric Association.

Berkowitz CD: Child abuse and neglect. In Tintinalli JE, Kelen GD, Stapczynski JS (eds): *Emergency medicine: a comprehensive study guide*, cd 6, New York, 2004, McGraw Hill, pp. 1847–1850.

Borg K: Self-harm and danger to others. In Adams JG, Barton ED, Collings J et al (eds): *Emergency medicine*, ed 1, Philadelphia, 2008, Saunders, pp. 2057–2062.

Brown J, Hamilton G: Breaking bad news: notifying the living of death. In Tintinalli JE, Kelen GD, Stapczynski JS (eds): *Emergency medicine: a comprehensive study guide*, ed 6, New York, 2004, McGraw-Hill, pp. 1832–1834.

Feldhaus KM: Female and male sexual assault. In Tintinalli JE, Kelen GD, Stapczynski JS (eds): *Emergency medicine: a comprehensive study guide*, ed 6, New York, 2004, McGraw-Hill, pp. 1850–1854.

Hutzler JC, Rund DA: Behavioral disorders: emergency assessment and stabilization. In Tintinalli JE, Kelen GD, Stapczynski JS (eds): *Emergency medicine: a comprehensive study guide*, ed 6, New York, 2004, McGraw-Hill, pp. 1812–1815.

Isaacs E: The violent patient. In Adams JG, Barton ED, Collings J et al (eds): *Emergency medicine*, ed 1, Philadelphia, 2008, Saunders, pp. 2047–2056.

Jotte RS: Addiction. In Adams JG, Barton ED, Collings J et al (eds): *Emergency medicine*, ed 1, Philadelphia, 2008, Saunders, pp. 2075–2083.

Kang CS, Harrison BP: Anxiety and panic disorders. In Adams JG, Barton ED, Collings J et al (eds): *Emergency medicine*, ed 1, Philadelphia, 2008, Saunders, pp. 2063–2067.

Marshall RAC: Conversion disorder, psychosomatic illness, and malingering. In Adams JG, Barton ED, Collings J et al (eds): *Emergency medicine*, ed 1, Philadelphia, 2008, Saunders, pp. 2069–2074.

Rund DA: Behavioral disorders: clinical features. In Tintinalli JE, Kelen GD, Stapczynski JS (eds): *Emergency medicine: a comprehensive study guide*, ed 6, New York, 2004, McGraw-Hill, pp. 1807–1812.

Sackeyfio AH, Gottlieb SJ: Anorexia nervosa and anorexia bulimia. In Tintinalli JE, Kelen GD, Stapczynski JS (eds): *Emergency medicine: a comprehensive study guide*, ed 6, New York, 2004, McGraw-Hill, pp. 1822–1825.

Salber PR: Intimate partner violence and abuse. In Tintinalli JE, Kelen GD, Stapczynski JS (eds): *Emergency medicine: a comprehensive study guide*, ed 6, New York, 2004, McGraw-Hill, pp. 1854–1858.

Taliaferro EH: Abuse in the elderly and impaired. In Tintinalli JE, Kelen GD, Stapczynski JS (eds): *Emergency medicine: a comprehensive study guide*, ed 6, New York, 2004, McGraw-Hill, pp. 1858–1860.

Questions and Answers

1. You are evaluating a 19-year-old man who has been brought in to the emergency department by his family for "acting strangely." The patient told his family that he was getting top secret information "from Martians." The family has always thought the patient was eccentric and on examination you also find the patient to have grossly disorganized behavior and speech. You diagnose the patient as having schizophrenia because:

   a. through further questioning he also meets criteria for a mood disorder
   b. he has a stable level of functioning at work and with self-care
   c. he has had the presence of delusions and disorganized behavior and speech for 1 week without treatment
   d. he has had continuous signs of inability to experience pleasure for at least 6 months
   e. he recently started abusing cocaine after he was started on anti-anxiety medicine that was abruptly discontinued

2. You meet a 27-year-old man in the emergency department wearing a batman outfit who tells you he is "going to save Gotham." He has just jumped off a one-story building and on evaluation he is found to have no severe traumatic injuries. In further discussion you learn from the patient and his family that he recently has "maximized his credit card limit with shopping sprees," "talks faster than you can comprehend," and he has been having "one-night stands" with multiple partners. You feel confident in his diagnosis of mania because you also learn:

a. he is planning on writing an epic novel
b. he sleeps all the time
c. he is using methamphetamines
d. he has been having the symptoms for 1 week

3. You have an 18-year-old diabetic girl (only on insulin) who was brought into the emergency department against her will after a hypoglycemic episode. The patient initially told the EMS crew that she refused to come to the hospital because she gets anxious at the hospital. You evaluate the patient and manage her sugar appropriately and there are no further diabetes-related issues. The patient tells you she feels intensely anxious because she feels like she will "never get out of the hospital." The patient tells you she "avoids the hospital at all costs" because she will "never escape." In addition to diabetes-related hypoglycemia you suspect she has:

a. panic attack
b. social phobia
c. agoraphobia
d. anxiety disorder caused by a general medical condition
e. generalized anxiety disorder

4. You evaluate a 35-year-old female patient in the emergency department who has intractable pain and vomiting from gastroparesis. You learn from the patient that she has a hard time feeling good about herself with feelings of emptiness. One month ago she was admitted for mutilating herself. The interview and physical examination are complete and the patient will not let you leave the room because she needs you to know her entire history with the disease. After you communicate your intent to treat her symptoms, she showers you with praise and affection as her favorite doctor. After your treatment plan is complete and her symptoms improve, the patient demands to see you and throws a temper tantrum for abandoning her as you now plan on discharging her from the hospital. The patient is exhibiting signs of:

a. antisocial personality disorder
b. narcissistic personality disorder
c. dependent personality disorder
d. histrionic personality disorder
e. borderline personality disorder

5. You meet a 19-year-old girl with a history of seizures. She casually states that she is about to "catch a seizure" and shows you a tremor in her left hand that gets more intense until her whole body is involved. You note that the patient's head moves side to side, she has uncoordinated movements of the extremities which you can stop, and she has wild pelvic thrusting, which requires more people to assist in her care. The patient's episode is complete and she has no post-ictal phase and she seems unconcerned about the whole experience. You make a diagnosis of pseudo-seizure which is under the category of:

a. somatization disorder
b. conversion disorder
c. factitious disorder
d. malingering
e. Munchausen's syndrome

6. You evaluate an 83-year-old man who presents to the emergency department from an assisted-care home for a "change in mental status." The patient has a history of Alzheimer's dementia and the nursing note only states that he is "acting bizarre" for a few days. You know that he is suffering from delirium rather than a progression of his dementia because:

a. he is not able to learn new information or to recall previously learned information
b. he has a failure to carry out motor activities despite having intact motor function
c. he has an inability to focus attention and has perceptual disturbances (e.g., hallucinations or delusions)
d. he fails to recognize or identify objects
e. he has a language disturbance and cannot plan, organize, or sequence

7. You meet a 22-year-old male medical student who presents to the emergency department telling you he may have a subarachnoid hemorrhage that he has researched while studying in school. The patient has chronic headaches and is preoccupied with what will happen to his career if it is left untreated. He has seen other physicians for this and has had "normal diagnostics" and received "lots of medicines" but his symptoms only come back. Your examination is normal and you diagnose the patient as having:

a. hypochondriasis
b. somatization disorder
c. body dysmorphic disorder
d. conversion disorder
e. narcissistic personality disorder

8. You are approached by a nurse who tells you to quickly see a violent patient. You proceed and see a young male being held down by two police officers. You learn that the patient has been in substance abuse rehabilitation but you don't know what drugs he previously abused. The drug treatment center did send a note stating that he had a seizure moments before they called the police and that he has had no access to acutely ingesting anything. The patient is tachycardic, hypertensive, tremulous, diaphoretic, and having hallucinations. The patient yells that he is "fighting off demons" (who are the officers). For rapid tranquilization, you choose to administer:

a. haloperidol
b. risperidone
c. lorazepam
d. phenytoin

9. You are taking care of 16-year-old teenage girl who is brought in by her parents after referral from her primary medical doctor for weight loss of unknown origin. She is 5 feet 4 inches tall and weighs 80 lbs. The patient has an intense fear of being overweight despite your attempts at convincing her she is under her expected weight. Furthermore, you learned that she has missed three menstrual cycles and the laboratory studies from her doctor's office show hypercholesterolemia and carotenemia. You are certain of her diagnosis because:

   a. she has parotid or submandibular gland swelling
   b. she has perception disturbance in body weight, shape, or size
   c. she is using laxatives
   d. she has loss of dental enamel or scars on the knuckles of the hand
   e. she refuses to maintain a body weight of at least 85 pounds.

10. You evaluate a 74-year-old man who presents to the emergency department after a suicide attempt. You know he is considered high risk for suicide completion because:

    a. he is married
    b. he has no past medical history
    c. he was accidentally discovered by a neighbor during the attempt
    d. he is employed at a fast-food restaurant
    e. he is deeply religious in a faith where suicide is considered taboo

11. Which of the following is characteristic of a grief reaction?

    a. chronic and less severe depressed mood present most of the day, more days than not for 2 years
    b. denial, anger, bargaining, guilt, and acceptance
    c. persistent sad mood or pervasive loss of interest in usual activities, lasting for at least two weeks characterized by low self-esteem
    d. one or more episodes of elated mood with a history of deflated mood

12. Pseudocyesis is classified as what type of disorder:

    a. somatization
    b. body dysmorphic disorder
    c. factitious disorder
    d. hypochondriasis
    e. conversion disorder

13. **Which** drug therapy is first-line for active catatonia?

    a. haloperidol
    b. risperidone
    c. cyclobenzaprine
    d. lorazepam

14. X-rays that are suggestive of child abuse include:

    a. more than one fracture in the same stage of healing

    b. "buckle" fractures
    c. metaphyseal chip fractures
    d. C2-C3 pseudo-subluxation

15. The most common psychiatric illnesses diagnosed in children, adolescents, and adults are:

    a. mood disorders
    b. thought disorders
    c. factitious disorders
    d. personality disorders
    e. neurotic disorders

16. "Positive" symptoms for schizophrenia include:

    a. flat affect
    b. loose associations
    c. poverty of speech (alogia)
    d. inability to experience pleasure (anhedonia)
    e. lack of motivation (avolition)

17. Alcohol withdrawal is characterized by:

    a. sweating, tremors, tachycardia (autonomic hyperactivity)
    b. global confusion
    c. hallucinations
    d. seizures

18. Which diagnosis has features that are **not** feigned:

    a. drug-seeking behavior
    b. body dysmorphic disorder
    c. Munchausen syndrome
    d. malingering
    e. Munchausen by proxy

19. Obsessive–compulsive neurotic disorder is characterized by:

    a. anxiety-provoking obsessive thoughts
    b. anxiety-calming repetitive compulsions
    c. pervasive impairment in interpersonal relationships
    d. all of the above

20. A patient who has 2 months of social withdrawal, pervasive impairment in self-care and interpersonal relationships, and positive or negative psychotic symptoms has the following diagnosis:

    a. schizophreniform disorder
    b. brief psychotic disorder
    c. schizotypal disorder
    d. schizoid personality disorder
    e. schizophrenia

---

1. **Answer: d**

The *DSM-IV (Diagnostic and Statistical Manual of Mental Disorders IV)* criteria for schizophrenia include the following: (1) Mood disorder or schizoaffective disorder with psychotic features have been ruled out. (2) A sharp deterioration from prior baseline level of functioning such as in work, grooming, or interpersonal relationships. (3) The presence of two or more positive symptoms: hallucinations, delusions, grossly disorganized speech or behavior (or catatonic behavior); and negative symptoms such as flattened affect, poverty of speech, **inability to experience pleasure,** or inability to perform goal-directed activities. (4) Symptoms not caused by substance abuse, medications, or a general medical condition. (5) Symptoms of continuous signs (including prodromal/negative symptoms) **for at least 6 months.**

2. Answer: a

This patient is having a *manic episode.* The *DSM-IV* criteria for manic episode include the following: (1) three or more of the following seven general categories of symptoms that have persisted: inflated self-esteem or grandiosity, insomnia, **increase in goal-directed activity (writing a novel)** or psychomotor agitation, pressured speech, flight of ideas, excessive hedonistic and pleasurable activities (money and sex), and easy distraction to trivial stimuli; (2) at least 2 weeks of persistently elevated, expansive, or irritable mood; (3) symptoms not caused by substance abuse, medications, or a general medical condition; (4) disease process is severe enough to cause impairment in social and occupational settings or hospitalization; and (5) symptoms do not meet criteria for a "mixed episode" (e.g., bipolar disorder).

3. Answer: c.

Agoraphobia is anxiety and subsequent avoidance of situations or places which escape or help may be difficult. **Panic attack** is a short period of sudden onset of intense worry, fear, and terror accompanied by feelings of impending doom. **Social phobia** is significant anxiety provoked by exposure to social or performance situations leading to avoidance behavior. **Anxiety disorder caused by a general medical condition** is associated with anxiety as a direct physiologic consequence of a general medical condition. In this patient, the diabetes has no relevance to the patient's anxiety. **Generalized anxiety disorder** is associated with at least 6 months of persistent and excessive anxiety.

4. Answer: e

Borderline personality disorder is characterized by poor self-image and emptiness, impulsiveness, instability of personal relationships alternating between idealization and devaluation, inability to control intense anger, efforts to avoid abandonment, and mood instability. **Antisocial personality disorder** is characterized by a pattern of reckless disregard and deceitfulness, violation, and lack of remorse toward others. **Dependent personality disorder** is characterized by a pervasive and excessive need to be taken care of that leads to fear of separation and need for approval. **Histrionic personality disorder** is characterized by excessive emotionality and attention-seeking behavior using inappropriate seduction and overdramatization. **Narcissistic personality disorder** is characterized by a selfish and inflated self-importance or grandiosity and the need for admiration or entitlement.

5. Answer: b

A **conversion disorder** is characterized by a sudden-onset dramatic single symptom that typically is painless and neurologic in origin. The symptoms are not under voluntary control of the patient and there is no pathophysiologic explanation for the disease. The disorder has a gender predilection toward women, and patients may show a lack of concern (la belle indifference) regarding the body dysfunction. **Somatization disorder** involves pain at different sites, that is, gastrointestinal, genitourinary and neurologic symptoms that are not intentionally produced or explained by a medical condition. **Factitious disorder** involves signs and symptoms that are intentionally produced in the absence of external incentives. **Malingering** involves signs and symptoms of disease that are intentionally produced, motivated by external incentives (e.g., time off from work). **Munchausen's syndrome** is a rare type of factitious disorder where patients exaggerate symptoms of a previously diagnosed illness or those difficult to disprove. They have a compulsion to feign illness and often undergo lengthy and advanced workups and finally refuse discharge ("career medical imposter").

6. Answer: c

Delirium is defined as an acute, rapid global impairment of cognitive dysfunction due to an underlying condition and involves disturbances in consciousness (focusing attention), cognition (disorientation and memory deficits), and perception (hallucinations or delusions). **Dementia** is defined as a gradually progressive deterioration of cognitive function involving memory impairment (choice **a**), apraxia (choice **b**), agnosia (choice **d**), aphasia, or disturbances in executive functioning (choice **e**).

7. Answer: a

Hypochondriasis has four features. (1) The patient's symptoms are typically disproportionate to physical examination findings of organic disease; (2) a preoccupation with one's body; (3) a compulsive insistence on being labeled as "sick" and subsequently crippled; (4) continuous and unsatisfactory pursuit of medical care and opinion with a history of intervention yet eventual return of symptoms. **Somatization disorder** involves pain at different sites; gastrointestinal, genitourinary, and neurologic symptoms that are not intentionally produced or explained by a medical condition. **Body dysmorphic disorder** is a preoccupation with an imagined defect in physical appearance. **Conversion disorder** involves sensory or motor symptoms not feigned and not medically explainable. **Narcissistic personality disorder** is characterized by self-centered behavior and pervasive grandiosity.

8. Answer: c

Lorazepam, a benzodiazepine, would be the first-line treatment for psychotic agitation in this patient who likely is suffering from alcohol withdrawal. **Haloperidol**

is the most widely used medication for rapid tranquilization in the United States and is effective against tension, anxiety, and hyperactivity; however, it should not be used a sole agent in alcohol withdrawal. **Risperidone** is an atypical antipsychotic agent with a broad spectrum of response with fewer side effects than haloperidol but it requires a dissolvable oral formulation that would be technically difficult in the above patient. Additionally, it would not treat the apparent withdrawal seizures. **Phenytoin,** an anticonvulsant, would not be the first-line medication in alcohol withdrawal seizures and would not be effective in this patient's agitation and state of sympathetic overdrive.

9. Answer: e

The patient has **anorexia nervosa** characterized by the following: refusal to maintain minimum body weight expected for age and height leading to body weight at least 15% below expected; an intense fear of becoming overweight even when underweight; perception disturbance in body weight, shape, or size; and absence of at least three consecutive expected menstrual cycles. **Bulimia** is characterized by the following: a minimum average of two binge eating episodes per week for at least 3 months; lack of control over behavior during binge episodes; perception disturbance in body weight, shape, or size; and self-induced vomiting, use of laxatives, dieting and fasting, and excessive exercising. Choices **b** and **c** fit both eating disorders and are not specific for anorexia nervosa.

10. Answer: c

This patient is at high risk for completion of suicide because of being elderly and male. If he was **accidentally discovered during the attempt, this would increase his suicide risk.** Other factors include suicidal ideation with a clear plan, a history of previous attempts, possession of weapons, or attempt with violent and lethal means. Signs and symptoms of suicide risk include patients who are in poor interpersonal relationships with lots of conflict; separated, widowed, or divorced; medically or mentally debilitated; unemployed or in legal trouble; with a family history of suicide; or with a belief system where suicide is not taboo.

11. Answer: b

A **grief reaction** is characterized by the features in choice **b.** Pathologic grief lasts for 8 months or beyond. Choice **a** is the definition of dysthymic disorder; **c** is the definition of major depressive disorder; and **d** is the definition of bipolar disorder.

12. Answer: e

Pseudocyesis is a **conversion disorder** related to pregnancy (including amenorrhea) without positive gestation where the patient is not feigning the belief or symptoms. Choices **a, b,** and **d** represent other

psychosomatic disorders, whereas in **c** the patient is feigning symptoms.

13. Answer: d

Benzodiazepines are the first-line therapy for active catatonia. Choices **a** and **b** are antipsychotic medications that treat other schizophrenia subtypes more effectively. Choice **c,** a muscle relaxer, does not "relax" catatonic immobility.

14. Answer: c

Metaphyseal chip fractures are commonly seen from the whiplash and shearing associated with shaking a child with flailing extremities. Fractures of child abuse are multiple and in different stages of healing so **a** is less common. Choice **b** is present in expected pediatric falls and **d** is a pediatric normal radiographic variant.

15. Answer: e

Neurotic or **anxiety disorders** are the most common psychiatric illnesses diagnosed in children, adolescents, and adults. The first-line pharmacologic therapy is benzodiazepines (e.g., lorazepam).

16. Answer: b

Loose associations represent disorganized thought, a "positive" symptom. Other positive symptoms include delusions, hallucinations, disorganized speech and behavior, or catatonia. Choices **a, c, d,** and **e** represent "negative" symptoms. Antipsychotic pharmacotherapy is generally better at treating positive symptoms than negative symptoms.

17. Answer: a

Alcohol withdrawal occurs 6 to 8 hours after alcohol cessation in susceptible patients. The other answer choices are defined as components of delirium tremens. Choice **c** occurs 1 day after cessation, **d** occurs 1 to 2 days after cessation, and **b** occurs 3 to 5 days after cessation. Withdrawal is treated with benzodiazepines and supportive care.

18. Answer: b

Psychosomatic disorders are not feigned, and the patient cannot control the symptoms. Choices **a, c, d,** and **e** are **factitious disorders** and have symptoms that are feigned.

19. Answer: d

All choices are characteristic of obsessive–compulsive neurotic disorder.

20. Answer: a

Schizophreniform disorder has psychotic features for 1 to 6 months. Choice **b** has symptoms less than 1 month. Choice **e** has symptoms for greater than 6 months. Choices **c** and **d** are personality disorders that are maladaptive and pervasive patterns of behavior but do not share the psychotic features of **a, b,** and **e.**

Acute and chronic renal failure

- Acute renal failure: a rapid decline in glomerular filtration rate (GFR) such that there is a 50% increase in serum creatinine from patient's baseline or a 50% decline in creatinine clearance
- Acute renal failure is divided into pre-renal, intrinsic, and postrenal failure
  - Prerenal failure is related to hypovolemia
  - Intrinsic failure relates to injury to the kidney itself from infection, nephrotoxic medications, or any agent or process that damages the kidney itself
  - Postrenal failure results from mechanical obstructions
- Chronic renal failure: over months to years, renal function is progressively lost such that hemodialysis (HD) or kidney transplant is required

SIGNS AND SYMPTOMS

- General: shortness of breath, fatigue, lethargy, edema, dysrhythmia
- Prerenal: decreased urine output, thirst, orthostatic hypotension, dizziness
- Intrinsic: skin infections, sepsis, hypotension, rhabdomyolysis
- Postrenal: mechanical obstructions (hypertrophic prostate obstruction or pelvic cancers)

DIAGNOSIS

- Urine microscopy
- BUN/creatinine ratio >20 = prerenal failure
- ECG: Demonstrates evidence of metabolic or electrolyte abnormality (e.g., hyperkalemia)
- Electrolyte disturbances: hyperkalemia, uremia, hypocalcemia, hyperphosphatemia
- CXR: May demonstrate fluid overload and/or infiltrate
- In intrinsic failure: kidney biopsy will help identify etiology of acute renal failure
- In postrenal failure: imaging such as intravenous pyelography, ultrasound (US), or computed tomography (CT) may be used to diagnose obstruction

TREATMENT

- IV fluid resuscitation with careful monitoring of urine output—especially if oliguric/anuric acute renal failure
- Identify and/or remove nephrotoxic offenders (new medications, treat infections)
- If acidosis, severe hyperkalemia, volume overload, uremia, or certain medications are involved, hemodialysis is a consideration
- Foley catheter if postrenal failure secondary to outflow obstruction

Complications of renal dialysis

- May include: consequences of delayed or missed treatments, fluid shifts, excessive volume removal (over dialysis), fistula infections, clots, or malfunctions.

SIGNS AND SYMPTOMS

- Missed dialysis: shortness of breath, congestive heart failure symptoms, hyperkalemia, dysrhythmias, cardiac arrest, weakness, fatigue, seizures, altered mental status, hyporeflexia, paresthesia or tetany, pleuritic chest pain, hypotension

- Over dialysis: hypotension, dizziness, syncope
- Infection at the catheter site (usually *Staphylococcus*): fever, warmth, erythema, tenderness to palpation, or loss of thrill over fistula
- Clots of fistula: loss of thrill over fistula
- Bleeding from fistula after dialysis

DIAGNOSIS

- Clinical
- Electrolyte disturbances
- ECG (hyperkalemia, dysrhythmias, pericarditis)
- CXR (volume overload, pericardial effusion findings)
- Ultrasound (cardiac if concern for pericarditis or tamponade or of fistula if concern for clot)

TREATMENT

- Gentle volume resuscitation if hypovolemic
- Urgent/emergent dialysis if volume overloaded or significant electrolyte derangements
- Electrolyte repletion as necessary
- Fistula infections may be treated with vancomycin and can maintain therapeutic levels up to 1 week after administration
- Clots of fistula typically treated by interventional radiology with thrombolysis and/or balloon angioplasty
- Bleeding from fistula: elevate nonocclusive focal pressure. If immediately after dialysis, protamine and/or DDAVP can be used to counteract the heparin used during HD

Glomerular disorders

GLOMERULONEPHRITIS

- Cause often unknown; however, known etiologies include systemic diseases, infections, drugs, and primary renal diseases
- Based on presentation: classifications include acute or chronic nephritic syndrome, rapidly progressive glomerulonephritis, idiopathic renal hematuric syndrome, and nephrotic syndrome

SIGNS AND SYMPTOMS

- Proteinuria, hematuria are the most common
- Edema caused by sodium retention and low albumin
- Hypertension
- Congestive heart failure
- Renal failure
- Autoimmune: fever, rash, arthritis

DIAGNOSIS

- 24-hour urine collection for protein and electrolytes
- Calcium—expect hypocalcemia in nephritic patients
- If infection suspected as etiology, cultures, complement levels, viral studies
- If autoimmune suspected as etiology, connective tissue markers (ANA, RF)

TREATMENT

- Supportive care
- Identify and treat the underlying cause when possible
- Fluid and sodium restriction
- Loop diuretics
- Dialysis as needed for severe volume overload, hyperkalemia

NEPHROTIC SYNDROME

- Caused by primary renal or systemic diseases
- Results in increased permeability of glomerular capillary barrier to plasma proteins
- Edema caused by sodium retention and low albumin
- Low albumin causes reduced plasma volume, leading to orthostatic hypotension and possibly shock
- Increased risk for thromboembolism

SIGNS AND SYMPTOMS

- Often asymptomatic
- Proteinuria
- Pitting edema
- Hypertension
- Hyperlipidemia
- Microscopic hematuria
- Postural hypotension

DIAGNOSIS

- Urinalysis positive for large amounts of protein
- Urine microscopy shows casts and cellular elements
- Renal biopsy is definitive test

TREATMENT

- IV hydration if clinically dehydrated
- Sodium restriction
- Loop diuretics to create controlled gentle diuresis
- Glucocorticosteroids
- ACE inhibitor
- Thromboembolism prophylaxis

Infection

CYSTITIS

- A urinary tract infection limited to the bladder with no upper tract signs or symptoms
- Most common organism *Escherichia coli*

SIGNS AND SYMPTOMS

- Dysuria, frequency, hesitancy, and hematuria
- May present as altered level of consciousness in the elderly

DIAGNOSIS

- Urinalysis demonstrating >10 WBC/HPF
- Urine dipstick demonstrating leukocyte esterase and/or nitrites
- Urine culture

TREATMENT

- Based on local resistance patterns
- Trimethoprim–sulfamethoxazole (TMP-SMX) resistance rates are increasing
- 3- to 5-day duration of treatment for uncomplicated cystitis
- Nitrofurantoin or cephalexin in pregnancy
- Phenazopyridine for treatment of symptoms, particularly dysuria

PYELONEPHRITIS

- Typically an ascending urinary tract infection starting from a cystitis
- Involves infection of the kidney structures
- Most commonly *E. coli*. Some *Staphylococcus saprophyticus*

SIGNS AND SYMPTOMS

- Symptoms of cystitis
- Costovertebral angle (CVA) tenderness or flank pain
- Fevers, malaise, body aches, rigors or chills
- Nausea and vomiting possible

DIAGNOSIS

- Clinical
- UA, urine culture

TREATMENT

- Oral outpatient therapy acceptable in uncomplicated cases in an otherwise healthy immunocompetent patient
- Parenteral antibiotics for complicated cases, including inability to tolerate oral medications, comorbid conditions, extremes of age, immunosuppressed state, and pregnancy
- Treatment based on local resistance patterns
- Treatment duration typically 7 to 14 days

Hernias

- Defined as an organ protruding through the wall that contains it
- Types of hernias: femoral, inguinal (direct and indirect), obturator, umbilical, incisional, and Spigelian (anterior abdominal wall)

SIGNS AND SYMPTOMS

- Pain and swelling at site of hernia
- Persistent pain, inability to reduce the hernia, fever, and/or vomiting may suggest the hernia is strangulated, incarcerated, or obstructed

DIAGNOSIS

- Clinical

TREATMENT

- Manual reduction

- Emergent surgical consultation if evidence of acute strangulation or incarceration
- General surgery follow-up if reducible

Male genital tract

INFLAMMATION/INFECTION

Balanitis/balanoposthitis

- **Balanitis:** Inflammation of the glans penis
- **Balanoposthitis:** balanitis with involvement of the foreskin (Fig. 15-1)
- Often seen in uncircumcised men with diabetes, poor personal hygiene, or morbid obesity
- Infectious causes include bacterial and viral causes as well as candidal species, *Gardnerella vaginalis*, *Treponema pallidum*, and trichomonal species

SIGNS AND SYMPTOMS

- Penile discharge or itching
- Tenderness or erythema of the glans penis or foreskin
- Phimosis
- Stenosis at meatus

DIAGNOSIS

- Clinical

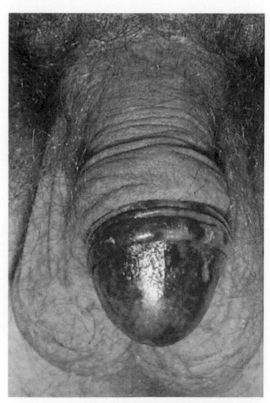

Figure 15-1. Candidal balanoposthitis. (From Korting GW: *Practical dermatology of the genital region*, Philadelphia, 1981, Saunders, p 159.)

TREATMENT

- Instruct patients to retract the foreskin daily and soak in warm water to clean penis and foreskin
- Obtain finger-stick glucose to evaluate for diabetes
- Culture any discharge
- **Pediatrics:** Topical antibacterial or antifungal, depending on etiology
- Adult men: Topical clotrimazole or oral fluconazole if candida is suspected

Epididymitis/orchitis

- Inflammation of the epididymis (epididymitis), testicle (orchitis), or both (epididymo-orchitis)
- Common in young men resulting from sexually transmitted diseases and in older men because of obstructive pathology (benign prostatic hypertrophy, cancer, urethral strictures)

SIGNS AND SYMPTOMS

- Progressive pain and swelling of epididymis and/or testicles
- Erythema of scrotal skin, dysuria, fever, and/or penile discharge

DIAGNOSIS

- Physical examination
- Doppler ultrasound
- UA
- Urine/urethral chlamydia/GC testing
- CBC may show mild leukocytosis

TREATMENT

- Antibiotics to cover chlamydia and gonorrhea if young adult, presuming STD etiology
  - 1. Ceftriaxone and doxycycline or
  - 2. Oflaxacin and tetracycline
- Antibiotics to cover prostatitis or bacteria associated with infection after instrumentation in older men, provided STD etiology less likely based on history
  - 1. Ciprofloxacin, augmentin or ceftriaxone
- Analgesia
- Scrotal elevation

Fournier gangrene (Fig. 15-2)

- Gangrene of the scrotum and perineum
- Aggressive, swiftly advancing necrotizing infection
- Because of poor hygiene of the perineal or rectal areas, skin breakdown, penile or scrotal infections, urinary catheters
- Polymicrobial infection with bacterial toxins and necrosis contributing to toxic clinical presentation
- Risk factors include diabetes, alcoholism, morbid obesity, recent abdominal surgery, and immunocompromised states

SIGNS AND SYMPTOMS

- Toxic appearance
- Nausea, vomiting

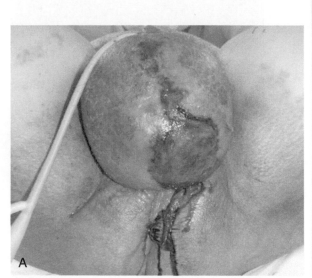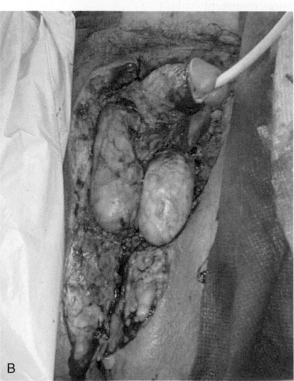

Figure 15-2. Fournier gangrene of the scrotum. **A,** Surface appearance of scrotum and perineum showing area of frank necrosis. **B,** Extent of soft tissue debridement required to achieve margins of viable tissue. Note that the testes within their tunica vaginalis compartment are spared. (From Wein AJ, Kavoussi LR, Novic AC et al: *Campbell-Walsh urology,* ed 9, Philadelphia, 2007, Saunders.)

- Pain out of proportion initially, then progressive anesthesia
- Skin may show discoloration, watery discharge, bullae, crepitus, or necrosis

DIAGNOSIS

- Clinical examination

TREATMENT

- Systemic resuscitation
- Broad-spectrum antibiotics
- Immediate surgical or urologic consultation for debridement
- Hyperbaric therapy in some cases

Prostatitis

- Bacterial infection of the prostate, which may be acute or chronic
- Bacterial speciation varies, depending on acute vs chronic infection and age

SIGNS AND SYMPTOMS

- Dysuria, frequency, hematospermia, suprapubic or testicular pain, pain with defecation, and/or urinary retention
- If acute infection, fevers, myalgias, tender prostate on palpation that may be boggy or firm

DIAGNOSIS

- Urinalysis and urine culture
- Prostate exam

TREATMENT

- Antibiotics
  - 1. Acute infection—outpatient treatment
    - <35 years old: ceftriaxone and doxycycline
    - >35 years old: ciprofloxacin
  - 2. Acute infection—inpatient:
    - Ampicillin/sulbactam, ceftriaxone, or piperacillin/tazobactam
  - 3. Chronic infection—outpatient:
    - Ciprofloxacin for 4 weeks
- Stool softeners
- Pain control
- Indwelling Foley catheter if urinary retention

Urethritis

- Most frequently caused by sexually transmitted diseases, including chlamydia, gonorrhea, *Ureaplasma urealyticum,* or occasionally trichomonas, candida, or herpes
- Consider coinfection with other STDs

SIGNS AND SYMPTOMS

- Urethral discharge, dysuria and pyuria

DIAGNOSIS

- Gonorrhea and chlamydia by urethral swabs or urinary tests

TREATMENT

- Chlamydia
  - Azithromycin or doxycycline
- Gonorrhea
  - Ceftriaxone IM

STRUCTURAL DISORDERS

Paraphimosis

- Glans entrapped by retracted foreskin
- Usually results from failure to manually retract foreskin but may be secondary to trauma

SIGNS AND SYMPTOMS

- Foreskin pulled back, pain, glans swelling, focal cellulites
- Urinary retention is possible

DIAGNOSIS

- Clinical

TREATMENT

- Multiple approaches to reduce glans swelling (ice, compression, topical sugar for osmotic effect, hyaluronidase injection at prepuce) to facilitate manual reduction
- Manual reduction method by upward traction on foreskin with downward pressure on glans
- Dorsal slit to foreskin if manual retraction fails
- Urology consult for circumcision, which may be immediate or as outpatient
- Admit for cellulitis or necrosis of penis

Phimosis

- Unable to retract foreskin to expose glans
- Etiologies include trauma, recurrent balanoposthitis or diaper dermatitis, inadequate circumcision

SIGNS AND SYMPTOMS

- Narrowed opening of the foreskin, dysuria, balanoposthitis, and/or acute urinary retention

DIAGNOSIS

- Clinical

TREATMENT

- Evaluate for obstruction
  - **Nonobstructive:** urology follow-up
  - **Obstructive:** place catheter or perform suprapubic aspiration. If vascular compromise, urology consultation and urgent dorsal slit incision

Priapism

- Penile erection without sexual stimulation that is painful and prolonged
- High-flow priapism often caused by trauma

- Low-flow priapism caused by hematologic disorders associated with sludging of blood (sickle cell disease, leukemia, polycythemia)
- Other etiologies include pharmacologic or idiopathic

SIGNS AND SYMPTOMS

- Persistent erection
- May include urinary retention

DIAGNOSIS

- History and clinical presentation

TREATMENT

- Pharmacologic:
  - Terbutaline 0.25 to 0.5 mg SC or 5 mg PO every 4 hours
  - Phenylephrine: dilute 1 mg in 100 mL saline. In corpus cavernosum, inject 10 mL boluses
  - Epinephrine: dilute 1 mg in 100 mL saline. In corpus cavernosum, inject 1 to 3 mL boluses
  - Pseudoephedrine: In corpus cavernosum, inject 60 to 100 mg
  - Intracavernous aspiration
  - Sickle Cell: exchange transfusion, PRBC transfusion or hyperbaric oxygen
  - Urologic consultation if detumescence does not occur

Prostatic hypertrophy (BPH)

- Noncancerous enlargement of the prostate associated with increasing age
- Growth rate is hormonally dependent on testosterone and dihydrotestosterone

SIGNS AND SYMPTOMS

- Complications of urination: frequency, urgency or hesitancy, weakened stream, incomplete emptying, straining, and/or nocturia

DIAGNOSIS

- History
- Digital rectal exam to palpate size of prostate
- Outpatient ultrasound and prostate-specific antigen (PSA) determination

TREATMENT

- Medical therapy
  - Alpha-1 adrenergic receptor blockers to reduce smooth muscle tone
  - 5-alpha reductase inhibitors: 5-alpha reductase metabolizes testosterone to dihydrotestosterone, which is known to stimulate prostate growth
- Surgical therapy:
  - There are multiple approaches and techniques, all of which involve reducing the size of the prostate

Torsion of testis

- A true urologic emergency—may result in loss of testicle and infertility

- Bimodal distribution of frequency, which includes the first year of life and puberty
- High risk in those with undescended testis
- Usually caused by abnormal anatomy—tunica vaginalis normally attaches low and to the posterior lateral side of testicle
- **Bell clapper deformity:** Higher insertion point of the tunica allows the testicle to rotate freely in the scrotum
- Twisting causes venous congestion and ultimately arterial compromise, resulting in testicular ischemia

SIGNS AND SYMPTOMS

- Extreme, sudden onset of pain, nausea, and vomiting
- Absence of urinary symptoms
- History of similar pain in the past that resolved spontaneously
- Scrotal pain, swelling, tenderness, firmness to touch, transverse or high-riding lie, absence of cremasteric reflex

DIAGNOSIS

- Clinical
- Doppler US study. If diagnosis is suspected clinically do not delay intervention to obtain US

TREATMENT

- Manual detorsion may be attempted, but definitive treatment will be surgical
- Immediate urologic evaluation with surgical exploration and potential bilateral orchiopexy

Torsion of the appendix testis

- The appendix testis is a remnant of the müllerian duct, and is present in >90% of testicles
- Located at the superior pole of the testicle
- Torsion of the appendix testis must be differentiated from testicular torsion, which is a true emergency

SIGNS AND SYMPTOMS

- Onset of pain may be acute or subacute
- Pain is located at the superior pole of the testicle, and the rest of the testicle is nontender
- Absence of systemic or urinary symptoms
- Scrotum is usually normal in appearance, although some swelling can occur
- Normal testicular lie, and intact cremasteric reflex
- "Blue dot sign"—characteristic blue dot visible at superior pole of the testicle in about 25%

DIAGNOSIS

- Testicular torsion must be ruled out—this can be done clinically if the diagnosis of torsion of the testicular appendage is completely obvious, otherwise must consider radiologic studies and urologic consultation
- Color Doppler ultrasonography—generally faster and more accessible
- Radionuclide imaging

TREATMENT

- Pain control, ice, scrotal support
- Urologic follow-up
- Surgery can be considered for intractable pain
- Emergent urologic consult if diagnosis is unclear and torsion remains a possibility

TUMORS

Testicular masses

- Most common cancer in men aged 15 to 35 years
- Often misdiagnosed as epididymitis, may be asymptomatic with gradual onset

SIGNS AND SYMPTOMS

- Painless, firm, and/or indurated testicle, or palpable mass
- May have abdominal pain and lymphadenopathy
- Hematospermia and pain to testicle may occur secondary to hemorrhage from within tumor

DIAGNOSIS

- Palpable, nontender, firm, intratesticular mass on clinical exam
- Transillumination of scrotum to evaluate if mass is cystic or solid
- US may reveal mass as well as acute hydrocele, which sometimes accompanies this clinical presentation
- Alpha-fetoprotein level may be elevated
- Urine pregnancy test is positive in setting of some germ cell tumors

TREATMENT

- Urgent urologic referral to evaluate for surgical exploration or orchiectomy

Prostate

- Prostate cancer commonly occurs after the age of 50 and is the result of mutating prostate cells that multiply in an uncontrolled fashion
- Most cases of prostate cancer are slow-growing

SIGNS AND SYMPTOMS

- May present completely asymptomatically
- Urinary hesitancy or retention, or decreased stream
- Acute spinal cord compression may be a complication of untreated or undiagnosed metastatic prostate carcinoma

DIAGNOSIS

- Elevated PSA level
- Abnormal contour of prostate on digital rectal exam

TREATMENT

- Surgery: prostatectomy, transurethral resection of the prostate (TURP), cryosurgery
- Radiation or hormonal therapy

Nephritis

HEMOLYTIC UREMIC SYNDROME (HUS)

- Usually noted in pediatric population between 6 months and 4 years in the setting of recent diarrheal illness from *E. coli* and *Shigella* that produce cytotoxins that damage renal endothelium, resulting in HUS
- *E. coli* O157:H7, a leading cause of HUS, is transmitted in contaminated food and water, but has also been found in unpasteurized foods
- Person-to-person spread occurs, particularly within families or day care centers

SIGNS AND SYMPTOMS

- Fever
- Bleeding (gastrointestinal bleeding, epistaxis, vaginal bleeding, hematuria)
- Abdominal pain
- Change in vision
- May have neurologic changes, including seizures, aphasia, paresthesias, change in mental status, confusion, or lethargy

DIAGNOSIS

- Thrombocytopenia, fever, renal dysfunction, hemolytic anemia
- CBC (anemia and thrombocytopenia) and peripheral blood smear shows schistocytes
- Prothrombin time (PT), partial thromboplastin time (PTT) are normal
- Normal DIC panel
- BUN/creatinine ratio elevated
- UA: proteinuria and red blood cells
- Blood cultures
- CT of the brain

TREATMENT

- Generally supportive, with intravenous fluids as needed
- Electrolyte repletion
- In cases of significant kidney failure or anuria, dialysis may necessary

STRUCTURAL DISORDERS

Calculus of urinary tract

- Commonly occur in the 3rd to 5th decade of life with a genetic predisposition
- Stone composition usually from calcium combined with oxalate and phosphate or struvite (magnesium–ammonium–phosphate often associated with urea-splitting bacterial infections)
- Struvite calculi often form in renal pelvis, resulting in staghorn calculus
- Most difficult areas of passage include the calyx, ureteropelvic junction, ureterovesicular junction
- Urinary tract diameter is smallest at the ureterovesicular junction

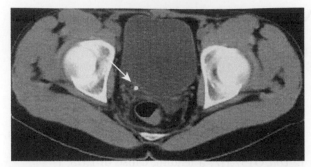

Figure 15-3. Computed tomography (CT) scan demonstrating ureteral calculus. Noncontrast CT showing a calculus (*arrow*) at the right vesicoureteral junction. (From Feehally J, Floege J, Johnson RJ: *Comprehensive clinical nephrology,* ed 3, St. Louis, 2007, Mosby.)

- 90% of stones are radio-opaque on plain radiographs

SIGNS AND SYMPTOMS

- Presence of calculi is usually painless until it starts to travel down the ureter, into the bladder, and out the urethra
- Acute onset of severe flank pain, may radiate to groin
- Urinary frequency or urgency, hematuria

DIAGNOSIS

- Urinalysis—microscopic to gross hematuria suggests nephrolithiasis; however, absence of blood does not rule out diagnosis
- BUN/creatinine to evaluate renal function
- Urine pregnancy test
- Non-contrast CT abdomen is preferred imaging modality (Fig. 15-3)
- Intravenous pyelogram or ultrasound imaging are other imaging options for those who are not CT candidates

TREATMENT

- Pain control, including NSAIDs, narcotics
- Tamsulosin (Flomax) 0.4 mg PO daily
- If urinalysis shows evidence of infection, urine culture should be sent and antibiotics initiated
- Urology consult for all febrile patients with obstructing stones, or those with obstruction and only one kidney. Also consider admission for intractable pain or vomiting

Obstructive uropathy

- A mechanical obstruction leading to inability to void
- Common causes of obstruction include prostate hypertrophy, prostate cancer, prostatitis, urethral strictures, bladder calculi or blood clots, and stool impaction

SIGNS AND SYMPTOMS

- Inability to urinate or incomplete emptying of the bladder
- Suprapubic abdominal discomfort or distension

DIAGNOSIS

- History
- Digital rectal exam to evaluate for prostatitis, enlarged prostate or stool impaction
- Bladder ultrasound

TREATMENT

- Bladder catheter or Coude catheter
- If unable to pass into the bladder via urethra, suprapubic aspiration of urine and catheter placement may be necessary in conjunction with urology consultation

POLYCYSTIC KIDNEY DISEASE (PCKD)

- An autosomal dominant genetic disorder involving progressive formation of multiple cysts in the kidneys
- There is a high incidence of congenital berry aneurysms with PCKD
- Cysts may not be confined only to kidneys. Liver and other solid organ cysts have been known to occur

SIGNS AND SYMPTOMS

- Flank pain, hypertension, dysuria

DIAGNOSIS

- Renal insufficiency progressing to end-stage renal disease
- Urinalysis may show evidence of urinary tract infection. Up to half of those with PCKD will have a urinary tract infection during their lifetime. The most common infections are an infected cyst and acute pyelonephritis
- CT renal scan or renal ultrasound
- Genetic testing

TREATMENT

- Appropriate antibiotic coverage for urinary tract infection flora
- Stringent control of blood pressure may slow formation of cysts and progression of disease
- End-stage renal disease associated with PCKD requires either hemodialysis or kidney transplant

KIDNEY TUMORS

- Renal cell carcinoma, arising from the renal tubule, is the most common renal cancer of adults

SIGNS AND SYMPTOMS

- Flank pain, hematuria, abdominal mass

DIAGNOSIS

- CT renal or renal ultrasound

TREATMENT

- Surgery, which may be followed by chemotherapy and/or radiation therapy

BIBLIOGRAPHY

Centers for Disease Control and Prevention, Workowski KA, Berman SM: Sexually transmitted diseases treatment guidelines, 2006, *MMWR Recomm Rep* 55:1–94, 2006.

Cohen HT, McGovern FJ: Renal cell carcinoma, *N Engl J Med* 353:2477–2490, 2005.

Hodde L: Emergency department evaluation and management of dialysis patient complications, *J Emerg Med* 10(3):317–334, 1992.

Javier I, Escobar JL II, Eastman ER et al: Selected urologic problems. In Marx JA (ed): *Rosen's emergency medicine: concepts and clinical practice*, ed 5, St. Louis, 2002, Mosby, pp. 1414–1421.

Marcozzi D, Suner S: The nontraumatic acute scrotum, *Emerg Med Clin North Am* 19:547–568, 2001.

Moake JL: Thrombotic microangiopathies, *N Engl J Med* 347:589–600, 2002.

Mulhall JP, Hong SC: Priapism: diagnosis and management, *Acad Emerg Med* 2:810–816, 1996.

Nelson WG, Marzo AM, Isaacs WB: Prostate cancer, *N Engl J Med* 349:366–381, 2003.

O'Donnell JA II: Phimosis and paraphimosis. In Barkin RM, Caputo GL, Jaffe DM, Knapp JF, Schafermeyer RW, Seidel JS (eds): *Pediatric emergency medicine*, ed 2, St. Louis, 1997, Mosby, pp. 1152–1153.

O'Reilly PH, Philippou M: Urinary tract obstructions, *Medicine* 35:420–422, 2007.

Press SM, Smith AD: Incidence of negative hematuria in patients with acute urinary lithiasis presenting to the emergency room with flank pain, *Urology* 45:75, 1995.

Rabinowitz R, Hulbert WC Jr: Acute scrotal swelling, *Urol Clin North Am* 22:101–105, 1995.

Schneider R: Acute scrotal pain. In Wolfson AB, Hendey GW, Hendry PL et al (eds): *Hardwood-Nuss' clinical practice of emergency medicine*, ed 4, Philadelphia, 2005, Lippincott Williams & Wilkins, pp. 420–428.

Sinert R: Acute renal failure. In Tintinalli JE, Kelen GD, Stapczynski JS (eds): *Tintinalli emergency medicine*, ed 5, New York, 2000, McGraw-Hill, pp. 611–614.

Sklar AH, Caruana RJ, Lammers JE, Strauser GD: Renal infections in autosomal dominant polycystic kidney disease, *Am J Kidney Dis* 10(2):81–88, 1987.

Vilke GM: Fournier's gangrene. In Schaider JJ, Hayden SR, Wolfe RE et al (eds): *Rosen & Barkin's 5-minute emergency medicine consult*, ed 3, Philadelphia, 2007, Lippincott Williams & Wilkins, pp. 428–429.

Vilke GM, Harrigan RA, Ufberg JW, Chan TC: Emergency evaluation and treatment of priapism, *J Emerg Med* 26(3):325–329, 2004.

Questions and Answers

1. A 65-year-old man who just finished hemodialysis was noted to be hypotensive and was brought to the ED. You administered a bolus of IV fluid without improvement. Which of the following is the most likely cause of his persistent hypotension?
   a. volume overload
   b. hyperkalemia
   c. hypermagnesemia
   d. pericarditis

2. Which of the following is a feature of nephrolithiasis?
   a. 10% of the time kidney stones are present on kidney, ureter, and bladder (KUB) x-ray
   b. kidney stones are most likely to cause obstruction at the ureterovesicular junction
   c. the absence of blood in urine rules out nephrolithiasis
   d. calcium oxalate often forms stones in the renal pelvis resulting in staghorn calculi

3. A 12-year-old boy presents to the ED with complaints of right testicular pain, which began gradually about 4 hours prior to arrival. On physical examination, his tenderness is localized to only the superior pole of the testicle, his cremasteric reflex is intact, and he has a blue dot visible near the superior pole of the testicle. His scrotum is not edematous or erythematous, and he has no nausea, vomiting, or abdominal pain. The most appropriate course of action for this patient is:
   a. emergent orchiopexy
   b. color Doppler ultrasonography of the testicle
   c. ice, scrotal support, NSAIDs, and close urologic follow-up
   d. ciprofloxacin 250 mg PO two times a day for 7 days

4. Which of the following is an absolute indication for admission and urologic consultation in the patient with an obstructing ureteral stone?
   a. hydronephrosis
   b. fever
   c. stone size >3 mm
   d. hematuria

5. A 42-year-old morbidly obese man presents with an inability to retract the foreskin of his penis. He notes the foreskin balloons up when he urinates. He denies fevers, chills, flank pain, abdominal pain, dysuria, nausea, or vomiting. On examination you note a morbidly obese male with a protuberant abdomen, no abdominal or flank pain, and a partially retractible foreskin that exposes inflammation of the glans penis that appears irritated with white cheese-like discharge. Urinalysis shows no evidence of

leukocyte esterase or nitrites. Finger stick glucose is 120. This patient needs treatment with:

a. Metformin 500 mg PO two times a day
b. ciprofloxacin 500 mg PO two times a day for 10 to 14 days
c. topical clotrimazole to affected area two times a day
d. cephalexin 500 mg PO TID for 5 days

6. An 82-year-old man has an indwelling Foley catheter since he fractured his right femur 2 weeks ago. He has had surgery, but is largely bed bound, as he is still unable to bear full weight on his right leg. He has been taking narcotics for pain control. He is on no other medications. He reports increasing abdominal distension over the last few days and has noted severe suprapubic abdominal pain since the morning when his Foley catheter stopped draining urine. He presents in severe discomfort. T = 98.6° F, heart rate 80 beats/min, blood pressure 140/80 mmHg. Bedside ultrasound reveals a severely distended bladder. The next thing to attempt is:

a. suprapubic needle aspiration of bladder
b. removal of Foley catheter
c. prostatic massage
d. rectal exam to evaluate for stool impaction

7. Which of the following is true of hemolytic uremic syndrome (HUS)?

a. thrombocytopenia, fever, renal dysfunction, macrocytic anemia
b. prothrombin time (PT), partial thromboplastin time (PTT) are abnormal
c. D-dimer and fibrinogen, fibrin are elevated
d. peripheral blood smear shows schistocytes

8. Testicular torsion is usually due to abnormal insertion of which of the following?

a. tunica albuginea
b. tunica vaginalis
c. tunica vasculosa
d. tunica adventitia

9. Which of the following is most concerning for testicular cancer?

a. palpable tender, firm, intratesticular mass on clinical examination
b. painless hematospermia
c. acute hydrocele on ultrasound
d. alpha-fetoprotein level is normal

10. Which of the following is a feature of phimosis?

a. unable to pull foreskin forward to cover glans
b. it is common with adequate circumcision
c. narrowed opening of the foreskin
d. manual reduction method by upward traction on foreskin with downward pressure on glans

11. A 3-year-old boy with no past medical history is brought in by parents for fever and fussiness. He has never had any symptoms like this before and is up to date on all his shots. Mom notes a significant decrease in the amount of urine he is making in his diapers but it does not smell foul. He does attend day care and recently got over having several days' worth of diarrhea after attending a picnic 1 week ago. Vital signs are T = 99.9, HR 140. Labs reveal WBC = 8000/mL, hemoglobin = 8 g/dL, platelets = 50,000/mL, creatinine = 1.6. Urinalysis reveals microscopic hematuria. Possible treatment plan includes:

a. outpatient treatment with supportive care and oral rehydration therapy
b. plasma exchange
c. antibiotics
d. platelet transfusion

12. A 42-year-old woman presents to the ED after dialysis, noting that her fistula is bleeding. She denies fevers, chills, dizziness, or lightheadedness. Which of the following is the most reasonable initial approach to address her bleeding fistula?

a. protamine
b. elevate arm and apply firm, nonocclusive pressure
c. DDAVP
d. cryoprecipitate

13. Which of the following electrolyte derangements is consistent with chronic renal failure?

a. hyperkalemia
b. hypercalcemia
c. hypophosphatemia
d. hypomagnesemia

14. Which of the following is an appropriate treatment for priapism?

a. terazosin 0.25 to 0.5 mg SC or 5 mg PO every 4 hours
b. phenylephrine: dilute 1 mg in 100 mL saline injected in corpus cavernosum, in 10 mL boluses
c. epinephrine: 10 mg in corpus cavernosum, inject 1- to 3-mL boluses
d. ice, compression, topical sugar for osmotic effect, hyaluronidase injection at prepuce

15. A BUN/creatinine ratio of >20 is most suggestive of which of the following?

a. urinary retention
b. intrinsic renal failure
c. pre-renal (hypovolemic) renal failure
d. kidney stone

16. Which of the following is a common finding associated with nephrotic syndrome?

a. vomiting
b. gross hematuria
c. pitting edema
d. flank pain

17. A 24-year-old woman presents to the ED with a chief complaint of urinary pain for 2 days. She denies fevers, chills, nausea, vomiting, or flank pain. She has an allergy to cephalosporins and penicillin. Physical exam reveals a T 98.6° F, heart rate of 68 beats/min (bpm), and a blood pressure of 130/85 mmHg. Urinalysis reveals presence of leukocyte esterase and nitrites. Urine microscopy shows WBC 11-20 cells/hpf. Urine pregnancy test is positive. Possible treatment plan includes:

    a. ciprofloxacin 250 mg PO two times a day for 3 days
    b. cephalexin 500 mg PO TID for 7 days
    c. nitrofurantoin 100 mg PO two times a day for 7 days
    d. trimethoprim/sulfamethoxazole (TMP/SMX) DS one tablet PO two times a day for 3 days

18. A 48-year-old man with a past medical history significant for arthritis, chronic renal failure, and hypertension, who is taking lisinopril and hydrochlorothiazide, is brought in by paramedics. He is hypertensive with acute left flank pain. On physical examination, he has bilateral palpable masses in his upper abdomen. Urinalysis reveals gross hematuria. This patient likely has:

    a. metastatic disease
    b. hepatosplenomegaly
    c. polycystic kidney disease
    d. Fournier gangrene

19. A 68-year-old man presents with progressive pain and swelling of his left testicle. He describes a heaviness and fullness to that testicle, and has noted some redness to his left scrotum. He notes some dysuria and reports subjective fevers. He has not been sexually active in the past 6 months and denies any penile discharge. This patient should be treated with:

    a. ceftriaxone 250 mg IM once and doxycycline 100 mg PO two times a day for 10 days
    b. ciprofloxacin 500 mg PO two times a day for 10 days
    c. vancomycin 1 g IV every 6 hours for 10 days
    d. penicillin VK 500 mg PO every 6 hours for 10 days

20. A homeless, alcoholic, diabetic man presents toxic in appearance. He is nauseated and vomiting and complaining of abdominal pain. Vitals show a temperature of 102° F, HR = 135 bpm, BP = 90/55 mmHg. On examination, his abdomen is diffusely tender especially in the lower quadrants and suprapubic region. The skin of his perineum, scrotum, and penis is discolored, edematous, blistering, and there is crepitus. He is noted to be insensate in this area. Next immediate course of action includes:

    a. valcyclovir 1 g orally twice a day for 10 days
    b. immediate surgical consult

    c. incision and drainage of bullae
    d. ceftriaxone 2 g IV daily for 10 days

---

1. Answer: c

Hypermagnesemia (c) can cause hypotension. Given that this patient has just been dialyzed, it is highly unlikely that he is **volume overloaded (a)** or is suffering from **hyperkalemia (b)**. While **pericarditis (d)** is a complication of renal failure, it should not cause hypotension without significant effusion.

2. Answer: b

Kidney stones are most likely to cause obstruction at the level of the ureterovesicular junction as this is where the urinary tract is narrowest in diameter **(b)**. 90% of kidney stones are radio opaque and are likely to be present on KUB x-ray **(a)**. The absence in blood does not rule out nephrolithiasis **(c)**. In up to 15% of cases, microscopic hematuria is absent. Struvite stones are most often associated with staghorn calculi in the renal pelvis **(d)**.

3. Answer: c

This patient presents with a classic case of torsion of the appendix testis. He has no findings that would suggest testicular torsion, as he has no scrotal swelling or tenderness, a normal cremasteric reflex, no systemic symptoms, and a "blue dot" sign characteristic of *torsion of the appendix testis*. As such, he can be safely discharged with ice, scrotal support, pain medication, and close follow-up **(c)**. Antibiotics are not indicated **(d)**, and his presentation is not consistent with testicular torsion, so ultrasonography **(b)** and surgery **(a)** are not indicated.

4. Answer: b

Many patients with obstructing stones will have **stones larger than 3 mm in size (c)**, and most will have **hydronephrosis (a)**, but many will do well with close outpatient follow-up. **Hematuria (d)** is common with ureteral stones and should not be an indication for admission. All patients with obstructing ureteral stones and **fever (b)** need emergent urologic consultation and admission to the hospital.

5. Answer: c

This patient presents with balanitis likely secondary to inability to provide adequate personal hygiene secondary to phimosis and body habitus. Treatment includes **topical antifungal (c)** or a one-time dose of oral antifungal fluconazole 150 mg. **Metformin (a)** is used in the treatment of diabetes, and although this patient may be at risk, his glucose level is less suggestive of this diagnosis. **Ciprofloxacin (b)** is a reasonable choice in the treatment of cystitis but the urinalysis does not suggest urinary infection. **Cephalexin (d)** is a reasonable choice if this presentation was concerning for a bacterial infection.

6. Answer: d

This patient presents with **stool impaction (d)** likely from his use of narcotics, immobility, and lack of a bowel regimen. Disimpaction may immediately remedy this obstructive uropathy. If there was no stool impaction, it may be reasonable to irrigate the indwelling Foley catheter to disrupt what may be occluding its lumen. If bladder irrigation through the Foley is not successful, it may be prudent to **remove the Foley (b)** and replace with another indwelling catheter. If there is no resolution of urinary retention, it may be necessary to **aspirate urine from the bladder with a suprapubic approach (a)**. Prostatic **massage (c)** is not helpful in the setting of urinary retention.

7. Answer: d

Peripheral blood smear **(d)** will show **schistocytes** as the result of hemolytic anemia. Patients will characteristically demonstrate thrombocytopenia, fever, renal dysfunction, and hemolytic anemia—not **macrocytic anemia (a)**. PT, PTT will be normal in the setting of HUS **(b)**. D-dimer, fibrinogen, and fibrin are sent to diagnose DIC, in which case these would be elevated—in the setting of HUS, these levels will be normal **(c)**.

8. Answer: b

The **tunica vaginalis (b)** usually inserts low and on the posterior lateral side of testicle. This is not the case in torsion as it is attached at a higher insertion point such that the testicle can rotate freely in the scrotum. Twisting of the testicle causes venous congestion and ultimately arterial compromise, resulting in testicular ischemia. **Tunica albuginea (a)** is the fibrous covering of the testes that lies under the tunica vaginalis. The **tunica vasculosa (c)** is the vascular plexus layer of the testes. **Tunica adventitia (d)** is the outermost layer of a blood vessel.

9. Answer: c

A **new or acute finding of hydrocele (c)** on ultrasound is concerning for testicular cancer, especially in the setting of a palpable NON-tender, firm, intratesticular mass on clinical exam. A **tender mass on clinical examination (a)** tends to favor epididymitis as testicular cancers are more characteristically nontender. **Painless hematospermia (b)** is often more associated with prostatitis. With testicular cancer, hemorrhage within the tumor will often result in painful hematospermia **(b)**. **Alpha-fetoprotein (d)** may be elevated in the setting of testicular cancer but this is not always reliable.

10. Answer: c

A **narrowed opening of the foreskin (c)** is characteristic of phimosis. Inability to pull foreskin forward to cover the glans **(a)** is consistent with *paraphimosis*. An adequate circumcision **(b)** would obviate phimosis but an inadequate circumcision may contribute to phimosis. Manual reduction **(d)** describes the method to reduce a paraphimosis.

11. Answer: a

This patient has *hemolytic uremic syndrome* likely from eating undercooked food that contained *Escherichia coli* serotype 0157:H7. Pediatric patients often do well with **supportive care (a)**. If there is evidence for renal failure, then early dialysis is a consideration. **Plasma exchange (b)** is the treatment of choice for the most severe of cases. Treatment with **antibiotics (c)** is not effective except if *Shigella dysenteriae* is suspected. **Platelet transfusion (d)** is not recommended as this patient is not hemorrhaging and it could exacerbate the thrombotic process.

12. Answer: b

The most reasonable initial approach in this case is the most conservative one. **Elevating the arm and applying firm, nonocclusive pressure** will stop the bleeding in many cases **(b)**. Occlusive pressure risks clotting of the AV fistula. If the bleeding does not stop using conservative means, it would be reasonable to give **protamine, DDAVP,** or **cryoprecipitate (a, c, d)** in an attempt to stop the bleeding.

13. Answer: a

Hyperkalemia is the most common life-threatening electrolyte derangement in renal failure **(a)** as it may lead to cardiac dysrhythmias and death. **Hypocalcemia** not hypercalcemia **(b)** is expected in end-stage renal disease because of the decrease in 1,25-dihydroxyvitamin D synthesis in the kidneys. With decreased urine excretion, **hyperphosphatemia** not hypophosphatemia is expected **(c)**. **Hypermagnesemia** not hypomagnesemia **(d)** is seen in chronic renal failure such that antacids and laxatives are contraindicated in these patients.

14. Answer: b

Phenylephrine (b) is an appropriate treatment for priapism. **Terazosin (a)** is used for benign prostatic hypertrophy. Instead, terbutaline 0.25 to 0.5 mg SC or 5 mg PO every 4 hours is another appropriate treatment. **Epinephrine (c)** is an appropriate choice but 1 mg (not 10 mg) must first be diluted in 100 mL of normal saline then injected into the corpus cavernosum in 1 to 3 aliquot boluses. **Ice, compression, sugar,** and **hyaluronidase** injection **(d)** is a treatment for *paraphimosis*.

15. Answer: c

Pre-renal (hypovolemic) renal failure is often marked by a BUN/creatinine ratio of >20 **(c)**. **Intrinsic renal failure, urinary retention,** and **kidney stones (a, b, d)** generally present with considerably lower BUN/creatinine ratios.

16. Answer: c

Many patients with nephrotic syndrome are asymptomatic. However, common findings associated with nephrotic syndrome include **pitting edema (c)**, postural hypotension, proteinuria, hypertension, hyperlipidemia, and microscopic hematuria. **Vomiting, gross hematuria,** and **flank pain (a, b, d)** are not typical presenting signs and symptoms of nephrotic syndrome.

17. Answer: c

This patient presents with *acute cystitis*. Given that she is pregnant, there are two outpatient choices for therapy, which are cephalexin **(b)** and **nitrofurantoin (c).** She has an allergy to cephalosporins, which eliminates **cephalexin** as a therapeutic choice. IF she were not pregnant, **ciprofloxacin (a)** would be a reasonable first-line choice. **TMP/SMX** DS is also a reasonable choice in a nonpregnant patient; however, resistance has been increasing, and 3-day courses of antibiotics are insufficient in pregnancy.

18. Answer: c

This patient suffered from a ruptured kidney cyst associated with **polycystic kidney disease (c)** resulting in acute flank pain and gross hematuria. Acute onset of pain with hematuria is an uncharacteristic presentation of **metastatic disease (a).** Although polycystic kidney disease can result in cystic disease of other solid organs, **hepatosplenomegaly (c)** would not likely represent

the bilateral masses resulting from PCKD on exam. **Fournier gangrene (d)** is a polymicrobial infection with bacterial toxins and necrosis that starts in the scrotum/perineum that presents with a toxic clinical presentation.

19. Answer: b

This patient has *epididymitis*. Given his age and history, antibiotic coverage with **ceftriaxone** and **doxycycline (a)** for sexually transmitted disease is unlikely to be helpful. Coverage for common urinary tract pathogens using **ciprofloxacin** is the best course of action **(b) vancomycin** and **penicillin (c, d)** do not cover the most common urinary tract pathogens and are thus incorrect.

20. Answer: b

This patient has *Fournier gangrene* and is critically ill. **Immediate surgical consult** for wide debridement is critical **(b).** Broad-spectrum antibiotics are required to cover the most likely culprits (*Streptococcus, Staphylococcus, Enterococcus, E. coli* or *Clostridium*); however, **valacyclovir (a)** is an inappropriate choice and **ceftriaxone (d)** does not ensure broad enough coverage. **Incision and drainage** is an insufficient intervention, as this will require wide debridement of affected tissues with clear margins.

16 | Thoracic/Respiratory

Tracy Leigh LeGros | Heather Murphy-Lavoie |
Pierre Detiege | Terence Hauver

Asthma and reactive airways disease

- **Definition:** A chronic disorder of bronchoconstriction, bronchial edema, obstruction, mucus plugging, increased secretions, inflammation, and hyperresponsiveness. Although previously considered reversible, reversibility may be "incomplete" due to airway remodeling
- **Pathophysiology:** Involves extrinsic-mediated and intrinsic-mediated immune responses, as well as significant airway remodeling
- **Extrinsic (IgE-mediated) asthma:** Inhaled allergens bind to IgE molecules that are bound to mast cells lining the tracheobronchial tree
  - **Characteristics:** accounts for <10% of cases; usually develops early in life
  - **Associations:** sensitivity to inhaled allergens, family history of allergic disease, increased IgE levels, positive allergen skin testing, and blood eosinophilia
- **Intrinsic (infection-induced) asthma:**
  - **Characteristics:** most common type; the inciting allergen usually remains unidentified. It is more severe, perennial, and has a limited response to bronchodilator therapy
  - **Associations:** less of a correlation with family history, low or normal IgE levels, and negative skin testing
  - **Symptoms:** The classic triad is that of cough, dyspnea, and wheezing. Also chest tightness, worsening of symptoms at night, or with exposure to environmental factors
- **Progression of symptoms:** prolonged expiratory phase, tachypnea, tachycardia, anxiety, hypertension, and perhaps diaphoresis with altered mental status. Accessory muscle use may ensue, with retractions, tripod positioning, and pulsus paradoxus (>12 mmHg drop in systolic blood pressure on inspiration)
- **Silent chest:** an ominous sign indicating extensive mucous plugging and/or insufficient air movement
- **Asthma triggers:**
  - **Respiratory infections:** commonly induce bronchospasm. Many viruses inflame the mucosa, enhancing airway reactivity
  - **Drugs:** particularly aspirin and nonsteroidal anti-inflammatory (NSAIDs)
  - **Aspirin-exacerbated respiratory disease (AERD):** AERD consists of a triad of aspirin sensitivity, asthma, and nasal polyps. Symptoms

include profuse rhinorrhea, conjunctival injection, periorbital edema, and at times scarlet flushing. It occurs more commonly in women and is a common cause of fatal asthma (may be a contributor in up to 25% of asthma-related intubations)

- **Occupational dusts, mold, and fumes:** patients are without symptoms on weekends, holidays, and vacations. However, they develop wheezing at work
- **Exercise:** usually occurs 5 to 20 minutes following exercise and is related to pulmonary parenchymal temperature changes. Cold, dry environments worsen symptoms. Warm, humid environments are less irritating
- **Gastroesophageal reflux:** commonly reported and thought to be vagally mediated secondary to microaspiration
- **Menstruation-associated asthma:** affects 30% to 40% of women with asthma, hormonal fluctuations are the presumed etiology
- **Psychological stressors:** trigger airway reactivity, probably through vagal stimulation
- **Risk factors for asthma-related deaths:**
  - History of sudden or severe exacerbations
  - Prior intubations or ICU admissions
  - Two or more ED visits or hospitalizations within one year
  - Use of more than 2 metered dosed inhalers (B_2-agonists) in a month
  - Current or recent withdrawal from systemic steroids
  - Serious psychiatric or psychosocial problems
  - Illicit drug use (inhaled cocaine or heroin)
- **Additional associations:** African Americans who live within the inner city and are between the ages of 15 to 34. They often die at night, either outside or on the way to the hospital and within 24 hours of symptom onset

DIAGNOSIS

- Medical history, physical examination, and serial measurements of objective lung function (spirometry)
- **Management:**
  - **Objective measurements of function:** the FEV_1 and PEFR should be interpreted as a % predicted to account for difference in age, sex, and height
  - **Forced expiratory volume in 1 second (FEV_1):** An initial FEV_1 of <1 L (<30% of predicted) indicates severe obstruction
  - **Peak expiratory flow rate (PEFR):** An initial PEFR <100 L/minute (<20% of predicted) indicates severe obstruction
  - **Pulse oximetry:** may be useful in assessing and following oxygenation. A saturation of <91% indicates severe obstruction or coincident pulmonary disease (e.g., pneumonia)
  - **Arterial blood gas (ABG):** is indicated in those with prolonged or severe attacks but should not delay treatment. Hypercapnia, severe hypoxemia, and/or metabolic acidosis usually do not occur

until the PEFR or the FEV_1 is <25% of predicted. Elderly and very young patients may decompensate earlier. Hypoxemia represents ventilation–perfusion mismatch and when coupled with an increasing $PaCO_2$ indicates impending respiratory failure

- **Nasal capnography:** is noninvasive means of monitoring bronchospasm severity (more studies needed)

TREATMENT

- **Supplemental oxygen:** should be given to all patients, as most are hypoxic. Their condition may worsen initially with bronchodilator therapy (increased ventilation–perfusion mismatch). The goal is to keep oxygen saturations >90% (95% in pregnant women and those with heart disease)
- **Inhaled beta 2-adrenergic agonists:** are a key component of initial treatment. They act on small airways, with an onset of action within 5 minutes. They are available in continuous nebulizations (preferred in ED) and metered dose inhalers (MDIs). Spacers improve drug delivery. Albuterol is preferred due to beta 2-specificity
  - **Mechanism of action** bronchodilate by increasing cAMP, decreasing mediator release from mast cells and basophils, and increasing mucociliary clearance
  - **Caution:** isoproterenol has been associated with some asthmatic deaths and may cause paradoxical bronchospasm
- **Subcutaneous injection of beta agonists:** may be effective for patients who cannot use inhaled devices effectively, are in extremis, those for whom initial treatments with aerosol beta-adrenergic agents fails, or if there is a substantial delay in treatment with aerosolized agents. Both epinephrine and terbutaline have greater beta effects, but terbutaline has a longer duration of action. Use with caution in the elderly, or those with coronary disease or hypertension
- **Inhaled anti-cholinergic agents:** work in large central airways; onset usually 30 minutes; use in patients who continue to wheeze after optimal treatment with beta-agonists. There is an added effect when used with beta-agonists. Examples include ipratropium bromide (preferred agent), atropine, and glycopyrrolate
  - **Mechanism of action:** antagonize acetylcholine at the postganglionic parasympathetic receptor (also decrease cGMP), reducing vagally mediated bronchoconstriction in larger airways
  - **Caution:** aerosolized atropine sulfate and glycopyrrolate have fallen out of favor because of high incidence of anticholinergic side effects
- **Corticosteroids:** should be administered to any patient whose airway obstruction is not promptly resolved by inhaled beta-adrenergic agents. Patients receiving them early require fewer admissions and sustain fewer relapses. Underutilization is associated with an increase in fatal outcomes. Onset of action is gradual, usually 3 hours and

peaking at 6 to 12 hours. Oral and intravenous administration have equivalent efficacy. Inhaled corticosteroids are irritating and can stimulate cough reflex or bronchospasm (not for acute use)
- **Mechanism of action:** increases responsiveness of beta-adrenergic receptors in the smooth muscle of the airways, limits inflammatory cell activation and recruitment, and disrupts arachidonic acid metabolism and synthesis of leukotrienes and prostaglandins
- **Caution:** Because the effects of corticosteroids may not be noted for hours, vigorous treatment with beta-adrenergic agents must be continued. Hydrocortisone promotes sodium retention and potassium excretion. Other side effects include hyperglycemia, hypokalemia, fluid retention, weight gain, mood alterations, rare psychosis, hypertension, peptic ulcer disease, aseptic necrosis of the femur, and rare allergic reactions
- **Magnesium sulfate:** an effective bronchodilator that has been shown to decrease the need for admission
  - **Mechanism of action:** it prevents histamine release from mast cells and opposes the action of acetylcholine. It directly inhibits bronchial smooth muscle contraction. Bronchodilation occurs within 2 to 5 minutes, but the effects dissipate rapidly
  - **Caution:** Side effects include nausea, vomiting, muscle weakness, loss of reflexes, respiratory depression, hypotension, sensation of warmth, and malaise. It is effective in severe exacerbations but not FDA-approved in the United States for the treatment of asthma
- **Noninvasive positive pressure ventilation (CPAP or BiPAP):** reduces the work of breathing and improves oxygenation in those with respiratory failure. No trials thus far related to the treatment of asthma
  - **Mechanism of action:** reduces muscle fatigue by increasing functional residual capacity and lung compliance and supplying some inflation pressure during inspiration
- **Other agents and actions to consider:**
  - **Methylxanthines:** not for acute use; consider only for patients in status who do not respond to optimized aggressive therapy or those maintained on theophylline who have subtherapeutic levels. Examples include theophylline and aminophylline
    - **Mechanism of action:** unclear
    - **Caution:** use alone or with beta-adrenergic agonists during acute episodes is associated with increased side effects and little effect on bronchospasm. They have a narrow therapeutic-toxicity window and may cause life-threatening cardiac dysrhythmias or seizures. Additional side effects include headache, nausea, vomiting, abdominal cramps, diarrhea, nervousness, tremor, confusion, hyperglycemia, hypokalemia, hypophosphatemia, hypomagnesemia, leukocytosis, respiratory alkalosis or metabolic acidosis. Numerous medications significantly alter theophylline levels (check drug interactions)

- **Halothane:** potent bronchodilator with a rapid onset of action. Side effects include cardiac dysrhythmias and cardiopulmonary shunting
- **Heliox:** an 80:20 or 70:30 mixture of helium and oxygen, it is sometimes given for those with respiratory acidosis to decrease turbulent flow. Helium is of low density and lowers airway resistance and decreases the work of breathing. It also increases the diffusion of CO_2 to improve gas exchange. Effects may be seen within 20 minutes of treatment. Should not be used if hypoxia exists
- **Leukotriene antagonists-inhibitors:** still under investigation. May be useful for long-term maintenance therapy
- **Intravenous montelukast:** one recent study demonstrated efficacy when paired with inhaled beta-adrenergic agonists
- **Treatment regimens based on symptom severity:**
  - **Moderate symptoms (FEV1 or PEFR >50%):** inhaled beta 2-agonist by nebulizer (three doses in first hour) + O_2 (ensure saturation >90%) + oral corticosteroids if no immediate response or if patient has recently taken oral corticosteroids
  - **Severe symptoms: (FEV1 or PEFR <50%):** inhaled high-dose beta 2-agonist + anticholinergic by nebulization (every 20 minutes or continuously for 1 hour) + O_2 (saturation >90%) + oral corticosteroids
  - **Impending or actual respiratory arrest:** intubation and mechanical ventilation + nebulized beta 2-agonist and anticholinergics + intravenous corticosteroids. The need for intubation occurs in 2% of patients. Between 10% and 30% require ICU admission
- **Criteria for intubation:** Primarily based on patient's clinical condition. ABG is a diagnostic aid that may show progressive hypoxemia and acidosis; respiratory fatigue, cyanosis, apnea, or mental status changes
- **Mechanical ventilation adjuncts:**
  - **Ketamine:** disassociative anesthetic with bronchodilator effects
  - **Benzodiazepines:** sedation that induces histamine release (avoid)
  - **Propofol:** rapid-onset deep sedation that has bronchodilator properties and may obviate the need for muscular paralysis
  - **Pancuronium:** paralytic that does not induce histamine release
  - **Permissive hypercapnia:** mechanical ventilation in which the patient is given rapid inspiratory flow rate, reduced respiratory frequency, and prolonged expiratory phase. This is done to reduce "auto-PEEP [positive end-expiratory pressure]," a phenomenon wherein expiratory airflow obstruction results in air trapping and higher lung volumes, continuously increasing intrathoracic pressure, decreasing venous return, and resulting in hypotension
  - **Anesthetic gases:** for critically ill, intubated asthmatic patients with persistent hypoxemia, it

may be necessary to administer isoflurane or halothane in the operating theater. Isoflurane has lower arrhythmogenic and hypotensive side effects

- **Criteria for discharge:** good response, with an FEV1 or PEFR > 70%, with response sustained for 60 minutes following last treatment without distress and normal physical examination
  - **Education:** Define goals of well controlled asthma, including: how medications work, how to use an inhaler, what constitutes worsening of asthma, when to adjust doses of medications, and when to seek additional care. Development of a written asthma action plan (daily instructions on management) also improves outcomes. Ensure proper follow-up
  - **Control of environmental factors and triggers:** Attempt to eliminate exposure to allergens (animal dander, cockroaches), as well as indoor and outdoor pollutants (perfumes, smoke, chemical household products)
  - **Medications:** albuterol MDI with spacer, and oral steroid prescription with consideration for inhaled steroid MDI to be started if prompt follow-up within 1 to 3 days with the primary doctor is not ensured
- **Criteria For admission:** FEV1 or PEFR <70% with mild to moderate symptoms; condition deteriorates; return for further therapy within days after discharge; dyspneic patients with significant hypoxemia (PaO$_2$ <60), hypercapnia, or acidosis; patients with continued abnormal vital signs after therapy; unreliable patients
- **Complications:** include pneumothorax, pneumomediastinum, subcutaneous emphysema, rib fractures, and costochondral strain. Cough syncope is rare and is usually noted in the moderately obese, middle-aged, male patient
- **Prognosis:** is generally good for 50% to 80%, especially for those with mild disease. However, asthma has high morbidity. In the United States, >4,000 deaths annually are attributed to asthma

Chronic obstructive pulmonary disease (COPD)

- **Definition:** a spectrum of chronic respiratory illnesses (chronic bronchitis, emphysema, and asthma) characterized by a cough, sputum production, dyspnea, airflow limitation, and impaired gas exchange. It is an abnormal inflammatory response in the small airways and lung parenchyma to noxious particles and gases. COPD is usually asymptomatic until the 5th or 6th decade of life
- **Epidemiology:** affects >15 million Americans yearly; mortality rate >50% within 10 years of diagnosis. COPD is the fourth-leading cause of death in the United States. A patient >65 years old requiring ICU admission for a COPD exacerbation has a 1-year mortality risk of 59%

- **Pathophysiology:** The inflammatory response involves the recruitment of neutrophils, macrophages, and cytotoxic T lymphocytes. Inflammation of the small airways results in increased resistance and airflow limitation. Alveolar hypoventilation results in hypoxemia and hypercarbia. VQ mismatching occurs, promoting further hypoxia, increasing physiologic dead space, and further exacerbating hypoventilation, hypercarbia, and hypoxemia. Moreover, destruction and coalescence of alveoli occurs, reducing gas-exchange surface area. This chronic airway obstruction results in right-sided heart failure, pulmonary hypertension, and cor pulmonale
- **Risk factors:** tobacco use is most predominant (80% to 90%), although 5% to 10% have never smoked. Only 15% of smokers acquire clinically significant COPD. Environmental pollution, cystic fibrosis, passive smoke inhalation, occupational exposure, and repeated respiratory infections are additional risk factors. Genetic factors may also be involved (alpha 1-antitrypsin deficiency)
- **Predictors of disability and death:** the single best indicator is a FEV$_1$
- **Triggers for exacerbations:**
  - Respiratory infections
  - Medical noncompliance or underdosing of medication
  - Weather changes
  - Drugs: beta-adrenergic blockers, sedatives
  - Cardiac dysrhythmias and left ventricular dysfunction
  - Noxious stimuli: exposure to allergens, irritants, mold, or continued smoking
- **Triggers for acute decompensation:**
  - Spontaneous pneumothorax: higher complication and mortality than non-COPD
  - Pulmonary embolism
  - Congestive heart failure
  - Respiratory infections
  - Acidosis: renal and/or hepatic failure (overwhelm limited reserve)

DIAGNOSIS

- **Physical examination highlights:**
  - Use of accessory muscles, tripod posture, tachycardia, tachypnea, JVD with expiration, retractions, muscle wasting, pulsus paradoxus, peripheral edema, dyspnea, hyperresonance to percussion
  - Confusion, somnolence, irritability: may be signs of hypercapnia and hypoxemia (impending respiratory failure)
- **Ancillary testing:**
  - **Pulse oximetry/ABG:** pH is single best lab marker to gauge severity of disease (reflects speed and degree of PaCO$_2$ changes)
  - **Chest radiograph:** usual findings include bullae and a flattened diaphragm. Additional findings include increased anteroposterior (AP) diameter, retrosternal airspace, and parenchymal lucency. The best use of chest x-ray (CXR) is to rule out

other diseases (pneumonia, pneumothorax, atelectasis, mass, or congestive heart failure [CHF])

- **Electrocardiogram:** findings include right atrial enlargement, right axis deviation, right ventricular hypertrophy, poor R-wave progression, low voltage, multifocal atrial tachycardia, and/or right ventricular hypertrophy/strain (cor pulmonale). Acute ischemic patterns (ACS) may be a triggering or complicating factor even in a COPD attack
- **FEV1 and/or PEFR:** measurements of airflow do not always yield accurate assessment of illness severity, but may be useful in judging response to therapy. In contrast to asthmatic patients, COPD patients do not typically demonstrate a marked change

TREATMENT

- **Oxygen:** critical treatment as hypoxemia is the major life threat. Maintain PaO_2 >60 mmHg or pulse oximetry 90% to 92%. Controlled O_2 therapy (Venturi mask) is preferred. In the acutely hypoxemic patient, supplemental oxygen is paramount and far outweighs the risk of hypercarbia caused by blunting of the hypoxemic drive in a chronic CO_2 retainer. Long-term ambulatory oxygen therapy is also the only treatment demonstrated to prolong life
- **Treatment of dysrhythmias:** like rapid atrial fibrillation, usually reflect coexisting heart disease worsened by acute hypoxemia
- **Beta 2-adrenergic agonists:** initial agent of choice (via nebulizer); however, effectiveness is dependent in part on the disease reversibility
- **Anticholinergics:** slower onset of action but has an additive effect when given with beta 2-agonists; the drug of choice for chronic disease, especially in those who respond poorly to beta-agonists
- **Corticosteroids:** useful in acute exacerbations. Even those who do not initially respond, when stable, may benefit from steroid administration. Patients with current or recent steroid use, require them in the emergency department. Oral and intravenous routes have similar efficacy
- **Methylxanthines:** widely used before the advent of inhaled beta 2-agonists and steroids. Caution though, because of narrow therapeutic window and associated with adverse effects, including nausea, cardiac dysrhythmias, and rarely, seizures. Not for use in an acute exacerbations. May be required in patients maintained on theophylline, as guided by drug levels
- **Magnesium sulfate:** bronchodilatory effects and may be an adjunct in those with severe exacerbations, provided they have normal renal function
- **Noninvasive positive pressure ventilation:** should be considered for those with moderate exacerbations, absence of nausea/vomiting, and normal mental status. It decreases the work of breathing, need for endotracheal intubation, hospital mortality, and shortens hospital stays

- **Endotracheal intubation:** required for those who fail to respond to acute interventions and begin to show signs of respiratory failure, such as mental status changes with worsening hypoxemia and acidosis
- **Complications:** hypotension or cardiovascular collapse from decreased venous return, sympathetic tone, and/or the administration of sedatives
- **Correcting ventilatory hypotension:** if hypotension does not resolve with IV fluids, temporarily disconnect the endotracheal tube (ETT) from the ventilator to relieve the excess positive intrathoracic pressure
- **Ventilator settings:** mechanical ventilation should be adjusted to allow longer expiratory time and a low tidal volume (5 to 7 mL/kg). Ventilatory frequency may be gradually increased to allow for resolution of the acidosis and pH normalization. Extrinsic PEEP may be added to nearly equal intrinsic or auto-PEEP. This will stent open the airways and reduce gas trapping
- **Paralytics:** short-term paralytics with sedation will eliminate dyssynchrony between the patient and ventilator and reduce the risk of hyperinflation
- **Mucolytics:** no evidence of acute efficacy
- **Antibiotics:** 50% of COPD exacerbations are caused by bacterial infections. Most involve *Haemophilus influenzae, Moraxella catarrhalis,* and *Streptococcus pneumoniae*
- **Criteria for discharge:** permitted with good response to therapy and with vital signs and pulmonary function approaching baseline. Maximize bronchodilator therapy and continue steroid treatments
- **Criteria for admission:** poor response to outpatient therapy, severe limitation of function, inability to engage in activities of daily living due to dyspnea, comorbid conditions, worsening respiratory failure, and/or new/progressive cor pulmonale

Bronchitis

- **Definition:** self-limited inflammation of the bronchi
  - **Acute bronchitis:** acute cough (<2 weeks) without prior lung disease and without clinical findings of pneumonia
  - **Chronic bronchitis:** cough with sputum production most days of the month for at least 3 months of the year for 2 consecutive years
- **Etiologies:** Usual causes include influenza A and B, parainfluenza, coronavirus (types 1 to 3), rhinovirus, adenovirus, respiratory syncytial virus (RSV), and human metapneumovirus. Less common causes (5% to 25%) include *Mycoplasma pneumoniae* (bullous myringitis), *Chlamydia pneumoniae,* and *Bordetella pertussis*
- **Symptoms:** cough (>5 days), usually with sputum production. The cough usually lasts 10 to 20 days. A fever is not usual and suggests either influenza or pneumonia. The strongest positive predictor for

acute bronchitis is cough and wheezing. The strongest negative predictor is nausea. There is significant overlap in symptomatology between bronchitis and asthma. In fact, approximately 33% of those with bronchitis also have asthma. The patient may also have symptoms including: malaise, rhinorrhea, sore throat, wheezing, myalgias, dyspnea, and chest pain

- **Risk factors for chronic bronchitis:** elderly, structural lung disease or poor lung function, other comorbid conditions, and those with frequent exacerbations requiring steroid use

DIAGNOSIS

- This is a clinical diagnosis. Chest radiographs are not indicated in previously healthy adults unless the cough has been present more than 3 weeks, clinical evidence of pneumonia is found, or the patient is elderly

TREATMENT (ACUTE BRONCHITIS MANAGEMENT)

- **Antibiotics:** The overprescription of antibiotics is the major issue to be addressed with the treatment of acute bronchitis. Although this disease is usually caused by a virus, 60% to 70% of patients are given antibiotics. At best, antibiotics may decrease sputum production and increase the return to work by a day or less. Moreover, even in those with atypical bacterial etiologies, antibiotic treatment does not affect outcome and is more likely to cause adverse side effects
- **Indications:** Only pertussis has shown any clinical responsiveness to antibiotics, and suspicion of pertussis is the only indication for antibiotics. If given, macrolides are first choice as they are active against mycoplasmal and chlamydial organisms as well as *B. pertussis*
- **Misconception:** Some clinicians suspect bacterial pathogens such as Streptococcus, Haemophilus, Staphylococcus, Moraxella, or even gram-negative bacilli. However, in adults, these pathogens do not cause "acute bacterial bronchitis," except in those with airway compromise (i.e., tracheostomy, intubation)
- **Supportive treatment:** Most patients with acute bronchitis have associated symptoms of the common cold, and will benefit from supportive care. These include analgesics (NSAIDs, aspirin), antipyretics (acetaminophen), antitussives (debatable efficacy), expectorants, ipratropium, and nasal decongestants. Beta-adrenergic agonists are not effective for coughs <4 weeks in duration unless airway obstruction (wheezing) is present (excluding cough-variant asthma). Steroids and mucolytics have unproven efficacy

TREATMENT (EXACERBATION OF CHRONIC BRONCHITIS MANAGEMENT)

- Approximately 66% are bacterial in origin, with Haemophilus, Streptococcus, and Moraxella the most common etiologies. Prescribe antibiotics to those patients with increased dyspnea and increased sputum purulence and/or volume. Use doxycycline, cephalexin, amoxicillin–clavulanate, or a fluoroquinolone
- **Complications:** <5% of patients with bronchitis develop pneumonia. Residual sequelae are rare for acute bronchitis

Bronchiolitis

- **Definition:** A virally induced bronchiolar inflammation, occurring usually in the spring and winter months in those 2 months to 2 years of age. It is usually self-limited and is the most common lower respiratory infection in infants. It is also the leading cause of hospitalization in those <1 year old (more than 80% are less than 6 months old)
- **Epidemiology:** RSV is responsible for 70% of bronchiolitis (80% to 100% in winter epidemics). Infection is by respiratory droplets, and familial transmission rates are approximately 45% (higher in day care). Annual incidence is 11% in those <1 year old
  - Other causes include adenovirus (11%), which has a more virulent presentation, and parainfluenza, which usually begins earlier in the year; outbreaks occur every other year. Mycoplasma, enterovirus, influenza, rhinovirus, and chlamydia are less common agents

SIGNS AND SYMPTOMS

- Disease severity is directly related to the size and maturity of the infant. Early symptoms mimic viral upper respiratory infections (URIs; rhinorrhea, cough, and low-grade fever). Other common symptoms include:
  - Tachypnea: 50 to 60 bpm (most common finding)
  - Fever: 38.5° to 39° C
  - Expiratory wheezing
  - Mild conjunctivitis or pharyngitis
  - Otitis media
  - Nostril flaring/grunting/chest wall retractions
  - Post-tussive vomiting
  - Irritability/poor feeding
- **Risk factors:** gestational age <37 weeks, age <3 months, chronic pulmonary disease, congenital heart disease, immunodeficiency, congenital and anatomical defects of the airways, and neurological disease
- **Environmental risks:** passive smoking, crowded dwellings, day care, concurrent birth siblings, older siblings, and high altitude

DIAGNOSIS

- Purely clinical; tests are of little value

TREATMENT

- **Nursing care:** respiratory support, adequate hydration, saline nasal drops and nasal bulb suction, humidified oxygen, apnea monitoring,

cardiopulmonary monitoring (with pulse oximetry), and frequent clinical reassessment
- **Proper positioning:** have the child sit in parent's arms or in position of comfort
- **Severe symptoms:** require supplemental O_2, intubation, and assisted ventilation
- **Do not:** "deep" suction lower pharynx or larynx or give chest physiotherapy

TREATMENT

- Little evidence for any useful drug treatment
- Antibiotics are of no use (most cases viral)
- The exception would be a patient with a concomitant otitis media (occurs commonly)
- Beta agonists produce only modest and transient improvement, but may be continued as an outpatient if the child responded to them in the ED. There is no proven role for epinephrine, ipratropium, ribavirin, and immunoglobulin agents
- Steroids are controversial. The benefit may be small, and must be weighed against the adverse events
- Several studies have shown that a combination of dexamethasone and salbutamol results in better outcomes than either agent alone
- **Criteria for discharge:** Patients can be managed as outpatients if they do not appear ill (without nasal flaring, retractions, grunting) and are adequately hydrated. The caretakers should be able to continue oral hydration and nasal bulb suctioning and should have been educated regarding expected clinical course
- **Criteria for admission:**
  - <3 months old
  - Respiratory rate >60 breaths/minute
  - Oxygen saturation <95%
  - Prematurity
  - Cardiopulmonary disease
  - Immunodeficient
  - Lethargy, toxic appearance, poor feeding, dehydration
  - Apneic episodes
  - Parent unable to care for child at home
- **Prognosis:** Bronchiolitis symptoms last for 7 to 10 days and most patients do well. Significant morbidity is rare. Hospitalization is required in 2%. Intubation is needed in 3% to 7%. The risk of death for a healthy infant is <0.5%. However, this risk rises in those with heart disease (3.5%) or chronic lung disease (3.45%)

Bronchopulmonary dysplasia (BPD)

- **Definition:** Bronchopulmonary dysplasia is also known as **neonatal chronic lung disease,** and is a significant preterm newborn respiratory illness. It occurs in those preterm infants treated with supplemental O_2 and positive-pressure ventilation. It is most common in those <1250 g (usually <1000 g) born between 22 and 32 weeks' gestation

Pathophysiology

- Not fully elucidated
- **Toxic factors:** combine to disturb normal lung alveolarization, resulting in decreased surface area for gas exchange
  - **Developing pulmonary vasculature:** is damaged, resulting in significant pulmonary dysfunction
  - **Prolonged supplemental oxygenation:** results in free radical formation with resultant cell damage
  - **Prolonged ventilation:** may result in pulmonary infections and barotrauma
  - **End result:** increased airway resistance, airway reactivity, and airway obstructions, as well as decreased lung compliance

SIGNS AND SYMPTOMS

- Tachypnea, tachycardia, retractions, grunting, nasal flaring; they also frequently desaturate and have significant weight loss within the first 2 weeks of life
- **Risk factors:**
  - In utero infections
  - Family history of atopy/asthma
  - Polymorphisms in surfactant protein B
  - Elevated levels of tumor necrosis factor–alpha
  - Atelectasis
  - Hypertension
  - Patent ductus arteriosus
  - Pneumonia
  - Subglottic stenosis
  - Tracheomalacia
  - Genetic abnormalities
- **Mortality risks**
  - Increasing duration of mechanical ventilation
  - Elevated mean airway pressures
  - Bacterial sepsis during previous month
  - Decreasing oxygen saturation
  - Small for gestational age

TREATMENT

- The treatment necessary to recruit alveoli and prevent atelectasis (CPAP + ventilation) in immature lungs may paradoxically cause lung injury and inflammatory changes
  - **Supportive care:** supplemental O_2 and continuous monitoring with pulse oximetry. Consider also transcutaneous or end-tidal CO_2 monitoring
  - **Chest x-rays:** can be used to determine the severity of BPD. Chest films usually demonstrate hyperinflation, atelectasis, pulmonary edema, and interstitial emphysema
  - **Steroids:** low-dose, short-term dexamethasone therapy is best in selected cases (those with increased ventilatory requirements at age 1 month)
  - **Optimization of nutrition:** adequate nutrition may facilitate weaning from mechanical ventilation. Infants with BPD have increased energy needs. Early parenteral nutrition helps obviate catabolic state
  - **Furosemide:** Diuretics are often used to prevent or treat volume overload

- **Surfactant therapy and vitamin A supplementation**
- **Bronchodilators:** may improve lung compliance by decreasing airway resistance. Beta agonists in combination with ipratropium bromide may be more effective than either agent alone
- **Methylxanthines:** used to improve diaphragmatic contractility; they increase respiratory drive, decrease pulmonary vascular resistance, and have a mild diuretic effect
- **Gentle mode ventilation:** synchronized intermittent mechanical ventilation has been shown to be effective, as has positive-pressure ventilation with various forms of nasal CPAP
- **RSV prophylaxis:** with palivizumab, a monoclonal antibody
- **Influenzae and pneumococcal vaccinations**
- **Complications:** BPD infants are at increased risk for respiratory infections, especially RSV, pulmonary barotrauma (volume trauma). In addition, these patients have high rates of rehospitalization, especially in the first year. Persistent abnormalities in pulmonary function studies are common. Moreover, abnormal neurological and muscular development occurs, as well as slow growth
- **Prognosis:** those with severe BPD have a higher risk of death, usually from respiratory failure, overwhelming pulmonary hypertension with cor pulmonale, or sepsis. Death increases with duration of mechanical ventilation. Retinopathy of prematurity is also a risk for those on prolonged supplemental oxygen. Those with mild disease usually do well. However, those with severe disease have significant pulmonary dysfunction, as well as abnormalities in neurodevelopment and growth

Foreign body aspiration

- **Definition:** Airway aspiration of a foreign body (FB) most commonly occurs in children (75%). FB aspiration is most common in those 6 months to 4 years old, with the peak at 2 years and a steep decline after age 3 years. Adults over 60 or those with potential abnormalities of deglutition (mental retardation, alcoholism, psychiatric disease, neurological and neuromuscular disorders) are also at higher potential risk
  - **Food:** is the most common FB aspirated: peanuts, grapes, raisins, hot dogs, popcorn, and carrots
  - **Non-edible FBs:** balloons/doctors' gloves (most common fatal FB), plastic toys or parts, pins, needles, jewelry, pencils, dental hardware, and teeth
- **Types:** The severity of the aspirations depends on whether it results in a complete or partial obstruction
  - **Complete obstructions:** occur above the carina and can rapidly lead to death
  - **Partial obstructions:** are not completely occlusive or occur distal to the carina
  - **Right main stem bronchus:** Most partial FB aspirations result in right main stem bronchus obstructions. This occurs for several reasons, including that the right main stem is larger than the left, the take-off angle from the trachea is smaller on the right, and airflow is greater on the right side

SIGNS AND SYMPTOMS

- **Complete obstructions:** cannot speak or cough, obvious respiratory distress, pantomime choking, and rapidly deteriorate without treatment
- **Partial obstructions:** may present many days to weeks later, often complaining of wheezing, persistent cough, and/or recurrent pneumonia

DIAGNOSIS

- **Screening radiographs:** of the chest (AP, lateral, inspiratory/expiratory) and soft tissue of the neck. Order portable studies if possible to keep the patient close at hand. If the patient cannot comply with obtaining inspiratory/expiratory films (look for hyperinflation of the involved lung) (Fig. 16-1), bilateral decubitus chest films can be obtained.

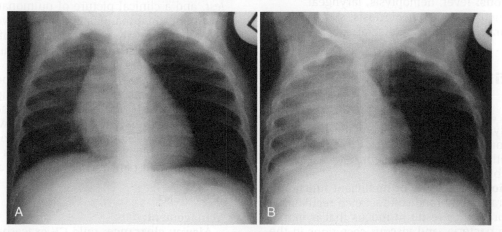

Figure 16-1. Inspiratory **(A)** and expiratory **(B)** x-rays of an 8-year-old boy with a left airway foreign body (peanut). No foreign object is visible on plain films, but the expiratory film shows overinflation of the left lung with mediastinal shift to the contralateral side. (From Rakel RE: *Textbook of family medicine,* ed 7, Philadelphia, 2007, Saunders.)

Fluoroscopy (more sensitive) may be necessary. However, as most FBs are radiolucent (85%), look for secondary signs of a retained FB. No radiographic studies are sensitive or specific enough to exclude a retained FB. If these studies are negative, but the index of suspicion remains high, bronchoscopy in the operating room (OR) is definitive

- **Obstructive emphysema:** hyperinflation on the affected side, occurs because the patient can inhale around the obstruction but cannot completely exhale
- **Mediastinal shift:** occurs on expiration (away from affected side)
- **Other secondary findings:** include pneumonia and atelectasis
- **Decubitus films:** will show that the affected lung will not collapse, even in the decubitus position

TREATMENT

- **General management ABCs**
- **Heliox** (80% helium/20% O_2): consider also in those with obstructing tumors as the decreased gas density may improve oxygenation. Be cautious when withdrawing heliox as the work of breathing substantially increases
- **Critical treatment:** for the acutely decompensating patient involves one of three pathways:
  - **Force FB out with maneuvers:** finger sweep (losing favor in all age groups), back blows, abdominal thrusts
  - **Laryngoscopy:** attempt to remove FB under direct visualization with Magill forceps. It may be possible to use the blunted (cut off) end of an ETT attached to wall suction with a meconium aspirator or a Y connector
  - **Control the airway:** the ETT may force the FB distally; surgical airway may be required if intubation fails. In children, the use of the laryngeal mask airway offers easy airway access, excellent visualization, and reliable airway management during bronchoscopy
- **Complications:** fever, hemoptysis, laryngeal swelling, pneumonia, bronchiectasis, strictures, pneumothorax, asphyxia, cardiac arrest

Cystic fibrosis (CF)

- **Definition:** autosomal recessive disorder that results in dysfunction of exocrine gland functions involving multiple organ systems. CF is the most common lethal inherited disease in Caucasians (1 in 3200 births)
- **Pathophysiology:** inactive or inefficient functioning of the CF transmembrane conductance regulator. These abnormalities result in mucus that is more adherent to bacteria, and viscous secretions in the respiratory tract, pancreas, GI tract, and sweat glands

SIGNS AND SYMPTOMS

- **Respiratory:** wheezing, paroxysmal coughing, post-tussive vomiting, recurring respiratory infections, bronchiolitis, pneumonia, pneumothorax, hemoptysis, digital clubbing, dyspnea on exertion, and recurrent sinusitis, rhinitis, and nasal polyps. By age 18 years, 80% of patients are permanently colonized by *Pseudomonas*
- **Water electrolyte balance:** increased sodium and chloride in sweat. During hot weather or during stress, the salt depletion and subsequent electrolyte abnormalities can be dramatic. The extreme chloride loss is compensated for by a rise in serum bicarbonate, which results in metabolic alkalosis. The patients present hyponatremic, hypokalemic, lethargic, and hypotensive. The treatment is normal saline and supplemental electrolyte correction
- **Gastrointestinal symptoms:** myriad
  - **Early:** meconium ileus (birth), meconium peritonitis
  - **Surgical:** distal intestinal obstruction, gallstones, scarring, adhesions, volvulus, intestinal atresia, intussusception, rectal prolapse, and perforation
  - **Chronic:** pancreatic insufficiency, fecal impaction, poor weight gain, salivary gland swelling, anorexia, malodorous greasy stools, flatulence, postprandial colicky pain, poor ability to absorb fat-soluble vitamins, jaundice, gastroesophageal reflux, GI bleeding, and failure to thrive early in life. Obstructive liver cirrhosis may occur because of the increased viscosity of bile, along with complicating esophageal varices, splenomegaly, hypersplenism, and passive liver congestion
- **Reproductive:** Males—delayed puberty and reduced fertility (azoospermia with agenesis of the vas deferens). They may also have undescended testicles, or hydroceles. Females—amenorrhea, though fertility is not as severely affected
- **Dermatologic:** many vitamin deficiencies, which lead to: dry skin (vitamin A) and cheilosis (vitamin B)

DIAGNOSIS

- Can be considered on the basis of a *positive sweat test*, and a clinical picture of pulmonary and gastrointestinal manifestations. Positive sweat test is neither perfectly sensitive nor specific, however
  - **Additional testing:** genotyping, semen analyses, and pulmonary function testing
  - **Radiographs:** Chest films show hyperinflation with peribronchial thickening and upper lobe bronchiectasis. More progressive disease results in flattened diaphragms, sternal bowing, thoracic kyphosis, pulmonary artery dilatation and right ventricular hypertrophy. Sinus films will demonstrate pansinusitis in almost all patients

TREATMENT

- **Management:**
  - **Airway clearance:** mild CF exacerbations can be treated by increasing the frequency of airway clearance measures. Chest physiotherapy using

high-frequency oscillator devices, noninvasive ventilatory mask therapy, postural drainage, bronchodilator therapy, and mucolytics are beneficial
- **Dornase alfa:** is an inhaled, aerosolized, purified solution of recombinant human DNAse. This enzymatic product improves pulmonary function
- ***Pseudomonas* prophylaxis:** chronic administration of azithromycin is recommended, as it has been shown to improve FEV1 in CF patients. Macrolide antibiotics have potent anti-inflammatory properties in addition to their antimicrobial effects
- **Acute Pseudomonal Exacerbations:** 80% of adults are permanently colonized with *Pseudomonas*. For acute infections, treatment is with an anti-pseudomonal penicillin or newer cephalosporin (ceftazidime, cefepime) combined with an aminoglycoside. Ensure that previous sputum cultures are reviewed and all last-known pathogens are covered
- **Complications:** hemoptysis, pneumothorax, vasculitis, heat stroke due to sweat dysfunction, mucocele and mucopyoceles (due to chronic sinusitis), eroding nasal polyps leading to CNS infections, portal hypertension, pulmonary hypertension, pancreatitis, liver failure, diabetes mellitus, cholecystitis, cholelithiasis, rickets, and osteoporosis
- **Prognosis:** CF is a disease marked by great heterogeneity of symptoms. The mean life span is 37 years, and it is the severity of the pulmonary manifestations that portends ultimate survival. Persistent lower airway infections with inflammation are the major cause of morbidity and mortality. It is a progressive disease, beginning with bronchitis, then bronchiolitis, bronchiectasis, cor pulmonale, and finally end-stage lung disease. Pulmonary involvement occurs in 90% and end-stage lung disease is the usual cause of death

Acute upper airway disorders

CROUP

- Heterogeneous group of illnesses affecting the larynx, trachea, and bronchi. Also called laryngotracheobronchitis, laryngotracheitis, and spasmodic croup. The overall result is inflammation in the larynx and subglottic airway
- **Incidence:** peak incidence in fall and winter; it is the most common cause of infectious airway obstruction in children, with a peak at age 2 years
- **Epidemiology:** Parainfluenza virus (75%), RSV, influenza A and B, other viruses less common. *M. pneumoniae* also a consideration

SIGNS AND SYMPTOMS

- Coryza, **barky cough,** hoarseness, inspiratory stridor, clear lungs, low-grade fever, symptoms

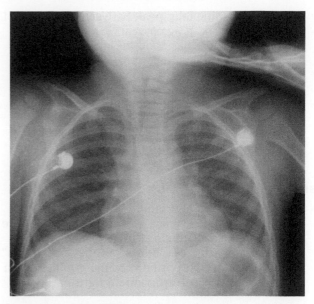

Figure 16-2. Radiograph of an airway of a patient with croup, showing typical subglottic narrowing ("steeple sign"). (From Kliegman RM, Behrman RE, Jenson HB, Stanton BF (eds): *Nelson textbook of pediatrics,* ed 18, Philadelphia, 2007, Saunders.)

worse at night; severe cases—biphasic stridor, nasal flaring, retractions, tachypnea, low oxygen saturations. Airway obstruction can occur (especially if child becomes agitated)

DIAGNOSIS

- Clinical, soft tissue neck radiograph (steeple sign) (Fig. 16-2)

TREATMENT

- **Supportive care:** with cool humidified air or oxygen
- **Racemic epinephrine:** via nebulizer (effects last 2 hours); should then get steroids too
- **Steroids:** corticosteroids (PO, IM, IV same); dexamethasone 0.15 to 0.6 mg/kg one dose; budesonide 2 mg via nebulization
- **Intubation:** for severe cases not responsive to treatment. Choose endotracheal tube smaller than typical for patient size
- **Outcomes:** majority receive supportive care, then discharged; observe for 2 to 4 hours after racemic epinephrine; <1% require intubation; rare bacterial secondary infections (bacterial tracheitis or pneumonia) can occur
- **Spasmodic croup:** Similar clinical picture except lack fever, sudden onset, shorter duration (may resolve prior to arrival), recurrent, possible allergic component

EPIGLOTTITIS

- Rapid progressive infection of the epiglottis and adjacent tissues usually caused by bacterial infection. Also called supraglottitis. Tissue cellulitis with inflammation and swelling leads to airway obstruction

- **Incidence:** traditionally peak between the ages of 1 and 5 years; peak at age 3 years. Since vaccinations, there has been an increase in older child and adult cases (mean age 46 years)
- **Etiology:** Most cases were secondary to *Haemophilus influenzae* type B. Since childhood vaccinations (early 1990s) dramatic decline in cases. As of now, there is no predominant pathogen (*H. influenza* type A, F, non-typeable *Haemophilus parainfluenza, S. pneumoniae, Staphylococcus aureus,* beta-hemolytic streptococci

SIGNS AND SYMPTOMS

- The onset is acute and rapidly progresses from a URI. Patients appear toxic, with a fever, severe sore throat, dysphagia, drooling, and possible stridor and respiratory distress. Beware of the "hot potato" voice and the tripod position, as these patients can progress to airway obstruction and arrest

DIAGNOSIS

- Clinical, must have a high index of suspicion. Examination may show a red, edematous epiglottis. Instrumentation may precipitate complete obstruction. Lateral neck x-ray on inspiration may show "thumb-sign" of an enlarged epiglottis (Fig. 16-3); criterion standard is direct visualization

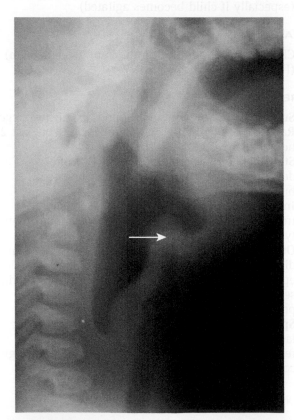

Figure 16-3. Lateral neck radiograph of a 4-year-old child with acute epiglottitis. Note characteristically distended hypopharynx and "thumbprint" edematous and aryepiglottic folds *(arrow)*. (From Long SS, Pickering LK, Prober CG (eds): *Principles and practice of pediatric infectious diseases,* ed 3, Philadelphia, 2008, Churchill Livingstone.)

TREATMENT

- Supportive care includes continuous monitoring, limiting anxiety-provoking procedures, and sitting in position of comfort
  - Immediate ENT/Anesthesia involvement
  - **Airway control:** intubation—consider fiberoptics, usually in operating suite with preparation for tracheostomy if necessary
  - **Broad-spectrum antibiotics:** ceftriaxone, ampicillin/sulbactam, piperacillin/tazobactam, nafcillin, vancomycin
  - **Steroids:** dexamethasone 0.6 mg/kg/day
  - **Outcomes:** most patients have a complete recovery if treated prior to airway obstruction; sepsis is rare, but hypoxic brain injury is a risk if airway not secured prior to obstruction

PERTUSSIS

- An acute, highly contagious respiratory infection caused by *B. pertussis,* a gram-negative coccobacillus. Pertussis is also called "whooping cough." Pertussis means violent cough
- **Incidence:** prevalent worldwide. Transmission via respiratory droplets. In the United States, the childhood vaccine (1940s) contributed to >90% reduction in morbidity and mortality. Cyclic variations in infection rates (peaks every 3 to 4 years) that increases cases in adolescents and adults
- **Vaccine:** acellular vaccine since early 1990s (eliminated risk of encephalopathy). Neither vaccine nor infection confers lifelong immunity. Susceptible 6 to 10 years after either

SIGNS AND SYMPTOMS

- **Catarrhal phase:** 1 to 2 weeks with URI symptoms
- **Paroxysmal phase:** 2 to 4 weeks, paroxysms of coughing in staccato fashion followed by quick inhalation producing "whoop." Possible diaphoresis and cyanosis during episode but nontoxic in between. Infants may have apneic episodes
- **Convalescent phase:** residual cough may last weeks to months

DIAGNOSIS

- Clinical; testing not widely available; perform PCR or culture secretions if <3 weeks' symptoms; perform PCR + serology if symptoms >3 weeks

TREATMENT

- Mainly supportive, consider admission in those <1 year old
  - **Antibiotics:** shortens course if used within 1st week, may decrease transmission if used within 4 weeks (macrolide or TMP-SMX)
  - **Steroids:** may help critically ill infants
  - **Beta-agonists:** do not reduce paroxysmal coughing
  - **Outcomes:** highest risk in infants <6 months (not vaccinated yet)

UPPER RESPIRATORY INFECTION

- Class of infections affecting any part of the upper respiratory tract, including rhinitis, sinusitis, pharyngitis, epiglottitis, laryngitis, tracheitis, bronchitis. Most common infectious illness in the general population and a frequent cause of missed work or school and frequent cause of visits to physicians. Occur year round. They spread person to person via inhaled respiratory droplets or contact of hand contaminated with pathogen to nose or eyes. Presentation varies by location or inflammatory reaction
- **Types:**
  - **Common cold:** children 3 to 8/year; adults 2 to 4/year; elderly 1/year
  - **Influenza:** varies between 5% and 20% of population each season
  - **Viruses:** cause most URIs—rhinovirus, enterovirus, adenovirus, parainfluenza virus, influenza, Epstein–Barr, coronavirus, and others
  - **Pharyngitis:** viral or bacterial (group A strep in 5% to 15%)

SIGNS AND SYMPTOMS

- Rhinorrhea, nasal congestion, cough, sneezing, sinus pressure, headache, sore throat, fever, myalgias, fatigue, malaise, nausea, vomiting, diarrhea, conjunctivitis, halitosis, rash/exanthem

DIAGNOSIS

- Clinical; laboratory tests generally not indicated, except in specific cases
  - **Group A strep test:** rheumatic fever
  - **Mononucleosis:** activity restrictions to avoid spleen rupture
  - **Rapid influenza test:** may decrease unnecessary antibiotic use
  - **Cultures:** for extended duration or progressively worsening symptoms (MRSA pneumonia after influenza infection)
  - **Imaging:** usually not indicated unless atypical findings on exam or prolonged symptoms. CXR for abnormal lung exam or hypoxia; CT sinuses if symptoms beyond 4 weeks

TREATMENT

- Supportive care
  - **Bacterial pharyngitis:** penicillin or macrolide
  - **Peritonsillar abscess:** clindamycin, second- to third-generation cephalosporin, ampicillin/sulbactam + ENT consultation
  - **Retropharyngeal abscess:** broad-spectrum antibiotics + ENT consultation
  - **Bacterial sinusitis:** penicillin, macrolide, doxycycline, TMP-SMX, fluoroquinolone
  - **Epiglottitis or pertussis:** (see specific sections)
  - **Cold medicines:** avoid cold medicines in children under 6 years old
  - **Aspirin:** avoid in children and adolescents with fever (Reye syndrome)

Airway obstruction

- **Definition:** any process that partially obstructs, completely obstructs, or functionally obstructs the flow of air into the lungs. A life-threatening emergency
- **High-risk patients:** much more common in children because of anatomical difference
  - **Tongue:** disproportionately large compared to adults; protrudes back into posterior oropharynx
  - **Airway:** smaller caliber; more prone to hypotonia of airway structures; epiglottis large in proportion to adults
  - **Prominent occiput:** causes flexion of head on c-spine
- **Causes:**
  - **Infectious:** epiglottitis, croup, bacterial tracheitis, retropharyngeal abscess, peritonsillar abscess, mononucleosis
  - **Foreign body:** nuts, grapes, small pieces of a toy
  - **Trauma:** can cause soft tissue swelling or hematoma; burn injury can cause edema to airway structures
  - **Anaphylaxis or angioedema**
  - **Laryngospasm or vocal cord dysfunction**
  - **Congenital conditions:** macroglossia, micrognathia, laryngomalacia, subglottic stenosis

SIGNS AND SYMPTOMS

- **Increased work of breathing:** tachypnea, nasal flaring, retractions, use of abdominal muscles for breathing
- **Stridor:** partial obstruction; high-pitched and inspiratory (supraglottic); biphasic (glottic or tracheal); expiratory (subglottic or lower tracheal)
- **Lower airway:** hoarseness, coughing, wheezing
- **Infectious:** fever, mental status changes
- **Severe:** decreased respiratory rate and bradycardia
- **Aphonia:** complete obstruction

DIAGNOSIS

- Clinical; requires rapid assessment for complete obstruction or imminent respiratory failure. Obtain history related to symptom onset, speed of progression, fever, choking episode, exposures, prior conditions, congenital abnormalities

TREATMENT

- **Patient position:** do not convert partial obstruction to complete. Avoid laying flat, anxiety-provoking procedures. Keep in position of comfort
- **Imaging:** should not delay or interfere with airway management. May help in epiglottis, croup, some foreign bodies
- **Partial obstruction:** immediate consultation for controlled intubation possibly in OR with setup for tracheostomy
- **Complete obstruction:** with foreign bodies requires an attempt to dislodge with back blows (infants) or abdominal thrust (children /adults). Remove with

Magill forceps if visible. If tracheal FB, may need to intubate and advance ETT into right main stem bronchus, then pull ETT back into position
- **Intubation:** bag-valve mask with pop-off valve closed if high pressure needed; use most experienced physician available with backup from ENT or anesthesiology; have fiberoptic and cricothyrotomy set up

Tracheostomy

- **Definition:** a surgical procedure creating an opening in the cervical trachea for the purpose of access to the tracheobronchial tree
- **Indications:**
  - Prolonged mechanical ventilation
  - Facial or neck trauma; larynx fracture
  - Airway obstruction (supraglottic or glottic): infection, edema, neoplasm, foreign body, congenital abnormality
  - Severe sleep apnea
- **Situations**
  - **Emergent** (slash): patient in *extremis,* very rare, typically a cricothyrotomy is done instead (faster)
  - **Urgent:** patient in acute respiratory distress but not *extremis,* able to get to a controlled environment (the operating suite) and the expectation of success with typical airway techniques is low. (double setup: intubation and tracheostomy)
  - **Elective:** patient generally intubated with anticipation of prolonged course or difficulty weaning from the ventilator
- **Procedure:** considered a surgical procedure and generally outside the scope of EM
  - **Tubes:** metal (Jackson), plastic (Shiley), silicone, or nylon; most include an outer cannula, inner cannula, and an obturator
    - **Cuffed:** allows for positive-pressure ventilation, may prevent aspiration, cuff contributes to pressure necrosis
    - **Uncuffed:** allows for speaking when patient occludes tube with finger, less pressure damage to trachea, must be replaced if patient needs to be bagged or placed on ventilator
    - **Size:** no. 6 Shiley for women, no. 8 Shiley for men
    - **Outer cannula:** remains in place
    - **Inner cannula:** can be removed to clean or in case of sudden obstruction (mucus plug). Connector to ambu-bag
    - **Obturator:** for ease and atraumatic insertion of outer cannula
  - **Post-procedure care:** initial tube kept in place 5 to 7 days; stoma mature by 1 week
  - **Frequent suctioning:** but limited to length of tube
  - **Wound site care:** initially protected with petroleum or iodine-soaked gauze, then kept clean and dry
  - **Education:** patient and family should be taught use of (and have) saline, suction machine, suction catheters, cleaning with hydrogen peroxide/saline. They should also be trained to remove and replace both inner and outer cannulas. Need replacement tube at home
- **Complications**
  - **Apnea:** loss of hypoxic drive
  - **Bleeding:** at wound edge (20% ED visits); treat with pressure or cauterization
  - **Barotrauma:** pneumothorax, pneumomediastinum, subcutaneous emphysema
  - **Traumatic injury:** recurrent laryngeal nerve, great vessels, esophagus
  - **Mucus plugging:** remove inner cannula and suction
  - **Infection:** cellulitis, wound infection, tracheitis
  - **Tube displacement:** use obturator to replace, consider one size smaller or use endotracheal tube
  - **Soft tissue:** tracheo-innominate erosion or fistula (prolonged or severe bleeding due to communication with innominate artery); tracheomalacia or stenosis; tracheoesophageal or tracheocutaneous fistulas; granulation tissue, scarring leading to obstruction; false tract from failed attempt to replace
- **Replacing/changing tracheostomy tube**
  - **Equipment needed**
    - Matched size tracheostomy tube and 1 to 2 sizes smaller
    - Obturator, red rubber catheter, or fiberoptic scope (guide)
    - Oxygen supply
    - Water-soluble lubricant
    - Wall suction and suction catheters
    - 10-mL syringe, tracheostomy collar or some other securing device
    - Ambu-bag and intubation equipment
  - **Procedure:**
  - Pre-oxygenate
  - Remove tube: following curved contour
  - Replace with lubricated outer cannula with obturator in place
  - Do not force; if resistance is met (risk creating false passage)
  - Red rubber catheter: can change over using this device
  - Fiberoptics: may aid placement in difficult situations
  - Confirm placement: breath sounds, end-tidal CO_2, or x-rays
  - Secure with ties or tracheostomy collar; one finger breadth between collar and neck

Tumors

BREAST TUMORS

- Tumors of the breast include benign and malignant masses and inflammatory breast cancer. Challenge to distinguish from other breast lumps such as cyst and abscess. Breast cancer is the most common cancer in women (one in nine over a lifetime). Breast cancer can occur in men (1% of all breast cancer)

- **Benign masses:** or changes affect up to 60% of women; account for 80% of all palpable masses; typically smooth, mobile, firm, rubbery, tender
  - **Fibrocystic change:** nodular, lumpy to palpation; may be tender; usually worse premenstrual time each month
  - **Fibroadenoma:** is a proliferative process in a single duct unit usually 2 to 3 cm but may vary in size and during menses in young women; may be multiple and spontaneously resolve or calcify after menopause
  - **Phyllodes tumor:** giant fibroadenoma that averages 5 cm in women 40 to 50 years old
- **Malignant masses:** more common in the upper, outer quadrant
  - **Risk factors:** family history, age, early menarche, late menopause, nulliparity, high-fat diet, oral contraceptive pills, estrogen replacement
  - **Presentation:** more likely hard, irregular, adherent to surrounding tissue, nontender; skin changes include edema, dimpling, and ulceration; bloody nipple discharge and palpable lymph nodes in axilla suggestive
- **Types:**
  - **Ductal carcinoma:** most common type; initially a localized, palpable mass that metastasizes to the lung, liver, brain, and bone
  - **Lobular carcinoma:** second most common; occurs diffusely throughout breast without mass initially; has a high rate of multifocality and bilaterality once it is invasive; more commonly metastasizes to the bone
  - **Paget disease of breast:** cancer of the epithelium of the nipple–areola complex; presents as a chronic eczematous rash; 1% of all breast cancer
- **Other types:** medullary, mucinous, tubular, papillary
  - **Inflammatory breast cancer**
  - **Pathophysiology:** symptoms due to tumor infiltration in dermal lymphatics causing inflammation and congestion
  - **Signs and symptoms:** erythema, edema, warmth, tenderness, breast enlargement; "orange-peel" skin changes and nipple retraction
    - **History:** ask about onset, change in size, pain, changes with cycle, skin changes, nipple discharge, fever, risk factors
    - **Clinical examination:** not accurate in determining cancer; a full examination should look for signs of metastasis. With the patient supine and with arm behind head, visualize for skin changes, small circular palpation, cover all four quadrants, gentle examination for posterior areola mass and nipple discharge, examine neck and axilla for lymph nodes. Ultrasound can aid in diagnosis of cyst and abscess. In men, malignant masses are usually retro-areolar and painless. Gynecomastia more likely tender and in adolescents
  - **Treatment:** infection should be treated with appropriate antibiotics; surgery consult or referral for abscess drainage; masses with any suspicion should be referred for mammography, ultrasound, and surgical referral

CHEST WALL TUMORS

- Masses can arise in any bone, soft tissue, cartilage or pleura
- **Osteosarcoma/Other bone tumors:** usually occur in rapidly growing long bones
- **Lipoma:** most common soft tissue tumor; these are slow-growing, benign fatty tumors that are asymptomatic, soft, lobulated, and mobile. They should be resected for any symptoms or for cosmetic reasons
- **Chondrosarcoma:** malignant tumor of cartilaginous origin; with increasing incidence after age 40 years. Can be located in sternum, ribs, or other bones
  - **Symptoms:** dull pain, worse at night, possible local swelling. Symptoms usually occur for 1 to 2 years prior to diagnosis. Can cause pathologic fracture. Pain with cartilaginous tumors suggests malignancy
  - **Diagnosis:** radiographs (lucent lesion with some calcification and well circumscribed) supplemented with CT scan
  - **Treatment:** resection, poor response to chemotherapy or radiation therapy
- **Malignant mesothelioma:** malignant neoplasm that originates from pleura; occurs in 1 in 100,000 population annually. Presents as a lobulated tumor with local spread to chest wall, lung, and mediastinum
  - **Etiology:** associated with exposure to asbestos (peak use 1930s to 1960s). The latent period between exposure and mesothelioma is 35 to 40 years
  - **Symptoms:** dyspnea, chest pain, cough, weight loss, increased sputum production
  - **Diagnosis:** chest radiograph may show a pleural effusion, mass, plaque-like or nodular pleural thickening. There may also be evidence of prior asbestos exposure (calcified pleural plaques, commonly at the bases). Patient should also have a CT of the chest and be referred for biopsy
  - **Treatment:** difficult to treat, usually fatal within 18 months of symptom onset
- **Localized fibrous tumor of the pleura:** a localized mesothelioma, unrelated to asbestos exposure. There are benign and malignant forms (7:1 ratio)
  - **Presentation:** firm soft-tissue mass >5 cm, anywhere in chest pleura; 50% have pedicles or a broad base
  - **Symptoms:** most patients are asymptomatic, occasionally cough, dyspnea, vague chest pain. Malignant form may have hemorrhage or necrosis in mass
  - **Diagnosis:** usually incidental finding on chest x-ray or CT of the chest. Follow-up biopsy for histopathologic exam to confirm
  - **Treatment:** resection has good outcome

PULMONARY TUMORS

- Heterogenous group of neoplastic masses of both benign and malignant nature that develop from pulmonary tissues. Solitary pulmonary nodules found at a rate of 1 to 2/1000 chest radiographs (30% are found to be malignant)

- **Benign lung tumors:** approximately 2% to 5% of primary lung tumors are benign and typically do not involve local tissue invasion or spread to other sites
  - **Types**
  - **Hamartomas (chondroadenomas):** most common benign lung tumor that develops in the peripheral lung and consists of epithelial, fat, and cartilage tissues
  - **Mucous gland adenomas (bronchial cystadenomas):** mass consisting of columnar cell-lined cyst
  - **Sclerosing hemangioma:** develops from terminal bronchiolar cells and contain solid areas, papillary structures, sclerotic areas, and areas of blood
  - **Others types:** chondromas, fibromas, lipomas, hemangiomas, teratomas
  - **Symptoms:** cough, pseudo-asthmatic wheezing, hemoptysis, dyspnea
  - **Diagnosis:** often incidental finding on chest x-ray (popcorn calcification characteristic of benign lesions)
  - **Complications:** most related to lung obstruction (atelectasis, postobstructive pneumonia)
  - **Treatment:** follow with serial chest x-ray or CT for change in size. Surgical resection if symptomatic and to confirm not it is not malignant
- **Carcinoid lung tumors:** initially considered benign, now felt to be the least aggressive form of bronchopulmonary neuroendocrine tumors. Represents 10% of all carcinoid tumors (GI most common location). Slow growing and rarely metastasize. No known causative agent
  - **Atypical carcinoid tumors:** intermediately aggressive and can metastasize. Up to 33% of patients are asymptomatic
    - **Symptoms:** usually arise from tumor size (atelectasis, postobstructive pneumonia, hemoptysis)
    - **Systemic symptoms:** neuroendocrine tumors can produce biologically active peptides and hormones
  - **Carcinoid syndrome:** serotonin flushing, tachycardia, bronchoconstriction, diarrhea, and hemodynamic instability. This syndrome is less common in carcinoid lung tumors than in those arising from the GI tract
  - **Treatment:** only treatment is surgical resection
- **Malignant lung tumors (lung cancer)**
  - **Incidence/epidemiology:** leading cause of cancer deaths in men and women; second-leading cancer behind prostate (men) and breast (women). Tobacco smoking leading cause (risk 13 times higher than nonsmoker)
  - **Non–small cell lung cancer:** 75% of all lung cancer. Divided into three groups
    - **Adenocarcinoma:** arise from bronchial mucous glands. Represents 35% to 40% of all lung cancer and is the most common form of lung cancer in nonsmokers. Is usually peripheral but can be multifocal (bronchoalveolar form)

- **Squamous cell carcinoma:** is usually central and may appear as a cavitary lesion. It represents 25% to 30% of all lung cancer and is associated with hypercalcemia from parathyroid-like hormone production
- **Large-cell carcinoma:** typically presents as a large peripheral mass and is associated with gynecomastia and galactorrhea. Represents 10% to 15% of all lung cancer
- **Pancoast tumor:** a superior pulmonary sulcus tumor growing at the thoracic inlet that is defined by location rather than histology
  - **Incidence/epidemiology:** 1% to 3% of all lung cancer; most are squamous-cell carcinoma or adenocarcinomas; originates in the extreme periphery and extends extra-pulmonary invading the chest wall, ribs, vertebrae, or mediastinum
  - **Characteristic clinical picture:** because it affects intercostal nerves, lower nerve roots of brachial plexus, the stellate ganglion, or the sympathetic nerve chain, many symptoms are possible
    - **Pain:** in shoulder, chest wall, vertebral border of scapula, arm and hand along the ulnar distribution
    - **Horner syndrome:** ptosis, miosis, anhidrosis
    - **Weakness:** in the ipsilateral hand
  - **Radiographic studies:** chest x-ray shows apical mass (Fig. 16-4), pleural thickening or plaque and possible bone destruction in superior ribs.

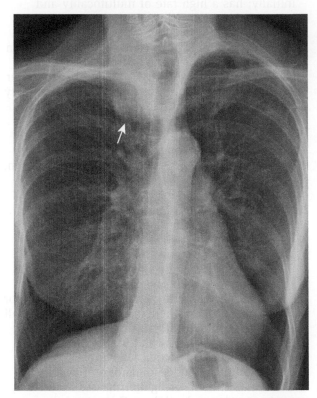

Figure 16-4. Pancoast tumor. This woman presented with deep shoulder pain. The PA radiograph of the chest, obtained after radiographs of the shoulder suggested apical mass, confirmed a mass in the apex of the lung *(arrow)* with destruction of the underlying bone. Because of the possibility of such a tumor, the lung apex is included. (From Weissman BN: *Imaging of arthritis and metabolic bone disease*, Philadelphia, 2008, Mosby.)

A CT of the chest is needed to identify invasion in the vertebral column, chest wall, mediastinum, and brachial plexus

- **Oat cell (small-cell) lung cancer:** most aggressive form of lung cancer as it grows rapidly and has early widespread metastasis (65% to 70% at diagnosis). Represents 13% of new lung cancer cases. Less than 5% are asymptomatic at presentation. May produce a variety of hormones that cause paraneoplastic syndromes. Syndrome of inappropriate antidiuretic hormone secretion (SIADH) is most common. Ectopic ACTH production (Cushing syndrome) occurs as well

Costochondritis

- **Definition:** benign, inflammatory process involving the costal cartilages and the costochondral or costosternal joints. It usually occurs in women (66%) and in those more than 40 years old. Infectious etiology is rare, but possible in intravenous drug users
- **Signs and symptoms:** almost always involves more than one joint (3rd, 4th, and 5th joints) and may mimic cardiac, pulmonary, or esophageal pathology. The pain is highly localized, and usually sharp at costochondral junctions. It is reproducible with light palpation. The pain is exacerbated by respiration, cough, or other movement of chest wall
- **Diagnosis:** clinical, no imaging or laboratory testing is indicated
- **Treatment:** NSAIDs and analgesics; local steroid injection can be performed if symptoms persist

Mediastinitis

- **Definition:** infectious process involving the mediastinal space; course is rapidly progressive and mortality approaches 20% despite appropriate treatment. It is termed *descending necrotizing mediastinitis* when due to extension from the retropharyngeal space or another ENT source
  - **Epidemiology:** there is a 6:1 male to female ratio; average age at presentation is 35
  - **Etiologies:** esophageal perforations (>90%); iatrogenic due to invasive procedures (75%); Boerhaave syndrome (rare); tracheal perforation; local spread of infection from adjacent structures
  - **Chronic mediastinitis:** associated with a more indolent course and less morbidity; usually because of tuberculosis, histoplasmosis, or another granulomatous disease
- **Signs and symptoms:** toxic appearance; fever and chills; pleuritic anterior or substernal chest pain; dyspnea; dysphagia or anterior neck pain
- **Diagnosis:** WBC usually markedly elevated; chest x-ray may show mediastinal widening or free air; CT or MRI of chest is usually definitive and necessary; needle aspiration of mediastinal space can also be performed

- **Treatment:** early airway control if deterioration is anticipated; broad-spectrum antibiotics, to include anaerobic coverage; surgical exploration, debridement and drainage is required

Pleural effusion

- **Definition:** an abnormal fluid collection within the pleural space; two categories
  - **Transudates:** due to systemic states of either increased hydrostatic pressure or decreased oncotic pressure; 90% are due to CHF; other common causes include nephrotic syndrome, glomerulonephritis, renal failure, hypoalbuminemia, and cirrhosis
  - **Exudates:** due to disorders of the pleura itself or inflammatory conditions; the most common cause is pneumonia; other causes include malignancy, lupus and other connective tissue disorders, and pancreatitis
  - **Special case:** a pulmonary embolism may cause either a transudative or an exudative effusion and is an often overlooked etiology
- **Types of effusions:**
  - **Parapneumonic effusion:** one associated with a pneumonia, pulmonary abscess, or bronchiectasis
  - **Empyema:** is an effusion characterized by frank pus
  - **Hemothorax:** is an effusion composed primarily of blood; the hematocrit of the effusion must be greater than 50% of the peripheral hematocrit
  - **Chylothorax:** contains chyle from a disrupted thoracic duct
  - **Loculated effusion:** results when pleural adhesions are present
  - **Massive effusion:** is usually >1.5 L and is most often due to malignancy
- **Signs and symptoms:** pleuritic chest pain, cough, dyspnea (usually occurs once the volume of the effusion is >500 mL), referred pain to ipsilateral shoulder, decreased breath sounds over the effusion, decreased tactile fremitus, dullness to percussion (which shifts with change in position), possible friction rub
- **Diagnosis:**
  - **Chest x-ray:** at least 250 to 500 mL must be present before an effusion is visible on upright PA view; unilateral haziness of the entire lung field may be seen on supine view; lateral decubitus view is the most sensitive plain film and can detect 5 to 10 mL of pleural fluid
  - **Ultrasound or CT scan:** can detect as little as 5 mL and can differentiate between pleural effusion and pleural thickening
  - **Thoracentesis:** indicated for a new effusion or an effusion of unclear etiology. Relative contraindications are coagulopathy and adhesions. A post-thoracentesis chest x-ray should be obtained to exclude pneumothorax

- **Pleural fluid analysis**
  - **Light criteria:** effusion is exudative if the following apply:
    - Pleural fluid protein/serum protein >0.5
    - Pleural fluid LDH/serum LDH >0.6
    - Pleural fluid LDH >2/3 of normal serum LDH
  - **Transudates:** no further fluid analysis needed
  - **Additional studies for exudates:** Gram stain and culture for aerobic, anaerobic, fungal, and mycobacterial organisms; cytology for malignancy
  - **Empyema:** markedly elevated WBCs, pleural fluid with pH <7.0 and decreased glucose
  - **Esophageal rupture or pancreatitis:** elevated pleural fluid amylase
  - **Tuberculosis:** elevated adenosine deaminase
  - **Bloody effusion:** in the atraumatic setting suggests pulmonary infarction or a malignancy
- **Treatment:** identification and treatment of the underlying etiology is key
- **Pleuritic pain:** responds well to NSAIDs
- **CHF effusion:** usually responds well to diuresis
- **Symptomatic effusion:** may be drained by needle thoracentesis
- **Tube thoracostomy:** usually required for resolution of: persistent effusion, complicated parapneumonic effusion, hemothorax, or empyema

Pleuritis

- **Definition:** refers to any inflammatory condition of the pleura
  - **Etiologies:** pulmonary embolism, uremia, pleural effusion, pneumonia, pneumothorax, tuberculosis
- **Signs and symptoms:** pleuritic chest pain (pleurisy) is the hallmark; dyspnea or fever, if present, are usually due to the associated underlying condition; may or may not have an associated pleural effusion
- **Diagnosis:** clinical; a chest x-ray or other imaging may be performed to exclude pneumonia, effusion, or other significant causes
- **Treatment:** pain symptoms may be treated with NSAIDs; treatment of any underlying etiology is key

Pneumomediastinum

- **Definition:** presence of free air within the mediastinum; may have an associated pneumothorax
  - **Etiologies:** strenuous activity, vigorous Valsalva maneuvers; breath-holding during marijuana or crack cocaine use; asthma; Boerhaave syndrome; iatrogenic esophageal perforation, foreign body aspiration (children), and trauma
  - **Spontaneous pneumomediastinum:** usually benign and self-limited
  - **Tension pneumomediastinum:** jugular vein distention, hypotension, and cardiovascular collapse

- **Signs and symptoms:** retrosternal chest pain, dyspnea, tachypnea, hoarseness, odynophagia, and may have subcutaneous emphysema. *Hamman sign* is the "crunching" sound auscultated over heart during systole—is rare but specific for pneumomediastinum
- **Diagnosis:** chest x-ray is usually diagnostic; CT scan of chest can detect minute amounts of free mediastinal air and often required to evaluate for the etiology. Esophagram should be performed if Boerhaave syndrome is suspected, preferably with Gastrografin. Bronchoscopy or esophagoscopy may be required to identify the source of significant or persistent pneumomediastinum
- **Treatment:**
  - **Supplemental oxygen:** speeds resorption for spontaneous pneumomediastinum
  - **Hospital admission:** most patients should be admitted for hemodynamic monitoring and serial evaluations
  - **Invasive procedures:** intubation, tube thoracostomy, or mediastinotomy are only rarely required as hemodynamic compromise is rare
  - **Broad-spectrum antibiotics and surgery:** required for Boerhaave syndrome and other traumatic etiologies
  - **Prognosis:** dependent on etiology

Spontaneous pneumothorax (PTX)

- **Primary spontaneous PTX:** occurs without a history of pulmonary pathology; usually due to the rupture of small, apical, subpleural blebs
  - **Associations:** most common in tall young males; slight association with atmospheric pressure changes, tobacco use, Marfan syndrome, and mitral valve prolapse
  - **Presentation:** usually occurs at rest rather than with exertion and has a 30% recurrence rate. These often have a delayed presentation because of the mild nature of the symptoms and slow rate of progression. Rarely progresses to tension PTX
- **Secondary spontaneous PTX:** associated with prior pulmonary pathology
  - **Associations:** COPD (most common underlying condition); AIDS (*Pneumocystis* pneumonia)
  - **Presentation:** usually has a higher mortality; often occurs bilaterally; usually results in marked dyspnea
- **Catamenial pneumothorax:** rare—secondary to ectopic endometrial tissue within the pleural space; occurs within 72 hours of onset of menses
- **Signs and symptoms:** can be sudden in onset
  - Pleuritic chest pain
  - Dyspnea: severity is correlated with the size of PTX
  - Tachycardia: most common physical examination finding
  - Breath sounds: decreased or absent with hyperresonance to percussion

- **Diagnosis**
  - **Chest radiograph:** thin line representing the visceral pleura is visible parallel to chest wall with absence of lung markings distal to this pleural edge; deep sulcus sign (Fig. 16-5) may be seen even on supine images; apical lordotic or an end-expiratory view may improve detection
  - **Ultrasound:** best visualized anteriorly in mid-infraclavicular region; will see a loss of "slide

sign" and loss of "comet tail" appearance on affected side
  - **CT scan of chest:** usually not required but is extremely sensitive for even miniscule PTX; also best way to quantitate volume
  - **ECG:** axis deviation, decreased QRS voltage, T-wave inversions
- **Treatment**
  - **High-flow supplemental oxygen:** for use in all patients; helps speed resorption fourfold over

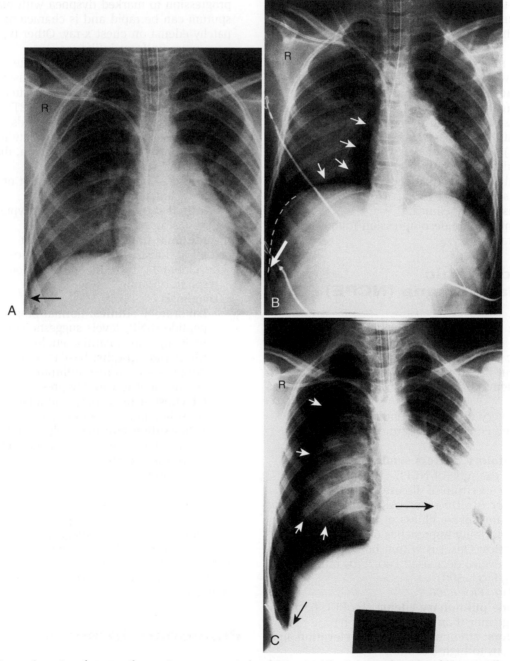

Figure 16-5. Deep sulcus sign of pneumothorax. On a posteroanterior chest x-ray **(A),** the costophrenic angle is normally acute *(arrow).* In a supine patient, a pneumothorax will often be anterior, medial, and basilar. On a subsequent supine film **(B),** the dark area along the right cardiac border and lung base appeared larger *(small arrows),* and the costophrenic angle much deeper and more acute than normal *(large arrow).* These findings were not recognized and, as a result, a tension pneumothorax developed in the same patient **(C)** with an extremely deep costophrenic angle *(large black arrow),* an almost completely collapsed right lung *(small white arrows),* and shift of the mediastinum to the left *(blackarrow over heart).* (From Mettler FA: *Essentials of radiology,* ed 2, Philadelphia, 2005, Saunders.)

room air; can be primary treatment for healthy patients with <20% spontaneous PTX (with repeat CXR in 6 hours)

- **Simple needle aspiration:** for use in healthy patients with a larger spontaneous PTX (>20%); has a success rate approaching 60%; placement of a catheter with attached stopcock or Heimlich valve for repeated aspirations may also be used
- **Tube thoracostomy:** warranted for persistent primary PTX, secondary PTX, or an associated pleural effusion; 20 to 28F tube is usually sufficient in the absence of trauma. Ventilator patients, those on noninvasive positive pressure ventilation, or those undergoing air transport will require chest tubes for expected enlargement of the PTX
- **Prognosis:** majority resolve within 1 week; the remainder will require pleurodesis or thoracoscopy
- **Tension pneumothorax**
  - **Clinical features:** vital sign instability (hypotension, tachypnea, tachycardia [although bradycardia may ensue as hypoxia and instability progress]), hypoxia, jugular venous distension, tracheal deviation away from the side of the PTX, decreased breath sounds and hyperresonance over the side of the PTX
  - **Diagnosis:** ideally clinical
  - **Treatment:** needle decompression followed by tube thoracostomy

Noncardiogenic pulmonary edema (NCPE)

- **Definition:** the accumulation of fluid and protein within the alveolar space in the absence of a cardiogenic etiology; usually due to some derangement in the permeability of the alveolar-capillary membrane rather than increased capillary pressure
- **Etiologies:** very diverse; depending on etiology, there may be concomitant cardiogenic pulmonary edema
- **Acute respiratory distress syndrome** (ARDS): prototypical example of NCPE
- **Definition:** a spectrum of diseases from mild (acute lung injury or ALI) to severe ARDS that can be due to virtually any severe illness or injury; despite treatment, mortality approaches 60%
- **Characteristics:** Onset is within hours to days of the inciting event; decreased PaO_2/FIO_2 ratio
  - **ALI:** PaO_2/FIO_2 <300
  - **ARDS:** PaO_2/FIO_2 <200
- **High-altitude pulmonary edema** (HAPE): occurs at elevations greater than 2500 m (8000 ft)
  - **Risk factors:** strenuous exertion at elevation and rapid ascent to high elevation
  - **Treatment:** immediate descent to lower altitude is required; supplemental oxygen and perhaps hyperbaric oxygen therapy are essential; drug therapy includes acetazolamide, nifedipine, and dexamethasone

- **Neurogenic pulmonary edema:** develops within hours of a neurologic injury and usually resolves in 2 to 3 days
  - **Associations:** acutely increased intracranial pressure; a frequent complication of status epilepticus, closed and penetrating head trauma, intracerebral hemorrhage and subarachnoid hemorrhage
  - **Treatment:** no treatment specific
- **Opiate overdose:** NCPE occurs within 2 hours of ingestion, or treatment with naloxone in chronic abusers. Usually resolves within 48 hours. The progression to marked dyspnea with pink frothy sputum can be rapid and is characterized by patchy edema on chest x-ray. Other types of NCPE have more uniform infiltrates
- **Reperfusion pulmonary edema:** after thrombolytics for pulmonary embolism
- **Reexpansion pulmonary edema:** after decompression of large or chronic PTX
- **Decompression sickness:** "the bends"
- **Other causes:** renal failure, salicylate toxicity, negative-pressure pulmonary edema, drowning, fat emboli, and toxic inhalations
- **Signs and symptoms:** sudden onset of symptoms is very characteristic of NCPE
  - **Cardinal signs:** tachycardia, tachypnea, and dyspnea are nearly universal
  - **Additional findings:** hypoxia that can progress to frank cyanosis; rales, either focal or diffuse; the development of frothy and/or bloody sputum; respiratory failure
- **Diagnosis**
  - **Laboratory studies:** normal brain natriuretic peptide (BNP) levels suggests NCPE; elevated BNP suggests a cardiac etiology
  - **Chest radiographs:** basilar edema that progresses to diffuse infiltrates; cardiac enlargement is variably present
  - **CT chest scan:** widespread airspace consolidation, more prominent basally
  - **Echocardiogram:** may help to differentiate cardiogenic from noncardiogenic etiology
  - **Swan-Ganz catheter:** may also help by determining the pulmonary alveolar wedge pressure
  - NCPE: ≤18 mmHg
  - Cardiogenic: >18 mmHg
- **Treatment:** mainstay is diagnosis and correction of the underlying etiology; supplemental oxygen, careful fluid management, and positive pressure ventilation or endotracheal intubation may be required

Pulmonary infections

LUNG ABSCESS

- **Etiologies:** may be a rare complication of pneumonia in the antibiotic era; commonly complicates aspiration pneumonia *Klebsiella;*

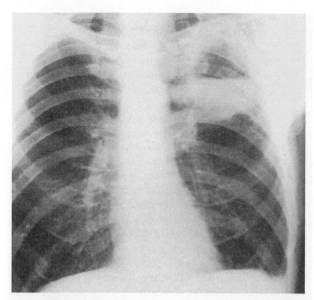

Figure 16-6. A single parenchymal cavity with an air-fluid level typifies an anaerobic (putrid) lung abscess. Most often these lesions are located in the dependent, aspiration-prone lung segments (e.g., the posterior segments of the right or left upper lobes) or the superior segment of the right lower lobe. This patient has a small left empyema as well. (From Mason RJ, Broaddus VC, Murray JF: *Murray and Nadel's textbook of respiratory medicine,* ed 4, Philadelphia, 2005, Saunders.)

tuberculosis; bacterial, fungal, or parasitic infection; neoplasm; and various inflammatory conditions
- **Risk factors:** elderly, alcoholism, seizures, esophageal motility disorders, depressed gag reflex, and a depressed level of consciousness
- **Signs and symptoms:** indolent course, fever, cough, night sweats, weight loss, and pleuritic chest pain
- **Diagnosis:** chest radiograph shows dense consolidation with an *air fluid level inside a cavitary lesion,* usually in the basal segments of the lower lobes or posterior segments of the upper lobes (Fig. 16-6)
- **Treatment**
  - **Intravenous antibiotics:** will successfully treat 85% to 90% of lung abscesses; piperacillin/tazobactam; metronidazole + ceftriaxone; moxifloxacin; intravenous antibiotics until no longer febrile, then oral antibiotics for another 4 to 8 weeks
  - **Drainage:** will usually occur spontaneously from communication of the abscess with the tracheobronchial tree; 10% will require surgical intervention
  - **Risk factors for failure of medical treatment:** recurrent aspiration, large cavity (>6 cm), prolonged symptoms prior to presentation, abscess associated with obstructing lesion, thick-walled cavities, underlying serious comorbidity, and the development of an empyema

ASPIRATION PNEUMONIA

- **Etiology:** oropharyngeal flora aspirated into lungs, may be complicated by chemical pneumonitis from aspiration of sterile but irritating gastric contents; represents the majority of nursing home-acquired pneumonia
- **Risk factors:** same as for lung abscess
- **Signs and symptoms:** may have witnessed episode of aspiration prior to pneumonia developing; other symptoms include cough, tachypnea, fever
- **Elderly patients:** may have mental status change, vomiting, or lethargy without the more classic symptoms
- **Diagnosis:** clinical picture is the key. Chest radiograph usually shows unilateral focal or patchy consolidations in the lower or dependent lung fields. The right lower lobe is most common if patient is upright when aspiration occurs
- **Treatment:** Piperacillin/tazobactam; metronidazole + ceftriaxone; moxifloxacin

ATYPICAL PNEUMONIA:

- Milder disease ("walking pneumonia")
- *Mycoplasma* pneumonia: subacute respiratory illness with cough, retrosternal chest pain, sore throat, and headache; more common in younger patients
  - **Chest radiographs:** patchy infiltrates, hilar adenopathy,
  - **Extrapulmonary manifestations:** are rare but include bullous myringitis, rash, neurologic symptoms, arthritis, arthralgias, and renal failure
- *Chlamydia* pneumonia: very common, often asymptomatic and more common in younger patients. Can be associated with adult-onset asthma
  - **Symptoms:** usually mild subacute illness with a sore throat, mild fever, and a nonproductive cough; occasionally symptoms may be more severe
  - **Chest radiograph:** patchy subsegmental infiltrates
- *Legionella* pneumonia: a spectrum of presentations, from a benign and self-limited illness to frank multisystem organ failure
  - **Symptoms:** usually a mild, nonproductive cough with fever, relative bradycardia
  - **Associated GI symptoms:** nausea, vomiting, diarrhea, and abdominal pain
  - **Associated diseases:** pancreatitis, sinusitis, myocarditis, and pyelonephritis
  - **Risk factors:** smoking, chronic lung disease, transplant patients, elderly, and immunosuppression. It is the most common atypical infection in the elderly (10% of CAP)
  - **Chest radiograph:** patchy infiltrates; may have hilar adenopathy or effusion

BACTERIAL PNEUMONIAS

- *Streptococcus* pneumonia (pneumococcus): most common cause of pneumonia in most populations

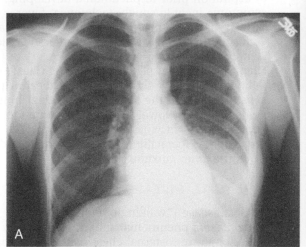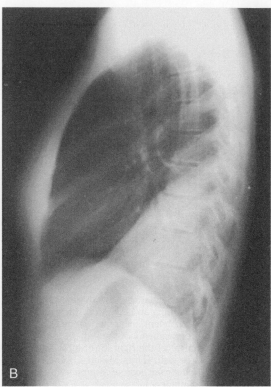

Figure 16-7. **A,** Posteroanterior film showing dense left lower consolidation consistent with bacterial pneumonia, in this case caused by *Streptococcus pneumoniae*. **B,** Lateral film of a patient with left lower lobe pneumococcal pneumonia. (From Mandell GL, Bennett JE, Dolin R: *Principles and practice of infectious diseases,* ed 6, Philadelphia, 2005, Churchill Livingstone.)

(HIV patients, alcoholics, children, and the elderly); stroking chills; rust-colored sputum
- **Chest radiograph:** lobar segmental pneumonia, parapneumonic effusion in 25%; round infiltrate is rare (Fig. 16-7)
- ***Staph. aureus* pneumonia**
  - **Associations:** chronic lung disease, aspiration, alcoholism, laryngeal cancer, nursing home patients, and immunocompromised patients
  - **Chest radiograph:** extensive multilobar involvement, empyema, effusions
- ***Pseudomonas* pneumonia:** an uncommon CAP that presents as a severe illness with cyanosis and confusion
  - **Risk factors:** prolonged hospitalizations, mechanical ventilation, neutropenia, cystic fibrosis, burns, central venous catheters, high-dose steroid therapy, structural lung disease, nursing home residents, and HIV patients
  - **Chest radiograph:** bilateral lobar infiltrates, occasional empyema
- ***Klebsiella* pneumonia:**
  - **Risk factors:** alcoholism and other aspiration risk patients, elderly, and those with chronic lung disease
  - **Chest radiograph:** lobar infiltrate, may have abscesses
- ***Haemophilus influenzae:*** incidence has decreased secondary to vaccinations

- **Risk factors:** alcoholism, elderly, chronic lung disease, immunocompromised, diabetics, and sickle cell disease
- **Chest radiograph:** pleural effusions and multilobar infiltrates
- **Diagnosis of bacterial pneumonia:** clinical picture and chest radiograph; sputum Gram stain and culture, and blood cultures, are insensitive however
- **Treatment of bacterial pneumonia:**
  - **Outpatient antibiotics:** doxycycline, macrolide, or fluoroquinolone—impacted by comorbidities and likely pathogens
    - **Azithromycin:** fewer GI side effects and easier dosing schedule than erythromycin or clarithromycin
    - **Fluoroquinolones:** should be reserved for patients with known resistant organisms, treatment failures, or patients at high risk for *Pseudomonas*
  - **Duration of treatment:** recommended is 3 to 5 days after resolution of fever (typically 7 to 14 days), with the exception of azithromycin
  - **Hospital admission:** 75% of pneumonia patients do not require admission. Admission is indicated for supplemental oxygen requirement, respiratory compromise, shock, inability to tolerate oral antibiotics, depressed mental status, age >65 years or <3 months, AIDS, alcoholism, extensive lung involvement; consider use of "CURB-65" and "PORT" scores to support unclear disposition decisions

FUNGAL PNEUMONIA

- Rare
- *Histoplasma capsulatum* pneumonia:
  - **Endemic areas:** found in soil contaminated with bat or bird dung, most often in caves and endemic to the Ohio, Missouri, and Mississippi River valleys
  - **Course:** often resolves without treatment; rarely disseminates unless the patient is immunocompromised
  - **Treatment:** refractory or severe cases can be treated with itraconazole, ketoconazole, or amphotericin
- *Coccidioides immitis* pneumonia: San Joaquin Valley Fever
- **Endemic areas:** inhaled soil from central California
  - **Course:** the pneumonia may be accompanied by meningitis, bone involvement, erythema nodosum, and erythema multiforme
  - **Treatment:** mild cases can be treated with fluconazole; more severe cases may require itraconazole or amphotericin
- *Blastomyces dermatitidis* pneumonia:
  - **Endemic areas:** inhaled soil in clustered in states adjacent to the Mississippi and Ohio rivers and the Great Lakes region
  - **Course:** pulmonary infection is asymptomatic in up to 50% of patients; mortality is 2% in the immunocompetent patient but 40% in patients with AIDS
  - **Treatment:** mild to moderate cases can be treated with itraconazole; reserve amphotericin for severe cases
- **Opportunistic fungal pathogens:** *Candida* species, *Aspergillus* species, *Mucor* species, *Cryptococcus neoformans*

VIRAL PNEUMONIA

- May be preceded by mild URI or viral syndrome; consider concomitant bacterial infections in more severe cases
- **Pediatric etiologies:** RSV is most common in those <5 years old; parainfluenza is the second most common pathogen
- **Adult etiologies:** most severe cases are complicated influenza infections, especially in the elderly
- **Signs and symptoms:** cough, coryza, tachypnea, fever
- **Diagnosis:** chest radiograph shows hyperexpanded lungs with patchy bronchial infiltrates; nasal swabs may identify viral pathogens
- **Treatment:** mostly supportive care:
  - **Aerosolized ribavirin:** for infants and children with severe RSV
  - **Amantadine:** may be helpful for influenza A
  - **Acyclovir:** is indicated for varicella pneumonia

PULMONARY TUBERCULOSIS (TB)

- **Etiology:** *Mycobacterium tuberculosis* is slow-growing aerobic rod/bacillus with acid-fast properties (AFB)

- **Primary infection:** organisms are inhaled, and most are killed by host defenses. Some may survive and be transported to regional lymph nodes and form granulomas/tubercles. Organisms may remain dormant for years (latent infection)
- **Location:** these organisms survive best in the high oxygen concentrations of the apical and posterior segments of the upper lobes. May also be found in the superior segments of the lower lobes, renal cortex, meninges, long bones, and vertebrae
- **Ghon complex:** caseation necrosis and calcification of hilar lymph nodes that occurs with primary infection
- **Signs and symptoms**
  - **Primary Infection:** usually asymptomatic but may lead to a positive PPD test in the immunocompetent individuals
  - **Reactivation tuberculosis:** characterized by prolonged fever, malaise, weight loss, night sweats, cough, and/or hemoptysis
  - **Miliary tuberculosis:** usually occurs in the immunocompromised, multiorgan seeding, splenomegaly, hepatomegaly, diffuse lymphadenopathy, anemia, hyponatremia, thrombocytopenia, and leucopenia
- **Diagnosis:**
  - **Sputum stain and Culture:** for AFB
  - **Lymph node/tissue biopsy:** for AFB
  - **Chest radiograph:** cavitary lesions predominantly upper/apical lung fields (Fig. 16-8)
- **Treatment:**
  - **Reactivation TB:** Four-drug therapy with isoniazid (INH), rifampin, pyrazinamide, ethambutol, plus vitamin B_6 to mitigate toxicity; treatment for 8 weeks followed by two-drug therapy for 18 weeks is the most common regimen
  - **New seroconversion:** consider for 9 months of INH therapy

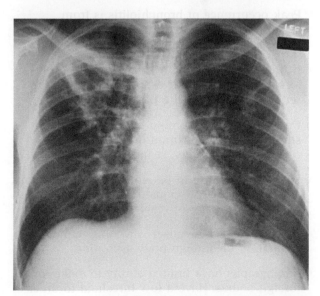

Figure 16-8. Frontal-view chest film showing upper lobe cavitary lesion typical of endogenous reactivation tuberculosis. (From Mason RJ, Broaddus VC, Murray JF: *Murray and Nadel's textbook of respiratory medicine,* ed 4, Philadelphia, 2005, Saunders.)

SEPTIC EMBOLI

- **Associations:** endocarditis and infective thrombophlebitis
- **Signs and symptoms:** fever, malaise, weakness, weight loss, new murmur, cough, and petechial rash
- **Diagnosis:**
  - **Chest radiograph:** multiple scattered areas of round infiltrates
  - **Blood cultures:** at least three sets should be drawn prior to antibiotic administration; any indwelling lines should be exchanged and cultured
  - **Echocardiogram and vascular ultrasound:** may identify source of emboli
- **Treatment:** broad-spectrum IV antibiotics, such as vancomycin and gentamicin

PEARLS

- Hypoxemia is not common for most acute exacerbations of asthma. A saturation of < 91% generally correlates with severe hypoxemia.

- Chronic obstructive pulmonary disease (COPD) patients do not reverse as rapidly as asthmatics. Have a lower threshold for admission.

- Never withhold oxygen from a hypoxemic COPD patient. The benefits of appropriate oxygenation far outweigh the risk of hypercapnia.

- Bronchitis is a self-limited process. Acute cases do not require antibiotics. Reserve antibiotics for those with COPD or evidence of chronic bronchitis.

- Bronchodilators are efficacious in bronchitis if wheezing is present.

- Peak occurrence of bronchiolitis is from November to February, and respiratory syncytial virus (RSV) is the primary causative agent.

- If bronchoscopy fails to locate the suspected foreign body, consider esophageal impaction with obstruction of the trachea.

- Consider retained foreign body in those who store things in their mouths: repairmen, construction workers, seamstresses.

- Suspect aspiration in patients with head trauma, altered level of consciousness, missing teeth, and any wheezing or respiratory difficulty.

- Children with new-onset wheezing mandate evaluation for foreign body aspiration.

- Radiographs have limited ability to detect most foreign bodies. Have a low threshold to order advanced testing for the stable patient, or have the patient evaluated directly in the operating theater.

- Patients on anticoagulants may present with spontaneous hematoma formation, resulting in partial or complete airway obstruction.

- Change a metal tracheostomy tube to a plastic cuffed tube with an inner cannula to connect patient to a ventilator and avoid an air leak.

- The latent period from asbestos exposure and malignant mesothelioma is 35 to 40 years.

- Malignant lung tumors can cause paraneoplastic syndromes (syndrome of inappropriate antidiuretic hormone secretion [SIADH], Cushing syndrome, others).

- Pancoast tumors may present with arm pain, upper extremity neurologic symptoms, Horner syndrome, and chest wall/periscapular pain.

BIBLIOGRAPHY

Adams J, Stark A: Outcome of infants with bronchopulmonary dysplasia. UpToDate. Available at http://utdol.com/online/content/topic.do?/topicKey = neonatal/17767.

Bartlett J: Acute bronchitis. UpToDate. Available at http://utdol.com/online/content/topic.do?topicKey = pc_id/5499&selectedTitle = 72.

Bartlett J: Aspiration pneumonia in adults. UptoDate. Available at http://utdol.com/online.

Bartlett J: Lung abscess. Up to Date. Available at http://utdol.com/online.

Bhimji S: Pancoast tumor. Available at http://www.emedicine.com.

Brandler E, Sinert R: Mediastinitis. Available at http://www.emedicine.com.

Colucci: Noncardiogenic pulmonary edema. Available at http://www.utdol.com/online.

Dee EK: Mesothelioma, malignant. Available at http://www.emedicine.com.

Driscoll W: Bronchopulmonary dysplasia. Available at http://www.emedicine.com/ped/TOPIC289.HTM.

Fanta C: Treatment of acute exacerbations of asthma in adults. UpToDate, Available at http://utdol.com/online/content/topic.do?topicKey = asthma/12318.

Gilbert DN, Moellering RC, Eliopoulos GM, Sande MA (eds): *The sanford guide to antimicrobial therapy 2008*, ed 38, Sperryville, VA, 2008, Antimicrobial Therapy.

Fauci AS, Braunwald E, Kasper DL et al: *Harrison's principles of internal medicine*, ed 17, New York, 2008, McGraw-Hill.

Heffner JE: Diagnostic evaluation of a pleural effusion in adults. Available at http://www.utdol.com/online.

Hide G: Chondrosarcoma. Available at http://www.emedicine.com.

Hoare Z, Lim W: Pneumonia: update on diagnosis and management, *Br Med J* 332:1077–1079, 2006.

Khan AN, Irion KL, Kasthuri RS, MacDonald S: Pulmonary edema, noncardiogenic. Available at http://www.emedicine.com.

Light RW: Primary spontaneous pneumothorax in adults. Available at http://www.utdol.com/online.

Lindman JP: Tracheostomy. Available at http://www.emedicine.com.

Litonjua A, Weiss S: Risk factors for asthma. UpToDate, Available at http://utdol.com/online/content/topic.do?topickey = asthma/0597.

Loftis LL: Emergent evaluation of acute upper airway obstruction in children. Available at http://utdol.com.

Louden M: Bronchiolitis. Available at http://www.emedicine.com/emerg/topic365.htm.

Lutfiyya MN, Henley E, Chang LF, Reyburn SW: Diagnosis and treatment of community-acquired pneumonia, *Am Fam Physician* 73:442–450, 2006.

17. Which of the following is true about lung cancer?
    a. carcinoid lung tumors metastasize early in the clinical course
    b. small-cell carcinoma is the most common and most aggressive
    c. adenocarcinoma is the most common in nonsmokers
    d. squamous-cell carcinoma is frequently associated hypercalcemia due to SIADH

18. A 68-year-old woman presents with weight loss, painful right breast enlargement, edema, and nipple retraction. On examination, the right breast is noted to be warm and tender but no palpable mass is evident. The patient reports taking two courses of antibiotics but "neither worked," and is requesting a stronger antibiotic. Proper management includes:
    a. close follow-up for mammogram and biopsy
    b. arrange for outpatient intravenous antibiotic therapy for breast cellulitis that failed oral antibiotic therapy
    c. warm compresses to the area until an abscess forms, then return to ED for incision and drainage
    d. workup for superior vena cava syndrome causing breast edema

19. A 48-year-old man presents to emergency room complaining of dizziness, feeling flushed, and diarrhea. His HR is 112 bpm and his BP is 188/105 mmHg. On chest x-ray, he is noted to have a 3-cm left lung mass. His symptoms are likely due to secretion of:
    a. antidiuretic hormone
    b. serotonin
    c. parathyroid-like hormone
    d. adrenocorticotropic hormone (ACTH)

20. A 65-year-old woman presents to the ED complaining of constant chest pain for 2 weeks, radiating to the back and left arm. Patient denies dyspnea or cough. Patient is noted to have left hand weakness, ptosis, and miosis. Her studies are likely to show:
    a. left breast mass with brain metastasis
    b. mediastinal mass with pericardial effusion
    c. large central left lung mass with popcorn calcification
    d. left apical lung mass with bony erosion

21. The most common cause of acute mediastinitis is:
    a. penetrating trauma
    b. esophageal perforation
    c. post-sternotomy complications
    d. inferior extension of Ludwig angina
    e. superior extension of an intra-abdominal infection

22. A 35-year-old man presents complaining of pleuritic anterior chest pain for the past 8 hours. He had several episodes of vomiting after binge eating and drinking last night but had been otherwise well. He also complains of shortness of breath and pain in the anterior neck. His vitals signs are T = 101.4° F, BP = 135/87 mmHg, HR = 124 bpm, RR = 20/minute, O_2 saturation = 99% on room air. Other than his ill appearance and distress, the physical examination is unremarkable. The most important actions to take in this patient's management are:
    a. IV antiemetics, proton pump inhibitor therapy, and CT of the abdomen and pelvis with PO and IV contrast
    b. Stat chest x-ray, electrocardiogram, and echocardiogram
    c. IV fluids, IV glucagon, and if symptoms are not relieved, GI consultation for immediate esophagogastroduodenoscopy
    d. broad-spectrum antibiotics, esophagram, and immediate general surgery consultation

23. The most common cause of transudative pleural effusions is:
    a. cirrhosis
    b. systemic lupus erythematosus
    c. congestive heart failure
    d. nephrotic syndrome
    e. pneumonia

24. The most common cause of an exudative pleural effusion is:
    a. cirrhosis
    b. nephrotic syndrome
    c. congestive heart failure
    d. malignancy
    e. pneumonia

25. A 65-year-old man with a history of chronic hypertension and congestive heart failure presents with complaints of gradually worsening shortness of breath and exercise intolerance. Vital signs are BP = 145/95 mmHg, HR = 104 bpm, T = 97.8° F, RR = 22/minute, O_2 saturation = 96%. The patient's renal function and brain natriuretic peptide (BNP) level are at baseline and his ECG pattern is unchanged from baseline. Chest x-ray reveals a large right sided pleural effusion. Subsequent thoracentesis yields ~500 mL of clear straw-colored fluid, with laboratory tests suggestive of transudative effusion. The patient's symptoms are improved. Repeat chest x-ray reveals no pneumothorax and the effusion is markedly improved. What are the most appropriate therapy and management of this patient?
    a. increase oral diuretic therapy and discharge to home with close primary care follow-up
    b. admit for IV diuresis and repeat thoracentesis in 12 hours

c. admit for serial enzymes, echocardiogram, and further cardiac evaluation
d. admit for IV antibiotics and observation until cultures from the pleural fluid are negative
e. place 38Fr chest tube and consult CT surgery for pleurodesis

26. A healthy 27-year-old man presents complaining of sudden onset of substernal chest pain. The pain is pleuritic in nature and started approximately 4 hours ago, immediately after heavy marijuana use. He denies fever, shortness of breath, or other complaints. Vital signs are: BP = 110/70 mmHg, HR = 106 bpm, T = 99.0° F, RR = 20/minute, O_2 saturation = 98% on room air. He is in no distress. His chest x-ray reveals pneumomediastinum. Which of the following physical examination findings is most specific for this patient's condition?
    a. decreased tactile fremitus
    b. Hamman sign
    c. decreased breath sounds
    d. subcutaneous emphysema
    e. hyperresonance to percussion

27. Bilateral spontaneous pneumothoraces are most commonly seen in which of the following conditions?
    a. *Pneumocystis* pneumonia
    b. Marfan syndrome
    c. catamenial pneumothorax
    d. anorexia nervosa
    e. tuberculosis

28. A healthy 33-year-old man with no significant past medical history presents with 2 days of anterior left-sided chest pain, which is pleuritic in nature, and shortness of breath. He is 6 feet 2 inches, 205 pounds, and vital signs are: BP = 112/74 mmHg, HR = 88 bpm, T = 98.6° F, RR = 22/minute, O_2 saturation = 98% on room air. A chest x-ray reveals a left-sided pneumothorax, with an estimated volume of 40% to 45%. What is the best management of this patient?
    a. No intervention necessary, patient may be safely discharged to home
    b. repeat chest x-ray in 12 hours
    c. needle aspiration and repeat chest x-ray in 12 hours
    d. tube thoracostomy with 22Fr chest tube
    e. tube thoracostomy with 36Fr chest tube and surgical consult for pleurodesis

29. Visualization of small pneumothoraces may be aided by which of the following chest x-ray views in addition to a normal PA chest view on inspiration:
    a. supine AP
    b. upright lateral
    c. supine lateral
    d. upright end-expiratory

30. A 25-year-old woman presented via EMS after being found comatose with markedly depressed respirations and cyanosis. She was given naloxone en route with improvement in her mental status and return of normal respiratory function. She admits to IV drug abuse but denies other significant past medical history. While she is being observed in the ED for continued somnolence, she develops dyspnea, cough productive of frothy, pink-tinged sputum, and decreased O_2 saturations and quickly requires mechanical ventilation. Which of the following findings is most consistent with this disease process?
    a. PaO_2/FIO_2 = 300
    b. basilar rales
    c. elevated BNP levels
    d. pulmonary artery wedge pressure = 15 mmHg
    e. jugular venous distention

31. Which of the following chest radiographs is most consistent with *Mycobacterium tuberculosis*?
    a. multiple round infiltrates
    b. dense lobar consolidation
    c. apical cavitary lesion
    d. bilateral interstitial infiltrates

32. Which of the following antibiotic regimens is most appropriate for outpatient management of community acquired pneumonia?
    a. ampicillin
    b. cephalexin
    c. azithromycin
    d. ciprofloxacin

33. Which of the following chest radiographs is most consistent with an atypical pneumonia?
    a. multiple round infiltrates
    b. dense lobar consolidation
    c. apical cavitary lesion
    d. patchy subsegmental infiltrates

34. Which of the following populations is most at risk for an aspiration pneumonia?
    a. children less than 5 years old
    b. adults more than 55 years old
    c. chronic alcoholics
    d. HIV positive

35. Which of the following treatments is most appropriate for lung abscess today?
    a. piperacillin/tazobactam
    b. gentamicin
    c. trimethoprim/sulfamethoxazole
    d. cefazolin

36. A 50-year-old woman presents to the emergency department complaining of a 5-day history of cough productive of rusty colored sputum,

shaking chills, and fever. If her pneumonia is caused by the pneumococcus, which of the following is most likely to be seen on her chest x-ray?

a. multiple round infiltrates
b. dense lobar consolidation
c. apical cavitary lesion
d. bilateral interstitial infiltrates

37. An 85-year-old nursing home patient presents with mental status changes, tachypnea, low-grade fever and a cough of 1 month's duration. Chest radiograph shows a dense consolidation with an air fluid level inside a cavitary lesion in the right lower lobe. Which of the following is most likely to predispose to failure of medical management?

a. recurrent aspiration
b. A 3-cm cavity
c. thin-walled cavitary lesion on CT
d. absence of empyema

38. A 20-year-old college student presents complaining of nonproductive cough, sore throat, retrosternal chest pain, low-grade fever, mild dyspnea, and general malaise for 5 days' duration. His chest radiograph shows patchy infiltrates and hilar adenopathy. Which of the following pathogens is most likely responsible for his pneumonia?

a. Pneumococcus
b. *Legionella*
c. influenza
d. *Mycoplasma*

39. A 70-year-old man presents with chest pain, dry cough, fever, nausea, vomiting, and diarrhea for 1 week. BP = 100/60 mmHg, HR = 76 bpm, RR = 24/minute, T = 101.6° F, oxygen saturation of 92% on 3 L of oxygen by nasal cannula. His chest radiograph shows a patchy infiltrate with a small left pleural effusion. Which of the following is the most likely atypical infection in this patient?

a. *Mycoplasma*
b. *Chlamydia*
c. *Legionella*
d. *Hemophilus*

40. Residents of the San Joaquin Valley in central California are at special risk for

a. Lyme pneumonia
b. *Coccidioides immitis* pneumonia
c. histoplasma pneumonia
d. *Blastomyces dermatitidis* pneumonia

---

1. Answer: c

Many factors are associated with risk for an asthma-related death, including sudden or severe exacerbations, prior intubations (or ICU admissions), multiple ED visits within 1 year, use of more than two meter dose inhalers (MDI) (beta 2 agonists) in a month, serious psychiatric or psychosocial problems, and illicit drug use. These other choices are diseases that are in the differential diagnosis of asthma.

2. Answer: a

Asthma treatment regimens are based on symptom severity. This patient is classified as severe by her symptoms. Intravenous corticosteroids are usually reserved for impending or actual respiratory arrest, and offer no advantage over orally administered agents. Hydration has not been proven efficacious.

3. Answer: b

PND is a finding in CHF, which is a great mimicker of COPD. **Pursed lip breathing** is a form of self-PEEP that patients with COPD use to elevate pressures inside small collapsible airways. **Respiratory alternans** (respiratory paradox) occurs when the weakened diaphragm of COPD patients is passively sucked upward during inspiration because the intercostals muscles are doing the work of breathing. In normal individuals, the abdomen moves outward during inspiration. **Kussmaul sign** is JVD occurring during inspiration and is found in COPD as well as other cardiovascular disease states. **Pulsus paradoxus,** another finding in COPD, is an inspiratory reduction in systolic pressure of >10 mmHg.

4. Answer: c

Pneumothoraces are best seen on upright or decubitus chest films; they can be difficult to detect on supine films, such as are performed on sick, ventilated patients. A radiolucency in the area of the costophrenic angle suggests pneumothorax in these patients.

5. Answer: d

Bronchitis is a self-limited inflammation of the bronchi, usually occurring during the winter months. The strongest positive predictors for acute bronchitis are a cough and wheezing. Many signs and symptoms are those of common URIs and colds. These include malaise, rhinorrhea, sore throat, myalgias, dyspnea, and chest pain.

6. Answer: a

This patient has acute *bronchitis*. Antibiotics are not indicated, as 70% are caused by viruses. Supportive treatment is the rule. Beta agonists are not effective for coughs <4 weeks unless obstruction (wheezing) is present. Steroids and mucolytics are unproven treatments.

7. Answer: c

Bronchiolitis is a virally induced bronchiolar inflammation occurring in those 2 months to 2 years of age. It is the most common lower respiratory tract infection in infants. **RSV** is responsible for 70% of infections, and is spread by respiratory droplets.

Other causes include **adenovirus,** parainfluenza, *Mycoplasma,* enterovirus, influenza, **rhinovirus,** and *Chlamydia.* **Parvovirus B19** is the cause of erythema infectiosum (Fifth disease).

8. Answer: e

This healthy, full-term infant has *bronchiolitis.* The mainstay of treatment is **supportive care.** He should receive adequate hydration, saline nasal drops, nasal bulb suction, humidified oxygen, apnea monitoring, and cardiac monitoring with pulse oximetry. **Antibiotics** are of no use, as most cases are viral. Beta agonists produce only modest and transient relief. There is no proven role for epinephrine, ipratropium, **ribavirin,** or **immunoglobulin.** The role of **corticosteroids** is controversial.

9. Answer: d

It is very difficult to directly identify an aspirated foreign body on a chest radiograph. Most foreign bodies (85%) are radiolucent, and secondary signs must be sought. There may be **hyperinflation on the affected side,** as a ball-valve phenomenon occurs during inspiration. The patient can inhale air around the obstruction, but cannot exhale past it. Additionally, there is **mediastinal shift away from the affected side. Pneumonia** and **atelectasis** are other secondary findings. However, on a decubitus film, the **obstructed and dependent lung fails to collapse in the decubitus position** as a result of hyperinflation.

10. Answer: c

Histoplasma infection is linked to the **Mississippi, Ohio,** and **Missouri River Valley** regions.

11. Answer: d

Humidified air may help and should not hurt; **dexamethasone** will decrease inflammation over time and **racemic epinephrine nebulized** will decrease inflammation rapidly but will wear off in 2 hours so the patient should be **observed** for return of symptoms **(d).** Only the very worse croup cases need **intubation (a). IV medications** may upset the child and make symptoms worse **(b).** Symptoms may return so **prompt discharge** without observation is not recommended after racemic epinephrine **(c).**

12. Answer: b

Haemophilus influenza **type B** was the classic causative pathogen for epiglottitis prior to vaccination against it **(a).** *Bordetella pertussis* is a highly contagious gram-negative coccobacillus that is prevalent worldwide **(b).** The **beta-hemolytic streptococcus** causes bacterial pharyngitis among other diseases **(c). Rhinovirus** causes viral URI **(d).**

13. Answer: c

This child has classic symptoms of *epiglottitis,* which is an airway emergency. **Laying the child flat** and placing a **mask** over his face will cause anxiety and efforts should be made to keep the child as comfortable as possible **(a). Laboratory studies** are not essential to the diagnosis and the **IV puncture** may upset the child **(b). Preparing for a difficult airway** and possible placement of a tracheostomy is important. Intubation should be done in operating suite with a setup for tracheostomy if needed **(c). Instrumentation** of the throat may worsen swelling and cause complete obstruction **(d).**

14. Answer: c

Without the inner cannula, the patient is at risk for an obstruction of the **outer cannula** that would necessitate removal of the tube. Also the inner cannula has a connector to adapt to a bag-valve-mask or to the ventilator **(a).** With an **uncuffed metal tube** you are unable to give positive pressure ventilation **(b).** An **endotracheal tube** can be a temporary tube until the appropriate-sized tube can be located and placed **(c). Never force a tube** or risk bleeding and the possible creation of a false passage **(d).**

15. Answer: a

Benign masses are more likely to be **tender** than malignant masses **(a).** Malignant mass are typically **indurated (d),** adherent to surrounding tissue **(b),** and **irregular (c).**

16. Answer: c

After asbestos exposure, there is a long latent period **(a)** of typically **35 to 40 years (c),** which is why cases are still being diagnosed despite the reduction in use of asbestos **(b).** Mesothelioma is difficult to treat and usually fatal 1 to 2 years after diagnosis **(d).**

17. Answer: c

Carcinoid lung tumors are the least aggressive lung cancers and **rarely metastasize (a). Small-cell carcinoma** is the **most aggressive** but **not the most common.** Non-small-cell lung cancer is the most common **(b). Adenocarcinoma** is the **most common in nonsmokers (c). Squamous-cell carcinoma** is associated with **hypercalcemia** from secretion of **parathyroid-like hormone (d).**

18. Answer: a

The patient is older, is not lactating, and has failed to respond to antibiotics. She may have *inflammatory breast cancer,* which is difficult to distinguish from infection **(a).** Diagnosis is made by **mammography** and **biopsy.** Symptoms probably are not infectious, so she should **not simply receive outpatient antibiotics**—intravenous or oral—at this point **(b).** Breast abscess **incision and drainage** are probably best handled by surgery **(c). Superior vena cava syndrome** usually causes facial and upper extremity edema bilaterally **(d).**

19. Answer: b

Antidiuretic hormone causes SIADH and hyponatremia **(a). Serotonin** causes carcinoid syndrome (b). **Parathyroid-like hormone** causes hypercalcemia (c). **ACTH** secretion causes Cushing syndrome, and although he is hypertensive, the rest of the clinical picture is one of *carcinoid syndrome* (d).

20. Answer: d

The patient has symptoms consistent with a *Pancoast tumor*. **Apical lung cancer** is the most common cause and tumor spreads into the **chest wall** and **ribs (d)**. **Breast cancer** with **metastasis to the brain** causes neurologic deficits or changes in mental status (a). A mass with **popcorn calcification** is typically a benign lung tumor and most are asymptomatic (c).

21. Answer: b

Esophageal perforations, whether spontaneous or secondary to other etiologies, cause more than 90% of acute mediastinitis.

22. Answer: d

Although many of the actions above may be beneficial, the onset of anterior chest pain, dyspnea, and fever soon after multiple episodes of vomiting is highly suggestive of acute mediastinitis due to *Boerhaave syndrome*. This condition warrants aggressive therapy with **antimicrobials** and **surgical exploration** to prevent the high morbidity and mortality associated with delay in therapy. Although **CT** will help diagnose the condition (and if done, should include the chest), it will create a significant delay in therapy; **antiemetics** and **proton pump inhibitor therapy (a).** are of little benefit. The condition is less likely to be pericarditis with the associated vomiting episodes, so **echocardiography** is not a priority (b). **IV glucagon** and **esophagogastroduodenoscopy** (c) are indicated for impacted esophageal food bolus.

23. Answer: c

Congestive heart failure causes the great majority of simple transudative effusions. **Pneumonia (e)** and **lupus (b)** are associated with exudative effusions. The remaining choices (a, d) are known, but less common, etiologies of transudates.

24. Answer: e

Pneumonia is the most common cause of exudative effusion, followed by **malignancy (d)**. While effusions due to **CHF (c)** are more common, they are transudative, as are **cirrhosis (a)** and **nephrotic syndrome (b)**.

25. Answer: a

CHF is the most common cause of pleural effusions. Simple transudative effusion of known cause may be managed with **therapeutic thoracentesis** and **diuresis** in the absence of fever, empyema, loculations, or other complicating factors. For chronic, gradually developing effusions, **repeat thoracentesis (b)** is rarely needed soon after the initial drainage. As the patient does not have any evidence of cardiac decompensation, **c** is not the best answer. **d** is

incorrect because the effusion is unlikely to be infectious and **antibiotics** are not warranted. **Chest tube** and **pleurodesis (e)** are likewise not indicated.

26. Answer: b

The chest x-ray reveals pneumomediastinum secondary to breath-holding during marijuana use. **Hamman sign,** a distinctive crunching sound heard over the heart during systole, is specific to pneumomediastinum and pneumopericardium. In contrast, the other signs are found in a number of conditions, including pneumothorax, but are frequently not present in *spontaneous pneumomediastinum*.

27. Answer: a

AIDS patients with *Pneumocystis* pneumonia are predisposed to pneumothoraces, which may even be bilateral and have significant associated mortality.

28. Answer: c

Choices **a** and **b** are incorrect as only pneumothoraces <20% should be expectantly managed. This medium-sized, spontaneous pneumothorax in a stable, healthy male without prior illness can be **aspirated** and if there is **no recurrence,** the patient may **safely be discharged** to home. For moderate-sized pneumothoraces (20% to 60%), needle aspiration alone is successful in greater than 50% of cases. Therefore **d** and **e** are incorrect as they are unnecessarily invasive. Catheter placement with attached stopcock or Heimlich valve would be another acceptable, minimally invasive treatment.

29. Answer: d

End-expiratory films may make detection of a pneumothorax easier. **Supine views (a, c)** often obscure pneumothorax. **Lateral views (b)** are more sensitive for effusion, but not for pneumothorax.

30. Answer: d

This represents a case of *opiate-induced noncardiogenic pulmonary edema*. The **wedge pressure is characteristically normal** in NCPE. Although the **PaO$_2$/FIO$_2$ ratio** is low, a value of **300 (a)** suggests a much less severe form of pulmonary edema—acute lung injury (ALI). **Basilar rales (b)** are much more typical of cardiogenic pulmonary edema. NCPE almost always presents with diffuse edema on chest x-ray and physical examination. **c** and **e** are incorrect as elevated **BNP** and **jugular venous distention** suggest heart failure.

31. Answer: c

While *Mycobacterium tuberculosis* infection can present with a variety of radiographic findings (including normal chest radiograph in the immunocompromised host), the classic presentation is an **apical cavitary lesion.**

32. Answer: c

Most community-acquired pneumonia should be treated with a **macrolide** to cover atypical organisms as well as pneumococcal pneumonia. Fluoroquinolones such as **ciprofloxacin** have inadequate coverage of community-acquired pneumonia; newer-generation fluoroquinolones, though often reserved for patients with suspected resistant organisms, treatment failures, or high risk of *Pseudomonas* infection, are more efficacious.

33. Answer: d

Atypical pneumonias are more likely to have **patchy subsegmental infiltrates** and hilar adenopathy.

34. Answer: c

Chronic alcoholics are most at risk for aspiration pneumonia. Other at-risk populations include those with chronically depressed mental status, esophageal motility disorders, elderly (>65 years old), and seizures.

35. Answer: a

The Sanford guide offers **piperacillin/tazobactam** as first-line for suspected aspiration or lung abscess, which can be due to multiple bacterial species, including anaerobes, gram-positive, and gram-negative species.

36. Answer: b

Bacterial pneumonia is more likely to have **lobar segmental infiltrates** and effusions on chest radiograph. Atypical pneumonia is more likely to have patchy subsegmental infiltrates and hilar adenopathy on chest radiograph.

37. Answer: a

Risk factors for failure of medical management of lung abscess include **recurrent aspiration,** large cavity (**>6 cm**), prolonged symptoms prior to presentation, abscess associated with obstructing lesion, **thick-walled cavities,** underlying serious comorbidity, or development of **empyema.**

38. Answer: d

This clinical picture is most consistent with an atypical pneumonia caused by *Mycoplasma.* It is characterized by a subacute respiratory illness with cough, retrosternal chest pain, sore throat, and headache. It is more common in younger patients.

39. Answer: c

Legionella is the most common atypical organism in elderly patients with pneumonia, representing 10% of community acquired pneumonia in this patient population. It is often associated with gastrointestinal symptoms and can be complicated by pancreatitis, sinusitis, myocarditis, and pyelonephritis.

40. Answer: b

Answers **c** and **d** are associated with the Midwestern river valleys (Ohio, Missouri, Mississippi, and the Great Lakes region). **Lyme disease (a)** does not cause pneumonia.

Analgesics

ACETAMINOPHEN

- Common formulation of many analgesics, cough and cold products
- Elimination half-life 3 to 4 hours
- Toxic metabolite (*N*-acetyl-*p*-benzo-quinone imine [NAPQI]) produced though cyp450
- Induced by chronic alcoholism and other p450 inducers
- NAPQI conjugates with glutathione
- Overdose depletes glutathione
- Potential acute toxic dose $\sim$150 mg/kg
- Alcoholics, malnourished, and chronically ill more susceptible to toxicity

SIGNS AND SYMPTOMS

- Early, <12 to 24 hours—anorexia, nausea and vomiting
- Quiescent phase—relative lack of symptoms
  - Begin to see elevation of transaminases
- Late, usually >48 hours—fulminate hepatic failure; elevation of transaminases, coagulopathy, renal insufficiency (elevated prothrombin time [PT]/international normalized ratio [INR]/partial thromboplastin time [PTT], elevated creatinine, metabolic acidosis)
- Recovery or transplant

DIAGNOSIS

- Recommended testing: complete blood count, electrolytes, blood urea nitrogen (BUN), creatinine, transaminases, coagulation profile, acetaminophen level
- Begin *N*-acetylcysteine treatment for:
  - 4-hour acetaminophen level ≥150 mcg/mL
    - Nomogram only useful following single acute overdose with known time of ingestion; it is not useful in chronic or repeated ingestions (Fig. 17-1)
  - Elevated transaminases with history of potentially toxic ingestion
  - Any elevated acetaminophen level with unreliable history or unknown time of ingestion

TREATMENT

- Consider early activated charcoal in the alert patient
- *N*-acetylcysteine
  - Serves as a glutathione precursor
  - Optimum dosing within 8 hours of ingestion
  - Oral loading dose 140 mg/kg
  - IV loading dose 150 mg/kg
  - Anaphylactoid reactions may occur in IV dosing
- Safe in pregnancy

---

*Toxidromes and toxicologic syndromes (e.g., anticholinergic toxidrome; opioid toxidrome; anticonvulsant hypersensitivity; serotonin syndrome; neuroleptic malignant syndrome)

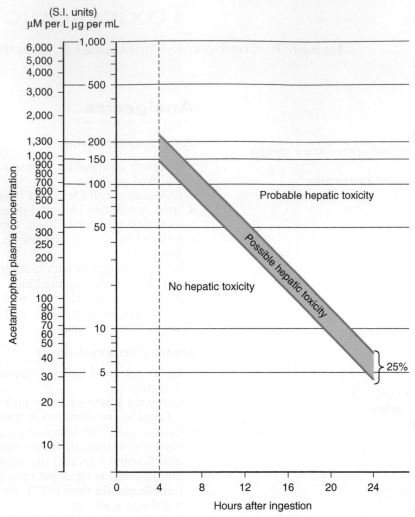

Figure 17-1. Rumack-Matthew nomogram for acetaminophen poisoning, a semilogarithmic plot of plasma acetaminophen concentrations vs time. Cautions for the use of this chart: (1) The time coordinates refer to time after ingestion. (2). Serum concentrations obtained before 4 hours may not represent peak concentrations. (3) The graph should be used only in relation to a single acute ingestion. This nomogram is not useful for chronic exposures, nor has it been validated for use after ingestions involving sustained-release acetaminophen products. (4) The lower solid line 25% below the standard nomogram is included to allow for possible errors in acetaminophen plasma assays and estimated time from ingestion of an overdose. (From Rumack BH, Hess AJ [eds]: *Poisindex, Denver, Micromedix,* 1995. Adapted from Rumack BH, Matthew H: Acetaminophen poisoning and toxicity, *Pediatrics* 55:871–876, 1975.)

NONSTEROIDAL ANTI-INFLAMMATORY DRUGS (NSAIDs)

- Inhibit the enzyme cyclooxygenase (COX1 and COX2))
- Decrease prostaglandin synthesis
- Common ingredients in analgesics, cough and cold products

SIGNS AND SYMPTOMS

- Toxicity in therapeutic dosing
  - Gastrointestinal (GI) bleeding
  - Renal insufficiency
  - Aseptic meningitis
  - May precipitate bronchospasm in asthmatics
- Acute overdose
  - Most common symptoms: abdominal pain, nausea, vomiting

- High doses—generally greater than 400 mg/kg ibuprofen
  - Central nervous system (CNS) depression, acidosis, cardiovascular collapse
- Hepatic and renal damage may occur
- Mefenamic acid may cause seizures in overdose

DIAGNOSIS

- Drug levels are not readily available
- Consider complete blood count, electrolytes, BUN, creatinine, acetaminophen, aspirin, coagulation profile, and liver enzymes

TREATMENT

- Antacids may be used for GI upset
- Asymptomatic or minimally symptomatic (GI upset) patients with no co-ingestion can be medically cleared after 4 to 6 hours of observation.

OPIATES AND RELATED NARCOTICS

- Typical agents: fentanyl, heroin, hydrocodone, hydromorphone, meperidine, methadone, morphine, oxycodone, propoxyphene

SIGNS AND SYMPTOMS

- CNS depression
- Respiratory depression
- Miosis
- Propoxyphene, tramadol, or meperidine may *not* cause miosis
- Propoxyphene is a potent sodium channel blocker (prolongs QRS complex)
- Risk of noncardiogenic pulmonary edema
- Withdrawal:
  - Anxiety, abdominal pain, lacrimation, myalgias, piloerection, vomiting, diarrhea

DIAGNOSIS

- Clinical
- Urine drug screen
  - High incidence of false negatives if screening only for opiates (e.g., morphine, codeine)

TREATMENT

- Respiratory support as needed
- Naloxone
  - Initial dose 0.4 mg diluted in 10 mL NS and given slow intravenous (IV) push
    - Synthetic opioids may need larger doses
  - If patient does not respond to 10 mg then unlikely opioid overdose (OD)
  - Caution in polydrug ingestion as naloxone may unmask another drug
  - Administration may produce acute withdrawal
  - Half-life 45 to 60 minutes—much shorter than most oral opioids
    - Risk of resedation, especially in patients with renal failure or who have taken opioids with long elimination half-lives (e.g., methadone)
- Clonidine has been used to attenuate withdrawal symptoms

SALICYLATES

- Found in a variety of prescription and over-the-counter products
- Therapeutic levels 10 to 30 mg/dL (100 to 300 mg/L)
- Therapeutic half-life 2 to 4.5 hours (hepatic metabolism)
  - Enzymes saturated in overdose (Michaelis–Menten kinetics)
- Absorption may be delayed
  - Enteric coated tablet, concretion formation, pylorospasm

- Weak acid—more of the salicylate compound in unionized form at lower pH
- Uncouples oxidative phosphorylation

SIGNS AND SYMPTOMS

- **Acute overdose**
  - Early: tinnitus, hyperpnea/tachypnea (primary respiratory alkalosis), GI distress
  - Progression to: metabolic acidosis, altered mental status
  - Late findings: renal insufficiency, pulmonary edema, cerebral edema, hyperthermia
- **Chronic ingestion**
  - Altered mental status, tinnitus, metabolic acidosis, pulmonary edema, hyperthermia
  - May resemble congestive heart failure (CHF), pneumonia, or sepsis

DIAGNOSIS

- Salicylate level
  - Serial levels every 2 hours until levels decline
- Complete blood count, electrolytes, BUN, creatinine, coagulation profile, liver enzymes
- Mixed respiratory alkalosis and metabolic acidosis
  - No anion gap early following overdose, large anion gap later in toxicity
  - May have metabolic alkalosis component secondary to vomiting

TREATMENT

- Administration of activated charcoal may be beneficial even late in presentation
  - Concretions and pylorospasm may slow aspirin passage through stomach
- Replace fluid loss
- Alkalinize the urine for levels >40 mg/dL
  - Ion traps salicylate in the blood compartment and urine compartment
- Avoid sedatives as this may result in a precipitous drop in pH (loss of respiratory alkalosis)
  - Intubation may result in similar consequence if ventilator rate not high enough
- Definitive therapy—hemodialysis
  - Indicated for:
    - Pulmonary edema
    - Cerebral edema
    - Renal insufficiency
    - Marked acid–base or electrolyte disturbance
    - Clinical deterioration despite supportive care and urinary alkalinization
    - Salicylate levels greater than 100 mg/dL (1000 mg/L)

Methyl salicylate—oil of wintergreen

- 5 mL of pure oil of wintergreen equals approximately 7 g of aspirin
- Quickly absorbed from the stomach
- Precipitous acidosis and altered mental status

Alcohols

ETHANOL

- Concentration varies with product
- Contained in mouthwashes, cooking extracts, medicinal syrups/elixirs
- As tolerance varies, clinical presentation may correlate poorly with blood levels
- Chronic use downregulates GABA (γ-aminobutyric acid) receptors and upregulates NMDA (*N*-methyl-*d*-aspartate) receptors

SIGNS AND SYMPTOMS

- **Acute intoxication**
  - Slurred speech, ataxia, CNS depression
  - Hypotension/myocardial suppression may be present in extreme intoxication
  - Hypoglycemia
    - More common in children and malnourished adults
- **Chronic use**
  - Gastritis, pancreatitis, hepatotoxicity, neurologic disorder (cortical atrophy, peripheral neuropathy, Wernicke encephalopathy, Korsakoff psychosis)
- **Alcoholic ketoacidosis**
  - Nausea, vomiting, tachycardia, hypotension
  - Likely has precipitating illness
    - Pancreatitis, hepatitis, gastritis

DIAGNOSIS

- **Acute intoxication**
  - Clinical
  - Blood ethanol levels
  - Presence of an osmolar gap without significant anion-gap acidosis
  - Average adult metabolism: 15 to 20 mg/dL/hour
- **Alcoholic ketoacidosis**
  - Usually low blood ethanol levels
  - Anion-gap metabolic acidosis
    - May have osmolar gap
  - Ketosis—predominance of beta-hydroxybutyrate
  - Blood glucose not significantly elevated
- **Acute withdrawal**
  - Tachycardia, tremors, hypertension, agitation
  - Hallucinations
  - Seizures
  - Delirium tremens

TREATMENT

- Supportive therapy for acute intoxication
- Volume replacement and glucose for alcoholic ketoacidosis
- Thiamine, magnesium, folic acid
- Benzodiazepines first-line for ethanol withdrawal and withdrawal seizures
  - Consider propofol or barbiturates for refractory seizures

GLYCOLS

- Contain two OH groups

TABLE 17-1   **Molecular Mass of Alcohols and Their Contribution to the Osmolal Gap**

Alcohol	Molecular weight (daltons)	Osmolal contribution (mOsm/kg H_2O) per 100 mg/dL	Anion gap elevated
Diethylene glycol	106	9	(+)
Ethanol	46	22	−
Ethylene glycol	62	16	+
Isopropyl alcohol	60	17	−
Isobutyl alcohol	74	14	−
Methanol	32	34	+
Propylene glycol	76	13	−

Ethylene glycol

- Primary ingredient in most brands of antifreeze
- Metabolized by alcohol and aldehyde dehydrogenase to glycoaldehyde, acidic by-products, and oxalate
- Oxalate precipitates with calcium to form calcium oxalate crystals
  - Calculate osmol gap (Table 17-1)
  - Calculate anion gap

Propylene glycol

- Common diluent for phenytoin and lorazepam
- Metabolized to lactic acid

Polypropylene glycol

- High-molecular-weight forms (bowel irrigation) are not readily absorbed and essentially not toxic
- Low-molecular-weight forms may cause mild acidosis

SIGNS AND SYMPTOMS

- CNS depression, slurred speech, ataxia
- Progression to renal failure
- May have focal neurologic deficits

DIAGNOSIS

- Classically: osmolar gap with anion-gap metabolic acidosis
  - Absence of osmolar gap does not rule out toxicity
- Presence of fluorescence on face or clothes under Wood lamp for antifreeze products
  - Urine fluorescence not sensitive or specific
- May have calcium oxalate crystals in urine
  - Monohydrate—needle shaped
  - Dehydrate—envelope shaped
- Blood levels are specific but may not be readily available

TREATMENT

- Fomepizole (4-methylpyrazole) or ethanol block metabolism of parent compound
- Cofactors thiamine and pyridoxine enhance metabolism to nontoxic metabolites (glycine and ketoadipate respectively)

- Definitive treatment—hemodialysis
  - Indicated for:
    - Moderate to severe acidosis
    - Ethylene glycol level >50 mg/dL—not an absolute indication
    - Renal failure
    - Focal neurologic findings

METHANOL

- "Wood alcohol"
- Component of solvents, chafing dish fuel, windshield washer fluid
- Metabolized by alcohol and aldehyde dehydrogenase to formaldehyde then formic acid, respectively
- Mildly intoxicating—much less so than ethanol
  - May not have significant signs of inebriation
- Long half-life
  - Acidosis may be delayed

SIGNS AND SYMPTOMS

- May have latent period of 12 to 24 hours
- May present with inebriation
- Gastritis, nausea, vomiting, visual disturbance (classic description "snowfield vision"), seizures, coma
- Basal ganglia infarcts or hemorrhage

DIAGNOSIS

- Classically: osmolar gap with anion gap metabolic acidosis
  - Absence of osmolar gap does not rule out toxicity
- Funduscopic examination may have disc or retinal edema
- Blood levels specific but may not be readily available

TREATMENT

- Fomepizole (initial dose 15 mg/kg) and ethanol prevent metabolism of methanol to formaldehyde
- Folic acid as cofactor may enhance conversion to CO_2 and H_2O
- Alkalemia favors formation of less toxic conformation
  - Sodium bicarbonate may be beneficial for acidemia
- Definitive treatment: hemodialysis
  - Indicated for:
    - Methanol concentration >50 mg/dL
    - Renal failure
    - Visual deficit
    - Metabolic acidosis

ISOPROPYL

- "Rubbing alcohol"
- Reportedly 2 to 3 times more intoxicating than ethanol
- Metabolized to acetone: osmolar gap *without* anion-gap acidosis

SIGNS AND SYMPTOMS

- Inebriation: slurred speech, nausea, vomiting, gastritis (may be hemorrhagic), CNS depression
- Hypotension in large ingestions
- Hypoglycemia may occur

DIAGNOSIS

- Fruity breath odor (acetone)
- Osmolar gap *without* high anion-gap acidosis
- Ketonemia and ketonuria
- Blood levels specific but may not be readily available

TREATMENT

- Supportive care
- Fluid resuscitation
- Fomepizole (4-methylpyrazole) *not* indicated
- Dialysis may be used in severe cases (myocardial suppression/ hypotension)

Anesthetics

LOCAL

- **Amide-linked**
  - Bupivacaine
  - Lidocaine
  - Prilocaine
  - Have the letter "i" in the root
- **Ester-linked**
  - Benzocaine
  - Procaine
  - Tetracaine
  - Benzonatate
  - Cocaine
- Bind to sodium channels and inhibit nerve conduction
- Allergic reactions more common with ester-linked
- Benzonatate is used as an antitussive agent
- Systemic toxicity may result when these agents are misused in the following examples:
  - Inadvertent intravenous administration (i.e., during nerve blockade)
  - Supratherapeutic dosing for local anesthesia (i.e., lidocaine without epinephrine: greater than 5 mg/kg; lidocaine with epinephrine greater than 7 mg/kg)

SIGNS AND SYMPTOMS

- **Local toxicity**—may include prolonged anesthetic effects
  - Spinal anesthesia may result in diaphragm paralysis
- **Systemic toxicity**—Acute onset of perioral paresthesias, confusion, muscle twitching, slurred speech with possible progression to seizures and dysrhythmias
  - Hypotension may occur secondary to peripheral vasodilation and decreased cardiac contractility

- Methemoglobinemia
  - Most frequently from benzocaine, also reported with prilocaine, lidocaine, and tetracaine

DIAGNOSIS

- Based on history and symptoms
- Drug levels are generally only available for cocaine and lidocaine
- Methemoglobinemia can be diagnosed with co-oximetry

TREATMENT

- Airway support
- Seizures may be treated with benzodiazepines
- Standard resuscitation procedures for cardiac arrest
- Cardiopulmonary bypass has been used for refractory cases
- Lipid emulsions have been used to treat systemic toxicity
- Treatment of significant methemoglobinemia with methylene blue

INHALATIONAL ANESTHETICS

- **Halogenated hydrocarbons**
  - Examples: halothane, isoflurane, sevoflurane, enflurane
  - Well-absorbed through lungs
  - Potency correlates with lipid solubility
- **Nitrous oxide**
  - Used as a propellant in some food products
    - Whipped cream ("whippets")
  - One of several inhalants of abuse
  - Chronic use causes functional B_{12} deficiency

SIGNS AND SYMPTOMS

- Halogenated hydrocarbons
  - Acute toxicity related to hypoxia
  - Halothane has been associated with hepatotoxicity
- Nitrous oxide
  - Acute toxicity related to hypoxia
  - Alerted mental status, syncope, in extreme cases cardiac arrest
  - Chronic use leads to peripheral neuropathy, megaloblastic anemia, and bone marrow suppression

Anticholinergics

- Antagonists of the muscarinic acetylcholine receptor
- Typical agents
  - Antihistamines
  - Antipsychotics
  - Tricyclic antidepressants
  - Tropane alkaloids
    - Various plants (e.g., Jimson weed, Belladonna)
  - Antispasmodics

SIGNS AND SYMPTOMS

- Act as "antimuscarinic" agents
- Mydriasis
- Dry mucous membranes
- Dry axillae
- Mumbling speech
- Hallucinations
- Flushing
- Temperature elevation
- Urinary retention
- Diminished bowel sounds
- Mnemonic: "Blind as a bat, dry as a bone, red as a beet, mad as a hatter, full as a flask, hot as a hare"

DIAGNOSIS

- Primarily clinical

TREATMENT

- Symptomatic
- Benzodiazepines for agitation
- Physostigmine may be a potential "antidote"
  - Contraindicated in patients with wide QRS on electrocardiogram (ECG) (i.e., tricyclic antidepressant [TCA] poisoning)—may cause asystole
  - Adverse effects—cholinergic toxidrome "sludge" symptoms

Cholinergic

- Nerve agents
- Organophosphorous insecticides (e.g., malathion, diazinon, dichlorvos, chlorpyrifos, parathion)
- Carbamates insecticides (e.g., carbaryl, aldicarb)
- *Inocybe* and *Clitocybe* mushrooms
- Methacholine, pilocarpine, bethanechol

SIGNS AND SYMPTOMS

- Mnemonic: DUMBELS (Diarrhea, Urination, Miosis, Bradycardia, Bronchorrhea, Bronchoconstriction, Emesis, Lacrimation, Salivation)

DIAGNOSIS

- Primarily clinical
- Plasma (butyryl or pseudo)-cholinesterase levels—not readily available
- RBC cholinesterase levels—more specific, not readily available

TREATMENT

- Atropine (reverses muscarinic symptoms)
  - Initial adult dose 2 mg IV often need repetitive dosing
  - End point drying of secretions and ease of ventilation
- Oximes (pralidoxime)
  - Helps reverse both nicotinic and muscarinic symptoms
  - Prevents "aging" of organophosphates
  - Not indicated in known carbamate poisoning
  - Initial adult dose 2 g IV

Anticoagulants

WARFARIN (COUMADIN)

- Majority of toxicity results during chronic therapeutic use
- Inhibits vitamin K epoxide reductase and vitamin K quinone reductase
  - Inhibits synthesis of vitamin K–dependent coagulation factors—II, VII, IX, X

SUPERWARFARINS

- Brodifacoum, bromadoline, chlorophacinone, difenacoum, diphacinone
- Increased affinity for vitamin K epoxide and quinone reductase
- Lipid soluble—markedly increases half-life
- Anticoagulant effects may last for months

SIGNS AND SYMPTOMS

- Ecchymosis, gingival bleeding, evidence of GI bleeding (hematemesis, melena), hematuria, intracranial hemorrhage
- Anticoagulant effects may begin within 12 hours; however, peak effects are generally not seen until 2 to 3 days
- Single unintentional acute ingestion of warfarin or superwarfarin
  - May develop slight elevation in INR
- Acute overdose following chronic warfarin use
  - Preexisting therapeutic decrease in vitamin K–dependent factors
  - Significant elevation in INR may occur
- Single intentional acute ingestion of warfarin
  - Generally asymptomatic
  - May have minimal elevation in PT and PTT
- Intentional overdose of superwarfarin products
  - Anticoagulant effects may begin 2 to 3 days later and persist for months

DIAGNOSIS

- **Single acute ingestion**
  - Baseline PT/INR followed by PT/INR at 48 hours
  - Normal INR at 48 hours rules out significant ingestion
- **Acute on chronic ingestion**
  - Baseline PT/INR followed by PT/INR at least daily
- **Acute superwarfarin ingestion**
  - Baseline PT/INR followed by PT/INR at 48 hours
  - Brodifacoum levels are available from specialized laboratories
  - Factors II, VII, IX, and X levels are decreased

TREATMENT

- Vitamin K_1 allows for carboxylation of dependent factors and restores factor function

- Does not provide effect for at least 6 hours
- Active hemorrhage may require fresh frozen plasma
  - Contains active clotting factors
- Prophylactic vitamin K not recommended after acute ingestion

HEPARIN

- Unfractionated heparin
- Low-molecular-weight heparin
  - Enoxaparin, dalteparin
- Intentional overdose is rare

SIGNS AND SYMPTOMS

- Coagulopathy
- Thrombocytopenia (heparin induced thrombocytopenia [HIT])

DIAGNOSIS

- HIT—thrombocytopenia, history of heparin exposure
- Bruising, gingival bleeding, epistaxis

TREATMENT

- Discontinue the agent
- Protamine sulfate
  - 1 mg neutralizes 100U heparin
  - Adverse reactions: anaphylactic, anaphylactoid reactions, pulmonary hypertension
  - Unproven for LMWH

Anticonvulsants

VALPROIC ACID

- Used as an anticonvulsant, mood stabilizer, migraine prophylaxis, and treatment of chronic pain
- Branched-chain carboxylic acid
- Delayed absorption with divalproex (Depakote)
- Therapeutic serum level ~ 50 to 150 mg/L

SIGNS AND SYMPTOMS

- **Acute overdose**
  - GI upset
  - CNS depression
  - May cause miotic pupils
  - Nystagmus generally not a prominent finding
  - Bone marrow suppression may occur and be delayed by 3 to 5 days
  - High serum level, approximately >850 mg/L, may result in metabolic acidosis.
- **Complications associated with therapeutic dosing**
  - Hyperammonemia with or without encephalopathy
  - Transaminitis
  - Pancreatitis
  - Fulminate hepatic failure
  - Coagulopathy

DIAGNOSIS

- Valproic acid level
  - Serial levels in 2 hours to evaluate for continued absorption
- Other useful laboratory studies
  - Complete blood count, electrolyte panel, hepatic profile, BUN and creatinine, coagulation panel, lipase
- An ammonia level is indicated in the encephalopathic patient taking valproic acid
  - Primary hyperammonemia

TREATMENT

- Supportive therapy and respiratory support as needed
- At high serum levels >850 mg/L, valproic acid and metabolic derangements are amenable to hemodialysis
- Carnitine supplementation
  - Consider for large overdoses (serum level >450 mg/L), hyperammonemia with encephalopathy and hepatic dysfunction
  - Typical dosing 100 mg/kg IV divided three times a day up to 3 g per day

PHENYTOIN

- Anticonvulsant, rarely used as an antidysrhythmic agent
- Decreases activity of neuronal sodium channels
- Erratic absorption following oral administration
- Parenteral preparations formulated with propylene glycol
  - Maximum infusion rate 50 mg/minute
  - Rapid infusion may lead to cardiovascular collapse
  - Fosphenytoin infusion may be infused 2 to 3 times faster
- Metabolism saturable at therapeutic doses
  - Michaelis–Menten kinetics—goes to zero order

SIGNS AND SYMPTOMS

- Nystagmus
  - Prominent finding even at therapeutic levels
- Ataxia
- Tremor
- Dysarthria
- Nausea
- Vomiting
- Confusion
- CNS depression
- Therapeutic dosing may result in hypersensitivity reactions (e.g., anticonvulsant hypersensitivity syndrome, Stevens–Johnson syndrome)
- Gingival hyperplasia is a side effect
- Avoid in pregnancy secondary to fetal hydantoin syndrome
- Adverse cardiovascular effects are rare after oral overdose
- Rapid infusions of IV phenytoin are associated with myocardial suppression and cardiovascular collapse (primarily due to propylene glycol present)

- Extravasation of phenytoin is associated with tissue necrosis
  - "Purple glove syndrome"

DIAGNOSIS

- Phenytoin level
  - Therapeutic levels 10 to 20 mg/dL
  - Serial levels every 2 hours until declining

TREATMENT

- Primarily supportive
- Consider charcoal for those presenting promptly with adequate airway protection
- Admit for moderate to severe symptoms or for increasing blood levels
- For cardiovascular compromise following intravenous infusion
  - Discontinue infusion; administer fluids and vasopressors as needed
- Medical clearance should be based on clinical appearance and falling phenytoin level

CARBAMAZEPINE

- Uses: antiepileptic, treatment of trigeminal neuralgia and chronic pain
- Erratic absorption
- Therapeutic range: 4 to 12 mg/dL
- Cyclic ring structure may give false positive on TCA screen
- Oxcarbamazepine considered a prodrug
  - Carbamazepine levels not accurate for oxcarbamazepine dosing

SIGNS AND SYMPTOMS

- Nystagmus
- Ataxia
- Mydriasis
- Tachycardia
- CNS depression
- Seizures
- Anticholinergic findings are usually present
- May cause syndrome of inappropriate antidiuretic hormone secretion (SIADH)
- Therapeutic dosing may result in anticonvulsant hypersensitivity syndrome

DIAGNOSIS

- Carbamazepine level
  - Serial levels every 2 hours until declining
- Monitor electrolyte panel, BUN, and creatinine for presence of SIADH

TREATMENT

- Admit symptomatic patients to a monitored bed
  - Risk of seizures
- Activated charcoal absorbs carbamazepine
- Seizures
  - First-line therapy: benzodiazepines
  - Second line: propofol or barbiturates

- Medical clearance should be based on clinical appearance and falling carbamazepine levels

PHENOBARBITAL

- Anticonvulsant and sedative–hypnotic
  - Chronic treatment of epilepsy or IV formulation for acute status epilepticus
- Enhance activation of neuro-inhibitory GABA channels
- Inducer of cytochrome p450
- Therapeutic range 20 to 40 mg/dL

SIGNS AND SYMPTOMS

- CNS depression
- Slurred speech
- Respiratory depression
- Coma
- Hypotension
  - More commonly associated with large oral ingestions or IV loading
- Cutaneous bullae (known as "barbiturate burns")
- Extreme intoxication may result in loss of primitive reflexes (may resemble brain death)

DIAGNOSIS

- Urine drug screens may reveal presence but not specific for acute overdose
  - Serum levels correlate better with symptoms
  - Serial levels every 2 hours until declining
- Monitor creatine phosphokinase (CPK) for evidence of rhabdomyolysis

TREATMENT

- Respiratory support as needed
- Fluids and vasopressor support as needed for hypotension
- Aggressive hydration for rhabdomyolysis
- Alkalinization of the urine can increase excretion of phenobarbital

OTHER ANTICONVULSANTS

- Lamotrigine
- Tiagabine
- Levetiracetam
- Topiramate
- Gabapentin

SIGNS AND SYMPTOMS

- Ataxia, nystagmus, CNS depression, nausea and vomiting common
- Myoclonus or seizures may occur
- Lamotrigine associated with Stevens–Johnson syndrome
- Topiramate may cause non–anion-gap metabolic acidosis

DIAGNOSIS

- History of exposure

TREATMENT

- Supportive care

Anticonvulsant hypersensitivity

- Aromatic anticonvulsants
- Carbamazepine
- Phenobarbital
- Phenytoin
- Familial history

SIGNS AND SYMPTOMS

- Most common in first few months of therapy
- Fever, rash, malaise
  - May have liver, renal, and cardiac involvement
- May develop toxic epidermal necrolysis

DIAGNOSIS

- History of offending agent
- Familial history of anticonvulsant hypersensitivity

TREATMENT

- Discontinue anticonvulsant agent
- Methylprednisolone
- Cross-reactivity to other aromatic anticonvulsants

Antidepressants

CYCLIC (Fig. 17-2)

- Low therapeutic index
- Highly lipophilic
- Typical agents:
  - Amitriptyline
  - Nortriptyline
  - Imipramine
  - Desipramine
  - Doxepin

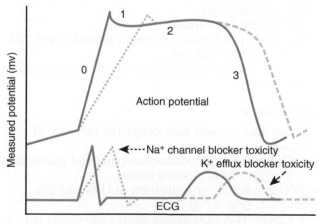

Figure 17-2. Cardiac style action potential with corresponding electrocardiographic tracing. Dotted line indicates the changes associated with Na+ channel blocker toxicity. Dashed line indicates the changes associated with K+ efflux blocker activity. (From Holstege CP, Eldridge DL, Rowden AK: ECG manifestations: the poisoned patient, *Emerg Med Clin N Am* 24(1):160, 2006.)

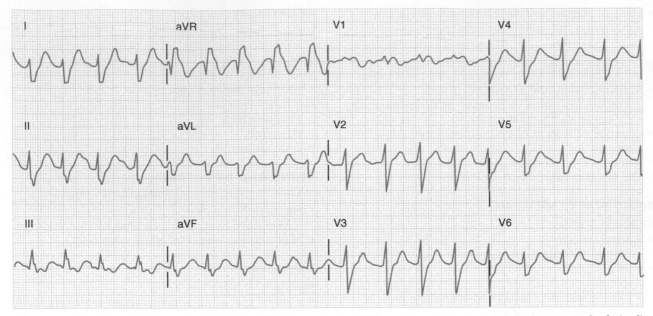

Figure 17-3. Na+ channel blocker poisoning. 12-lead ECG demonstrating QRS complex widening and tachycardia as a result of tricyclic antidepressant overdose. Note amplitude of R wave in lead aVR >3 mm.

- Amoxapine
- Maprotiline
- May have active metabolites
- Anticholinergic
  - Anticholinergic effects may delay absorption
- Proconvulsant
- Dysrhythmogenic
  - Cardiac sodium and potassium channel blockade
- Peripheral alpha-adrenergic blockade

SIGNS AND SYMPTOMS

- CNS depression
- Tachycardia
- Hypotension
- Seizures
- QTc prolongation
- QRS prolongation
- Ventricular dysrhythmia
- May have precipitous decline in mental status and progression to seizures
- Clinical picture in massive overdose may resemble brain death

DIAGNOSIS

- Urine drug screens may detect the presence of TCAs
  - Cyclobenzaprine, carbamazepine, and quetiapine may give false positive results.
- ECG is integral for evaluation of QRS and QTc intervals (Fig. 17-3)
  - Classic TCA ECG shows sinus tachycardia with a QRS duration >100 milliseconds with terminal R wave in lead aVR (>3 mm) and S wave in lead I; usually occur together but can occur in isolation
  - Compare to baseline ECG as either may pre-exist
  - QRS duration greater than 100 milliseconds is associated with an increased risk of seizures

- QRS duration greater than 160 milliseconds is associated with an increase risk of ventricular dysrhythmia

TREATMENT

- Intravenous sodium bicarbonate therapy is indicated for QRS duration >100 milliseconds or terminal R wave >3 mm in lead aVR in setting of known or possible TCA overdose.
- First-line treatment for seizures is benzodiazepines
  - Second-line propofol or barbiturates
- Metabolic acidosis should be treated with sodium bicarbonate to decrease cardiotoxicity of the drug
- Ventricular dysrhythmias should be treated with sodium bicarbonate and standard resuscitation techniques
- Hypotension should be treated with intravenous normal saline
  - Give sodium bicarbonate in the presence of QRS prolongation, R wave >3 mm in lead aVR
  - Phenylephrine is first-line treatment for refractory hypotension
- Patients that have not developed symptoms within 6 hours can be medically cleared
- Symptomatic patients should be admitted
- Physostigmine is contraindicated for anticholinergic symptoms

MONOAMINE OXIDASE INHIBITORS (MAOIs)

- Primarily used for depression
- Inactivate the enzyme that metabolizes catecholamines in the CNS
- Selegiline selective for MAO-B receptor
  - No diet restriction

SIGNS AND SYMPTOMS

- **Acute overdose**
  - Symptoms may be delayed
  - Nausea, tremor, agitation, hypertension, hyperreflexia, dysrhythmia, seizures, and cardiovascular collapse
- **Tyramine reaction**
  - Indirect sympathomimetic
  - May occur with high-risk foods
    - Beer, fava beans, cheese, aged meats, red wine, yeast
  - Usually 15 to 90 minutes after ingestion
  - Hypertension, headache, flushing, diaphoresis, tachycardia
  - May lead to hypertensive emergency
- **Serotonin syndrome**
  - May occur with concomitant use of other pro-serotonergic drugs (i.e., selective serotonin reuptake inhibitors [SSRIs], TCAs, dextromethorphan, meperidine)
  - Signs and symptoms: restlessness, hyperreflexia, agitation, clonus, delirium, hyperthermia, autonomic instability, rigidity

DIAGNOSIS

- No specific drug levels are available
- History of medication or high-risk food ingestion and clinical syndrome of sympathetic and/or serotonergic overdrive

TREATMENT

- Treat hypertensive crisis, titrate IV vasodilators
  - Beta-blockers may lead to unopposed alpha effect
- Serotonin and sympathomimetic symptoms may be treated with benzodiazepines
- First-line treatment for seizures are benzodiazepines
- Treat hyperthermia with active cooling
- Monitor CPK, electrolytes, BUN, and creatinine
- Monitor even asymptomatic patients for 24 hours

SEROTONIN REUPTAKE INHIBITORS (SSRIs)

- **Typical agents**
  - Fluoxetine
  - Sertraline
  - Citalopram
  - Escitalopram
  - Paroxetine
  - Venlafaxine
  - Trazodone
  - Bupropion
- Block reuptake of serotonin into presynaptic terminal
- Nonselective agents may also affect norepinephrine and dopamine reuptake
- Primarily used as antidepressants.
- Bupropion used for smoking cessation
- Trazodone often used as a sleep aid

SIGNS AND SYMPTOMS

- CNS depression is common
- May cause seizures (more frequent reports with bupropion)
- Citalopram is associated with delayed-onset QTc prolongation
- Serotonergic symptoms
  - May present following acute ingestion of a single agent or polypharmacy with multiple pro-serotonergic agents
  - Restlessness, hyperreflexia, agitation, clonus, delirium, hyperthermia, autonomic instability

DIAGNOSIS

- History of ingestion
- Serotonin syndrome presents with constellation of symptoms:
  - Rigidity, hyperreflexivity and clonus in lower extremities greater than upper extremities, altered mental status, autonomic instability, and hyperthermia
- Urine serotonin levels not accurate in diagnosis
- QT prolongation may be evident following trazodone, venlafaxine or citalopram ingestions

TREATMENT

- Primarily supportive care
- Hypotension generally responsive to fluid bolus
- Consider magnesium for QT prolongation
- First-line treatment for seizures is benzodiazepines
- Cyproheptadine is "classic antidote" although rarely indicted

LITHIUM

- Primarily acts as a neurotoxin in overdose
- Cation—resembles sodium and potassium
- Therapeutic range 0.6 to 1.2 mEq/L
- Primarily excreted by the kidney
- States of sodium depletion or dehydration promote increased resorption

SIGNS AND SYMPTOMS

- Tremor
- Ataxia
- Nystagmus
- Nausea/vomiting
- Slurred speech
- Confusion
- Hyperreflexia/clonus
- Myoclonus
- Coma
- Seizures
- Nephrogenic diabetes insipidus (DI) possible

DIAGNOSIS

- Lithium level
  - Green top tubes will give false elevation (lithium heparin)
- May have decreased anion gap

- ECG
  - T-wave flattening/inversion, nonspecific ST changes, possible bradycardia
- Nephrogenic DI may result in:
  - Hypernatremia
  - Elevated BUN/creatinine

TREATMENT

- Sodium polystyrene sulfonate binds lithium and may be effective following acute overdose
  - Closely monitor serum potassium
- Optimize hydration and sodium status
- Monitor electrolytes frequently for development of DI
- Hemodialysis effectively removes lithium
  - Continuous renal replacement may prevent rapid fluid and electrolyte shifts
  - Indicated for:
    - Severe CNS depression
    - Lithium induced seizures
    - Patients with renal failure
    - No consensus for specific levels

Antiparkinsonism drugs

- Pro-dopaminergic agents
- Anticholinergic/antihistaminic agents
- MAO inhibitors/ catechol-O-methyl transferase (COMT) inhibitors

SIGNS AND SYMPTOMS

- Levodopa: agitation, CNS depression, movement disorders
- Amantidine: agitation, delirium, ataxia, possible anticholinergic symptoms
- Selegiline: see MAO-inhibitors
- Anticholinergic/antihistamine: see anticholinergic section

DIAGNOSIS

- Primarily clinical—assays are not readily available and of no utility in the acute setting
- Monitor for sympathetic excess (MAOIs) or anticholinergic toxidrome.

TREATMENT

- Primarily supportive
- Benzodiazepines for agitation and movement disorder
- Dopamine receptor antagonist may be considered for movement disorder, but should not be used in patients with pre-existing parkinsonism
- Titrate IV vasodilators for hypertension

Antihistamines and antiemetics

- "Classic" antihistamine and phenothiazines have anticholinergic side effects

- "Nonsedating" antihistamines and 5-HT$_3$ (serotonin) antagonists lack this effect.
- Used in cough and cold products and sleep aids
- May be abused for anticholinergic properties
- **"Classic" antihistamines**
  - Diphenhydramine
  - Dimenhydrinate
  - Chlorpheniramine
  - Meclizine
- **"Nonsedating"**
  - Loratadine
  - Fexofenadine
  - Cetirizine
- **Phenothiazines**
  - Prochlorperazine
  - Promethazine
- **5-HT$_3$ antagonists**
  - Ondansetron
  - Granisetron

SIGNS AND SYMPTOMS

- **"Classic" antihistamines**
  - CNS depression
  - Anticholinergic toxidrome
    - Mydriasis, mumbling speech, dry skin, decreased bowel sounds, urinary retention, hyperthermia, delirium
  - Seizures may occur
  - Diphenhydramine is associated with QRS and QT prolongation
- **Nonsedating antihistamines**
  - May lose selectivity in higher doses
- **Phenothiazines**
  - Anticholinergic toxidrome may occur
  - Extrapyramidal symptoms including dystonic reactions
  - May lower seizure threshold
  - Risk of QT prolongation
- **5-HT$_3$ antagonists**
  - Limited toxicity in overdose

DIAGNOSIS

- History and constellation of anticholinergic toxidrome
- Specific drug levels not readily available
- ECG may reveal QRS or QTc prolongation
- Monitor CPK for rhabdomyolysis

TREATMENT

- Benzodiazepines as needed for agitation
- Treat QRS prolongation >100 milliseconds with sodium bicarbonate
- Consider IV magnesium sulfate for QTc prolongation
- Benzodiazepines are first-line therapy for seizures
- Consider physostigmine as a diagnostic/treatment agent
  - Contraindicated in the presence of ECG abnormalities other than tachycardia

Antipsychotics

TYPICAL (CLASSIC)

- D_2 dopaminergic receptor antagonists
- Associated with greater risk of extrapyramidal symptoms
- May cause antihistaminic effects and alpha-1 adrenergic receptor blockade
- Typical agents: chlorpromazine, thioridazine, haloperidol, droperidol, fluphenazine

SIGNS AND SYMPTOMS

- **Acute intoxication**
  - CNS depression
  - Orthostatic hypotension
  - Tachycardia
  - Dose-dependent respiratory depression
  - QTc prolongation possible
  - Mild hyperthermia possible, especially in warm ambient temperatures
  - Phenothiazines may lower seizure threshold
- **Extrapyramidal symptoms** (EPS)
  - **Dystonic reactions**
    - Usually within 5 days of starting or changing dose
    - Normal mental status
    - Involuntary sustained muscle contraction
    - Most common in muscles of head and neck
    - Laryngospasm may be a life-threatening complication
  - **Akathisia**
    - Sensation of motor restlessness and anxiety
    - Agitation, constant movement
    - Generally occurs with initial dosing or early in treatment
  - **Tardive dyskinesia**
    - Persistent, involuntary orofacial movements
    - Generally irreversible
    - Most often develops after years of treatment
  - **Parkinsonism**
    - Rigidity (cogwheel)
    - Bradykinesia
    - Tremor
    - Postural instability
    - Often occurs within months of starting therapy
    - Reversible
- **Neuroleptic malignant syndrome** (NMS)
  - Altered mental status
  - Hyperthermia
  - Rigidity ("lead-pipe")
  - Autonomic instability
  - Typically evolves over several days
  - Typically within 2 weeks of initiating or escalating therapy, although may occur at any time during treatment

DIAGNOSIS

- **Acute overdose**
  - History
  - Orthostatic hypotension, tachycardia, may have miotic pupils
  - May have QTc prolongation
- **EPS symptoms**
- History of neuroleptic use along with characteristic symptoms
- **NMS**
  - CPK elevations in 98%
  - Leukocytosis
  - Constellation of symptoms
  - History of neuroleptic, dopamine antagonist or abrupt withdrawal of antiparkinsonian drugs (dopamine agonists)

TREATMENT

- **Acute intoxication**
  - Primarily supportive
  - Hypotension typically responds to fluid bolus
  - Direct alpha-adrenergic agents vasopressors of choice
    - Phenylephrine
    - Norepinephrine
  - Treat seizures with benzodiazepines
  - QTc prolongation may be treated with magnesium sulfate
    - Adult dose 2 g IV
- **Akathisia**
  - Reduction in antipsychotic dose
  - Anticholinergic agents
    - Diphenhydramine (25 to 50 mg IM/IV adults, children 5 mg/kg/day in divided doses every 4 to 6 hours)
    - Benztropine (1 to 2 mg IM/IV)
  - Benzodiazepines may be useful
- **Dystonia**
  - Anticholinergic agents
    - Diphenhydramine (25 to 50 mg IM/IV adults, children 5 mg/kg/day in divided doses every 4 to 6 hours)
    - Benztropine (1 to 2 mg IM/IV)
    - Generally need repeat dosing for 48 to 72 hours
  - Benzodiazepines
  - If continued use of neuroleptic is needed, consider continuing anticholinergic agent or switch to lower-potency or atypical antipsychotic
- **Parkinsonism**
  - Anticholinergic agents may decrease symptoms
    - Benztropine (1 to 2 mg IM/IV)
  - Dopamine agonists may be beneficial
  - Use low doses of typical agents or switch to atypical agent
- **Tardive dyskinesia**
  - Discontinue antipsychotic if possible
  - Often resistant to treatment
- **NMS**
  - Benzodiazepines
  - Hydration
  - Aggressive cooling for hyperthermia
  - Bromocriptine
    - Dose typically 2.5 to 10 mg three times a day in adults
    - Only available in oral formulation
  - Dantrolene
    - May relieve rigidity and help with hyperthermia

ATYPICAL

- Agents: clozapine, risperidone, olanzapine, quetiapine, aripiprazole
- Possess less risk of extra pyramidal symptoms

SIGNS AND SYMPTOMS (SIMILAR TO THAT SEEN WITH TYPICAL ANTIPSYCHOTICS, EXCEPT FOR MIOSIS)

- CNS depression
- Orthostatic hypotension
- Hypotension
- Tachycardia
- Miosis
- Possibility of QTc prolongation

DIAGNOSIS

- History with constellation of symptoms (miosis, hypotension, tachycardia, CNS depression, QTc prolongation)
- Specific drug levels not readily available

TREATMENT

- Hypotension generally fluid-responsive
  - Refractory hypotension be treated with a direct-acting alpha adrenergic agent (phenylephrine, norepinephrine)
- CNS and respiratory depression may require intubation
- Monitor QT interval
- Progressive CNS depression warrants admission to ICU

Bronchodilators

METHYLXANTHINES

- Examples: theophylline, theobromine, caffeine
- Act as phosphodiesterase inhibitors
- Adenosine receptor antagonists
- Michaelis–Menten kinetics in overdose (saturable)
- Therapeutic range 5 to 15 mcg/mL
  - Severe toxicity expected in acute overdose: >100 mcg/mL
  - Severe toxicity expected in chronic toxicity: >60 mcg/mL

SIGNS AND SYMPTOMS

- Nausea
- Tremors
- Persistent vomiting
- Agitation
- Tachycardia
  - Supraventricular dysrhythmias common
- Hypotension
- Seizures are common in severe overdose

DIAGNOSIS

- **Acute presentation**
  - Primarily based on history and clinical presentation

- Laboratory values may reveal hypokalemia, hyperglycemia
- Hypotension, tachycardia, with hypokalemia, hyperglycemia and metabolic acidosis very suggestive
- Theophylline levels are helpful in diagnosis
- **Chronic overdose**
  - Nausea and vomiting may not be as prevalent
  - Tachycardia common
  - Seizures may occur at lower serum levels

TREATMENT

- Fluid resuscitation
- Activated charcoal may be useful secondary to enteric recirculation of the drug
- Nonselective beta adrenergic blockers theoretically treat hypotension and tachycardia produced by beta adrenergic stimulation
- Hemodialysis effectively removes the drug
  - Should be considered for:
    - Life-threatening complications
    - Serum levels in acute overdose >80 to 100 mcg/mL
    - Serum levels in chronic overdose >40 mcg/mL

BETA-2 ADRENERGIC AGONISTS

- Albuterol
- Clenbuterol
- Terbutaline
- Specific activity at beta 2 receptor
  - Lose specificity in overdose
- Vascular, smooth muscle, and bronchial relaxation

SIGNS AND SYMPTOMS

- Agitation
- Tremor
- Tachycardia
- Hypotension

DIAGNOSIS

- Primarily based on history and clinical presentation
- Laboratory values may reveal hypokalemia, hyperglycemia
- Specific drug levels are not readily available

TREATMENT

- Fluid resuscitation
- Alpha adrenergic agonists are vasopressors of choice
- Hypokalemia is a result of intracellular shifts and generally does not require treatment

Carbon monoxide

- Leading cause of poisoning-related death in the United States
- Colorless, odorless, nonirritating, tasteless gas
- Product of incomplete combustion of carbon-containing materials

- Faulty gas appliances, poorly ventilated stoves, automobile exhaust fumes
- Affinity for hemoglobin 200 to 250 times that of O_2
- Fetal hemoglobin more affinity than adult hemoglobin
- Impairs oxyhemoglobin saturation and reduces oxygen delivery
  - Shifts oxyhemoglobin dissociation curve to the left
  - Tighter O_2 binding (left = latch)
- Binds to myoglobin
- Inhibits cytochrome oxidase

SIGNS AND SYMPTOMS

- Generally nonspecific
- Headache, fatigue, nausea, vomiting, flu-like illness (without the fever)
- Possible chest pain, syncope, seizures, hypotension, myocardial suppression
- Delayed neurologic sequelae
  - Onset of cognitive deficits days to weeks after CO exposure
  - Symptoms range from memory deficit, difficulty performing calculations, and personality disorder to Parkinsonism.

DIAGNOSIS

- Standard pulse oximetry gives falsely elevated readings
- Arterial blood gas may show normal PaO_2 and oxygen saturation
  - Oxygen saturation calculated from PaO_2
- Co-oximetry must be used to measure carboxyhemoglobin
  - Specific levels do not necessarily correlate with symptoms
- Metabolic acidosis may be present
- Elevated CPK and troponin are common
- ECG may show signs of ischemia

TREATMENT

- Removal from the source
- Oxygen
- Hyperbaric oxygen (HBO) reduces half-life from ~200 minutes on room air to 20 to 30 minutes
  - May reduce the incidence of delayed neurologic sequelae
  - As of this writing, the American College of Emergency Physicians consensus statement does not mandate use of HBO
  - Consider HBO for loss of consciousness, persistent neurologic deficits, hemodynamic compromise, and pregnant females.

PEARLS

- Rumack–Matthew nomogram only helpful in acetaminophen overdose when the time of ingestion is known and it is a single ingestion.

- Propoxyphene, tramadol, meperidine may not cause small pupils like opioids are expected to produce.

- Propoxyphene has opioid and sodium channel–blocker toxicologic potential and may be mixed with acetaminophen (Darvocet).

- Fever, altered mental status, agitation, and dilated pupils are characteristic of sympathomimetic and anticholinergic toxidromes; however, dry axillae (absence of sweating) favors anticholinergic toxicity.

- Be prepared for anaphylactoid reactions when administering protamine sulfate, vitamin K, or N-acetylcysteine intravenously.

- Clonidine can present like an opioid in overdose (bradycardia, depressed mental status, and small pupils).

- In treating patients with an anticholinergic toxidrome, physostigmine is contraindicated in the presence of ECG abnormalities (e.g., widened QRS complex; rightward deviation in the terminal 40 milliseconds of the frontal-plane QRS axis) other than sinus tachycardia.

- Hypotension and tachycardia, with hypokalemia, hyperglycemia, and metabolic acidosis are very suggestive of theophylline overdose; seizures may develop that are difficult to treat.

- Standard pulse oximetry may be falsely "normal" in carbon monoxide poisoning; co-oximetry of a venous or arterial blood sample is necessary.

- Topiramate may cause a non–anion-gap metabolic acidosis, and should be considered in the differential diagnosis of that acid–base disturbance.

BIBLIOGRAPHY

Aaron CK, Northrup K: Sympathomimetic syndrome. In Brent J, Wallace K, Burkhart K et al (eds): *Critical care toxicology: diagnosis and management of the critically poisoned patient*, ed 1, Philadelphia, 2005, Elsevier, pp. 383–392.

Bateman DN: Cholinergic syndromes. In Brent J, Wallace K, Burkhart K et al (eds): *Critical care toxicology: diagnosis and management of the critically poisoned patient*, ed 1, Philadelphia, 2005, Elsevier, pp. 271–280.

Belson MG, Watson WA: Nonsteroidal anti-inflammatory drugs. In Flomenbaum NE, Goldfrank LR, Hoffman RS et al (eds): *Goldfrank's toxicologic emergencies*, ed 8, New York, 2006, McGraw-Hill, pp. 573–579.

Berk WA, Henderson WV: Alcohols. In Tintinalli JE, Kelen GD, Stapczynski JS (eds): *Emergency medicine: a comprehensive study guide*, ed 6, New York, 2004, McGraw-Hill, pp. 1064–1070.

Boyer EW, Shannon M: The serotonin syndrome, *N Engl J Med* 352:1112–1120, 2005.

Braitberg G: Carbamazepine. In Brent J, Wallace K, Burkhart K et al (eds): *Critical care toxicology: diagnosis and management of the critically poisoned patient,* ed 1, Philadelphia, 2005, Elsevier, pp. 559–564.

Brent J, Klein LJ: Lithium. In Brent J, Wallace K, Burkhart K et al (eds): *Critical care toxicology: diagnosis and management of the critically poisoned patient,* ed 1, Philadelphia, 2005, Elsevier, pp. 523–532.

Bruno GR, Carter WA: Nonsteroidal anti-inflammatory drugs. In Tintinalli JE, Kelen GD, Stapczynski JS (eds): *Emergency medicine: a comprehensive study guide,* ed 6, New York, 2004, McGraw-Hill, pp. 1094–1097.

Burns MJ: Neuroleptic agents. In Brent J, Wallace K, Burkhart K et al (eds): *Critical care toxicology: diagnosis and management of the critically poisoned patient,* ed 1, Philadelphia, 2005, Elsevier, pp. 505–522.

Clark RF: Insecticides: organic phosphorus compounds and carbamates. In Flomenbaum NE, Goldfrank LR, Hoffman RS et al (eds): *Goldfrank's toxicologic emergencies,* ed 8, New York, 2006, McGraw-Hill, pp. 1497–1512.

Curry SC: Salicylates. In Brent J, Wallace K, Burkhart K et al (eds): *Critical care toxicology: diagnosis and management of the critically poisoned patient,* ed 1, Philadelphia, 2005, Elsevier, pp. 621–630.

Doyon S: Opioids. In Tintinalli JE, Kelen GD, Stapczynski JS (eds): *Emergency medicine: a comprehensive study guide,* ed 6, New York, 2004, McGraw-Hill, pp. 1071–1074.

Doyon S: Anticonvulsants. In Flomenbaum NE, Goldfrank LR, Hoffman RS et al (eds): *Goldfrank's toxicologic emergencies,* ed 8, New York, 2006, McGraw-Hill, pp. 731–745.

Eldridge DL, Holstege CP: Utilizing the laboratory in the poisoned patient, *Clin Lab Med* 26:13–30, 2006.

Eldridge DL, Van Eyk J, Kornegay C: Pediatric toxicology, *Emerg Med Clin North Am* 25:283–308, 2007.

Erickson TB, Thompson TM, Lu JJ: The approach to the patient with an unknown overdose, *Emerg Med Clin North Am* 25:249–281, 2007.

Evans CE, Sebastian J: Serotonin syndrome, *Emerg Med J* 24:20–21, 2007.

Flomenbaum NE: Salicylates. In Flomenbaum NE, Goldfrank LR, Hoffman RS et al (eds): *Goldfrank's toxicologic emergencies,* ed 8, New York, 2006, McGraw-Hill, pp. 550–564.

Furbee RB, Rusyniak DE: Antihistamines. In Brent J, Wallace K, Burkhart K et al (eds): *Critical care toxicology: diagnosis and management of the critically poisoned patient,* ed 1, Philadelphia, 2005, Elsevier, pp. 449–456.

Gorman D, Drewry A, Huang YL, Sames C: The clinical toxicology of carbon monoxide, *Toxicology* 187:25–38, 2003.

Greller HA: Lithium. In Flomenbaum NE, Goldfrank LR, Hoffman RS et al (eds): *Goldfrank's toxicologic emergencies,* ed 8, New York, 2006, McGraw-Hill, pp. 1052–1061.

Hahn IH, Nelson LS: Opioids. In Brent J, Wallace K, Burkhart K et al (eds): *Critical care toxicology: diagnosis and management of the critically poisoned patient,* ed 1, Philadelphia, 2005, Elsevier, pp. 611–620.

Harrigan RA, Brady WJ: Antipsychotics. In Tintinalli JE, Kelen GD, Stapczynski JS (eds): *Emergency medicine: a comprehensive study guide,* ed 6, New York, 2004, McGraw-Hill, pp. 1044–1047.

Hoffman RS: Methylxanthines and selective B2-adrenergic agonists. In Flomenbaum NE, Goldfrank LR, Hoffman RS et al (eds): *Goldfrank's toxicologic emergencies,* ed 8, New York, 2006, McGraw-Hill, pp. 989–1003.

Holstege CP, Dobmeier SG: Nerve agent toxicity and treatment, *Curr Treat Options Neurol* 7:91–98, 2005.

Hung OL, Nelson LS: Acetaminophen. In Tintinalli JE, Kelen GD, Stapczynski JS (eds): *Emergency medicine: a comprehensive study guide,* ed 6, New York, 2004, McGraw-Hill, pp. 1088–1093.

Jacobsen D, McMartin K: Methanol and formaldehyde poisoning. In Brent J, Wallace K, Burkhart K et al (eds): *Critical care toxicology: diagnosis and management of the critically poisoned patient,* ed 1, Philadelphia, 2005, Elsevier, pp. 895–901.

Juurlink D: Antipsychotics. In Flomenbaum NE, Goldfrank LR, Hoffman RS et al (eds): *Goldfrank's toxicologic emergencies,* ed 8, New York, 2006, McGraw-Hill, pp. 1039–1051.

Kao LW, Furbee RB: Drug-induced Q-T prolongation, *Med Clin North Am* 89:1125–1144, 2005.

Kao LW, Nañagas KA: Toxicity associated with carbon monoxide, *Clin Lab Med* 26:99–125, 2006.

Katz KD, Ruha A-M: Barbiturates. In Brent J, Wallace K, Burkhart K et al (eds): *Critical care toxicology: diagnosis and management of the critically poisoned patient,* ed 1, Philadelphia, Elsevier, 2005, pp. 547–552.

Katz KD, Wallace KL: Anti-Parkinson's medications. In Brent J, Wallace K, Burkhart K et al (eds): *Critical care toxicology: diagnosis and management of the critically poisoned patient,* ed 1, Philadelphia, 2005, Elsevier, pp. 583–596.

Kaufman B, Griffel M: Inhalational anesthetics. In Flomenbaum NE, Goldfrank LR, Hoffman RS et al (eds): *Goldfrank's toxicologic emergencies,* ed 8, New York, 2006, McGraw-Hill, pp. 1016–1023.

Kraut JA, Kurtz I: Toxic alcohol ingestions: clinical features, diagnosis, and management, *Clin J Am Soc Nephrol* 3:208–225, 2008.

Larson AM: Acetaminophen hepatotoxicity, *Clin Liv Dis* 11:525–548, 2007.

Lawrence DT, Kirk MA: Chemical terrorism attacks: update on antidotes, *Emerg Med Clin North Am* 25:567–595, 2007.

Lheureux P, Penaloza A, Zahir S, Gris M: Science review: carnitine in the treatment of valproic acid-induced toxicity—what is the evidence? *Crit Care* 9:431–440, 2005.

LoVecchio F: Phenytoin. In Brent J, Wallace K, Burkhart K et al (eds): *Critical care toxicology: diagnosis and management of the critically poisoned patient,* ed 1, Philadelphia, 2005, Elsevier, pp. 553–558.

Marshall H, Emerman CL: Theophylline. In Tintinalli JE, Kelen GD, Stapczynski JS (eds): *Emergency medicine: a comprehensive study guide,* ed 6, New York, 2004, McGraw-Hill, pp. 1098–1102.

Martin TG: Anticholinergic syndrome. In Brent J, Wallace K, Burkhart K et al (eds): *Critical care toxicology: diagnosis and management of the critically poisoned patient,* ed 1, Philadelphia, Elsevier, 2005, pp. 261–270.

Mills KC: Monoamine oxidase inhibitors. In Tintinalli JE, Kelen GD, Stapczynski JS (eds): *Emergency medicine: a comprehensive study guide,* ed 6, New York, 2004, McGraw-Hill, pp. 1039–1043.

Mills KC: Newer antidepressants and serotonin syndrome. In Tintinalli JE, Kelen GD, Stapczynski JS (eds): *Emergency medicine: a comprehensive study guide,* ed 6, New York, 2004, McGraw-Hill, pp. 1033–1038.

Mills KC: Tricyclic antidepressants. In Tintinalli JE, Kelen GD, Stapczynski JS (eds): *Emergency medicine: a comprehensive study guide,* ed 6, New York, 2004, McGraw-Hill, pp. 1025–1032.

Mills KC: Cyclic antidepressants. In Brent J, Wallace K, Burkhart K et al (eds): *Critical care toxicology: diagnosis and management of the critically poisoned patient,* ed 1, Philadelphia, 2005, Elsevier, pp. 475–484.

Mills KC: Monoamine oxidase inhibitors. In Brent J, Wallace K, Burkhart K et al (eds): *Critical care toxicology: diagnosis and management of the critically poisoned patient,* ed 1, Philadelphia, 2005, Elsevier, pp. 485–494.

Nelson LS: Opioids. In Flomenbaum NE, Goldfrank LR, Hoffman RS et al (eds): *Goldfrank's toxicologic emergencies,* ed 8, New York, 2006, McGraw-Hill, pp. 590–613.

O'Malley GF: Emergency department management of the salicylate-poisoned patient, *Emerg Med Clin North Am* 25:333–346, 2007.

Osborn HH: Phenytoin and fosphenytoin toxicity. In Tintinalli JE, Kelen GD, Stapczynski JS (eds): *Emergency medicine: a comprehensive study guide,* ed 6, New York, 2004, McGraw-Hill, pp. 1117–1121.

Perry HE, Shannon MW: Theophylline and other methyl xanthines. In Brent J, Wallace K, Burkhart K et al (eds): *Critical care toxicology: diagnosis and management of the critically poisoned patient,* ed 1, Philadelphia, 2005, Elsevier, pp. 457–464.

Raschke RA, Curry SC: Thrombolytics, heparin and derivatives, and antiplatelet agents. In Brent J, Wallace K, Burkhart K et al (eds): *Critical care toxicology: diagnosis and management of the critically poisoned patient,* ed 1, Philadelphia, 2005, Elsevier, pp. 701–710.

Reilly TH, Kirk MA: Atypical antipsychotics and newer antidepressants, *Emerg Med Clin North Am* 25:477–497, 2007.

Rowden AK, Norvell J, Eldridge DL, Kirk MA: Updates on acetaminophen toxicity, *Med Clin North Am* 89:1145–1159, 2005.

Rowden AK, Norvell J, Eldridge DL, Kirk MA: Acetaminophen poisoning, *Clin Lab Med* 26:49–65, 2006.

Rusyniak DE, Sprague JE: Toxin-induced hyperthermic syndromes, *Med Clin North Am* 89:1277–1296, 2005.

Schears RM: Barbiturates. In Tintinalli JE, Kelen GD, Stapczynski JS (eds): *Emergency medicine: a comprehensive study guide*, ed 6, New York, 2004, McGraw-Hill, pp. 1051–1054.

Schwartz DR, Kaufman B: Local anesthetics. In Flomenbaum NE, Goldfrank LR, Hoffman RS et al (eds): *Goldfrank's toxicologic emergencies*, ed 8, New York, 2006, McGraw-Hill, pp. 1004–1015.

Snodgrass WR: Valproic acid. In Brent J, Wallace K, Burkhart K et al (eds): *Critical care toxicology: diagnosis and management of the critically poisoned patient*, ed 1, Philadelphia, 2005, Elsevier, pp. 565–571.

Stork CM: Serotonin reuptake inhibitors and atypical antidepressants. In Flomenbaum NE, Goldfrank LR, Hoffman RS et al (eds): *Goldfrank's toxicologic emergencies*, ed 8, New York, 2006, McGraw-Hill, pp. 1070–1082.

Su M, Hoffman RS: Anticoagulants. In Flomenbaum NE, Goldfrank LR, Hoffman RS et al (eds): *Goldfrank's toxicologic emergencies*, ed 8, New York, 2006, McGraw-Hill, pp. 887–902.

Suchard JR, Curry SC: Oral anticoagulants. In Brent J, Wallace K, Burkhart K et al (eds): *Critical care toxicology: diagnosis and management of the critically poisoned patient*, ed 1, Philadelphia, 2005, Elsevier, pp. 695–700.

Tomassoni AJ: Antihistamines and decongestants. In Flomenbaum NE, Goldfrank LR, Hoffman RS et al (eds): *Goldfran''s toxicologic emergencies*, ed 8, New York, 2006, McGraw-Hill, pp. 785–793.

Wax PM: Anticholinergic toxicity. In Tintinalli JE, Kelen GD, Stapczynski JS (eds): *Emergency medicine: a comprehensive study guide*, ed 6, New York, 2004, McGraw-Hill, pp. 1143–1145.

Weaver LK, Hopkins RO, Chan KJ et al: Hyperbaric oxygen for acute carbon monoxide poisoning, *N Engl J Med* 347:1057–1067, 2002.

Wiener SW: Toxic alcohols. In Flomenbaum NE, Goldfrank LR, Hoffman RS et al (eds): *Goldfrank's toxicologic emergencies*, ed 8, New York, 2006, McGraw-Hill, pp. 1447–1459.

Wolf SJ, Lavonas EJ, Sloan EP, Jagoda AS: Clinical policy: critical issues in the management of adult patients presenting to the emergency department with acute carbon monoxide poisoning, *Ann Emerg Med* 51:138–152, 2008.

Yip L: Salicylates. In Tintinalli JE, Kelen GD, Stapczynski JS (eds): *Emergency medicine: a comprehensive study guide*, ed 6, New York, 2004, McGraw-Hill, pp. 1085–1087.

Yip L: Ethanol. In Flomenbaum NE, Goldfrank LR, Hoffman RS et al (eds): *Goldfrank's toxicologic emergencies*, ed 8, New York, 2006, McGraw-Hill, pp. 1147–1161.

Questions and Answers

1. A 46-year-old female presents to the emergency department with altered mental status. She is awake and answers questions with slurred speech; she has ataxia and horizontal nystagmus. Her vital signs are temperature (T) = 98.3° F, pulse (P) = 105 beats per minute (bpm), respiratory rate (RR) = 22/minute, blood pressure (BP) = 112/68 mmHg, O_2 saturation = 100%. Her electrolyte panel reveals a sodium of 138 mmol/L, a bicarbonate of 16 mmol/L, glucose of 110 mmol/L, and an anion gap of 19. Her salicylate level is undetectable. Her osmolar gap is 38. Initial management of this patient would include:

   a. alkalinization of the urine (150 mEq $NaHCO_3$ in 100 mL D5W run at 2 times maintenance)
   b. administration of fomepizole (15 mg/kg IV)
   c. administration of activated charcoal (1 g/kg PO)
   d. administration of atropine (2 mg IV)

2. Which of the following is an electrocardiographic feature of tricyclic antidepressant poisoning?

   a. T-wave inversions in the lateral leads
   b. bradycardia with first-degree atrioventricular block
   c. QRS prolongation with a prominent R wave in lead aVR and S wave in lead I
   d. ST segment elevation in lead II, III, and aVF

3. In the setting of acute tricyclic antidepressant poisoning, what "antidote" should be used for evidence of QRS prolongation on the electrocardiogram?

   a. sodium polystyrene sulfonate
   b. sodium bicarbonate
   c. activated charcoal
   d. lidocaine

4. A 26-year-old woman presents to the emergency department after an acute drug ingestion. She has miosis, lethargy, tachycardia, and mild hypotension. Her vitals are T = 97.8° F, P = 134 bpm, RR = 12/minute, BP = 84/58 mmHg, O_2 saturation = 96%. She has a past medical history of chronic back pain and is taking oxycodone, cyclobenzaprine and quetiapine to help her sleep. What is the most likely cause of this patient's hypotension?

   a. oxycodone
   b. cyclobenzaprine
   c. quetiapine
   d. clonidine

5. A 67-year-old man presents to the emergency department with altered mental status. His family members last saw him 2 days ago, at which time he was acting more confused than normal. Physical examination reveals muscle rigidity and diaphoresis, but no hyperreflexia or clonus. His vitals are T = 102.2° F, P = 122 bpm, RR = 22/minute, BP = 154/100 mmHg, O_2 saturation = 98%. The patient has a past medical history of schizophrenia and is taking niacin, fluoxetine, chlorpromazine, and simvastatin. The medication most likely to result in this syndrome is:

   a. niacin
   b. fluoxetine

c. chlorpromazine

d. simvastatin

6. A 17-year-old woman presents to the emergency department by EMS after ingestion of an over-the-counter sleep aid. She is lethargic, flushed, has large pupils, dry skin, and mucous membrane and absent bowel sounds. EMS states that she had a generalized tonic–clonic seizure in route. Vital signs are T = 100.7° F, P = 140 bpm, RR = 18/minute, BP = 98/60 mmHg, O_2 saturation = 100%. She has a wide complex rhythm on the cardiac monitor and the ECG reveals a wide complex tachycardia (QRS 128 milliseconds). The most appropriate treatment at this time would be:

   a. defibrillation

   b. administration of procainamide at 30 mg/minute to a maximum of 17 mg/kg

   c. synchronized cardioversion

   d. administration of sodium bicarbonate (1 to 2 mEq/kg bolus)

7. Patients with a history of anticonvulsant hypersensitivity syndrome may be safely started on what agent?

   a. carbamazepine

   b. phenytoin

   c. phenobarbital

   d. valproic acid

8. Chronic abuse of which agent may lead to peripheral neuropathy and anemia?

   a. nitrous oxide

   b. toluene

   c. methylenedioxymethamphetamine (MDMA)

   d. Psilocybin mushrooms

9. A tyramine reaction is associated with use of which agent?

   a. paroxetine

   b. phenytoin

   c. cocaine

   d. isocarboxazid

10. A 23-year-old man presents with acute cocaine intoxication. He is agitated and diaphoretic. Vital signs are T = 105.8° F, P = 130 bpm, RR = 28/minute, BP = 168/90 mmHg, O_2 saturation = 99%. His ECG shows sinus tachycardia with a QRS of 110 milliseconds, QTc of 420 milliseconds, and the presence of peaked T waves. The most important step in initial management is:

    a. administration of sodium bicarbonate (1 to 2 mEq/kg IV)

    b. administration of haloperidol 10 mg IV

    c. aggressive cooling

    d. administration of calcium gluconate (1 g IV)

11. Use of which agent may lead to the neuroleptic malignant syndrome?

    a. lithium

    b. fluoxetine

    c. levodopa/carbidopa

    d. diphenhydramine

12. A 46-year-old man presents 28 hours after self-poisoning with an unknown drug. He complains of nausea, vomiting, and abdominal pain. His vitals are T = 98.8° F, P = 110 bpm, RR = 20/minute, BP = 115/86 mmHg. Laboratory tests reveal a bicarbonate of 24 mmol/L with an anion gap of 12 mmol/L; AST is 1638 U/L, ALT is 970 U/L, PT is 28.5. What is the most common side effect of the appropriate antidote?

    a. hypokalemia

    b. inebriation

    c. CNS depression

    d. anaphylactoid reaction

13. A 56-year-old man presents after acute poisoning with an unknown drug. He is alert and oriented complaining of dyspnea, abdominal pain, and nausea and has vomited multiple times. He also complains of tinnitus following the ingestion. Vital signs are T = 98.6° F, P = 105 bpm, RR = 26/minute, BP = 124/88 mmHg, O_2 saturation = 100%. Laboratory analysis reveals a bicarbonate of 15 mmol/L, glucose of 86 mg/dL, sodium of 141 mmol/L, and chloride of 102 mmol/L, BUN is 20 mg/dL, creatinine 1.2 mg/dL. ABG reveals a pH of 7.48, $PaCO_2$ 12 mmHg and PaO_2 of 134 mmHg. Initial treatment of the most likely poisoning would include:

    a. administration of promethazine 50 mg IV

    b. hydration and administration of sodium bicarbonate infusion

    c. aggressive cooling techniques

    d. administration of bromocriptine

14. Hemodialysis is indicated for which of the following complications of salicylate toxicity?

    a. aspirin level greater than 70 mg/dL

    b. persistent vomiting

    c. hypokalemia

    d. CNS dysfunction

15. Hyperammonemia may be caused by which of the following agents?

    a. carbamazepine

    b. lithium

    c. valproic acid

    d. topiramate

16. The "antidote" for tropane alkaloid poisoning is associated with what side effect?

    a. pulmonary hypertension

    b. dry mucous membranes, urinary retention, decreased bowel sounds

    c. vomiting, diarrhea, salivation

    d. alkalemia and hypernatremia

17. Which of the following toxic alcohols may result in hypocalcemia?

  a. isopropyl alcohol
  b. methanol
  c. propylene glycol
  d. ethylene glycol

18. A 32-year-old construction worker is found unresponsive in an underground parking garage. He was last seen using a propane-powered saw to cut sections of concrete. The saw was not running when he was found. On physical examination, the patient has shallow respirations, pupils are midsize and reactive, and the patient withdraws to painful stimuli. Vitals are T = 98.6° F, P = 120 bpm, RR = 8/minute, BP = 98/62 mmHg, O_2 saturation = 98%. The most likely agent involved in this poisoning:

  a. binds hemoglobin with less affinity than oxygen
  b. shifts the oxyhemoglobin dissociation curve to the right.
  c. has the characteristic odor of "rotten eggs"
  d. results in a normal PaO_2 on ABG

19. After an endoscopy to remove an esophageal food impaction, your patient becomes dyspneic, with perioral cyanosis and an oxygen saturation reading of 85% on room air. Topical anesthetics were used for the endoscopy. A possible complication of appropriate treatment would be:

  a. methemoglobinemia
  b. flushing
  c. hypotension
  d. CNS depression

20. Following an ingestion of an over-the-counter sleep aid known to contain doxylamine, an 18-year-old boy presents to the emergency department with hallucinations, mumbling speech, agitation, dry skin, flushing, and tachycardia. He receives 2 mg of lorazepam, with significant improvement of his agitation. Thirty minutes later the patient again becomes agitated and begins banging his arms against the bedrails. An appropriate solution to this common cause of agitation in patients with this toxidrome is:

  a. administration of haloperidol
  b. administration of a fluid bolus to promote renal drug elimination
  c. administration of N-acetylcysteine
  d. placing a Foley catheter

1. Answer: b

Slurred speech, ataxia, and nystagmus, though nonspecific, are signs of *alcohol intoxication*. Both ethylene glycol and methanol are intoxicating substances (although methanol less so than ethylene glycol). Both substances also may cause an anion-gap metabolic acidosis with an elevated osmolar gap.

Fomepizole (b) blocks the enzyme alcohol dehydrogenase to prevent the formation of toxic by-products. Fomepizole does not remove the toxic by-product, therefore, dialysis may be necessary depending on the clinical situation. **Alkalinization of the urine (a)** is the appropriate treatment of salicylate toxicity, not toxic alcohols. **Activated charcoal (c)** does not bind toxic alcohols. **Atropine (d)** is the treatment for cholinergic poisoning, but would not be indicated in the treatment of toxic alcohols.

2. Answer: c

T-wave inversions in the lateral leads (a), though not specific, are a finding common to lithium toxicity. **Bradycardia with first-degree atrioventricular block (b)** may be found in overdose of calcium channel blockers and beta-blockers, but is not typical of TCA poisoning. **QRS prolongation with prominent R wave in aVR and S wave in lead I (c)** is a result of myocardial sodium channel blockade and is an indicator of toxicity in TCA poisoning. **ST-segment elevation in leads II, III, and aVF (d)** would be concerning for an inferior myocardial infarction.

3. Answer: b

QRS prolongation in the setting of acute poisoning is indicative of sodium channel blockade and should initially be treated with **sodium bicarbonate (b)** intravenous boluses (1-2 mEq/kg). **Sodium polystyrene sulfonate (a)** is useful in the treatment of hyperkalemia, but also binds lithium and may decrease absorption after an acute lithium overdose. **Activated charcoal (c)** may bind some sodium channel–blocking agents, therefore preventing absorption, but has not been proven to affect patient morbidity or mortality and is not a direct treatment of sodium channel blockade. **Lidocaine (d)** is a type Ib Vaughan–Williams antidysrhythmic that may be useful in the treatment of refractory wide complex dysrhythmias. Although it may be indicated for dysrhythmia in some overdose settings, **sodium bicarbonate (b)** has more utility in overcoming sodium channel blockade and therefore is the correct answer.

4. Answer: c

Quetiapine (c) is an atypical antipsychotic. In overdose, is causes peripheral alpha-1 adrenergic blockade leading to miosis along with possible hypotension and reflex tachycardia. **Oxycodone (a)** is a opioid and results in miosis along with dose-related hypotension and bradycardia. **Cyclobenzaprine (b)** features anticholinergic symptoms in overdose, leading to tachycardia, but dose not cause hypotension. Although the patient is not noted to be on **clonidine (d),** a clonidine overdose may resemble that of an opioid, causing miotic pupils along with CNS depression, *bradycardia,* and hypotension.

5. Answer: c

Niacin (a) is used in the treatment of hyperlipidemia and may result in cutaneous flushing; however, it does not result in rigidity or hyperthermia. **Fluoxetine (b)** is a selective serotonin reuptake inhibitor. Its use may result in serotonin syndrome, which presents as agitation, tachycardia, hyperreflexia, and clonus (particularly of the lower extremities), rigidity, hyperthermia, and autonomic instability. Although it can occur during therapeutic use of only one serotonergic agent, it more commonly presents after overdose of a serotonergic agent or when combining multiple agents with pro-serotonergic properties. *Neuroleptic malignant syndrome* usually occurs within 1 to 2 weeks of starting or escalating therapy on an antipsychotic medication such as **chlorpromazine (c)**, but may occur at any time during treatment. Symptoms include altered mental status, rigidity, autonomic instability, and hyperthermia. Patients generally do not have hyperreflexia or clonus. Creatine phosphokinase elevations are common. Contrary to the more rapid onset of serotonin syndrome, onset of neuroleptic malignant syndrome is typically over a few days. **Statins (d)** may cause elevations in CPK, along with muscle soreness, but do not cause rigidity, hyperthermia, or autonomic instability.

6. Answer: d

Over-the-counter sleep aids often contain diphenhydramine as the active ingredient. *Diphenhydramine is a sodium channel–blocking agent* that may cause seizures and QRS prolongation in overdose. In addition to decreasing dromotropy, sodium channel–blocking agents may also decrease inotropy, leading to impaired cardiac contraction and hypotension. **Sodium bicarbonate (d)** is first-line therapy for treating sodium channel blockade in the poisoned patient. Because tachycardic rhythms with QRS prolongation may resemble ventricular tachycardia, unstable patients may be treated with **cardioversion (c),** and coding patients should be treated with **defibrillation (a)** and standard advance life support guidelines; however, the rhythm may be refractory to these treatments secondary to the continued presence of the sodium channel blockade. Therefore, sodium bicarbonate should be administered concurrently with these actions in the setting of a patient poisoned with a sodium channel–blocking agent. **Procainamide (b)** has no role in the treatment of a poisoned patient.

7. Answer: d

Carbamazepine (a), phenytoin (b), and **phenobarbital (c)** are all aromatic anticonvulsants and all may be associated with anticonvulsant hypersensitivity syndrome. As there is significant cross-reactivity between the aromatic agents, a nonaromatic anticonvulsant should be used in patients with history of this syndrome. These nonaromatic agents include gabapentin, topiramate, levetiracetam, tiagabine, and **valproic acid (d).**

8. Answer: a

MDMA (c) has been associated with hyperthermia and hepatic damage, possibly from contaminants in the product, but does not cause anemia or peripheral neuropathy. **Toluene (b)** may cause leukoencephalopathy in chronic use and may also cause a metabolic acidosis. **Nitrous oxide (a)** results in a *functional B_{12} deficiency* and can cause peripheral neuropathy and megaloblastic anemia with chronic exposure. **Psilocybin** mushrooms **(d)** are not associated with chronic toxicity.

9. Answer: d

Symptoms of a tyramine reaction include headache, flushing, hypertension, diaphoresis, and tachycardia. These symptoms are similar to the sympathomimetic toxidrome produce by **cocaine (c)** toxicity. However, this syndrome specifically relates to the symptoms caused by ingestion of tyramine-rich foods produced when patients are taking MAO-A inhibitors such as **isocarboxazid (d).** **Paroxetine (a)** may interact with MAO inhibitors to produce serotonin syndrome. **Phenytoin (b)** is an anticonvulsant that may also be used as an antidysrhythmic agent. Rapid infusion may result in hypotension and cardiovascular collapse. Extravasation is associated with significant tissue necrosis and may cause the "purple glove syndrome" when given through a peripheral line.

10. Answer: c

All of the above therapies may be used in the treatment of this patient. *Sympathomimetic toxicity* usually causes hypokalemia secondary to activation of beta adrenergic receptors and the resulting shift of potassium into cells. Hyperkalemia, along with hyperthermia, is evidence of mitochondrial uncoupling as a result of extreme sympathomimetic toxicity. Hyperkalemia is suggested by peaked T waves on ECG. Elevated ambient temperatures along with hyperthermia have been directly linked to mortality in cocaine intoxication. **Aggressive cooling measures (c),** initially with evaporative techniques, which may progress to internal cooling measures, are the most important step to take initially to save this patient's life. Benzodiazepines blunt the sympathetic response and may improve tachycardia and hypertension and should be administered concomitantly with cooling; they are the treatment of choice for cocaine toxicity and agitation over **haloperidol (b),** which may also lower the seizure threshold. Cocaine is a sodium channel–blocking agent, and QRS prolongation in the setting of cocaine poisoning may be treated with **sodium bicarbonate (a),** but this is not the most important initial step. **Calcium gluconate (d)** is useful in stabilizing the myocardium and preventing dysrhythmia in the setting of hyperkalemia; however, it does not treat the route of the problem and is not the most important initial step to take.

11. Answer: c

Neuroleptic malignant syndrome (NMS) is characterized by altered mental status, rigidity, autonomic instability, and hyperthermia. It may be caused by use of a dopamine D_2 receptor–blocking agent (usually typical or atypical antipsychotics) or from abrupt withdrawal of a dopamine agonist (**levodopa/ carbidopa**) (**c**). **Lithium** (**a**) is associated with neurologic symptoms in overdose, including tremor, ataxia and hyperreflexia, and CNS depression, but does not cause NMS. **Fluoxetine** (**b**), especially in combination with other pro-serotonergic agents, may cause serotonin syndrome. **Diphenhydramine** (**d**) is associated with the anticholinergic toxidrome.

12. Answer: d

In a patient with delayed presentation following overdose, transaminitis and coagulopathy, even with a negative acetaminophen level, would be suggestive of *acetaminophen toxicity* and should prompt treatment with *N*-acetylcysteine. *N*-acetylcysteine, when given in the IV form, may result in **anaphylactoid reaction** (**d**), characterized by flushing, urticaria, angioedema and possible hypotension and bronchospasm. Generally, slowing the rate of infusion and use of antihistamines will prevent further symptoms. **CNS depression** (**c**) is not a side effect of *N*-acetylcysteine; it may be caused by another commonly used "antidote" often used in poisoned patients: benzodiazepines. **Hypokalemia** (**a**) may be caused by administration of sodium bicarbonate, especially when given in continuous infusion without supplemental potassium. **Inebriation** (**b**) may result from an ethanol infusion, an older therapy used to block alcohol dehydrogenase in the treatment of ethylene glycol and methanol poisoning. Fomepizole, a newer "antidote," does not cause inebriation but may prolong inebriation in already intoxicated patients.

13. Answer: b

The most likely poison involved in this case is *aspirin*. This patient has a primary respiratory alkalosis along with an anion-gap metabolic acidosis. Along with symptoms of vomiting and tinnitus, salicylates would best fit this clinical picture. The feeling of dyspnea is common and may come from direct stimulation of the respiratory center in the brainstem. As salicylates are weak acids, **alkalization of the serum** (**b**) and urine can "trap" the ionized form in the blood and urine, respectively. It is important to include potassium in the bicarbonate infusion (unless contraindicated) in order to avoid hypokalemia. **Promethazine** (**a**) is a useful antiemetic; however, less-sedating alternatives, such as ondansetron, would be preferred in salicylate poisoning to avoid masking CNS symptoms and respiratory depression. As this patient remains afebrile, **cooling techniques** (**c**) are not indicated at this time. **Bromocriptine** (**d**) is a dopamine agonist that may help reverse symptoms of neuroleptic malignant syndrome. Patients with neuroleptic malignant syndrome are expected to have altered mental status, rigidity, and hyperthermia.

14. Answer: d

Aspirin levels greater than 100 mg/dL are associated with a poor outcome and should lead to

hemodialysis; however, patients with **levels of only 70 mg/dL** may still do well with conservative therapy (**a**). **Persistent vomiting** is a common complication of aspirin poisoning, but does not warrant hemodialysis (**b**). **Hypokalemia** is a common complication of alkalinization therapy. Unless contraindicated (renal failure), sodium bicarbonate drips should have 40 mEq of KCl included to prevent hypokalemia. The presence of **hypokalemia** does not warrant hemodialysis (**c**). Cerebral edema is an end-organ effect of salicylate poisoning; the presence of **CNS dysfunction** is an indicator of cerebral edema and severe poisoning, and should prompt treatment with hemodialysis (**d**).

15. Answer: c

Secretion of vasopressin may be stimulated by **carbamazepine** leading to SIADH (**a**). **Lithium** (**b**) is associated with decreased aquaporin channel expression in the distal renal tubules, leading to nephrogenic diabetes insipidus. **Topiramate** (**d**) acts as a carbonic anhydrase inhibitor resulting in a non–anion gap metabolic acidosis. **Valproic acid** (**c**) may cause carnitine depletion leading to hyperammonemia.

16. Answer: c

Tropane alkaloids are present in a variety of plant species and result in the *anticholinergic toxidrome*. *Physostigmine* is an acetylcholinesterase inhibitor that increases levels of acetylcholine in the neuronal synapse to help overcome blockade of the muscarinic acetylcholine receptor. In patients not poisoned with anticholinergic drugs, or when given in excess, physostigmine may result in the *cholinergic toxidrome*, including **lacrimation, salivation, vomiting, diarrhea, bronchorrhea,** and **bronchoconstriction**. Therefore, the correct answer is (**c**). Protamine sulfate is the reversal agent for heparin overdose; it may cause anaphylactoid and anaphylactic reactions along with **pulmonary hypertension** (**a**). Atropine, often used to treat the cholinergic toxidrome, results in **dry mucous membranes, urinary retention,** and **decreased bowel sounds** (**b**) along with mydriasis. Sodium bicarbonate, used to treat poisoning with sodium channel–blocking agents, and to alkalinize the urine in salicylate poisoning, may result in **alkalemia** and **hypernatremia** (**d**).

17. Answer: d

Isopropyl alcohol (**a**) is metabolized to acetone. After ingestion, an osmolar gap without significant anion gap metabolic acidosis may be present. **Methanol** (**b**) is metabolized to formic acid, resulting in a high anion gap acidosis with an osmolar gap. **Ethylene glycol** (**d**) is also metabolized to acidic by-products, causing an osmolar gap with a high anion gap metabolic acidosis. Its metabolite, oxalic acid, chelates calcium and may result in hypocalcemia. **Propylene glycol** (**c**) is metabolized to lactic acid.

18. Answer: d

Patients found down in enclosed spaces should always be considered to have *carbon monoxide (CO) poisoning*. Symptoms of CO poisoning are generally nonspecific and include headache, nausea, vomiting, altered metal status, possible seizures, and coma. Primary treatment includes removal from the source and oxygen therapy. Carbon monoxide has a 200 times *greater* **affinity for hemoglobin than oxygen (a).** Binding of CO to the heme moiety causes the remaining oxygen molecules on the hemoglobin to bind more tightly. This results in a *left* **shift of the oxyhemoglobin dissociation curve (b).** Carbon monoxide itself is odorless. **Hydrogen sulfide** is often described as having the **odor of rotten eggs (c).** As carbon monoxide does not affect the amount of dissolved oxygen in the blood, the **PaO_2 is expected to be relatively normal in poisoning (d).**

19. Answer: a

Methemoglobinemia may be caused from the use of benzocaine, a topical anesthetic used in endoscopy. Symptoms of methemoglobinemia include cyanosis, dyspnea, headache, and dizziness. Because of light absorption characteristics of methemoglobin, oxygen saturations tend to gravitate towards 85%. Treatment of symptomatic methemoglobinemia consists of administration of *methylene blue*. However, methylene blue is an oxidizing agent that, when given in excessive amounts or in predisposed individuals (G6PD deficiency), **may cause/worsen methemoglobinemia (a)** or precipitate hemolysis. **Flushing (b)** is not a common side effect of methylene blue, but it may result from administration of *N*-acetylcysteine. **Hypotension** is also not a side effect of methylene blue; however, nitrites, used to induce methemoglobinemia in the setting of cyanide poisoning, may cause hypotension **(c).** Methylene blue is not known for causing **CNS depression (d).**

20. Answer: d

This patient is displaying symptoms of the *anticholinergic toxidrome*. Along with the above symptoms, *urinary retention* is a common manifestation and may result in agitation due to an overdistended bladder. **Placing a Foley catheter (d)** allows for decompression of the bladder and often results in a significant reduction in agitation. **Haloperidol (a)** has weak anticholinergic properties and is not the best option in this patient. *N*-acetylcysteine **(c)** may be necessary after overdose of some sleep aids if they contain acetaminophen as a coformulation; however, it would not help in this situation. **Saline diuresis (b)** has not proven to be beneficial following overdose and would likely worsen the patient's agitation if begun without placing a bladder catheter to relieve overdistention.

BETA-ADRENERGIC BLOCKERS

CALCIUM CHANNEL BLOCKERS

DIGITALIS GLYCOSIDES

OTHER ANTIHYPERTENSIVE AGENTS

Diuretics
Clonidine

CAUSTIC AGENTS

Alkali
Acids

COCAINE

CYANIDE

HYDROGEN SULFIDE

HALLUCINOGENS

Lysergic acid diethylamide (LSD)
MDMA ("Ecstasy")
Phencyclidine (PCP)
Jimson weed and angel's trumpet

HEAVY METALS

Lead
Arsenic
Mercury

INSECTICIDES, HERBICIDES,
AND RODENTICIDES

Insecticides
Herbicides
Rodenticides

HYDROCARBONS

ANTIDIABETIC AGENTS

Insulin
Sulfonylureas
Biguanides

INHALED TOXINS

IRON

ISONIAZID

MARINE TOXINS

Ciguatera
Scombroid

METHEMOGLOBINEMIA

MUSHROOMS/POISONOUS PLANTS

Castor bean (Ricinus communis)
Foxglove (Digitalis purpurea) and
  oleander
Jequirity Bean (Abrus precatorius)

Poison hemlock (Conium maculatum)
Water hemlock (Cicuta maculata)

NEUROLEPTICS

SEDATIVE/HYPNOTICS

STIMULANTS/SYMPATHOMIMETIC
  AGENTS

STRYCHNINE

LITHIUM

Beta-adrenergic blockers

- **Mechanism of toxicity** is blockade of beta-receptors, decreasing production of cAMP, and resulting decreased inotropy and chronotropy with beta-1 blockade and vasoconstriction, bronchospasm, and hypoglycemia with beta-2 blockade
- Certain beta-blockers also have other mechanisms of action
  - Sodium channel blockade (quinidine-like effect), prolongation of the QRS complex
    - Acebutolol, oxprenolol, pindolol, propranolol
  - Potassium channel blockade leading to prolongation of the QT interval—sotalol
  - Central nervous system (CNS) sedation— propranolol (highly lipid soluble and crosses the blood–brain barrier)

SIGNS AND SYMPTOMS

- Cardiovascular—bradycardia, hypotension, cardiac conduction delays/blocks, cardiogenic shock
- CNS—coma, seizures (propranolol)
- Metabolic—hypoglycemia
- Pulmonary—respiratory depression, bronchospasm

DIAGNOSIS

- Usually clinical, based on history and physical examination findings

TREATMENT

- Gastric decontamination
- Fluid administration
- Atropine, transcutaneous/transvenous pacemaker for unstable bradycardia
- Glucagon 0.05 to 0.15 mg/kg (3 to 10 mg for average-sized adult) then 1 to 5 mg/hour infusion (may cause vomiting)

- Catecholamines—norepinephrine, dopamine, and epinephrine
- Sodium bicarbonate for wide QRS complex
- For refractory hypotension/bradycardia, consider insulin–euglycemia therapy, cardiopulmonary bypass

Calcium channel blockers

- **Mechanism of toxicity** is blockade of calcium channels, decreasing the amount of intracellular calcium, which leads to reduced stimulus for smooth and cardiac muscle contraction

SIGNS AND SYMPTOMS

- Cardiovascular—hypotension, bradycardia, conduction blocks/delays, cardiogenic shock
- Metabolic—hyperglycemia

DIAGNOSIS

- Usually clinical, based on history and physical examination findings

TREATMENT

- Gastric decontamination
- Fluid administration
- Atropine, transcutaneous/transvenous for unstable bradycardia
- Calcium (should avoid if digoxin toxicity is possible)
  - Calcium chloride or gluconate (10 mL [0.15 mL/kg] of 10% solution over 5 minutes)
  - May repeat every 10 minutes as needed
    - Catecholamines—norepinephrine, dopamine, or epinephrine
    - Glucagon 0.05 to 0.15 mg/kg (3 to 10 mg for average-sized adult) then 1 to 5 mg/hour infusion
    - For refractory hypotension/bradycardia, consider insulin–euglycemia therapy, cardiopulmonary bypass

Digitalis glycosides

- **Mechanism of toxicity**
  - Inactivates the Na/K ATPase pump, responsible for maintaining the electrochemical membrane potential. When Na^+ accumulates intracellularly, it is exchanged for calcium via the sodium–calcium exchanger, which increases the intracellular and sarcoplasmic calcium resulting in increased inotropy
  - Increases vagal tone—decreases conduction through the sinoatrial (SA) and atrioventricular (AV) nodes
  - May result from digoxin, digitoxin (not available in U.S. currently), or digoxin-like substances/plants such as oleander, foxglove, squill or sea onion, lily-of-the-valley, and ouabain (these substances may be detected by serum immunoassays for digoxin)

SIGNS AND SYMPTOMS

- **Acute toxicity**—intentional or accidental ingestion
  - Gastrointestinal (GI)—nausea/vomiting
  - CNS—headache, dizziness, confusion, coma
  - Cardiac—bradydysrhythmias, AV block, and ventricular tachydysrhythmias
  - Electrolyte abnormalities—hyperkalemia
  - Markedly elevated digoxin concentration
- **Chronic toxicity**—typically elderly patients with renal insufficiency
  - GI—nausea, vomiting, diarrhea, abdominal pain
  - CNS—fatigue, weakness, confusion, delirium, coma, visual disturbances (yellow-green halos around lights)
  - Cardiac—bradydysrhythmias, AV block, ventricular tachydysrhythmias
  - Electrolyte—normal, decreased, or increased serum potassium, hypomagnesemia
  - Minimally elevated or "therapeutic range" digoxin concentration

DIAGNOSIS

- Based on history and physical examination findings and correlated with serum digoxin concentration, although levels may not clearly predict or exclude toxicity
  - Common precipitants: renal insufficiency, old age, drug–drug interactions (e.g., verapamil, quinidine, amiodarone, cyclosporine, NSAIDs all associated with increased digoxin levels)

TREATMENT

- Gastric decontamination (for acute ingestion)
- Fluid administration
- Bradydysrhythmias
  - Atropine, pacemaker, Fab fragments
- Ventricular tachydysrhythmias
  - Fab fragments, magnesium sulfate (2 to 4 g IV), lidocaine (1 mg/kg IV), electrocardioversion (may induce ventricular fibrillation; use as a last resort)
- Hyperkalemia
  - Avoid calcium gluconate or chloride
  - Treat with standard therapies, including Fab fragments, which lower the serum potassium by treating the poisoned Na/K ATPase pump
- Fab fragments (for dosing, see package insert)—onset of action 30 minutes to 1 hour
  - Simplified dose calculation: no. of vials = *serum digoxin level* (ng/mL) × *patient's weight* (kg)/100

Other antihypertensive agents

DIURETICS

- The most commonly prescribed antihypertensives

Thiazide and loop diuretics

- Toxicity is manifested by volume contraction and electrolyte abnormalities
- **Clinical manifestations**—hypotension, tachycardia, altered mental status (from poor perfusion), hyponatremia, hypokalemia, hypocalcemia (loop diuretics), hypomagnesemia, hyperuricemia (thiazide diuretics), hypochloremic metabolic alkalosis
- **Treatment**—volume replacement (usually with normal saline) and electrolyte repletion

CLONIDINE

- Alpha-2 receptor antagonist in the brain, which decreases sympathetic output
- **Clinical manifestations**—hypotension, bradycardia, altered mental status—from agitation, hallucinations to sedation, coma, apnea (especially in children), pupillary miosis
- **Treatment**—gastric decontamination, fluid administration, atropine (for bradycardia), vasopressor support; naloxone may be helpful

Caustic agents

- Most corrosive agents are either alkali or acidic

ALKALI

- Ingestion causes deep tissue injury **(liquefaction necrosis)**
- Higher risk of perforation

ACIDS

- Ingestion causes **coagulation necrosis,** creating eschar, which limits further tissue penetration

SIGNS AND SYMPTOMS

- Oral/facial burns, dysphonia, stridor, wheezing, chest pain, abdominal pain, vomiting, dysphagia, dyspnea/respiratory distress, stomach/esophageal necrosis, perforation, and hemorrhage

TREATMENT

- Airway evaluation and securing the airway early
- Dilution or neutralization not recommended, nor is gastric decontamination
- Endoscopy—consult early
- Steroids and antibiotics are controversial
  - Complications
    - Edema of the upper airway—larynx, epiglottis
    - Perforation; stricture formation (late complication)

Cocaine

- **Mechanism of toxicity**
  - Local anesthetic—inhibits fast sodium channels (prolongs QRS complex on electrocardiogram [ECG])
  - CNS stimulant—increases release, and prevents reuptake, of norepinephrine and dopamine

SIGNS AND SYMPTOMS

- CNS—agitation, seizures, intracranial infarctions and hemorrhage
- Pulmonary—pulmonary hemorrhage, barotrauma, pneumonitis, asthma, pulmonary edema
- Cardiac—hypertension, tachycardia, dysrhythmias
  - Sodium channel blockade can widen the QRS complex (similar to quinidine)
  - Cocaine-associated acute myocardial infarction
    - Incidence in patients presenting with chest pain ranges from 0.7 to 6%
    - Arises from vasoconstriction, but also from thrombus formation as well as premature coronary atherosclerosis, all related to cocaine use
- Rhabdomyolysis—can produce both traumatic and nontraumatic rhabdomyolysis, which can lead to renal failure

TREATMENT

- General supportive measures—cardiac monitoring with frequent vital signs
- Seizures, agitation should be treated with benzodiazepines
- Hyperthermia
  - Aggressive measures to decrease the temperature including cooling blanket, ice water lavage, ice packs, cool mist spray with fans, hydration, benzodiazepines and (if necessary) intubation with paralysis
- Chest pain
  - Evaluation for myocardial ischemia, pneumothorax (insufflation), aortic dissection (hypertension)
  - Patients suspected of acute coronary syndrome (ACS) should be treated similarly to those with traditional ACS with nitrates, morphine, and aspirin
  - Benzodiazepines should be given in addition as early management
  - Recommendations to avoid early beta-blocker administration are controversial and based on the concept that beta-blockers may theoretically lead to unopposed alpha-adrenergic stimulation and worsening coronary vasoconstriction
- QRS-complex prolongation
  - Administration of sodium bicarbonate boluses and alkalinization to a serum pH of 7.45 to 7.5
- Body "Packers" and "Stuffers"
  - Stuffers (people who ingest poorly packaged drugs in an attempt to evade police) are usually symptomatic on arrival to the emergency

department (ED). These patients can be given charcoal, treated if symptomatic and observed
- Packers (people who ingest large amounts of drugs in wrapped packages with the intent of smuggling) who are asymptomatic should be given charcoal followed by whole bowel irrigation with polyethylene glycol solution. If they become symptomatic, packet rupture should be suspected and immediate surgical consultation for emergent laparotomy should be obtained for packet removal in addition to treating the patient symptomatically, while awaiting surgery

Cyanide

- **Mechanism of toxicity**
  - Cyanide rapidly induces a noncompetitive inhibition of cytochrome oxidase c activity, resulting in anaerobic metabolism, cellular hypoxia, and lactic metabolic acidosis
- Clinical findings (initial ⇒ late)
  - Time course depends on the form, type of exposure, and concentration
- Inhalational exposure as well as ingestion of salt forms—onset is within minutes
- Agents requiring metabolic action or breakdown (e.g., sodium nitroprusside) may be delayed
  - Cardiovascular—tachycardia, hypertension, bradycardia, hypotension, asystole
  - CNS—headache, drowsiness, seizures, coma
  - Pulmonary—dyspnea, tachypnea, apnea

DIAGNOSIS

- Cyanide levels are not immediately available to guide clinical decisions, so maintain a high index of suspicion in victims of house fires with a severe metabolic acidosis
- Toxic cyanide levels correlate with lactate levels above 10 mmol/L in victims of house fires

TREATMENT

- 100% oxygen
- Two options: Cyanokit (hydroxocobalamin) or Cyanide Antidote Kit (nitrites and sodium thiosulfate)
- Cyanokit—recently approved by FDA for treatment of cyanide toxicity
  - Hydroxocobalamin given intravenously over 30 minutes
- Cyanide Antidote Kit
  - Nitrites
    - Amyl nitrite is inhaled (only to be given if IV access is unobtainable), sodium nitrite is IV
    - Induces methemoglobinemia, which is relatively contraindicated in persons with coexisting carboxyhemoglobin from smoke inhalation. Use with caution as it results in hypotension
  - Sodium thiosulfate IV
    - Safer than nitrites when diagnosis is not clear

Hydrogen sulfide

- **Sources**—colorless, flammable gas found in industry or as a natural by-product of organic decomposition (e.g., gases from sewer, manure)—sulfur "rotten egg" smell may be absent at high concentrations
- **Mechanism of toxicity** is similar to cyanide—binds cytochrome oxidase c, which disrupts oxidative phosphorylation, causing metabolic acidosis and lactate accumulation; also possesses irritant properties to mucous membranes

SIGNS AND SYMPTOMS

- Low concentrations—ocular/mucosal irritation ("gas eye"), delayed pulmonary edema, and corneal destruction
- Higher concentrations—rapid loss of consciousness, seizures, and death

DIAGNOSIS

- Usually based on history and clinical findings

TREATMENT

- Removal from exposure, decontamination, and 100% oxygen; administration of nitrites from the cyanide antidote kit can be given to promote methemoglobinemia (hydrogen sulfide binds more quickly to methemoglobin)

Hallucinogens

LYSERGIC ACID DIETHYLAMIDE (LSD)

- Chemically synthesized or obtained by hydrolysis of ergot alkaloids from the fungus *Claviceps purpurea*
- Serotonin receptor agonist ($5HT_2$)
- Rapidly absorbed, onset of effects in 30 minutes, peak effects in 4 hours, and duration of action is 8 to 12 hours
- Physiologic effects include mydriasis, as well as tachycardia, hypertension, and hyperthermia (all mild); facial flushing, nausea, piloerection, bruxism, increased muscle tension, and hyperreflexia may be seen
- Patients may present to the ED as a result of acute adverse psychological effects ("bad trip"), including anxiety, panic attacks, and paranoia
- Treatment involves minimizing external stimuli and reassurance; oral or parenteral benzodiazepines can be considered if the patient is extremely agitated or experiencing significant sympathomimetic stimulation

MDMA ("ECSTASY")

- MDMA (3,4-methylenedioxymethamphetamine, "Ecstasy") is a synthetic substituted amphetamine

- Indirect monoamine agonist causing release and inhibiting reuptake of 5-HT and dopamine
- MDMA is usually ingested in tablets at doses of 50 to 200 mg, with effects usually lasting 4 to 6 hours
- Rarely causes hallucinations but instead produces sensory effects (color perception, tactile sensation). Also euphoria, and increased social/sexual interest
- Common symptoms include sympathomimetic effects (vital sign elevations)
- Deaths have been reported with MDMA use, including fatal dysrhythmias and **intracranial hemorrhage.** A syndrome similar to serotonin syndrome has also been reported, including hyperthermia, seizures, disseminated intravascular coagulation, rhabdomyolysis, and renal failure. **Hyponatremia** can occur and may be a telltale sign of ingestion—either due to excessive water consumption or possibly inappropriate antidiuretic hormone secretion

TREATMENT

- Activated charcoal
- Hypertension and tachycardia usually respond to benzodiazepines
- Hyperthermia should be controlled with rapid cooling measures

PHENCYCLIDINE (PCP)

- Synthetic chemical structurally related to ketamine
- Acts as a glutamate antagonist at the *N*-methyl-D-aspartic acid (NMDA) receptor
- A variety of clinical effects usually lasting 4 to 6 hours can be seen
  - CNS stimulation or depression—may be physically violent, catatonic, or comatose
  - Nystagmus and hypertension (most common manifestations), diaphoresis, muscle rigidity, rhabdomyolysis, tachycardia, decreased response to painful stimuli, dystonic reactions, hypoglycemia, and hyperthermia

TREATMENT

- Benzodiazepines can be given for agitation and seizures if they occur
- Haloperidol has also been used in the treatment of agitation
- Evaluate for rhabdomyolysis and treatment with hydration and consideration of sodium bicarbonate
- Rapid cooling measures for hyperthermia

JIMSON WEED AND ANGEL'S TRUMPET

- From the *Datura stramonium* and *Datura candida* plants, which contain anticholinergic alkaloids
- Delirium, hallucinations, and seizures can occur along with other classic anticholinergic effects
- Physostigmine should be considered for severe anticholinergic symptoms

Heavy metals

LEAD

- **Mechanism of toxicity**
  - Absorption by respiratory and GI tract (skin absorption is negligible)
  - In the CNS, lead injures neuronal and microvascular tissue, and can cause cerebral edema and seizures. Decreases cyclic adenosine monophosphate (cAMP) and protein phosphorylation, which contribute to memory and learning deficits
  - Lead toxicity may also cause motor neuropathy, hemolysis (RBC basophilic stippling on peripheral smear), Fanconi syndrome (aminoaciduria, glycosuria, phosphaturia, and renal tubular acidosis), and elevations of transaminases
- **Clinical manifestations**
  - CNS
    - Acute—encephalopathy, seizures, altered mental status, papilledema, optic neuritis, ataxia
    - Chronic—headaches, irritability, depression, fatigue, mood and behavioral changes, memory deficit, sleep disturbance
  - Other effects include motor weakness (e.g., wrist drop), depressed/absent deep tendon reflexes [DTRs], GI effects (abdominal pain, diarrhea, constipation, vomiting), hypoproliferative and/or hemolytic anemia, basophilic stippling, and reproductive effects (decreased libido, sterility, spontaneous abortion, premature birth, decreased/abnormal sperm production)
  - Renal
    - Acute—Fanconi syndrome, renal tubular acidosis
    - Chronic—interstitial nephritis, kidney dysfunction, hypertension, gout

DIAGNOSIS

- History of exposure to lead or the combination of abdominal or neurologic dysfunction with hemolytic anemia should prompt testing
- Children presenting with encephalopathy should be tested
- Radiographic studies, especially of the long bones, reveal evidence of "lead lines"—horizontal, metaphyseal lead bands that represent failure of bone remodeling, not deposition of lead
- Blood lead concentration—capillary blood levels for screening; confirmatory venous blood testing

TREATMENT

- Severe toxicity
  - Attention to ABCs, seizures should be treated with benzodiazepines and phenobarbital
  - IF abdominal x-ray reveals evidence of radiopaque flecks consistent with lead, whole bowel irrigation should be started
  - Chelation therapy should be started in the ED before obtaining laboratory verification of

diagnosis when lead encephalopathy is strongly suspected
- British anti-Lewisite (BAL) 75 mg/m^2 IM every 4 hours for 5 days followed in 4 hours by CaNa$_2$EDTA 1500 mg/m^2 for 5 days as continuous IV infusion, or as 2 to 4 divided IV doses/day
- Symptomatic patients without encephalopathy and asymptomatic patients with lead levels greater than 75 mcg/dL in adults and 45 mcg/dL in children
  - 2,3-Dimercaptosuccinic acid (DMSA) (succimer) 350 mg/m^2 PO three times daily for 5 days then two times daily for 14 days
- Repeat levels should be rechecked 1 to 2 weeks after chelation for possibility of redistribution from tissues back into blood

ARSENIC

- Found in insecticides, rodenticides, herbicides, mining, smelting/refining, homeopathic medicines, kelp
- **Mechanism of toxicity**
  - Acute exposure produces dilation and increased permeability of small blood vessels, resulting in GI mucosal and submucosal inflammation and necrosis, cerebral edema and hemorrhage, myocardial tissue destruction, and fatty degeneration of the liver and kidneys
  - Chronic exposure causes peripheral neuropathy

SIGNS AND SYMPTOMS

- **Acute exposure**
  - Symptoms usually occur within 30 minutes to several hours postexposure and include vomiting, cholera-like diarrhea, hypotension, tachycardia, nonspecific ST-segment and T-wave changes, prolongation of the QT interval, torsades de pointes, acute encephalopathy, pulmonary edema, acute renal failure, and rhabdomyolysis
- **Chronic exposure**
  - Peripheral neuropathy (stocking glove, initially sensory then motor/sensory), skin rash, and nonspecific malaise and weakness follow a history of gastroenteritis occurring 1 to 6 weeks earlier
  - Skin findings—hyperpigmentation, hyperkeratosis of the palms and soles, morbilliform rash, and epidermoid cancer
  - Weakness, muscle aches, personality changes, periorbital and extremity edema, decreased hearing secondary to sensorineural damage. Chronic encephalopathy with delirium, hallucinations, disorientation, agitation, and confabulation resembling Korsakoff syndrome
  - Squamous cell and basal cell cancer, respiratory tract cancer, hepatic angiosarcoma, and possibly leukemia has been associated with chronic exposure

DIAGNOSIS

- Without known exposure, suspicion must be based on history, signs, and symptoms

- Definitive diagnosis is made on a specialized 24-hour urine collection

TREATMENT

- IV fluids to restore fluid volume; however, overhydration should be avoided as pulmonary and cerebral edema can occur
- Seizures should be treated initially with benzodiazepines
- Ventricular tachycardia should be treated according to ACLS protocols with avoidance of antidysrhythmics that prolong the QT interval (Class IA, IC, III)
- Whole bowel irrigation should be initiated if there is evidence of radiopaque materials
- Chronic toxicity should be directed toward prevention of further absorption of arsenic
- Chelation therapy with BAL (3 to 5 mg/kg IM every 4 hours for 2 days, then 3 to 5 mg/kg every 6 to 12 hours) should be started in symptomatic cases with known or suspected acute poisoning
- DMSA (succimer) can then be used as clinical condition stabilizes or in cases of chronic arsenic toxicity with the same dosing as in lead poisoning

MERCURY

- All forms are toxic but differ in routes of absorption, constellations of clinical findings, and responses of therapy
- **Organic**
  - Elemental—found in battery and thermometer manufacture, dentistry, jewelry and lamp manufacture, photography, mining, manufacture of scientific equipment. Absorbed primarily by inhalation of its vapor
  - Salts—found in taxidermy, fur processing, tannery work, chemical laboratories, manufacture of explosives, fireworks, disinfectants, button batteries, inks, and vinyl chloride. Absorbed primarily through the GI tract, they do not enter the CNS in significant amounts
- **Inorganic** (short-, long-chained alkyl and aryl compounds; e.g., methyl and ethyl mercury)
  - Found in seafood, embalming, manufacture of drugs, fungicides, bactericides, handling of pesticides, coated seeds, working with wood preservatives
  - Highly lipid-soluble compounds cross membranes—RBCs, CNS, liver, kidney and fetus
- **Mechanism of toxicity**
  - Binds with sulfhydryl groups affecting many different enzyme and protein systems

SIGNS AND SYMPTOMS

- Depend on form and route of administrations
  - In general, the neurologic, GI, and renal systems are predominately affected
  - CNS findings include **erethism**—a potpourri of neuropsychiatric maladies, including anxiety, depression, mania, irritability, sleep disturbances,

excessive shyness, and memory loss. Tremor is common
- Short-chained alkyls produce paresthesias, ataxia, muscular rigidity, or spasticity, and visual and hearing loss
- Chronic toxicity of elemental/organic forms may cause renal glomerular and tubular damage
- Acute elemental inhalational exposure produces pneumonitis, adult respiratory distress syndrome, and progressive pulmonary fibrosis with death
- Mercuric salts produce a profound corrosive gastroenteritis with abdominal pain, then cardiovascular collapse and acute renal tubular necrosis
- Children can develop **acrodynia**—an immune-mediated condition characterized by a generalized rash, fever, irritability, splenomegaly, and generalized hypotonia with particular weakness of the pelvic and pectoral muscles

DIAGNOSIS

- History, and typical physical findings, especially tremor
- Look for **erethism** or **acrodynia**
- With the exception of short-chained alkyls, a 24-hour urine mercury (after 5-day seafood-free diet) measurement should be obtained
- As short-chained alkyls are primarily secreted in bile, laboratory diagnosis should be obtained with whole-blood mercury levels

TREATMENT

- Ingestion of mercurial salts should be treated with aggressive GI decontamination including gastric lavage and activated charcoal
- BAL is the preferred chelator for mercuric salts and should be given 5 mg/kg IM once, then 2.5 mg/kg IM every 8 to 12 hours for 1 day then 2.5 mg/kg every 12 to 24 hours until clinical improvement occurs
- BAL is contraindicated in methyl mercury poisoning as it may worsen CNS symptoms
- DMSA is the chelator of choice in both cases of chronic or mild cases at doses of 10 mg/kg PO every 8 hours for 5 days then every 12 hours for 14 days

Insecticides, herbicides, and rodenticides

INSECTICIDES

- Four main classes—organophosphorous, carbamates, organochlorines, pyrethrins

Organophosphorous compounds (OPs)

- Absorption via inhalation, mucous membrane, transdermal, transconjunctival, and GI

- **Mechanism of toxicity**
  - Inhibit enzyme acetylcholinesterase leading to accumulation of acetylcholine in the CNS, autonomic nervous system, and neuromuscular junction
  - Compounds bind irreversibly over a variable amount of time (aging)—treatment must be administered before this process is complete

SIGNS AND SYMPTOMS

- Agent, quantity, and type of exposure vary—most are symptomatic within 8 hours, and nearly all within 24 hours
- CNS—anxiety, restlessness, emotional lability, tremor, headache, dizziness, mental confusion, delirium, hallucinations, seizures, coma
- Parasympathetic
  - **SLUDGE + Killer bees "B's"—S**alivation, **L**acrimation, **U**rination, **D**efecation, **G**I pain, **E**mesis, and **b**radycardia, **b**ronchorrhea, **b**ronchospasm *or*
  - **DUMBELS—D**efecation, **U**rination, **M**uscle weakness, **m**iosis, **B**radycardia, bronchorrhea, bronchospasm, **E**mesis, **L**acrimation, **S**alivation
- Neuromuscular junction—muscle fasciculations, weakness, and paralysis
- An intermediate syndrome may occur 1 to 4 days after acute poisoning
  - Paralysis of flexor neck muscles, cranial nerve palsies, proximal limb and respiratory muscles occurs. Symptoms resolve within 4 to 18 days
- Delayed neuropathy
  - Occurs 1 to 3 weeks after acute exposure

DIAGNOSIS

- Based on history and clinical findings along with confirmatory cholinesterase assays

TREATMENT

- Airway control, respiratory support, decontamination, prevention of further absorption, antidotes
  - Decontamination can be performed with water and soap
  - 100% oxygen by facemask, cardiac monitor, suction for secretions
  - If intubation is needed—use a nondepolarizing agent (succinylcholine is metabolized by plasma cholinesterase and prolonged paralysis may result)
  - Atropine can be titrated to drying of tracheobronchial secretions and can be started at 1 mg and given every 5 minutes
  - Pralidoxime regenerates acetylcholinesterase prior to aging, dose is 1 to 2 g for adults, 20 to 40 mg/kg (maximum dose 1 g) in children

Carbamates

- Similar in mechanism of toxicity to OPs; however, the effect is reversible and not permanent

- Symptoms of acute intoxication are similar but are shorter in duration
- Carbamates do not effectively penetrate the CNS and seizures do not occur
- Atropine should be used the same as for OP; pralidoxime use is controversial

Organochlorines

- Hexachlorocyclohexane (Lindane) is still used to treat scabies and lice infestations, seizures and CNS toxicity can develop with therapeutic use in children and the elderly
- Mechanism of toxicity is repetitive neuronal discharges following an action potential

SIGNS AND SYMPTOMS

- Mild poisoning presents with dizziness, fatigue, malaise, headache, irritability, delirium, tremulousness, myoclonus, and facial paresthesias
- Severe poisoning may present with seizures, coma, respiratory failure, and death

TREATMENT

- Oxygen, supportive care, and benzodiazepines for seizures

Pyrethrins

- Naturally occurring substances found in chrysanthemum—less toxic than previous compounds
- Commonly used as aerosols; inhalation is most common route of exposure
- **Mechanism of toxicity** is sodium channel blockade, causing repetitive neuronal discharge
- **Clinical findings**
  - Allergic hypersensitivity reactions are the most common effect manifesting as dermatitis, asthma, allergic rhinitis, hypersensitivity pneumonitis, or anaphylaxis
  - Upper airway irritation may occur with inhalation exposure
  - Systemic absorption may lead to paresthesias, hyperexcitability, tremors, seizures, muscle weakness, respiratory failure, dizziness, headache, vomiting, diarrhea, and fatigue. In severe poisoning, coma, muscle fasciculations, pulmonary edema, and seizures may occur

TREATMENT

- Supportive measures include removal from source, decontamination, and benzodiazepines for seizures

HERBICIDES

- Bipyridyl herbicides (e.g. Paraquat and Diquat)
- **Mechanism of toxicity**
  - Severe local irritant plus potent systemic toxin causing liver and renal necrosis followed by pulmonary fibrosis

SIGNS AND SYMPTOMS

- Local skin irritation/ulceration
- Upper respiratory tract exposure results in mucosal injury, cough, dyspnea, chest pain, pulmonary edema, epistaxis, and hemoptysis
- Ingestion causes GI mucosal lesions leading to abdominal pain and vomiting
- Severe ingestions can cause pulmonary edema, congestive heart failure, and renal failure in several hours, seizures, GI perforation and hemorrhage, and hepatic failure

DIAGNOSIS

- Largely history, although serum Paraquat concentrations may be used

TREATMENT

- Early and aggressive decontamination to limit absorption
- Use of low oxygen mixtures (less than 21% FiO_2) to prevent superoxide formation
- Gut decontamination with activated charcoal, diatomaceous Fuller earth (1 to 2 g/kg in 15% aqueous solution), or bentonite (1 to 2 g/kg in a 7% aqueous slurry) given every 4 hours
- Charcoal hemoperfusion can remove Paraquat and should be used as soon as possible

RODENTICIDES

- Long-acting anticoagulants are the most common type of exposure—single low-dose exposures do not cause any bleeding problems, toxicity requires a large single exposure or repeated exposure over several days
  - Onset of coagulopathy is 12 to 48 hours post-ingestion
  - In intentional ingestions, a baseline INR needs to be obtained, with a follow-up at 24 to 48 hours
  - If INR is greater than twice normal, then vitamin K should be given, and titrated daily to keep INR <2. Weeks to months of therapy may be needed

Hydrocarbons

- Common examples include fuels, lighter fluids, lamp oil, paints, paint removers, pesticides, medications, cleaning and polishing agents, spot removers, degreasers, lubricants, and solvents
- Toxicity of these compounds depends on the physical characteristics (volatility, viscosity, and surface tension), chemical characteristics (aliphatic, aromatic, or halogenated), presence of toxic additives (pesticides or heavy metals), route of exposure, and dose
- **Mechanism of toxicity**
  - Cause direct toxicity to the lung after pulmonary aspiration or systemic intoxication after ingestion, inhalation, injection, or skin absorption. Most hydrocarbons are irritating to the eyes and skin

- Chemical pneumonitis is caused by direct tissue damage and disruption of surfactant. Hydrocarbons with low viscosity and low surface tension are at the highest risk for aspiration
- Aliphatic hydrocarbons and simple petroleum distillates are poorly absorbed from the GI tract and cause little systemic toxicity unless aspirated
- Aromatic and halogenated hydrocarbons, alcohols, ethers, and ketones are well absorbed from the GI tract and can causes systemic toxicity

SIGNS AND SYMPTOMS

- Pulmonary aspiration
  - Immediate onset of coughing or choking that may progress in minutes to hours to a chemical pneumonitis—tachypnea, retractions, grunting, wheezing, hypoxia
- Ingestion
  - Abrupt nausea, vomiting, occasionally with hemorrhagic gastroenteritis
- Systemic toxicity
  - Symptoms are highly variable depending on compound
  - Commonly confusion, ataxia, headache, lethargy, coma, seizure, and respiratory arrest
  - Cardiac dysrhythmias may occur as a result of cardiac sensitization from halogenated and aromatic hydrocarbons
  - Hepatic and renal injury may occur, depending on the substance
- Injection
  - Local injection causes local tissue inflammation, pain, and necrosis

DIAGNOSIS

- Aspiration pneumonitis
  - Based on history of exposure and presence of respiratory symptoms such as coughing, tachypnea, and wheezing
  - If those symptoms are absent and chest x-ray is normal 4 to 6 hours postexposure, then it is unlikely that a significant pneumonitis will occur
- Systemic toxicity
  - Based on history of exposure and appropriate clinical findings

TREATMENT

- Aspiration pneumonitis
  - Basic supportive care, treat hypoxia and bronchospasm
  - Steroids and antibiotics have not been shown to influence outcome
- Ingestion
  - Supportive care
- Injection
  - For injections in fingertip or hand, especially those involving a high-pressure paint gun, consultation with a plastic or hand surgeon is essential, as prompt exploration, irrigation, and debridement are often needed

Antidiabetic agents

INSULIN

- Lower glucose by direct stimulation of cellular uptake and metabolism of glucose
- Not toxic when orally ingested
- Time to onset and duration of action depends of form of insulin administered

SIGNS AND SYMPTOMS

- Manifestations of hypoglycemia; agitation, confusion, coma, seizures, tachycardia, and diaphoresis

TREATMENT

- If patient hypoglycemic, concentrated glucose should be administered
  - Adults: dextrose 50%, 1 to 2 mL/kg
  - Children: dextrose 25% 2 to 4 mL/kg
  - Children <1 year old: dextrose 10% 5 to 10 mL/kg
- Repeated boluses as needed and infusions of 5% to 10% dextrose to keep glucose levels 60 to 100 mg/dL

SULFONYLUREAS

- Work by stimulating endogenous pancreatic secretion and secondarily by enhancing peripheral insulin receptor sensitivity and reducing glycogenolysis
- Onset of action typically 1 to 3 hours but may be delayed up to 16 hours, duration of action 12 to 24 hours
- Clinical manifestations are similar to hypoglycemia caused by insulin

TREATMENT

- Glucose (as above)
- Octreotide—Prevents insulin release from the pancreas
  - Adults: 50 to 100 mcg IV or SQ every 12 hours as needed
  - Children: 4 to 5 mcg/kg/day divided every 6 hours IV or SC
  - Patients should be monitored at least 12 hours after last dose to make sure rebound hypoglycemia does not occur
- Patients suspected of ingestion of sulfonylureas should be observed for a minimum of 24 hours

BIGUANIDES

- Works by decreasing hepatic glucose production and intestinal absorption of glucose, increases peripheral glucose uptake and utilization; *does not* cause hypoglycemia in overdose
- Can cause lactic acidosis, a rare but potentially lethal adverse reaction; risk factors include renal failure, alcoholism, and advanced age

SIGNS AND SYMPTOMS

- Lactic acidosis can initially present with nonspecific symptoms, including malaise, vomiting, and respiratory distress
- The mortality rate for severe lactic acidosis may be up to 50%

TREATMENT

- IV fluids and sodium bicarbonate for acidosis. Excessive sodium bicarbonate may worsen the acidosis
- Metformin is removed by hemodialysis which also improves the acidosis

Inhaled toxins

- *Simple asphyxiants* simply displace oxygen from the environment causing hypoxia, leading to death
- *Pulmonary irritants* are a group a chemicals that cause acute lung injury (ALI) when inhalation exposure occurs
- Determinants of toxicity include concentration of gas, duration of exposure, and most importantly water solubility
  - Highly water-soluble agents such as **ammonia** and **hydrochloric acid** have good warning properties and cause ocular, mucosal, and upper airway irritation, and with prolonged exposure, significant lower airway irritation/ALI
  - Poorly water-soluble agents such as **phosgene** have poor warning properties (little upper airway irritation) and prolonged exposure can cause significant delayed symptoms of noncardiogenic pulmonary edema. Phosgene smells of freshly mown hay
- Treatment is mostly supportive; oxygen and mechanical ventilation if needed

Iron

- **Mechanism of toxicity**
  - Potent catalyst in the production of oxidants that cause direct GI toxicity
  - Iron enters the mitochondria, where it inhibits oxidative phosphorylation, resulting in a metabolic (lactic) acidosis

SIGNS AND SYMPTOMS

- Amount of elemental iron ingested determines the toxicity, with various concentrations by product (12% to 33%)
- Moderate toxicity results from ingestions of 20 to 60 mg/kg, severe toxicity with ingestions >60 mg/kg. Patients may develop initial GI symptoms (vomiting, diarrhea), followed by a somewhat asymptomatic "latent phase," and finally, the "shock phase" with hypotension, third-spacing, acidosis, and coagulopathy. After 2 to 5 days,

hepatic failure may ensue and gastric outlet obstruction from fibrosis may occur weeks after ingestion
- The absence of GI symptoms for over 6 hours after ingestion virtually rules out significant toxicity

DIAGNOSIS

- Based on history of exposure, and presence of nausea, vomiting, diarrhea, hypotension
- Visible radiopaque pills on an abdominal x-ray also suggests significant ingestion
- Iron levels between 300 and 500 mcg/dL correlate with significant GI toxicity and mild systemic toxicity, and levels higher than 500 mcg/dL correlate with moderate systemic toxicity, levels higher than 1000 mcg/dL are associated significant morbidity

TREATMENT

- Treat shock with IV crystalloid fluids and replace volume with blood products as necessary
- Whole bowel irrigation should be strongly considered, especially if many pills are present on x-ray
- Deferoxamine—given in cases of significant clinical toxicity or iron levels over 500 mcg/dL
  - Intravenous route is preferred 10 to 15 mg/kg/hour infusion, can be titrated upwards (up to 45 mg/kg/hour) but hypotension can occur

Isoniazid

- **Mechanism of toxicity**—reduces the amount of GABA, leading to uninhibited electrical activity and seizures

CLINICAL MANIFESTATIONS

- Nausea, vomiting, slurred speech, ataxia, depressed sensorium, coma, respiratory depression, and seizures usually occur within 30 to 60 minutes
- Severe acidosis resulting from persistent seizures
- Hepatic injury can be seen and may be delayed by several days

DIAGNOSIS

- Usually based on history and clinical presentation
- Should be suspected in any patient with seizures that are unresponsive to conventional anticonvulsants

TREATMENT

- Airway protection and assist ventilation if necessary
- Treat seizures with benzodiazepines
- Pyridoxine (vitamin B_6)
  - If amount of isoniazid is known, give equal amount of pyridoxine
  - Give at least 5 g if ingested amount unknown

Marine toxins

- Several marine toxin ingestions with neurologic symptoms can result from foodborne poisonings

CIGUATERA

- Results from ingestion of warm-water bottom-dwelling fish from more than 500 different species, including barracuda, sea bass, parrot fish, red snapper, grouper, amber jack, kingfish, and sturgeon as the most common sources
- Ciguatoxin is elaborated from blue-green algae, protozoa, and free algae dinoflagellates that the fish ingest and becomes incorporated into the flesh, tissue, and viscera of larger fish
- **Mechanism of toxicity**—binds to sodium channels in tissues and increases sodium channel permeability

SIGNS AND SYMPTOMS

- 2 to 6 hours after ingestion of the fish (eaten fresh or properly prepared, frozen, by all methods), acute onset of diaphoresis, abdominal pain, vomiting, profuse diarrhea, myalgias, arthralgias, ataxia, and weakness with a variety of neurologic symptoms, including headache, sensation of loose painful teeth, peripheral dysesthesias/paresthesias, watery eyes, tingling of tongue, lips, throat, and perioral area, metallic taste, reversal of temperature discrimination, vertigo, and visual disturbances
- Cardiac symptoms include bradycardia and orthostatic hypotension
- GI symptoms usually resolve in 24 to 48 hours; however, cardiac and neurologic symptoms may persist for several days to weeks

DIAGNOSIS

- Based on history of ingestion of this type of fish, although laboratory confirmation can be obtained by enzyme-linked immunosorbent assay

TREATMENT

- IV fluids, activated charcoal can be considered
- Mannitol may produce a decrease in neurologic and muscular symptoms

SCOMBROID

- Results from ingestion of temperate or tropical dark meat fish, including marine tuna, albacore, bonito, mackerel, skipjack, mahi-mahi and amber jack, that was improperly stored after removal from the water
- Poisoning results from ingestion of histamine in the meat that is produced from bacteria on the surface of the fish
- Within several minutes to hours symptoms occur, including numbness, tingling, burning sensation of the mouth; dysphagia; headache; and a flush characterized by intense diffuse erythema of the face, neck, and upper torso. Occasionally patients get nausea, vomiting, dizziness, palpitations, abdominal pain, or diarrhea. Rare symptoms include pruritis, urticaria, angioedema, or bronchospasm
- Treatment includes IV fluids, and parenteral antihistamines such as diphenhydramine

Methemoglobinemia

- Oxidized form of hemoglobin (Fe^{3+}) that exists naturally in small amounts (<1%), reduced back to deoxyhemoglobin (Fe^{2+}) by enzymatic processes
- Unable to bind and carry oxygen, thereby reducing the oxygen content in the blood
- Acquired when normal mechanisms responsible for the elimination of methemoglobin are unable to deal with an exogenous oxidant stress, such as a drug or chemical agent
- Most common drugs/chemicals that cause methemoglobin are phenazopyridine, benzocaine (local anesthetic), and dapsone. Other agents include nitrates/nitrites, other local anesthetics, and sulfonamides

SIGNS AND SYMPTOMS

- Severity of symptoms depend on percentage of methemoglobin
- Patients with levels below 20% with normal hemoglobin levels are usually asymptomatic, although may have cyanosis at much lower levels
- Methemoglobin levels of 20% to 30%—anxiety, headaches, dizziness, nausea, tachypnea, tachycardia
- Methemoglobin levels of 50% to 60%—severely impair oxygen delivery to tissues resulting in coronary ischemia, dysrhythmias, coma, seizures, and lactic acidosis
- Levels >70% usually not compatible with life

DIAGNOSIS

- Should be considered in all patients who present with cyanosis that does not improve with oxygen
- The blood has a characteristic "chocolate-brown" color
- Pulse oximetry will often give false readings—usually between 80% and 85%. Confirmation is dependent on co-oximetry on a venous or arterial blood gas

TREATMENT

- Supportive measures with oxygen
- Methylene blue
  - Accelerates the enzymatic reduction of methemoglobin by NADPH–methemoglobin reductase, a normally minor enzymatic pathway
  - 1 to 2 mg/kg IV—effects may be seen in 20 minutes
  - Repeat dosing may be given but higher doses (7 mg/kg) paradoxically causes methemoglobinemia

Mushrooms/poisonous plants

- There are more than 5000 varieties of mushrooms of which about 50 to 100 are known to be toxic; divided into early toxicity (within 2 hours of ingestion) and delayed toxicity (6 hours to 20 days)
- If GI symptoms occur within 2 hours of ingestion, the clinical course will most likely be benign
  - Treatment is generally supportive with IV fluids and antiemetics
- Mushrooms containing muscarine can cause neurologic symptoms and muscarinic or cholinergic "SLUDGE" syndrome. Symptoms typically present within 30 minutes and spontaneously resolved within 4 to 12 hours. Treatment is mostly supportive; in severe cases, atropine can be administered for bradycardia and hypotension unresponsive to IV fluids
- Delayed onset of GI symptoms (>6 hours) may indicate a serious and potentially fatal course
  - Concern is either hepatotoxicity (*Amanita* or *Gyromeitra* spp.) or renal failure (*Cortinarius* or *Amanita smithiana*)
  - Elevations in transaminases may not occur until 24 to 48 hours after ingestion. Renal failure may not present until 3 to 20 days after ingestion
  - If hepatotoxic *Amanita* is suspected, then treatment includes high-dose penicillin, silymarin, *N*-acetylcysteine, and high-dose cimetidine should be considered after discussion with a toxicologist
  - There is no specific treatment for mushroom-induced renal failure
- There are hundreds of poisonous plants that have a wide variety of toxicities and it is not possible to discuss them all here. The following are the most highly poisonous plants

CASTOR BEAN (*Ricinus communis*)

- Contains ricin, a highly potent toxalbumin that inhibits protein synthesis and causes severe cytotoxic effects of multiple organ systems
- Symptoms include delayed hemorrhagic gastroenteritis, followed by delirium, seizures, coma, and death
- Whole bowel irrigation is suggested for GI decontamination to speed transit time

FOXGLOVE (*Digitalis purpurea*) AND OLEANDER

- Contains digitalis glycosides that are similar in action to digitalis
- Digoxin levels are not equivalent although there may be some cross-reactivity
- See digitalis section for clinical findings and treatment

JEQUIRITY BEAN (*Abrus precatorius*)

- Contains abrin, a toxalbumin, one of the most lethal naturally occurring toxins
- Symptoms include delayed hemorrhagic gastroenteritis, followed by delirium, seizures, coma, and death
- Treatment includes whole bowel irrigation similar to that for castor beans and supportive care

POISON HEMLOCK (*Conium maculatum*)

- Contains coniine alkaloids, which are similar to nicotine
- Symptoms occur 15 minutes to 1 hour after ingestion and include burning and dryness of the mouth, tachycardia, tremors, diaphoresis, mydriasis, profound muscle weakness, and seizures. In severe cases, ascending paralysis, rhabdomyolysis, acute renal failure, bradycardia, coma, and death occur
- Treatment includes GI decontamination, activated charcoal, and supportive care

WATER HEMLOCK (*Cicuta maculata*)

- Contains cicutoxin, the highest concentrations of which are in the root
- Mechanism of toxicity is by inhibition of noncompetitive GABA antagonists to GABA receptors
- Symptoms occur quickly and include nausea, vomiting, and abdominal pain, followed by delirium, seizures, and death. Seizures may be severe and resistant to conventional anticonvulsants
- Treatment includes GI decontamination and supportive care

Neuroleptics

- Group of medications used for the treatment of schizophrenia and other psychosis
- Older "typical" antipsychotics traditionally have been associated with severe adverse reactions, the newer "atypical" do cause similar reactions less commonly
- **Mechanism of toxicity**
  - Work by blocking reuptake of dopamine, mostly in the limbic system
  - Blockade of dopamine at the basal ganglia is responsible for the extrapyramidal symptoms
  - Typical antipsychotics also block to varying degrees alpha-adrenergic (hypotension), muscarinic (hyperthermia, tachycardia, papillary dilation), and histaminic (sedation) receptors
  - Atypicals block the same receptors at varying degrees, but also block serotonin receptors

(improve negative symptoms and cognitive dysfunction)

- **Clinical manifestations/adverse reactions**
  - **Dystonic reactions**—involuntary contractions that usually affect muscles of the neck (torticollis), jaw (trismus), trunk (opisthotonus), tongue, those around the eye
    - Treatment is diphenhydramine 25 to 50 mg IM or IV. Dose can be repeated in 15 to 30 minutes if symptoms partially resolve. Alternative is benztropine (Cogentin) 1 to 2 mg, which may be less sedating. Therapy should be continued with oral meds for 2 to 5 days
  - **Akathisia**—motor restlessness with anxiety; may be mistaken for worsening of underlying disorder
    - Treatment: discontinue/reduce dose, diphenhydramine may also improve symptoms
  - **Tardive dyskinesia**—involuntary movements associated with chronic therapy and older/"typical" agents
    - Symptoms include repetitive, choreoathetoid movements of the face, mouth, and tongue. Rarely, the arms and legs can be involved
  - **Overdose**
    - CNS—mild sedation to coma, seizures
    - Cardiovascular—tachycardia, hypotension, prolonged QT interval, ventricular dysrhythmia, torsade de pointes

Neuroleptic malignant syndrome

- Idiosyncratic, rare, potentially fatal reaction most commonly associated with antipsychotics, but other drug classes have been implicated
- Clinical features include hyperthermia, "lead pipe" muscle rigidity, autonomic lability, including hyper- and hypotension, tachycardia, pallor, vasoconstriction, diaphoresis, and altered mental status, including confusion, agitation, and coma
- Risk factors include age (young or middle-aged adults most common), concomitant condition of exhaustion, dehydration, or general debilitated state, and a history of the same
- No characteristic laboratory findings confirm the diagnosis; made from history of medication usage and clinical findings
- Treatment consists mostly of supportive care; rapid cooling is essential, critical care monitoring, muscle relaxation with benzodiazepines, dantrolene (a specific muscle relaxant) 1 to 2.5 mg/kg IV titrated to effect (10 mg/kg max cumulative dose)

TREATMENT

- GI decontamination if warranted
- Intravenous fluids for hypotension
- ECG should be obtained. If ventricular dysrhythmias arise, treat with type IB (e.g. lidocaine) and avoid Class IA (e.g. quinidine, disopyramide, procainamide). Wide complex tachycardias (QRS widening) should be managed

with intravenous sodium bicarbonate. Torsade de pointes should be treated with overdrive pacing and magnesium infusion

Sedative/hypnotics

- **Mechanism of toxicity**—almost all agents stimulate the activity at the GABA receptor, which is the primary inhibitory neurotransmitter in the brain

SIGNS AND SYMPTOMS

- Mild intoxication resembles ethanol intoxication with drowsiness, disinhibition, ataxia, slurred speech, and confusion
- Larger ingestions cause coma and rarely respiratory depression, with the exceptions below
- Barbiturates in larger overdoses produce profound sedation, hypothermia, respiratory depression, and hypotension

DIAGNOSIS

- Based on history and physical examination; does appear in urine toxicologic screens

TREATMENT

- GI decontamination and general supportive care
- Flumazenil is a selective antagonist of benzodiazepines and reverses the central nervous system findings. It is contraindicated in patients in whom elevated intracranial pressure is suspected. Recurrent toxicity may occur when flumazenil has worn off. It may precipitate withdrawal in patients who are habituated to benzodiazepines. Usage has caused generalized seizures in patients who have coingested other medications, particularly tricyclic antidepressants
- Urinary alkalinization can be considered in long-acting barbiturates (e.g., phenobarbital)

Stimulants/ sympathomimetic agents

- Includes both illicit drugs and prescription medications, including amphetamines and caffeine
- **Mechanism of toxicity**
  - Central nervous system stimulant
  - Enhancing release/preventing reuptake of excitatory neurotransmitters (norepinephrine and dopamine)

CLINICAL MANIFESTATIONS

- See "Cocaine" for details of cocaine toxicity
- **Amphetamines**
  - Hyperthermia, tachycardia, hypertension, acute myocardial infarction, aortic dissection, altered mental status, seizures, traumatic/nontraumatic rhabdomyolysis with sometimes-resultant acute renal failure

- **Caffeine**
  - Nausea/vomiting, diarrhea, tachycardia, tachypnea, agitation, electrolyte abnormalities (hypokalemia and hyperglycemia), seizures, dysrhythmias
  - Hypertension, tachycardia, seizures, coma, hyporeflexia, muscle fasciculations, weakness, and paralysis

DIAGNOSIS

- Based from history and constellation of physical findings

TREATMENT

- GI decontamination
- Key to therapy is rapid CNS sedation and close monitoring of vital signs
- Benzodiazepines should be given early and frequently for agitation, abnormal vital signs, and seizures
- Rapid cooling is essential
- Intravenous fluids to replace volume depletion

Strychnine

- Found as a rodenticide and as an adulterant in illicit drugs such as cocaine and heroin
- **Mechanism of toxicity**—competitively antagonizes the binding of glycine, causes increased neuronal excitability and exaggerates reflex-arcs, resulting in generalized seizure-like contractions of skeletal muscles

CLINICAL MANIFESTATIONS

- Muscular stiffness and cramps precede generalized muscular contractions. Extensor muscle spasms, and opisthotonus usually begin 15 to 30 minutes after exposure and are triggered by emotional or mild physical stimuli

DIAGNOSIS

- Based on history of rodenticide ingestion or recent intravenous drug use and presence of seizure-like generalized muscular contractions
- Treatment consists of limiting external stimuli (e.g., noise, touch). Benzodiazepines are first-line agents for treatment of spasm. For severe cases, nondepolarizing neuromuscular blockers may be used after intubation and mechanical ventilation. Symptoms usually improve within 24 hours

Lithium

- Acute toxicity arises from intentional ingestion whereas chronic toxicity may occur in patients with stable therapeutic doses with any state that causes dehydration, sodium depletion, or excessive sodium reabsorption
- Precise mechanism of toxicity not understood

CLINICAL MANIFESTATIONS

- **Acute toxicity**—Initially causes nausea and vomiting, systemic manifestations are minimal and may be delayed, levels will initially be high but will fall with equilibration into tissues
- **Chronic toxicity**
  - Usually present with systemic toxicity with levels that may be high normal or slightly above normal
  - Mild to moderate toxicity results in lethargy, muscle weakness, slurred speech, ataxia, tremor (often course), and myoclonic jerking
  - Severe toxicity may present with agitated delirium, coma, convulsions and hyperthermia
  - Nephrogenic diabetes insipidus (excessive free water loss due to impaired kidney response to antidiuretic hormone) is a complication of chronic therapy and may lead to dehydration and hypernatremia

DIAGNOSIS

- Should be suspected in any patient with known psychiatric history who presents obtunded, confused, or tremulous
- Supported with an elevated lithium level, although levels do not correlate with severity of toxicity

TREATMENT

- Consider gastric lavage for large recent ingestion, activated charcoal will not bind to lithium
- Intravenous fluids especially if dehydrated
- Hemodialysis removes lithium effectively
  - Indications for dialysis include severely altered mental status, seizures, or patients who are unable to excrete lithium. There is no specific level at which one needs dialysis

PEARLS

- Phencyclidine (PCP) toxicity frequently presents with altered sensorium and nystagmus.

- Hydrogen sulfide is unique in that it is a simple asphyxiant and a chemical irritant.

- MDMA or "ecstasy" toxicity may present with serotonin syndrome symptoms; beware associated intracranial hemorrhage and look for hyponatremia as a clue.

- Jimson weed ingestion presents with anticholinergic symptoms.

- *Erethisa* (mercury poisoning) is a constellation of neuropsychiatric symptoms.

- *Acrodynia* (mercury poisoning) features rash, fever, splenomegaly, and hypotonia (especially pelvic/pectoral muscles).

- Pralidoxime is the antidote for organophosphates; atropine is helpful.

■ Do not give calcium salts for bradycardia in suspected calcium channel blocker overdose unless you are sure there is no digitalis toxicity.

■ Phosgene gas smells like freshly mown hay.

■ Deferoxamine is used for iron toxicity.

■ Observe suspected sulfonylurea overdoses for 24 hours to monitor for hypoglycemia.

■ Loose/painful teeth, dysesthesias, and reversal of temperature discrimination are some of the unique and bizarre symptoms of ciguatera poisoning.

BIBLIOGRAPHY

Alapat P, Zimmerman J: Toxicology in the critical care unit, *Chest* 133:1006–1013, 2008.

Bellinger D: Lead, *Pediatrics* 113:1016–1022, 2004.

Brodkin E, Copes R, Mattman A et al: Lead and mercury exposures: interpretation and action, *Can Med Assoc J* 176:59–63, 2007.

Halpern J: Hallucinogens and dissociative agents naturally growing in the United States, *Pharmacol Ther* 102:131–138, 2004.

Kerns W: Management of beta-adrenergic blocker and calcium channel antagonist toxicity, *Emerg Med Clin North Am* 25:309–331, 2007.

McCord J, Jneid H, Hollander J et al: Management of cocaine-associated chest pain and myocardial infarction: a scientific statement from the American Heart Association Acute Cardiac Care Committee of the Council on Clinical Cardiology, *Circulation* 117:1897–1907, 2008.

Rischitelli G, Nygren P, Bougatsos C et al: Screening for elevated lead levels in childhood and pregnancy: an updated summary of evidence for the US Preventive Services Task Force, *Pediatrics* 118:e1867–e1895, 2006.

Tintinalli JE, Gabor GD, Stapnzynski JS (eds): *Emergency medicine: a comprehensive study guide*, ed 6, New York, 2004, McGraw-Hill.

Umbreit J: Methemoglobin—It's not just blue: a concise review, *Am J Hematol* 82:134–144, 2007.

Questions and Answers

1. Treatment for isoniazid-induced seizures includes:
   a. methylene blue
   b. calcium
   c. flumazenil
   d. pyridoxine
   e. Prussian blue

2. A 30-year-old man presents after referral to the Emergency Department after ingestion of a mushroom he found while he was in the forest. He looked in "a book" and is now concerned about what he ate. At what time period for onset of vomiting would you be concerned about a possibly hepatotoxic ingestion?
   a. 20 minutes
   b. >6 hours
   c. 2 to 3 hours
   d. 1 hour
   e. 4 hours

3. Organophosphate toxicity can present with all of the following EXCEPT:
   a. urinary retention
   b. bronchorrhea
   c. muscle fasciculations
   d. diaphoresis
   e. bradycardia

4. Treatment for cocaine-associated acute myocardial infarction includes all of the following EXCEPT:
   a. oxygen
   b. nitrates
   c. morphine
   d. beta-adrenergic blockers
   e. aspirin

5. A 34-year-old man was using a high-pressure paint gun when the gun slipped and he sustained a puncture wound to his left index finger. He complains of a moderate amount of pain in his hand but is otherwise asymptomatic. All of the following are appropriate treatment options EXCEPT:
   a. x-rays of the hand
   b. tetanus immunization
   c. wound irrigation and referral to a hand surgeon in 2 to 3 days
   d. intravenous pain medications
   e. digital block using a local anesthetic

6. Firefighters pull a 34-year-old homeless woman from a house fire. She is unconscious and hypotensive. You begin to order labs and contemplate your next treatment while assessing her ABCs. Which of the following is a marker for cyanide toxicity?
   a. lactate concentration greater than 10 mmol/L
   b. creatinine >3.3 mmol/L
   c. lactate concentration of 3 mmol/L
   d. carboxyhemoglobin level of 5%
   e. venous pH of 7.35

7. Sulfonylurea-induced hypoglycemia can be treated with:
   a. octreotide
   b. propranolol
   c. alprazolam
   d. fomepizole
   e. phenobarbital

8. An 84-year-old woman is brought into the Emergency Department complaining of feeling lightheaded and weak. Her medications include

hydrochlorothiazide, metoprolol, aspirin, and digoxin. Vital signs reveal: heart rate (HR) = 38 beats per minute (bpm), blood pressure (BP) = 92/68 mmHg, respiratory rate (RR) = 14/minute, and oxygen saturation = 94%. Physical examination is unremarkable except for decreased pulse rate and slightly delayed capillary refill. Laboratory results include a potassium of 6.4 mmol/L, BUN 54 mg/dL, Cr 2.6 mg/dL, and a pending digoxin level. All of the following would be acceptable treatments for this type of toxicity EXCEPT:

a. FAB fragments for elevated digoxin level
b. lidocaine for tachydysrhythmias
c. calcium for hyperkalemia
d. atropine for bradycardia
e. intravenous fluids for hypotension

9. Which of the following is a complication of chronic lithium toxicity:

a. hyperkalemia
b. diabetes insipidus
c. opisthotonus
d. Cushing syndrome
e. porphyria

10. A 5-year-old man is brought into the Emergency Department because his parents thought his skin looked "funny." When further questioned, they admit that he possibly got into some pills of his older sister's for a recent urinary tract infection. He appears comfortable on the bed in no acute distress. It appears that he has some perioral duskiness in addition to a grayish tint to his fingers and toes. His vitals signs are: HR = 140 bpm, RR = 30/minute, BP = 94/58 mmHg, and oxygen saturation = 85%. You place the child on oxygen, which does not improve the oxygen saturations. What is the most likely diagnosis?

a. sulfhemoglobinemia
b. carboxyhemoglobinemia
c. methemoglobinemia
d. sickle cell anemia
e. argyria

11. Which of the following is most consistent with neuroleptic malignant syndrome (NMS)?

a. occurs when two serotonergically active medications are combined producing toxicity
b. NMS is a rare non–dose-related idiosyncratic reaction
c. most commonly arises from the selective serotonin reuptake inhibitors class of medications
d. common symptoms include hyperthermia, hallucinations, urinary retention, and red, dry, skin
e. NMS should be treated with physostigmine

12. Digoxin antibody fragments should be considered in toxic ingestions of:

a. Jimson weed
b. Poison hemlock
c. foxglove
d. water hemlock
e. castor bean

13. A 2-year-old boy was witnessed by his mother to drink a portion of a bottle containing lamp oil, so she brought him into the Emergency Department. He coughed several times but did not vomit and now looks fine. What are the appropriate treatment options for this patient?

a. a chest x-ray in 4 to 6 hours, and if asymptomatic then discharge home
b. if asymptomatic, discharge home
c. intubation and mechanical ventilation for concern for chemical pneumonitis
d. administration of prophylactic antibiotics
e. administration of steroids to prevent development of fibrosis

14. A 67-year-old man presents to the Emergency Department after his wife found him slumped over in a bathroom with several empty pill bottles. He is currently being treated for hypertension and benign prostatic hypertrophy. His vitals signs are: HR = 34 bpm, BP = 82/46 mmHg, RR = 10/minute, oxygen saturation = 93%. He responds to questions and admits to taking pills but does not say which ones. His fingerstick glucose is 289 mg/dL. Which of the following agents are most appropriate for treatment?

a. metoprolol
b. hydralazine
c. methylene blue
d. insulin-euglycemia therapy
e. pyridoxine

15. A 34-year-old migrant field worker is brought into the Emergency Department after getting splashed on the arms and legs with an unknown pesticide. He is anxious, diaphoretic, bradycardic, and manifests profuse secretions. Which of the following treatments is appropriate for this type of poisoning?

a. irrigation with alcohol-based disinfectant
b. intubation with succinylcholine
c. administration of atropine until the maximum recommended dose of 0.04 mg/kg is reached
d. administration of pralidoxime to prevent aging of the pesticide
e. administration of atropine until the heart rate reaches a maximum of 120 bpm

16. Which of the following does **not** cause hallucinations?

a. LSD
b. Jimson weed
c. MDMA
d. hemlock
e. diphenhydramine

17. Which of the following is TRUE of iron ingestions?
    a. severe toxicity occurs with ingestions of 10 mg/kg
    b. absence of significant GI symptoms excludes clinically significant iron toxicity
    c. iron concentrations of <1000 mcg/dL do not result in toxicity
    d. deferoxamine should be used in all patients who present with ingestions greater than 20 mg/kg
    e. the percentage of iron formulations should be multiplied by 10 to calculate the elemental iron ingestion

18. A 3-year-old girl is brought into the Emergency Department by her parents because she would not wake up this morning. The girl had been taking a medication that the parents had obtained in India for treatment of gastrointestinal disorders. The parents report she has had increasing abdominal cramping, headaches, and altered mental status. In the Emergency Department she is somnolent. Vitals signs reveal HR = 140 bpm, RR = 10/minute, BP 104/76 mmHg, oxygen saturation = 92%. During your examination, she has a prolonged seizure for which you give midazolam and phenobarbital, and then intubate. A noncontrast head CT reveals diffuse cerebral edema. You suspect lead toxicity and a blood lead concentration returns at 120 mcg/dL. What is next most appropriate treatment?
    a. succimer
    b. BAL
    c. CaNa$_2$EDTA
    d. environmental investigation of the home
    e. activated charcoal

19. Which of the following is TRUE of scombroid marine toxicity?
    a. scombroid results from ingestion of histamine in fish
    b. it typically results from toxin elaborated from dinoflagellates
    c. the mainstay of treatment is mannitol
    d. results from ingestion of large bottom-dwelling fish such as sturgeon
    e. reversal of temperature discrimination is a typical symptom

20. A 20-year-old man was recently started on haloperidol for schizophrenia. He presents to the Emergency Department with diffuse muscle spasms, diaphoresis, and facial grimacing. His vitals signs are: HR = 140 bpm, BP = 180/100 mmHg, RR = 20/minute, and oxygen saturation = 98%. On examination, the patient is diaphoretic and has episodes of muscle spasms in his neck, face, and back. What is the next most appropriate action?

    a. activated charcoal 70 g
    b. scopolamine patch
    c. diphenhydramine 50 mg IV
    d. noncontrast head CT
    e. atropine 2 mg IV
    f. dantrolene 70 mg IV

---

1. Answer: d

Pyridoxine is the treatment for seizures caused by isoniazid that are not controlled by benzodiazepines. Isoniazid toxicity should be suspected in cases of recurrent or persistent seizures. If the amount of isoniazid is known, an equal amount of pyridoxine can be given. If the dose is unknown, 5 g should be given.

2. Answer: b

GI symptoms that occur for more than 6 hours post ingestion should be concerning for the possibility of a hepatotoxic mushroom ingestion and should be treated with high-dose penicillin, silymarin, *N*-acetylcysteine, and high-dose cimetidine after discussion with a toxicologist.

3. Answer: a

Urinary retention is a manifestation of *anticholinergic poisoning* not cholinergic poisoning as is seen in organophosphate poisonings.

4. Answer: d

Beta-adrenergic blockers are contraindicated in cocaine toxicity because of concern for unopposed alpha adrenergic receptor activity.

5. Answer: c

Patients with a high-pressure paint gun injury should have **immediate hand or plastic surgery consultation** for possible emergent surgical exploration, irrigation, and debridement. Often, the wound extends up the arm and extensive irrigation and debridement are needed.

6. Answer: a

Patient's who presents with hypotension and a lactic metabolic acidosis from a building fire should be suspected of having cyanide toxicity and should be treated with either the Cyanokit or the Cyanide Antidote Kit. A **lactate over 10 mmol/L** has been shown to correlate with cyanide toxicity.

7. Answer: a

Octreotide, in addition to glucose supplementation, is the treatment of choice for sulfonylurea toxicity, as it prevents insulin release from the pancreas.

8. Answer: c

Calcium should not be given to patients with hyperkalemia that are suspected to have digoxin toxicity. As digoxin blocks the Na/K-ATPase pump, intracellular calcium increases. Administering more calcium may overwhelm the myocytes and may increase the risk of ventricular dysrhythmias.

9. Answer: b

Nephrogenic diabetes insipidus is a possible complication of chronic lithium toxicity and is not seen in acute overdose.

10. Answer: c

This is a typical presentation for a patient presenting with **methemoglobinemia.** They often present with very few symptoms. Consideration for treatment of methemoglobinemia would be levels over 30% or patients who are symptomatic; the child probably ingested phenazopyridine; other drugs commonly linked with methemoglobinemia include nitrites/nitrates, dapsone, nitroglycerin, local anesthetics, and sulfa compounds.

11. Answer: b

Neuroleptic malignant syndrome is **a rare idiosyncratic reaction, and not dose related.** It is seen mostly with antipsychotic usage but has been seen with other classes of medications as well.

12. Answer: c

Foxglove contains digoxin-like compounds that are similar to pharmaceutical digoxin poisoning. Digoxin levels can be obtained but may not be representative of true levels.

13. Answer: a

If the child is currently asymptomatic, then a period of **observation of at least 4 to 6 hours is warranted** and if the **x-ray and examination are negative,** the child can be **discharged with close observation.** If the child is symptomatic or has findings on the chest x-ray suggestive of pneumonitis, then a longer period of observation is recommended. Steroids and antibiotics have not been shown to influence morbidity or mortality after *hydrocarbon ingestion.*

14. Answer: d

Consideration of **insulin-euglycemia therapy** should be given to patients with *possible calcium channel blocker overdose,* and this patient fits that toxidrome with hypotension, bradycardia, and hyperglycemia.

15. Answer: d

The concern for this patient would be exposure to an *organophosphate.* Decontamination should ideally be performed prior to patient transport but may need to be performed at the Emergency Department with copious amounts of soap and water. **Atropine** should

be given and titrated for drying of secretions; there is **no maximum dose or heart rate** for organophosphate toxicity. **Pralidoxime** is given to prevent the irreversible phosphorylation of pseudocholinesterase, which prevents potential reversal of symptoms.

16. Answer d

Hemlock does not cause hallucinations; all of the other substances will produce some degree of hallucinations in toxic levels.

17. Answer: b

Severe toxicity is usually seen with elemental iron ingestions of **>100 mg/kg. Lack of abdominal pain, vomiting, and diarrhea preclude significant iron toxicity.** When an iron concentration is obtained, levels of 300 to 500 mcg/dL correlate with moderate GI toxicity, and mild systemic toxicity and levels greater than 500 mcg/dL correlate with moderate systemic toxicity, levels greater than 1000 mcg/dL are associated significant morbidity. **Deferoxamine** should be considered in cases with **significant clinical toxicity** or in cases with iron concentrations **greater than 500 mcg/dL.**

18. Answer: b

Immediate treatment of *lead encephalopathy* should begin with chelation. **BAL** works both intra- and extracellularly to bind lead. **Succimer** is an oral chelator that can be used after the patient becomes stable. **CaNa$_2$EDTA** is another parenteral chelator that is used in conjunction with BAL. The first dose of CaNa$_2$EDTA is given 4 hours after administration of BAL because of evidence that CaNa$_2$EDTA alone may increase lead uptake into the brain. **Activated charcoal** will not bind to lead and does no play a role in the treatment of lead. **Environmental investigation** should be performed but is not the most immediate concern for this patient.

19. Answer: a

Scombroid toxicity is a result of ingestion of the parts of the fish that contain **histamine** elaborated from bacteria. Choices **b** through **e** all occur in *ciguatera poisoning.*

20. Answer: c

This patient presents with symptoms that are consistent with *acute dystonia* resulting from starting a new antipsychotic. Symptoms typically resolve shortly after administration of **IV diphenhydramine** or benztropine mesylate. Oral therapy should continue for several days and the medication should be discontinued.

Richard A. Harrigan | Matthew L. Tripp | Jacob W. Ufberg

Major/multi-system trauma

TRAUMA TRIAGE

- **High risk/possible benefit from trauma center care**
  - Glasgow Coma Scale (GCS) score < 14
  - Vital signs abnormal (e.g., systolic blood pressure [BP] < 90 mmHg; respiratory rate [RR] < 10 or > 29 breaths/min)
  - Severe injuries—penetrating injury to head, neck, torso, and proximal extremities; flail chest; significant trauma plus burns; two or more proximal long bone fractures; pelvic fractures; paralyzed extremity; limb amputation; paralysis
  - Other considerations for trauma center care—severe mechanism of injury (e.g., motor vehicle collision [MVC] with ejection, rollover, death to another in vehicle, or >20 minute extrication time, high-speed, significant intrusion; auto vs. pedestrian; auto vs. bicyclist; motorcycle collision >20 mph and/or victim thrown from bike; falls from height [>20 feet]; extremes of age [<5 or >55 years old]; comorbidities; medication issues [anticoagulants])

INITIAL TRAUMA EVALUATION: PRIMARY SURVEY → RAPID RESUSCITATION → SECONDARY SURVEY → FURTHER TESTING AND TREATMENT → DISPOSITION

- **Primary survey**
  - Goal—find and stabilize/treat life-threatening problems
  - **A** (airway with cervical spine control) **B** (breathing) **C** (circulation with hemorrhage control) **D** (disability due to neurologic issues) **E** (exposure)
  - Address life-threats as encountered (e.g., intubation for airway; chest decompression for tension pneumothorax)
  - Resume A-B-C-D-E if needed to stop and address an issue discovered along the progression
- **Secondary survey**
  - Rapid but thorough, with frequent reassessment of airway, vital signs, level of consciousness (primary survey issues)
  - Head-to-toe evaluation
  - Stage for further interventions/testing (temporizing packing; sutures, staples of rapidly bleeding lacerations; x-rays [cervical spine, chest,

pelvis—vs. CT evaluation after secondary survey]; nasogastric tube; bladder catheter; splinting; urine for blood/pregnancy testing, etc.)

CRITICAL ISSUES IN INITIAL TRAUMA ASSESSMENT

- **Airway/breathing (A and B)**
  - If airway obstructed → immediate intervention
  - Inspect airway for reversible causes (e.g., debris in mouth, tongue positioning, impingement due to fractured facial bones) and utilize positioning, airway adjuncts (e.g., oral airways) or definitive treatment (rapid sequence intubation [RSI]; surgical airway if RSI not possible) if necessary
  - Other anatomic areas of focus beyond oropharynx—neck (e.g., expanding hematoma, tracheal crush or transecting injury), chest (check respiratory rate, flail segment, asymmetry of breath sounds)—discussed in detail later in chapter
  - Intubation optimally via orotracheal RSI, with cervical spine immobilization when appropriate; nasotracheal intubation rarely indicated
  - Cricothyrotomy is surgical airway method of choice in adults (see Chapter 21, Procedures)
  - Cardiorespiratory compromise from suspected *tension pneumothorax* [neck veins distended, absent breath sounds on affected side, hypoxia, tracheal deviation]) requires definitive treatment (needle decompression/tube thoracostomy) before chest x-ray
- **Circulation (C)**—shock and hemorrhage control
  - Secure intravenous access with two large-bore IV lines and infuse crystalloid
  - Bedside ultrasound
  - External hemorrhage—initial treatment is direct manual pressure
  - Classes of hemorrhage—vital signs (VS) are relative to the individual's "normal" resting HR and BP, so the following classes are a general guide (Table 19-1)
  - Level of consciousness, skin color, capillary refill, and integrity of peripheral pulses are important in the assessment of the circulatory state
  - After crystalloid infusion, Type O blood is transfused in unstable patients suspected to be so due to hemorrhagic shock; type O-negative in women of childbearing age

- Watch for hypothermia, coagulopathy, acidosis in massive transfusion scenarios
- Massive transfusion may require concomitant transfusion of fresh frozen plasma (FFP) and platelets
- Colloid therapy does not appear to be more advantageous than crystalloid
- No clear indication (backed by randomized control trials) for recombinant Factor VIIa in the treatment of circulatory hemorrhage due to trauma as of yet
- **Disability (D)**—briefly survey consciousness, motor examination, and pupillary size in suspected head injury
  - GCS score—range 3 to 15; best response; eye opening (1 to 4)/verbal (1 to 5)/motor (1 to 6)—see head injury section
  - Protect/immobilize cervical spine when impaired mental status prevents clinical assessment in the proper scenario
- **FAST examination** (Focused Assessment with Sonography in Trauma) looking for free intraperitoneal fluid
  - Also useful in suspected *pericardial tamponade* (agitation, hypotension, distended neck veins, clear and equal breath sounds, and distant heart sounds)

Head trauma

GENERAL

- Leading cause of traumatic death in people younger than 25 years
- Categorization of traumatic brain injury (TBI)—minor (GCS score 14 to 15), moderate (GCS score 9 to 13) and severe (GCS score 3 to 8)
- Assume coincident cervical spine injury (see **Trauma II** Chapter 20) if can't exclude clinically and/or by mechanism of injury
- *SCALP* layers mnemonic (outer-to-inner layers)—**s**kin (dermis) → sub**c**utaneous tissue with blood vessels → galea **a**poneurosis → **l**oose areolar tissue (site of subgaleal hematomas) → **p**ericranium
- Skull consists of bones of varying thickness; thinnest is temporal
- Under skull are the 3 protective layers: *dura mater* (with dural venous sinuses), *arachnoid* with subarachnoid space (cerebrospinal fluid [CSF]

TABLE 19-1 **Classes of Hemorrhage**

	Class I	Class II	Class III	Class IV
Blood loss (mL)	<750	750-1500	1500-2000	>2000
Blood loss (%)	<15	15-30	30-40	>40
Pulse (bpm)	<100	100-120	120-140	>140
Blood pressure	Normal	Normal	Decreased	Decreased
Pulse pressure	Normal	Decreased	Decreased	Decreased

there), and *pia mater* (adherent to gray matter of brain)

- CSF produced in choroid plexi (mostly in lateral ventricles) and circulates through *ventricles* (lateral [1 and 2], third, and fourth) in the brain and *cisterns* (variety of names) surrounding the brain as well as subarachnoid space—ventricles and cisterns should be scrutinized on CT for blood and for effacement (mass effect) or closure (herniation/blockage of flow)

KEY PATHOPHYSIOLOGIC MECHANISMS IN TBI

- Cerebral blood flow [CBF] modified by physiologic milieu, including
  - Vasoconstriction (from hypertension, alkalosis, hypocarbia)
  - Vasodilation (from hypotension, acidosis, hypercarbia)
- Cerebral perfusion pressure [CPP] reliant on difference between circulatory inflow (estimated by mean arterial pressure [MAP]) and outflow (estimated by intracranial pressure [ICP]) as below:
  - $CPP = MAP - ICP$
- Optimal autoregulation of CBF depends upon CPP being between 50 and 150 mmHg; normal ICP is roughly 5 to 15 mmHg (65 to 195 mmH$_2$O)—so MAPs of 60 to 160 mmHg would be desirable for optimal perfusion
- Goal of temporary, controlled hyperventilation in clinical instances of increased ICP with herniation is to promote cerebral vasoconstriction
  - pCO$_2$ of 30 to 35 mmHg
  - Narrow margin of risk–benefit
  - The risk of hyperventilation is brain ischemia and should be reserved for temporization prior to emergent surgery or cases refractory to:
    - Head-of-bed elevation 30 degrees
    - Volume to keep MAP of 90 mmHg (or treat hypertension)
    - Oxygenation
    - Mannitol (onset 30 minutes; duration 6 to 8 hours)
- Rapid rise in ICP with brain compression can result in *Cushing reflex*—hypertension, bradycardia, respiratory disturbance

GLASGOW COMA SCALE SCORE AND TRAUMATIC BRAIN INJURY

- GCS and TBI—best response score used to risk-stratify patients after head injury (Table 19-2)
- **Mild TBI (GCS score 14 to 15)** has history of loss of consciousness (LOC), amnesia to event, altered mental status at time of event, and/or enduring/transient focal neurologic findings. Can be risk stratified in many ways, consider:
  - **Low-risk mild TBI**—GCS score 15, no LOC, amnesia, vomiting, or diffuse headache
  - Intervention: no imaging; observation

TABLE 19-2 **GCS and TBI: Best Response Score Used to risk-stratify patients after head injury**

Score	Eye opening	Verbal	Motor
1	None	None	None
2	To pain	Moans	Decerebrate
3	To speech	Nonsense	Decorticate
4	Spontaneous	Disoriented	Withdraws/ moves to pain
5	—	Alert/oriented	Localizes pain
6	—	—	Follows commands

- **Medium-risk mild TBI**—GCS score 15 with one of above
- Intervention: CT scan
- **High-risk mild TBI**—GCS score 14 or 15, with skull fracture and/or neurologic deficits; high risk includes coagulopathy, elderly, intoxicated, seizure disorder, postneurosurgical procedure
- Intervention: CT scan
- **Moderate TBI (GCS score 9 to 13)**—(<20% mortality) consider intubation, neurosurgical consultation, monitored unit in addition to CT scan
- **Severe TBI (GCS score <9)**—(roughly 40% mortality) CT scan and admission to intensive care unit in hospital with neurosurgical capabilities

SPECIFIC CLINICAL ENTITIES IN HEAD TRAUMA

- **Signs and symptoms** are as described above, and variable
- **Imaging** is almost always initially done with noncontrast CT
- **Disposition** involves neurosurgical consultation
- **Skull fractures** may be simple or complicated, and may or may not be associated with underlying TBI. Higher risk if intersect middle meningeal artery or dural venous sinus distribution, are open, result in intracranial air, or are depressed (through inner table). CT imaging obviates need for skull x-rays
  - **Basilar skull fractures** (Fig. 19-1) involve temporal bone; complications include hemotympanum, hearing loss, CSF leak/dural tear, cranial nerve entrapment, carotid injury (sphenoid)
  - Suspect with CSF otorhinorrhea, hemotympanum, raccoon eyes, Battle sign (mastoid ecchymosis), post-traumatic vertigo or hearing loss, and/or new cranial nerve palsy
  - All need CT, admission, consideration of antibiotics (risk for meningitis)
- **Cerebral contusion** is a brain bruise, often occurring in the frontal, temporal, or occipital regions. May be single, multiple, *coup* or *contrecoup* (or both), and may be associated with subarachnoid hemorrhage or other more severe injuries
  - May evolve over time
  - CT without contrast is the diagnostic test of choice

- Admission with observation and neurosurgical consultation is advisable
- **Subarachnoid hemorrhage (SAH)** (Fig. 19-2)
  - The most common CT abnormality after head injury

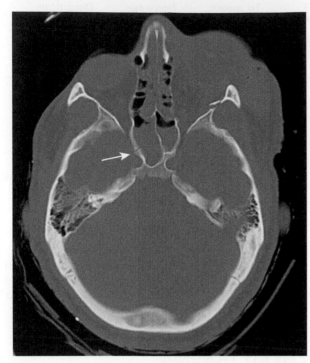

Figure 19-1. Basilar skull fracture.

- Amount of blood correlates inversely with GCS score and prognosis
- CT scan without contrast is the diagnostic test of choice
- Admission, nimodipine for vasospasm, and neurosurgical involvement is indicated
- **Subdural hematoma (SDH)** (Fig. 19-3)
  - More common in those with cerebral atrophy—such as the elderly and alcoholics, due to increased distance spanned by the bridging veins that may rupture after trauma
  - More common than epidural hematomas
  - Presentation may be delayed in part due to slower venous bleeding
  - They may be acute (<24 hours), subacute (24 hours to 2 weeks), or chronic
  - Acute SDH appears hyperdense on CT (and may cross the skull suture lines)
  - Subacute and chronic may be isodense or hypodense (to the adjacent brain tissue)
    - Isodense lesions are best detected by inferential findings (effacement, shift, compression of adjacent sulci/gyri) on noncontrast CT, and are better seen on contrast-enhanced CT or MR imaging
  - Management depends upon degree of brain injury rather than size of the SDH, as well as the chronicity—and is not always operative
- **Epidural hematoma (EDH)** (Fig. 19-4)
  - Form between the dura mater and the inner skull, and result from arterial bleeding after

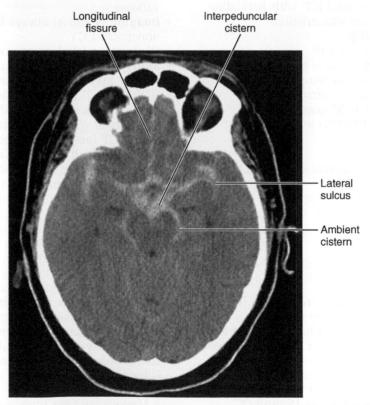

Figure 19-2. Subarachnoid hemorrhage in a 51-year-old man involved in a motor vehicle accident. In contrast to lens-shaped epidural hematomas and crescent-shaped subdural hematomas, subarachnoid hemorrhages spread through the cisterns and fissures surrounding the brain. (Courtesy Dr. Raymond F. Carmody, University of Arizona College of Medicine.)

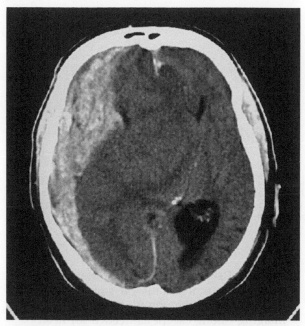

Figure 19-3. Non–contrast-enhanced computed tomography scan of acute right temporal subdural hematoma. There is acute bleeding as well as delayed bleeding, which explains mixed density. Mass effect is large, with midline shift measuring approximately 2.7 cm right to left. Right lateral ventricle has been obliterated. (From Marx JA, Hockberger RS, Walls RM, Adams J, Rosen P: *Rosen's emergency medicine: concepts and clinical practice*, ed 6, Philadelphia, 2006, Mosby.)

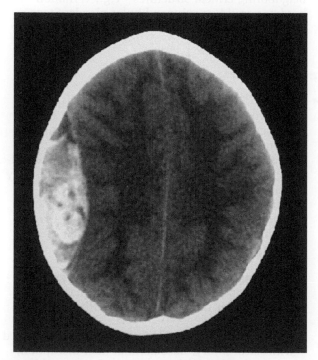

Figure 19-4. Non–contrast-enhanced computed tomography scan of acute epidural hematoma at level of right midconvexity. There is an associated mass effect and moderate midline shift. (From Marx JA, Hockberger RS, Walls RM, Adams J, Rosen P: *Rosen's emergency medicine: concepts and clinical practice*, ed 6, Philadelphia, 2006, Mosby.)

direct impact (or occasionally after tangential gunshot wounds to the head or blast injuries), or from dural tears and bleeding from the underlying dural venous sinus
- Time from onset to symptoms varies accordingly
  - Patients may or may not present with a "lucid interval" following head trauma and initial LOC
- As with SDH, outcome is worse if the presentation is coma
- EDH characteristically is biconvex and does not cross suture lines
- Management is usually operative.
- **Diffuse axonal injury**
  - Due to white matter/brain stem axonal disruption
  - It is defined as coma beginning immediately after head trauma and persisting at least 6 hours—without focal culpable lesions on CT
  - Injury severity is revealed by clinical progression
  - Outcome is guarded, and management is directed toward optimizing ICP and CPP in the neurosurgical intensive care setting
- **Concussion**
  - Is the clinical condition of head injury followed by (perhaps) LOC, (perhaps) with transient amnesia—and without evidence of causative intracranial abnormality on head CT
  - Headache and temporary confusion are common.
  - Type, severity, and duration of post-traumatic symptoms determine the severity of the concussion, and thus are outside the realm of EM
  - Concussion does not result in loss of memory for name, address, etc. and does not lead to confabulation
  - Follow-up visits should determine return to sports
  - *Post-concussive syndrome* (headache, nausea, irritability, difficulty with memory or concentration, sleep disturbance and mood alteration) is a possible complication
- **Brain herniation syndromes**—are emergent conditions that call for immediate treatment to decrease ICP, emergent CT imaging if possible, and consideration for ED skull trephination ("burr holes")
  - **Uncal**—temporal lobe uncus under medial tentorium; ipsilateral fixed/dilated pupil (CN III compression), followed by contralateral motor weakness/paralysis (with some variation)
  - **Central transtentorial**—due to midline lesions; bilateral pinpoint pupils, bilateral Babinski reflexes, increased motor tone—may progress to fixed/midrange pupils and decorticate posturing
  - **Cerebellotonsillar**—cerebellar tonsils through foramen magnum; pinpoint pupils, flaccid paralysis, rapid death
  - **Upward posterior fossa**—posterior fossa lesion causes herniation up through the tentorium; conjugate downward gaze, pinpoint pupils and rapid death

Facial trauma

EYE

- **Ruptured globe**—suspect with penetrating injury to eye or eyelid—usually causes pain and visual disturbance
  - **Physical examination**—shallow anterior chamber, hyphema, irregular pupil are clues; positive Seidel test (aqueous streaming of fluorescein on slit lamp) indicative
  - **Imaging**—CT scan
  - **Treatment**—protective eye shield; do not measure pressure; IV antibiotics, pain control, antiemetics if necessary; NPO; ophthalmology consultation
- **Lid lacerations/nasolacrimal apparatus disruption**—suspect with medial eyelid lacerations, especially medial to the punctum. All lid margin (medial or not) lacerations (>1 mm) best repaired by ophthalmology within 24 hours; 24 to 36 hours for lacrimal canalicular stenting and repair.
- **Retrobulbar hematoma**—after significant orbital trauma, especially in coagulopathic patient
  - **Physical examination**—proptosis, extraocular muscle limitation with pain, visual disturbance, binocular diplopia
  - **Imaging**—CT scan
  - **Treatment**—correct coagulopathy; ophthalmology consultation; consider lateral canthotomy (see Chapter 21, Procedures)
- **Traumatic lens dislocation or traumatic cataract** may occur after blunt or penetrating trauma; presentation may be immediate or delayed
  - **Signs and symptoms**—decreased vision, monocular diplopia, pain, inability to visualize retina on ophthalmoscopy, increased intraocular pressure. May have associated hyphema, vitreous hemorrhage
  - **Imaging**—CT scan
  - **Disposition**—ophthalmology consultation
- **Retinal detachment** may occur after trauma, when vitreous fluid oozes into a break between the inner sensory layer of the retina and the underlying pigmented (choroidal) layer
  - **Signs and symptoms**—flashing lights with cascade of floaters, visual loss is later (peripheral or central/macular, depending on site of detachment); afferent pupillary defect may occur, decreased intraocular pressure relative to unaffected eye, visual loss, confrontational defect—or may appear normal on ED examination
  - **Imaging**—none, although bedside ultrasound may be diagnostic
  - **Disposition**—if acute, urgent ophthalmology consultation (hours, not minutes)

NOSE/EAR

- **Septal hematoma** (Fig. 19-5)/**Auricular hematoma**—require ED treatment to prevent cartilage necrosis, "cauliflower ear"

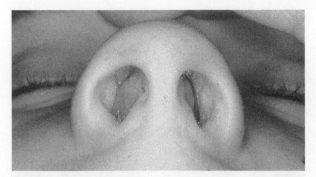

Figure 19-5. Bilateral septal hematoma in a 6-year-old child. There is obstruction of both sides of the nose. (From Cummings CW, Haughey BH, Thomas JR, Harker LA: *Otolaryngology: head and neck,* ed 4, Philadelphia, 2005, Mosby.)

- **Signs and symptoms**—pain, epistaxis, dark reddish-blue protuberant mass on septal surface or visible hematoma on pinna
- **Imaging**—none except as needed for head trauma
- **Treatment**—ED incision and drainage followed by anterior packing and sinusitis/toxic shock antibiotic prophylaxis (nose), or by aspiration and pressure dressing (ear)—check for reaccumulation

MOUTH

- **Lacerations** should be evaluated for violation of neighboring critical structures—e.g., vermilion border; parotid or submandibular glands; Stensen or Wharton ducts; facial nerve (buccal structures anterior to tragus)

FRACTURES

- **Orbit**
  - **"Blowout" (inferior wall)**—usually due to globe impact/increased intraorbital pressure causing fracture of thin inferior wall
    - **Signs and symptoms**—pain, swelling, upward-gaze diplopia (inferior rectus entrapment—may be self-limited), infraorbital paresthesia/anesthesia (infraorbital nerve traction), rarely enophthalmos, subcutaneous emphysema (sinus violated)
    - **Diagnosis**—CT/coronal views or plain radiography
    - **Treatment**—close follow-up 1 to 2 weeks; no driving/patch for comfort if diplopia; avoid sneezing or blowing the nose (orbital emphysema)
  - **Medial wall/lamina papyracea**—often associated with nasal injury, nasolacrimal duct disruption, or other midface fractures
    - **Signs and symptoms**—pain, swelling, exophthalmos, diplopia, and swelling/subcutaneous emphysema after sneezing/blowing nose may occur

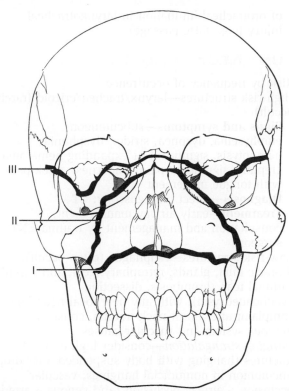

Figure 19-6. Le Fort I fracture is a horizontal fracture that separates the bone containing the maxillary dentition from the remainder of the craniofacial skeleton. The Le Fort II fracture is a pyramidol fracture that extends across the maxilla through the infraorbital rim and orbital floor up through the medial orbital wall and across the nasal root area, then across similarly the other side. The LeFort III fracture is the true craniofacial separation that includes fractures of the zygomatic arches and frontozygomatic areas, then crosses the lateral inferior and medial orbits and is completed across the nasal root. Note that all Le Fort fractures cross the nasal septum and pterygoid plates. (From Cummings CW, Haughey BH, Thomas JR, Harker LA: *Otolaryngology: head and neck,* ed 4, Philadelphia, 2005, Mosby.)

- **Diagnosis**—CT/coronal views
- **Treatment**—close follow-up (1 week) if isolated; avoid sneezing or blowing the nose
- **Midface**—often involve great forces and should prompt thorough search for complications and consideration of (at least) intracranial and cervical spine injury
  - **LeFort** (Fig. 19-6)
    - May be unilateral, bilateral, or asymmetric, and are best visualized by looking at the schematic in the figure
    - LeFort I and II fractures can be suspected by grasping the upper teeth and gums (maxillary arch) and pulling
    - If the upper teeth and hard palate move, suspect LeFort I
    - If the nose and upper teeth/palate move, suspect LeFort II
    - LeFort III is craniofacial dysjunction (face separated on stress from skull) and is often associated with CSF leak
  - **Diagnosis**—CT scan/coronal views

- **Treatment**—facial surgery/trauma surgery consultation; admission; antibiotic prophylaxis for sinus violation
- **Zygoma**—is tripartite (zygoma, maxilla, lateral orbit). Swelling and tenderness, perhaps enophthalmos and a step-off, are evident
  - **Diagnosis**—CT/coronal views; plain radiography with "bucket handle" view
  - **Treatment**—referral as outpatient for facial surgery follow-up
- **Mandibular**—may be isolated or multiple, including segments distant from the point of impact due to the ring shape of the bone
  - **Signs and symptoms**—pain, swelling, trismus, malocclusion, sublingual hematoma, visible intraoral fracture (open fracture), lower lip numbness (inferior dental nerve injury), positive "tongue blade" test
    - *Tongue Blade test:* Place a tongue blade between patient's clenched teeth and attempt to break it. If the patient is unable to hold the tongue blade, a fracture is more likely
  - **Diagnosis**—pantomography, mandibular series, facial CT
  - **Treatment**—open fractures require admission and IV antibiotics; otherwise consultation with orofacial surgeons for stabilization vs. admission

Neck trauma

PENETRATING NECK TRAUMA

- Calls for immediate airway assessment followed by work-up. Critical vascular structures, as well as the airway, esophagus, and the cervical spine testify to the complex nature of the region. Violation of the platysma constitutes penetrating neck trauma (at risk for injury to deeper, crucial structures)
- **Signs and symptoms** (emergent)—dyspnea, hoarseness (direct laryngeal trauma or recurrent laryngeal nerve injury), expanding hematoma, bruit, new neurologic finding, subcutaneous emphysema, or shock
- **Diagnosis**—proceeds after airway and circulation issues are stabilized, and is with respect to "zone" of injury (Fig. 19-7 and Table 19-3]
  - Early rapid sequence orotracheal intubation is recommended for penetrating neck injury with "hard signs" of vascular or airway injury (e.g., expanding hematoma, severe active bleeding, shock, bruit, cerebral ischemia/altered mental status, airway obstruction or impending airway obstruction) and preparation should be made simultaneously for alternative airway management (cricothyrotomy)
  - Potential of injury in any of these zones necessitates consultation with the appropriate surgical or trauma-surgical service
  - Unstable Zone 1 injuries will need CT surgery consultation as the approach is often thoracic.

- Zones 1 and 3 are usually evaluated nonoperatively unless unstable/obvious surgical indication.
    - Zone 1: angiographically/radiographically (pneumothorax); esophageal evaluation; as well as laryngoscopy/bronchoscopy if evidence of an airway injury
    - Zone 3: angiographically
- Zone 2 evaluation—debate between mandatory surgical neck exploration versus selected surgical approach based on diagnostic tests (vascular and esophageal evaluation); emerging role of helical CT angiography in select, stable patients
- **Treatment**
    - Anticipatory airway control
    - Early consultation
    - Remember: do not probe neck wounds; IV antibiotics for suspected esophageal injury; perils

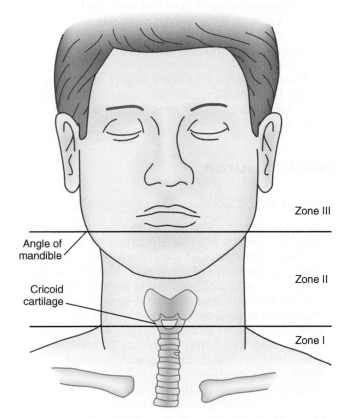

Figure 19-7. Zones of the neck. (From Marx JA, Hockberger RS, Walls RM, Adams J, Rosen P: *Rosen's emergency medicine: concepts and clinical practice,* ed 6, Philadelphia, 2006, Mosby.)

of orotracheal intubation in laryngotracheal injury (e.g., false passage)

BLUNT NECK TRAUMA

- Risk by frequency of occurrence
- High-risk structures—larynx/trachea/cricoid (rarely occult)
    - **Signs and symptoms**—subcutaneous emphysema, dyspnea, stridor, dysphonia, hemoptysis, significant or expanding hematoma, crepitus, significant pain/tenderness, neck pain with tongue movement
    - **Diagnosis**—direct laryngoscopy; CT
    - **Treatment**—early airway management; consultation and management by trauma/ENT surgeons
- Low-risk structures—esophagus (often occult), thoracic duct, glands, retropharyngeal, and vascular (intimal tear, thrombosis, dissection, pseudoaneurysm); with any new focal neurologic complaint after blunt neck trauma, consider nervous system and vascular causes
- *Hanging/strangulation*—consider high cervical fractures (hanging with body suspended after drop) uncommon in nonjudicial hangings; vascular occlusion > airway occlusion (and venous > arterial occlusion within vascular); thyroid cartilage/laryngeal/hyoid damage (cricoid rare); pulmonary edema/ARDS; cerebral edema
    - **Signs and symptoms**—ligature marks not universal, petechial hemorrhage (skin, conjunctiva, mucous membranes—*Tardieu spots*), neurologic deficits, coma, evidence of airway injury (as above)
    - **Diagnosis and treatment**—as above for blunt trauma

Thoracic trauma

GENERAL

- Complex compartment; assessment involves consideration of mechanism (penetrating vs. blunt), multiple structures (trachea, lungs, heart, great vessels, bony, esophageal, diaphragmatic, spine/neurologic)
- Thoracoabdominal injuries necessitate consideration of both compartments (diaphragmatic excursion makes point of entry and point of injury relative to diaphragmatic position)

TABLE 19-3 **Zones of Injury**

Zone 1	Zone 2	Zone 3
Sternal notch → cricoid	Cricoid → mandible angle	Mandible angle → skull base
■ Arteries (carotid, vertebral, subclavian)	■ Arteries (carotid, vertebral)	Arteries (carotid, vertebral)
■ Veins	■ Veins (jugular)	Veins (jugulars)
■ Lung apices	■ Trachea	Glands (parotid)
■ Trachea	■ Larynx	CN IX, XII
■ Esophagus	■ Pharynx	Spinal cord
■ Thyroid	■ Esophagus	
■ Thoracic duct	■ Nerves (vagus, rec. laryngeal)	
■ Spinal cord	■ Spinal cord	

BONY INJURY

- **Rib fracture**
  - **Signs and symptoms**—pain/tenderness, palpable crepitus/fracture; 4 to 9 most common
  - **Diagnosis**—x-ray (may be occult) and look for pneumothorax (PTX), hemothorax, and pulmonary contusion
  - **Treatment**—pain management; incentive spirometry; intercostal nerve block in selected patients
  - **Complicated rib fractures**—ribs 1 to 2 may portend more serious underlying injury when associated with other rib fractures (i.e., unless focal, direct blow); ribs 9 to 12 consider intra-abdominal injury (spleen, liver, kidney, as well as PTX), *flail chest* (2+ sites on 3+ ribs = flail chest segment; paradoxical movement of segment; risk for ventilatory failure)
- **Sternum fracture**
  - In MVC, restrained > unrestrained at risk for sternum fracture
  - Isolated fractures are benign; not associated with blunt aortic injury
  - Cardiac complications (e.g., contusion) about 1% to 6%; screen with ECG and troponin
  - Best seen on lateral x-ray; CT best for associated mediastinal injury
  - Treat associated conditions; analgesia for isolated fracture

PULMONARY INJURY

- **Pneumothorax (PTX)**—air in pleural space; can occur with penetrating > blunt thoracic trauma (rib fracture fragment or alveolar rupture due to increased pressure during inspiration/closed glottis)
  - Simple, communicating ("sucking chest wound"—lung collapse on inspiration), and tension (mediastinal shift away from wound with hemodynamic compromise)
  - **Signs and symptoms**—may be absent or subtle
    - Dyspnea, chest pain, tachypnea, tachycardia, distended neck veins, decreased or absent breath sounds, subcutaneous emphysema
    - Agitated/hypotensive/hypoxic/distended neck veins/in *extremis* → think tension
  - **Diagnosis**
    - Clinical, if signs of tension → needle decompression followed by tube thoracostomy *before* imaging
    - Chest x-ray (upright → apices; supine → extra-sharp heart border/deep sulcus sign) (Fig. 19-8)
    - CT very sensitive (clinical significance questionable for "occult PTX" seen only on CT—unless positive-pressure ventilation anticipated)
    - Ultrasound (absence of "sliding" of pleural layers past each other with breathing; horizontal lines or comet tails)
    - Penetrating chest trauma + negative chest x-ray = repeat chest x-ray in 3 hours (supplants "6-hour rule")

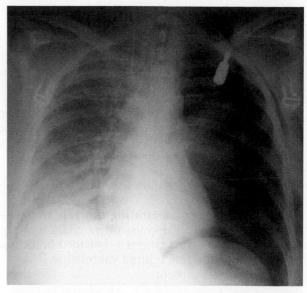

Figure 19-8. **Left-sided pneumothorax** seen on a supine chest radiograph demonstrating the deep sulcus sign and an unusually sharp left heart border. (From Adam A, Dixon AK, Grainger RG, Allison DJ: *Grainger and Allison's diagnostic radiology*, ed 5, Philadelphia, 2008, Churchill Livingstone.)

  - **Treatment**
    - Tube thoracostomy—not needle aspiration alone
    - Observation if isolated, asymptomatic, apical, <25% vs. observe only an occult PTX not undergoing positive-pressure ventilation/general anesthesia
- **Hemothorax (HTX)**—blood in the pleural space; penetrating or blunt mechanism—25% have PTX; more often from intercostal or mammary vessels than central vasculature
  - **Signs and symptoms**—similar to PTX
  - **Diagnosis**—blunted angles on upright chest x-ray approximates 200 to 300 mL; may appear as diffuse haziness on supine film, where larger volumes can be hidden
  - **Treatment**—tube thoracostomy with 36 to 40F tube; operative management if
    - 1000 to 1500 mL output immediately after tube placement
    - 200 mL/hr output for first 3 hours
- **Pulmonary contusion**—lung bruise with edema and hemorrhage but without laceration (Fig. 19-9)
  - **Signs and symptoms**—dyspnea, chest pain, hemoptysis, tachypnea, tachycardia, hypoxia (hypercarbic acidosis may develop); >80% have associated extrathoracic injury
  - **Diagnosis**—chest x-ray shows patchy infiltrate, always appears within 6 hours, lasts up to 72 hours; CT more sensitive
  - **Treatment**—supportive, limiting IV fluids, consider differential intubation and ventilation of unaffected/affected lung
- **Tracheobronchial injury**—penetrating and blunt trauma; can communicate with pleural space (PTX) or not (pneumomediastinum, air around bronchus,

occult/delayed); blunt more common cause of intrathoracic tracheobronchial injury (80% within 2 cm of carina)
- **Signs and symptoms**—significant air leak, hemoptysis, subcutaneous emphysema; Hamman crunch
- **Diagnosis**—chest x-ray (air around bronchus; pneumomediastinum; massive PTX); CT is better; suspect if persistent air leak (chest tube does not expand PTX and sustained bubbling of water-seal apparatus); bronchoscopy
- **Treatment**—intubate over scope if possible; high-frequency ventilation may be necessary to expand lung; surgery
- **Air embolism after penetrating thoracic trauma**—may occur with positive-pressure ventilation after chest wounds where air from a damaged bronchus enters the neighboring injured vasculature (risk clue: hemoptysis present)

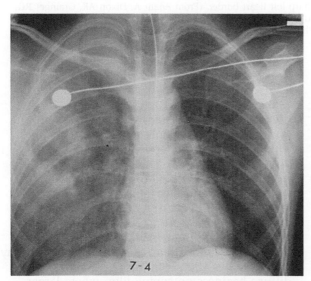

Figure 19-9. Chest film showing a pulmonary contusion. (From Townsend CM, Jr, Beauchamp RD, Evers BM, Mattox KL: *Sabiston's textbook of surgery,* ed 18, Philadelphia, 2007, Saunders.)

- **Signs and symptoms**—acute neurologic or dysrhythmic event after intubation for chest trauma
- **Diagnosis**—clinical
- **Treatment**—Trendelenburg positioning, ED thoracotomy to clamp injured pulmonary segment and aspirate air from heart/ascending aorta

CARDIOVASCULAR INJURY

- **Cardiac tamponade**—penetrating > blunt trauma; can temporarily prolong life by controlling hemorrhage but cause death when tamponade impedes diastolic function
  - **Signs and symptoms**—suspect when penetrating trauma in "the box" (right midclavicular line → left anterior axillary line, clavicles → xiphoid); Beck triad unreliable (hypotension, distended neck veins, muffled heart sounds); Kussmaul sign (neck veins distend paradoxically with inspiration); electrical alternans on monitor rare in acute tamponade
  - **Diagnosis**—clinical; FAST scan/transthoracic echocardiography (Fig. 19-10); transesophageal echocardiography if intubated; chest x-ray usually normal
  - **Treatment**—IV fluids; pericardiocentesis questionable; ED thoracotomy definitive in critical tamponade
- **Myocardial contusion**—blunt trauma resulting in cellular injury from focal hemorrhage in the cardiac muscle; less severe than *traumatic myocardial infarction*, which involves injury to the coronary artery and/or irreversible cellular death
  - **Signs and symptoms**—external evidence of chest trauma usual but not universal; chest pain; faster than expected tachycardia; mechanism important
  - **Diagnosis**—ECG (new conduction block [e.g., right bundle branch block], dysrhythmia, ST/T-wave changes); elevated troponins; echocardiography; no true criterion standard
  - **Treatment**—controversial; monitor and further evaluate those with significant ECG changes/elevated troponins; no aspirin/heparin

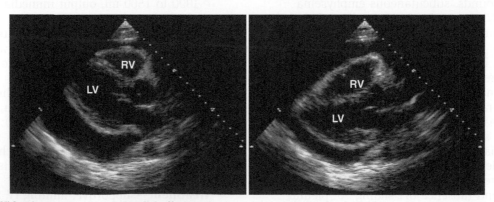

Figure 19-10. With a large amount of pericardial effusion, the heart has a swinging motion, which is an ominous sign of cardiac tamponade. When the left ventricular *(LV)* cavity is close to the surface *(left)*, the QRS voltage increases on the electrocardiogram, but it decreases when the LV swings away from the surface *(right)*, producing electrical alternans. *RV,* Right ventricle. (From Oh JK, Seward JB, Tajik AJ: *The echo manual,* ed 3, Philadelphia, 2006, Lippincott Williams & Wilkins. Used with permission of Mayo Foundation for Medical Education and Research.)

- **Blunt aortic injury**—mostly commonly injured thoracic vessel; suspect with high-speed MVC/fall from height (profound deceleration injuries); 80% to 90% of tears occur just distal to left subclavian artery; ascending aortic injury less common/usually associated with cardiac injury
  - **Signs and symptoms**—retrosternal, chest, or interscapular back pain; pseudo-coarctation syndrome (hypertension in arms with diminished femoral pulses); harsh systolic murmur (precordial or interscapular); physical examination unreliable and other injuries from severe mechanism may distract
  - **Diagnosis**—chest x-ray *may* show loss of aortic arch shadow, absence of aortopulmonary window, tracheal deviation to the right, widened paraspinal margins, displaced nasogastric tube, left apical pleural cap/hemothorax;
    - 12% of chest x-rays may be normal
    - Helical CT with contrast better test (and better than angiography); transesophageal ultrasound
  - **Treatment**—surgery (or surgical consultation and admission for "minimal aortic injury" on CT); blood pressure control (e.g., esmolol with systolic BP target of 100 to 120 mmHg)

ESOPHAGEAL INJURY

- Blunt or penetrating may cause perforation; may be rapidly fatal if missed; usually not isolated; presentation may be delayed or obscured by distracting injuries
  - **Signs and symptoms**—chest, back or epigastric pain, pleuritic, worse with swallowing; subcutaneous emphysema; Hamman sign (crunch on auscultation); toxic appearance later in course
  - **Diagnosis**—chest x-ray with pneumomediastinum, PTX, left-sided pleural effusion, wide mediastinum; initially water-soluble esophagram preferred because nonobscuring if endoscopy needed; CT
  - **Treatment**—early surgical consultation and repair; broad-spectrum IV antibiotics; volume

Abdominal trauma

PENETRATING ABDOMINAL TRAUMA

- Stab wounds (SW) > gunshot (GSW) wounds in frequency but not injury severity
- Liver > small bowel in frequency for SW but small bowel > large bowel > liver for GSW
- As in neck injury, do not probe penetrating abdominal wounds in the ED
- *Juxtadiaphragmatic injuries* prompt concern for thoracic as well as abdominal injury
- Also consider retroperitoneal, genitourinary, and spinal injury
- **Signs and symptoms**—serial examinations are important; hypotension seen initially is usually suggestive of solid organ or vascular injury

- Wounds in the lower thorax to the level of the greater trochanter, as well as back and flank are candidates for peritoneal violation
- **Diagnosis**—laboratory tests seldom diagnostic but serve as baseline; plain x-rays are helpful for foreign bodies (e.g., bullet fragments)
  - **Ultrasound**—FAST scan useful if positive (for hemoperitoneum and hemopericardium, vs. look-alikes—ascites and pericardial effusion, respectively) and when used serially in patients under surgical observation
    - Threshold debatable—probably 100 to 500 mL of free fluid
    - Misses retroperitoneal, solid organ, hollow viscus, and diaphragmatic injury
    - Negative FAST does not exclude serious injury
  - **CT scan**—most useful in retroperitoneal or flank wounds when the abdominal examination and apparent trajectory do not suggest peritoneal violation
  - **Diagnostic peritoneal lavage** (see Chapter 21, Procedures) is less useful in penetrating than blunt abdominal trauma *(see below)*, as threshold for surgical exploration is open to debate.
  - **Local wound exploration**—if anterior fascia not violated, peritoneum is intact; best left in the hands of experienced surgeons/traumatologists
- **Management**
  - **Surgical management**—in the form of observation, extended workup, local wound exploration, laparoscopy, laparotomy, etc.
    - *Laparotomy indications* include hemodynamic instability, peritoneal signs, evisceration, diaphragmatic injury, GI bleeding (rare), free air in the abdomen, implement *in situ*

BLUNT ABDOMINAL TRAUMA

- Spleen > > liver > bowel in injury frequency; MVC most common mechanism of injury; beware solitary lap belt for injury (worse than shoulder/lap); consider diaphragmatic rupture with abdominal compressive injuries.
- **Signs and symptoms**—hypotension seen initially is usually suggestive of solid organ or, less commonly, vascular injury; serial examinations are important in stable patients
- **Diagnosis**—laboratory tests seldom diagnostic but serve as baseline; plain x-rays are of limited utility (except chest x-ray)
  - **Ultrasound**—FAST scan useful if positive
  - **CT scan**—most useful diagnostic test in stable patient with blunt abdominal trauma; sees solid organs, hollow viscus and retroperitoneal well
  - **Diagnostic peritoneal lavage** (see Chapter 21, Procedures)—positive DPL in blunt trauma = (1) initial aspiration of 10 mL of frank blood; (2) after 1 L saline irrigation with at least 250 mL return: 100,000 RBC/mm^3, and 20,000 to 100,000 is indeterminate; (3) pelvic fracture complicates interpretation (false positive lavage, but frank

blood aspiration still compelling, should be performed open); misses retroperitoneal/lone hollow viscus injuries as would FAST
- **Management**
  - **Surgical management**—in the form of observation, extended workup, local wound exploration, laparoscopy, laparotomy, etc.
    - *Laparotomy indications* include hemodynamic instability attributable to the injury, peritoneal signs, diaphragmatic injury, GI bleeding (rare), free air in the abdomen

Pelvic, thoracolumbar, and hip trauma

PELVIC FRACTURES

- **General**
  - *Bony pelvis* consists of coccyx, sacrum, and innominate bones (consisting of ilium, ischium, and pubis) with stability maintained by ligaments, which may be disrupted in trauma—consider as anterior and posterior arches
  - Rich adjacent *vasculature* lies posteriorly and may be disrupted (along with marrow blood loss), causing retroperitoneal hematoma. Blood

loss in high-grade pelvic fractures is significant and a major contributor to mortality
- *Neurologic* structures include the cauda equina → lumbar and sacral plexi—trauma may cause bowel/bladder/genital dysfunction
- *Organs*: bladder, urethra, prostate, uterus, vagina, and lower colon
- **Signs and symptoms**
  - Pain, paresthesias (as above), gross hematuria, ecchymoses (e.g., perineal), leg length difference; use cautious compression of iliac crests/symphysis pubis for stability
  - Rectal examination for displaced prostate, blood, sensation, and tone; penile examination for blood at the meatus, sensation. Bony irregularity or fragments may be encountered on recto-vaginal examination
- **Diagnosis**
  - **Pelvic x-ray** includes AP, inlet/outlet views. Look for symmetry, and normal width of pubic symphysis (≤5 mm) and sacroiliac joints (2 to 4 mm) and various fractures
  - **CT**—imaging view of choice due to superior visualization of fracture and can detect hematoma, bladder integrity (CT cystography). Classification of pelvic fractures is varied and complex—one is the *Tile system* (Table 19-4)

TABLE 19-4 Pelvic Fractures—by Tile's classification

Tile's Type A: (Fig. 19-11) **Pelvic ring is *stable;* low-energy fractures** A1 Avulsion fracture, innominate A2 Stable iliac wing or ring fracture with minimal displacement A3 Transverse sacral/coccyx fracture	■ 33% all pelvic fractures ■ Heal well with rest, analgesia ■ Avulsion from muscle contraction ■ Iliac wing—check acetabulum ■ Superior/inferior pubic ramus—{1} ■ Sacral—upper differs from lower {2} ■ Coccyx—usually conservative treatment
Tile's Type B: **Pelvic ring is *partially stable*; high energy (rotation unstable; vertically stable)** B1 Unilateral open book B2 Lateral compression injury {3} (Fig. 19-12) B3 Bilateral, Type B	■ High-energy injuries ■ Frequent association with intraperitoneal injury, retroperitoneal hematoma ■ Double break in pelvic ring = serious injury ■ Pubic symphysis wide or adjacent fracture ■ Hinge = posterior SI joint vs. adjacent fracture ■ Neurologic and vascular injury ■ Rami: double fracture or overriding *anteriorly* ■ Sacral fracture/ligament disruption *posteriorly* ■ Pubic symphysis wide or adjacent fracture ■ Hinge = posterior SI joint vs. adjacent fracture ■ Neurologic and vascular injury
Tiles Type C: (Fig. 19-13) **Pelvic ring is *unstable* {4}; high energy (rotation and vertically)** C1 Unilateral C2 Bilateral (one side B, one side C) C3 Bilateral (both sides C)	■ Vertical shear forces → ligamentous and/or bone injury ■ Hemipelvis displaces posteriorly and/or rostrally ■ *Anteriorly*—symphyseal disruption or multiple pubic ramus fractures. ■ Significant neurologic, vascular injury
Highlights of pelvic fractures 1. **Isolate pubic ramus (A2)**—most common fracture of pelvis; seen often in elderly 2. **Transverse sacral (A3)**—upper fractures present with local and referred pain (gluteal, perirectal, posterior thighs) and neurologic injury is common. May need surgery to correct. Lower fractures may present similarly, but are usually without neurologic injury and usually do not need surgical fixation. 3. **Lateral compression fractures (B2)**—typically require lower fluid requirements in resuscitation than do AP compression and vertical shear injuries. 4. **Clues to Type C posterior arch injury**—look for signs of significant ligamentous injury (avulsion at L5 transverse process, ischial spine, lower lateral sacrum) or vertical translation (displacement of pubic ramus fracture; sacral foramina are asymmetric)	

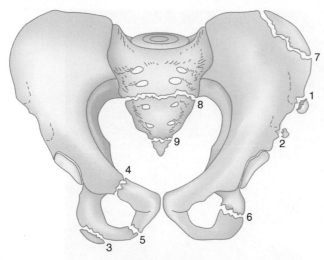

Figure 19-11. Fractures of individual pelvic bones. **1,** Avulsion of anterosuperior iliac spine; **2,** avulsion of anteroinferior iliac spine; **3,** avulsion of ischial tuberosity; **4,** fracture of superior pubic ramus; **5,** fracture of inferior pubic ramus; **6,** fracture of ischial ramus; **7,** fracture of iliac wing; **8,** transverse fracture of sacrum; **9,** fracture of coccyx. (From Marx JA, Hockberger RS, Walls RM, Adams J, Rosen P: *Rosen's emergency medicine: concepts and clinical practice,* ed 6, Philadelphia, 2006, Mosby.)

- **Treatment**
  - Complex pelvic fractures have high morbidity and mortality
    - Vertical shear mortality (Tile's C) = 25%
    - AP compression mortality 14% to 26%
    - Major blood transfusion possibilities—AP > vertical shear > lateral compression in one study
  - *Embolization* used to control hemorrhage
  - Early *orthopedic consultation* for operative fixation
    - Consider other significant injuries with significant pelvic fractures

THORACOLUMBAR SPINE FRACTURES

- Thoracolumbar junction second to cervical in frequency of spine injury
- Thoracic spine more stable than cervical, but neurologic findings common with fractures
- Lumbar cord terminates at L1; continues as conus medullaris → cauda equina; nerve roots are less often injured with lumbar spine fracture

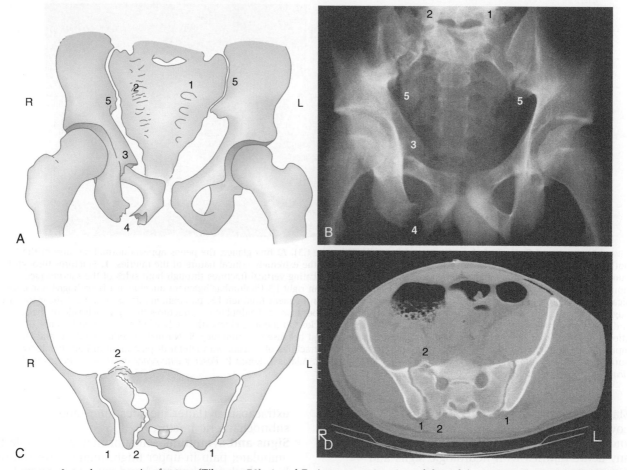

Figure 19-12. Lateral compression fracture (Tile type B2). **A** and **B,** Anteroposterior view of the pelvis. **1,** Normal sacral foraminal lines on the left; **2,** sacral foraminal lines on the right are indistinct and do not mirror the normal side, indicating the subtle second break in the pelvic ring; **3** and **4,** fractures of the superior and inferior pubic rami are overriding and displaced, indicating the lateral compression forces (there must be a second break in the pelvic ring); **5,** normal sacroiliac joints. **C** and **D,** Computed tomography scan of same pelvis. **1,** Normal sacroiliac joints; **2,** compression fracture of the sacrum through the foramen corresponding to the loss of definition of the foraminal lines in **A** and **B.** (From Marx JA, Hockberger RS, Walls RM, Adams J, Rosen P: *Rosen's emergency medicine: concepts and clinical practice,* ed 6, Philadelphia, 2006, Mosby.)

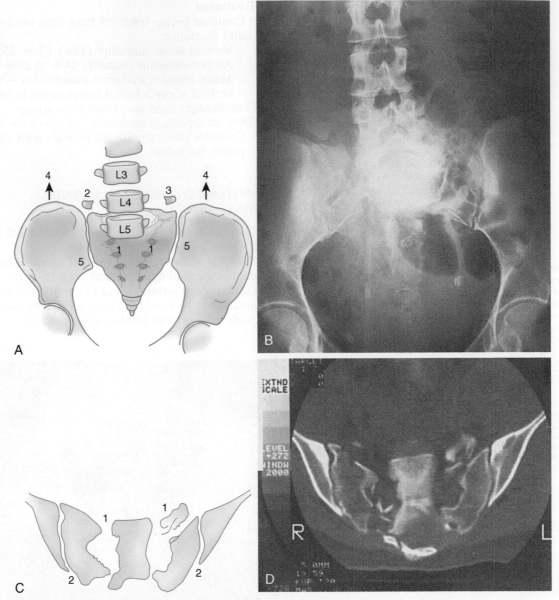

Figure 19-13. **A** and **B,** Vertical shear fractures bilaterally (Tile type C3). At first glance, the pelvis appears normal because of the smooth, uninterrupted arcuate line, but careful interpretation reveals the extremely critical nature of the injuries: **1,** Fractures through the sacrum—note loss of definition and symmetry of sacral foramina indicating vertical fractures through both sides of the sacrum (see computed tomography scan in **D**). **2,** Transverse process fragment from right L5 (iliolumbar ligament attachment) is pathognomonic for a vertical shear fracture through the right sacrum. **3,** Transverse process fragment from left L5, pathognomonic for a vertical shear fracture through the left sacrum. **4,** Both hemipelves are dislocated cephalad because of the double-ring fractures through each side of the sacrum. This dislocation explains why the L5 transverse processes appear so close to the iliac crests (the body of L5 is obscured because of rotational dislocation of the central free sacral fragment posteriorly and because of technique). **5,** Normal sacroiliac joints. **C** and **D,** Computed tomography scan of same pelvis. **1,** Bilateral comminuted fractures of sacrum with lateral displacement of both hemipelves; **2,** normal sacroiliac joints. (From Marx JA, Hockberger RS, Walls RM, Adams J, Rosen P: *Rosen's emergency medicine: concepts and clinical practice,* ed 6, Philadelphia, 2006, Mosby.)

- Major and minor fractures (Table 19-5)
- Low threshold for advanced imaging (e.g., CT) and spine consultation with acute bony injuries or any acute injuries with neurologic signs and symptoms

HIP FRACTURES

- Include those of the acetabulum and proximal femur; fractures can be considered intra- vs.

extracapsular (latter includes inter- and subtrochanteric fractures)
- **Signs and symptoms**—may or may not be able to ambulate; pain in upper thigh, inguinal region, or knee; look for shortened and externally rotated leg; if absent, proceed to gentle rotation of extended leg—if significant pain, proceed to imaging; if not, gentle range of motion of hip. Hypotension may occur with significant fractures, but other sources should be ruled out (e.g., spine,

TABLE 19-5 **Major and Minor Spine Fractures**

Wedge compression fracture (major/usually stable, but unstable until defined otherwise by CT)	■ Loss of anterior height on x-ray ■ CT defines posterior spine/canal involvement ■ Usually no neurologic deficit
Burst fracture (Fig. 19-14) (major/unstable)	■ Loss of anterior and posterior height on x-ray ■ CT defines stability
Chance fracture (Fig. 19-15) (major/unstable)	■ Classic—lap belt with high speed MVC ■ Spinous process, lamina, pedicles, vertebral body and transverse processes fractured
Flexion-distraction injury (major/unstable)	■ Loss of anterior height on x-ray ■ Spreading out of interspinous spaces posteriorly
Translation injury (major/unstable)	■ One vertebral body translates on adjacent segment(s) ■ Neurologic injury common
Spinous process fracture Transverse process fracture Pars interarticularis fracture	■ All minor and stable ■ CT evaluates related nonorthopedic injury as well as for possible major thoracolumbar spine fractures

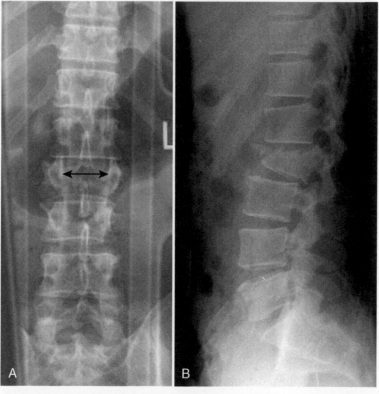

Figure 19-14. Lumbar burst fracture. **A,** Anteroposterior radiograph shows loss of height of L2 and widening of the pedicles are forced laterally *(double-headed arrow)* with body compression. **B,** Lateral view shows significant loss of height of L2 and marked posterior retropulsion of the posterior cortical bone nearly occluding the spinal canal. (From Browner BD, Levine AM, Jupiter JB, Trafton PG, Krettek C: *Skeletal trauma,* ed 4, Philadelphia, 2008, Saunders.)

abdominal, pelvic). Check neurovascular status distally
■ **Diagnosis**—AP and lateral x-ray; occult fracture better detected by CT or MR imaging.
■ **Management/treatment** (early)
  ■ **Acetabular**—affects weight bearing; associated with sciatic nerve injury. Orthopedic consultation/admission

■ **Femoral head**—uncommon in isolation and more often seen with dislocation; avascular necrosis (AVN) may result from dislocation; urgent reduction/orthopedic consultation, possible surgery
■ **Femoral neck**—associated with osteoporosis; proximal-to-distal classified subcapital (most common), transcervical, and basicervical; AVN

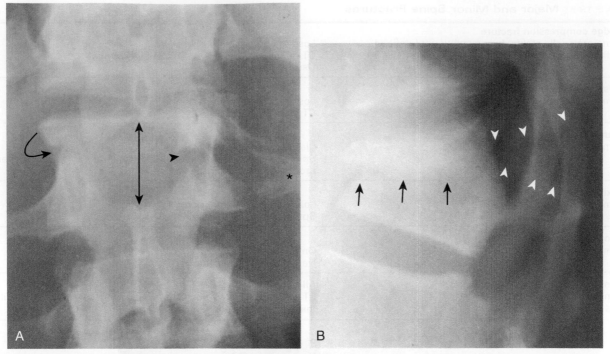

Figure 19-15. **Chance fracture of L1.** The frontal projection (**A**) shows a comminuted fracture of the left transverse process (*), transverse fracture of the left pedicle *(arrowhead)*, separation of the T12 and L1 laminae and spinous processes *(double arrow)* and a fracture of the right superolateral cortex of L1 *(curved arrow)*. In the lateral projection (**B**), the arrowheads indicate a distracted transverse fracture of the spinous process and laminae and the arrows indicate the horizontal fracture of the body with anterior wedging. (From Adam A, Dixon AK, Grainger RG, Allison DJ: *Grainger and Allison's diagnostic radiology*, ed 5, Philadelphia, 2008, Churchill Livingstone.)

may result. Orthopedic consultation, no traction (interferes with blood supply), surgery.

- **Trochanteric—greater** (avulsion of gluteus medius or direct impact) or **lesser** (avulsion of iliopsoas)
  - Generally have limping gait preserved
  - Amount of displacement of fracture fragment determines need for possible orthopedic surgery
  - May be discharged on crutches, weight bearing as tolerated, and with orthopedic follow-up
- **Intertrochanteric**—associated with osteoporosis; AVN less likely; traction and orthopedic consultation; surgery
- **Subtrochanteric**—associated with osteoporosis in elderly and high-energy injury in younger population; coincident large-volume blood loss possible; Hare or Sager traction splint; orthopedic consultation, surgery
- **Femoral shaft**—are not truly hip fractures; suggests high energy trauma in younger cohort; profound blood loss may occur; Hare or Sager traction splint; orthopedic consultation, surgery

HIP DISLOCATION

- Associated with high-energy injury (usually MVC) and suggests major trauma; approximately 80% to 90% are posterior; urgent reduction (hours) is key and the sooner, the better; look for associated

femoral neck/shaft fractures (precludes closed reduction of the hip dislocation)
- **Posterior dislocations**—leg presents shortened, adducted, and internally rotated; associated with acetabular and femoral head fractures; associated sciatic nerve injury (10%) and AVN (directly related to time to reduction)
- **Anterior dislocations**—leg presents abducted and externally rotated, with knee flexion if anteroinferior dislocations; associated with sciatic nerve injury and AVN
- **Hip prosthetic dislocations**—can occur with seemingly trivial mechanisms of injury (thus, a low threshold to image is key); resultant AVN not an issue but sciatic nerve injury is; prosthetic component disturbance and fracture of adjacent bone during reduction can occur

Genitourinary trauma

GENERAL

- Involves penetrating vs. blunt mechanisms as well as upper (renal, ureters) vs. lower tract (bladder, urethra) vs. genital injury; signs (e.g., hematuria) may be nonspecific and nonlocalizing
- **Signs and symptoms**—pain, swelling, local ecchymosis or hematoma, blood at the meatus (urethral injury → Foley catheter contraindicated), high-riding prostate (posterior urethral injury →

Foley catheter contraindicated), hematuria (gross vs. microscopic discussed below)
- **Diagnosis** and **Treatment**—discussed below

PENETRATING TRAUMA

- Suspicion for genitourinary (GU) injury by mechanism or clinical signs/symptoms should be imaged if stable; unstable patients can undergo the less-than-optimal single-image intravenous pyelogram while in the OR
- **Signs and symptoms**—are nonspecific and insensitive; hematuria or its absence lacks predictive value of injury to the upper tract
- **Diagnosis**—imaging is based on mechanism and proximity, and CT with IV contrast is best for possible upper tract injury; ureteral injury is rare
- **Treatment**—surgical consultation with likely intervention

BLUNT TRAUMA

- Causes GU injury far more commonly than penetrating
- Signs and symptoms again lack predictive value
- Gross hematuria or hemodynamic instability mandate imaging of some kind, depending upon mechanism and associated injury (e.g., deceleration—renal pedicle, pelvic fracture—bladder/urethra, straddle injury—urethra)—see below.
- **Management** involves GU consultation for operative vs. conservative treatment course depending upon the injury and associated trauma
- **Renal injury**
    - *Renal pedicle*—mechanism of rapid deceleration; renal artery thrombosis from intimal disruption most common; CT with IV contrast is the best study
    - *Renal contusion*—most common injury to kidney (>90%); best seen on CT with IV contrast. Presence of microscopic hematuria alone in the stable adult blunt trauma victim (including no episodes of hypotension) does not mandate imaging if renal contusion is suspected; outpatient follow-up ensuring clearing of the hematuria is recommended
    - *Renal laceration*—often causes perirenal hematoma; CT with IV contrast is the best study
    - *Renal pelvis rupture*—more rare; kidney fills through calyceal system then contrast extravasates on CT; if missed, presents with high fever, flank/abdominal pain, may be toxic in appearance
- **Bladder injury**—high association with pelvic fracture; includes contusion and rupture (extraperitoneal > intraperitoneal); cystography or CT cystography are the best studies
- **Urethral injury**—may be posterior (pelvic fractures) or anterior (direct trauma, straddle injury, pelvic fracture); retrograde urethrogram (Fig. 19-16) is best test
    - Very uncommon in women, as urethra is short

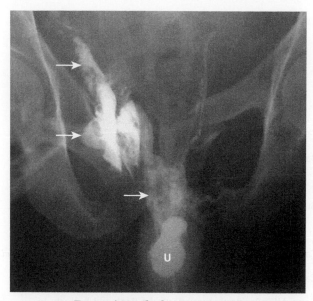

Figure 19-16. **Traumatic urethral injury.** Retrograde urethrogram shows opacification of the anterior urethra (U) and extravasation of contrast medium *(arrows)* from the urethra. (From Adam A, Dixon AK, Grainger RG, Allison DJ: *Grainger and Allison's diagnostic radiology,* ed 5, Philadelphia, 2008, Churchill Livingstone.)

PEARLS

- Ten percent of patients with stab wounds to the kidney will not have hematuria.

- In the trauma patient, blood at the meatus mandates retrograde urethrography before Foley catheter placement to assess for urethral laceration.

- Narrowing of the pulse pressure precedes frank hypotension in circulatory shock.

- Isolated microscopic hematuria in the stable adult blunt trauma victim does not mandate imaging, except in those with rapid deceleration injury or hypotension (transient or persistent).

- Subacute or chronic subdural hematoma may be isodense or hypodense to brain tissue on noncontrast CT; look for effacement, shift, and compression of adjacent sulci/gyri.

- Tangential gunshot wounds to the head (scalp injured; skull appears to be intact) are best evaluated with CT scan even in neurologically intact patients to exclude epidural hematoma from blast effect.

- Penetrating injury to the neck is defined as that which violates the platysma muscle; do not probe penetrating neck wounds.

- Hemothorax appears as a hazy hemithorax on supine chest films.

- With significant deceleration injury, remember blunt aortic and renal pedicle trauma.

■ Pelvic fractures with hypotension should spark interventional radiology consultation as well as orthopedic.

■ Ability to ambulate does not preclude the presence of a hip fracture.

BIBLIOGRAPHY

Baron BJ: Penetrating and blunt neck trauma. In Tintinalli JE, Kelen GD, Stapczynski JS (eds): *Emergency medicine: a comprehensive study guide*, New York, 2004, McGraw-Hill, pp. 1590–1595.

Buchman TG, Hall BL, Bowling WM, Kelen GD: Thoracic trauma. In Tintinalli JE, Kelen GD, Stapczynski JS (eds): *Emergency medicine: a comprehensive study guide*, New York, 2004, McGraw-Hill, pp. 1595–1613.

Cambridge TM, Small E, Bernhardt DT: Concussion [letter], *N Engl J Med* 356:1788, 2007.

Cantu RC, Herring SA, Putukian M: Concussion [letter], *N Engl J Med* 356:1787, 2007.

Conn AKT: Penetrating trauma to the flank and buttock. In Tintinalli JE, Kelen GD, Stapczynski JS (eds): *Emergency medicine: a comprehensive study guide*, New York, 2004, McGraw-Hill, pp. 1620–1622.

Cornwell EE: Initial approach to trauma. In Tintinalli JE, Kelen GD, Stapczynski JS (eds): *Emergency medicine: a comprehensive study guide*, New York, 2004, McGraw-Hill, pp. 1537–1542.

Cwinn AA: Pelvis. In Marx JA, Hockberger RS, Walls RM et al (eds): *Rosen's emergency medicine: concepts and clinical practice*, ed 6, Philadelphia, 2006, Mosby, pp. 717–734.

Eckstein M, Henderson S: Thoracic trauma. In Marx JA, Hockberger RS, Walls RM et al (eds): *Rosen's emergency medicine: concepts and clinical practice*, ed 6, Philadelphia, 2006, Mosby, pp. 453–488.

Gibbs MA, Newton EJ, Fiechtl JF: Femur and hip. In Marx JA, Hockberger RS, Walls RM et al (eds): *Rosen's emergency medicine: concepts and clinical practice*, ed 6, Philadelphia, 2006, Mosby, pp. 735–769.

Gin-Shaw SL, Jordan RC: Multiple trauma. In Marx JA, Hockberger RS, Walls RM et al (eds): *Rosen's emergency medicine: concepts and clinical practice*, ed 6, Philadelphia, 2006, Mosby, pp. 300–316.

Graham RH, Mulrooney BC: Cararact, traumatic. Available at www.emedicine.medscape.com/1211083.

Hasan N, Colucciello SA: Maxillofacial trauma. In Tintinalli JE, Kelen GD, Stapczynski JS (eds): *Emergency medicine: a comprehensive study guide*, New York, 2004, McGraw-Hill, pp. 1583–1590.

Heegaard WG, Biros MH: Head. In Marx JA, Hockberger RS, Walls RM et al (eds): *Rosen's emergency medicine: concepts and clinical practice*, ed 6, Philadelphia, 2006, Mosby, pp. 349–381.

Kirsch TD, Lipinski CA: Head injury. In Tintinalli JE, Kelen GD, Stapczynski JS (eds): *Emergency medicine: a comprehensive study guide*. New York, 2004, McGraw-Hill, pp. 1557–1569.

Larkin GL: Retinal detachment. Available at www.emedicine.medscape.com/798501.

Larson JL: Injuries to the spine. In Tintinalli JE, Kelen GD, Stapczynski JS (eds): *Emergency medicine: a comprehensive study guide*, New York, 2004, McGraw-Hill, pp. 1703–1712.

Levy F, Kelen GD: Genitourinary trauma. In Tintinalli JE, Kelen GD, Stapczynski JS (eds): *Emergency medicine: a comprehensive study guide*, New York, 2004, McGraw-Hill, pp. 1622–1629.

Mannucci PM, Levi M: Prevention and treatment of major blood loss, *N Engl J Med* 356:2301–2311, 2007.

Marx JA, Isenhour J: Abdominal trauma. In Marx JA, Hockberger RS, Walls RM et al (eds): *Rosen's emergency medicine: concepts and clinical practice*, ed 6, Philadelphia, 2006, Mosby, pp. 489–514.

McKay MP: Facial trauma. In Marx JA, Hockberger RS, Walls RM et al (eds): *Rosen's emergency medicine: concepts and clinical practice*, ed 6, Philadelphia, 2006, Mosby, pp. 382–398.

Meredith JW, Hoth JJ: Thoracic trauma: when and how to intervene, *Surg Clin North Am* 87:95–118, 2007.

Mitchell JD: Ocular emergencies. In Tintinalli JE, Kelen GD, Stapczynski JS (eds): *Emergency medicine: a comprehensive study guide*, New York, 2004, McGraw-Hill, pp. 1449–1464.

Neschis DG, Scalea TM, Flinn WR, Griffith BP: Blunt aortic injury, *N Engl J Med* 359:1708–1716, 2008.

Newton K: Neck. In Marx JA, Hockberger RS, Walls RM et al (eds): *Rosen's emergency medicine: concepts and clinical practice*, ed 6, Philadelphia, 2006, Mosby, pp. 441–453.

Rathlev NK, Medzon R, Bracken ME: Evaluation and management of neck trauma, *Emerg Med Clin North Am* 25:679–694, 2007.

Ropper AH, Gorson KC: Concussion, *N Engl J Med* 356:166–172, 2007.

Scalea TM, Boswell SA: Abdominal injuries. In Tintinalli JE, Kelen GD, Stapczynski JS (eds): *Emergency medicine: a comprehensive study guide*, New York, 2004, McGraw-Hill, pp. 1613–1620.

Schneider RE: Genitourinary system. In Marx JA, Hockberger RS, Walls RM et al (eds): *Rosen's emergency medicine: concepts and clinical practice*, ed 6, Philadelphia, 2006, Mosby, pp. 514–536.

Steele MT, Ellison SR: Trauma to the pelvis, hip, and femur. In Tintinalli JE, Kelen GD, Stapczynski JS (eds): *Emergency medicine: a comprehensive study guide*, New York, 2004, McGraw-Hill, pp. 1712–1726.

Questions and Answers

1. Transverse fractures to the upper segments of the sacral spine:
   a. present with lower back pain radiating to the anterior thigh
   b. commonly involve neurologic injury
   c. present with lower back pain radiating to the umbilicus
   d. usually heal well with conservative management (bedrest, analgesia, laxatives, and sitz baths)

2. Which of the following cases portends a high risk of injury severity and would benefit from early triage to trauma center care?

   a. 20-year-old fell off bicycle with wrist pain/swelling as the only complaint
   b. 80-year-old confused all day after fall in kitchen; takes metoprolol, warfarin, and gemfibrozil; awake, not speaking, lethargic, and moving all extremities symmetrically but randomly, without external signs of major trauma and normal vital signs
   c. 33-year-old with stab wound to the palm of the hand, with stable vital signs and normal neurovascular examination of the affected hand
   d. 44-year-old in MVC who had to be extricated from vehicle (7 minutes) after impact to his

door without significant intrusion; no loss of consciousness, complaining of neck, shoulder, and ankle pain with a normal screening neurological examination.

3. A 22-year-old male presents with a deep, knife-wound laceration to the medial upper arm, with significant bleeding noted on his clothes. His vital signs are: heart rate (HR) = 122 beats per minute (bpm), respiratory rate (RR) = 28/minute, blood pressure (BP) = 86/68 mmHg, and oxygen saturation = 99% on room air. He is diaphoretic and anxious, but cooperative. The distal extremity is slightly cool, with delayed capillary refill and a weak but detectable radial pulse. Initial management should include:

   a. manual direct pressure to the wound
   b. blind clamping of the brachial vessels with a Lauer clamp
   c. application of an arterial tourniquet to the arm proximal to the wound
   d. local exploration of the wound at the bedside to exclude arterial injury

4. The most common CT abnormality after traumatic brain injury is:

   a. diffuse axonal injury
   b. cerebral contusion
   c. subdural hematoma
   d. subarachnoid hemorrhage

5. In acute cardiac tamponade after stab wound to the chest, the chest x-ray can be expected to show:

   a. a water-bottle heart
   b. an enlarged right (more often than left) ventricular shadow on x-ray
   c. a normal cardiac silhouette
   d. concomitant pneumothorax

6. A 40-year-old woman presents with several slashes to the neck and upper arms after a knife fight. She has no significant past medical history, and her vital signs are normal. The injuries to her upper arms appear superficial, and her peripheral pulses are equal and full with normal capillary refill noted. On examination of the neck, violation of the _____ would suggest the potential for injury to vital neck structures (e.g., major vessels, nerves).

   a. platysma muscle
   b. sternocleidomastoid muscle
   c. dermal layer of skin
   d. deep cervical fascia

7. A 23-year-old man presents after being stabbed in the chest with an ice pick. Intravenous drug paraphernalia were found by police at the scene. He has no past medical history. On examination, his HR is 128 bpm, his RR is 30/minute, and his blood pressure is 68/48 mmHg. He is ashen, diaphoretic, and agitated. His pupils are 2 mm

bilaterally. His neck veins are slightly distended, and the trachea is mildly deviated to the left. His heart sounds are faint. His lungs sounds are audible bilaterally, but seem louder on the left. There is a small aperture stab wound at the midaxillary line in the right chest, without subcutaneous emphysema. His abdomen is soft. IV access is obtained. Emergency department management should include:

   a. rapid sequence endotracheal intubation → chest x-ray → tube thoracostomy for pneumothorax if evident
   b. nasotracheal intubation → chest x-ray → tube thoracostomy for pneumothorax if evident
   c. tube thoracostomy of the right chest → chest x-ray for assessment
   d. needle decompression of right chest → tube thoracostomy → chest x-ray for assessment
   e. naloxone 2 mg intravenously → assess response → chest x-ray → tube thoracostomy for pneumothorax if evident

8. After head injury, most significant extracranial hematomas form under the:

   a. subcutaneous layer
   b. galea aponeurosis
   c. prepontine cistern
   d. pericranium

9. A burst fracture of the first vertebral body of the lumbar spine after a jump from significant height:

   a. involves loss of anterior but not posterior height of the vertebral body on lateral x-ray
   b. is considered a stable fracture
   c. is also called a Chance fracture
   d. should be evaluated by CT scan to assess extent and stability

10. Radiographic signs suggestive of blunt aortic injury after severe deceleration injury in an MVC include:

    a. Hamman sign
    b. opacification of aortopulmonary window
    c. pneumomediastinum
    d. Westermark's sign

11. Which of the following causes cerebral vasoconstriction?

    a. hypocarbia
    b. hypercarbia
    c. hypotension
    d. hypotension and hypocarbia

12. A 44-year-old man awaiting head CT after blunt head trauma develops a progressively depressed level of consciousness. He smells of alcohol and is verbally unresponsive. His pupillary examination reveals the left to be round and reactive to light, but the right to be round, dilated and nonreactive. His gag reflex is intact. Motor examination reveals withdrawal to pain on the right side but flaccidity on the left. You suspect epidural hematoma and:

a. transtentorial central herniation
b. cerebellar tonsillar herniation
c. uncal herniation
d. thiamine deficiency

13. A 30-year-old male presents with a gunshot wound to the abdomen. He is awake, alert, but slightly agitated. His skin is mildly diaphoretic. His vital signs are: HR = 118 bpm, BP = 106/90 mmHg, RR = 26/minute, and oxygen saturation = 99% on room air. Physical examination reveals a single gunshot wound to the right upper quadrant of the abdomen with no exit wound noted; his breath sounds are equal and clear bilaterally. The rectal examination is negative for occult or gross blood. You estimate that he has lost _____ % of his blood volume.

a. <15
b. 15 to 30
c. 30 to 40
d. >40

14. Clinical evidence of a basilar skull fracture includes:

a. Cushing reflex
b. Post-traumatic hearing loss
c. Cullen sign
d. Unilateral fixed and dilated pupil with depressed mental status
e. Papilledema

15. A 23-year-old man presents after being punched in the left eye. He complains of pain, swelling, and vague numbness of his ipsilateral cheek and upper teeth. His midface is stable, but there is swelling and tenderness of the inferior orbital region and maxilla. There is no hyphema and the visual acuity is normal. It is important to test for _____ while he is gazing _____.

a. diplopia/downward
b. nystagmus/downward
c. diplopia/upward
d. nystagmus/upward

16. A patient has a stab wound to the neck from an ice pick, located between the sternocleidomastoid muscle and the larynx, with stable vital signs and no obvious airway or neurovascular compromise on initial evaluation. This constitutes a _____ injury and might best be managed by _____.

a. Zone I/angiography
b. Zone II/angiography
c. Zone I/surgical neck exploration
d. Zone II/surgical neck exploration
e. Zone III/surgical neck exploration and angiography

17. The threshold indication for urgent thoracotomy in the operating suite by the trauma surgeon in a patient with a stab wound to the right chest is _____ of blood through the chest tube immediately after placement.

a. 2000 mL
b. 1500 mL
c. 750 mL
d. 500 mL

18. Threshold findings reasonably consistent with a "positive" diagnostic peritoneal lavage in the setting of significant blunt abdominal trauma include:

a. any gross blood on aspiration
b. after 1 L saline infusion followed by ≥1 L return, >5000 RBC/mm³
c. after 1 L saline infusion followed by ≥500 mL return, >10,000 RBC/mm³
d. after 1 L saline infusion followed by ≥250 mL return, >100,000 RBC/mm³
e. after 1 L saline infusion, return of gross blood >250 mL

19. Which hip fracture has the highest association with major blood loss, perhaps even leading to shock?

a. trochanteric
b. femoral head
c. femoral neck
d. subtrochanteric

20. A 34-year-old man presents after an assault with fists and blunt objects; he reports "balling up" in the fetal position to protect himself. He has no past medical history, takes ibuprofen for knee pain, and is not intoxicated. There was no loss of consciousness. He complains of diffuse pain over the back and flanks, as well as the posterior thighs and upper arms. On examination, his vital signs are normal. The trachea is midline, the neck is nontender. His lungs are clear and the ribs are mildly tender on the left posterior thorax. The abdomen is soft and nontender. There is mild to moderate tenderness over the paraspinal back, flanks, posterior thorax, and arms, without significant bruising or swelling. There is swelling and point tenderness over his mid-forearm on the ulnar aspect. Workup includes an x-ray of the forearm (incomplete fracture of the ulna, midshaft), a chest x-ray (normal), and a urinalysis (no gross hematuria; on microscopy, 30 to 50 RBCs/HPF). In addition to splinting of the forearm fracture and analgesia, what is the most appropriate disposition?

a. admit for serial urinalyses
b. ED urologic consultation
c. intravenous pyelogram, single view
d. CT of the abdomen with IV contrast
e. discharge with outpatient follow-up to ensure clearing of the hematuria.

---

1. Answer: b

Transverse fractures to the upper sacrum (Tile's Type A3) are more severe than their lower sacral counterparts, which, like coccygeal fractures, usually heal well with **conservative management (d).** Upper sacral fractures **more often have neurologic injury** than do those of the lower sacrum **(b).** The pain **radiates to the buttocks and posterior thighs,** not the anterior thighs **(a)** or the umbilicus **(c).** CT imaging is superior for visualization and assessment for hematoma.

2. Answer: b

Altered mental status after a fall in a patient on warfarin portends possible significant head injury (e.g., subdural hematoma) that may need neurosurgical intervention. Trauma center care would be optimal to manage the potential major head injury, as well as to rule out other significant injuries from the fall. The other injuries need thorough assessment, but not early transfer to a trauma center.

3. Answer: a

External hemorrhage in the trauma bay is first treated with **manual direct pressure** while assessment and emergent resuscitation proceeds. **Blind clamping (b)** and **exploration** in search of nonvisible bleeding vessels **(d)** is not indicated in the initial trauma assessment. Use of a **tourniquet (c)** before direct pressure in cases such as this that do not involve amputation is not advisable.

4. Answer: d

Diffuse axonal injury (a) does not manifest characteristic abnormalities on the CT scan, although there may be deep structure hemorrhage (periventricular, white matter). While all others occur, **subarachnoid hemorrhage (d)** is the most common abnormality seen on head CT in the head trauma patient.

5. Answer: c

Unlike chronic, atraumatic pericardial effusions, which accumulate slowly and thus **enlarge the cardiac shadow on x-ray (a),** acute pericardial effusion with tamponade from trauma requires less blood volume and thus **does not alter the cardiac silhouette (c).** Although the right ventricle is penetrated more frequently than the left, the **right heart is not differentially affected on x-ray (b),** and although a **pneumothorax** may occur as well **(d),** it is not to be expected.

6. Answer: a

Violation of the platysma (a), which lies beneath the superficial fascia in the neck, does not guarantee injury to vital structures, but makes it a possibility. The **sternocleidomastoid muscle (b)** is encased by the investing layer of the deep cervical fascia and divides the anatomic anterior and posterior triangles of the neck—its location does not serve as a reliable marker of separation of vital from nonvital tissues. The **dermal layer of skin (c)** can be violated, and the vital structures remain safe if the platysma is not violated. The **deep cervical fascia (d)** has an investing layer, a deeper pretracheal layer, and an

even deeper prevertebral layer. It wraps around many of the crucial structures (e.g., carotid artery sheath).

7. Answer: d

The most likely diagnosis for this unstable patient is *tension pneumothorax in the right chest;* the drug issue is secondary and, moreover, this does not parallel an opioid toxidrome, so **naloxone is not indicated (e).** In unstable patients where tension pneumothorax is suspected, **treatment precedes the diagnostic chest x-ray (a and b),** and decompression of the pneumothorax is paramount **(c and d)**—even over intubation. The **chest can be most rapidly decompressed with a needle,** so choice **d** is the best answer.

8. Answer: b

Subgaleal hematomas (b) can be quite large; the layer beneath the tough fibromuscular galea is their site of formation because the blood can dissect easily through the loose areolar tissue that lies under the galea. Significant blood loss can occur from scalp lacerations through the dermis into the **subcutaneous layer (a),** but these bleed externally. The **pericranium (d)** is tightly adherent to the underlying bone. The **prepontine cistern (c)** is a CSF-filled *intra*cranial space located anterior to the pons (midbrain); it should be scrutinized for subarachnoid hemorrhage on CT scan.

9. Answer: d

Wedge compression fractures involve **loss of anterior height only on lateral x-ray (a)** and are more likely to be stable fractures than are *burst fractures;* a **Chance fracture (c),** classically associated with lap belt, high-speed MVC injuries, involves the posterior elements as well as the vertebral body. **Burst fractures should be considered unstable (b)** and are **best evaluated by CT scan (d)** if first detected on plain film.

10. Answer: b

Chest x-ray signs suggestive of aortic injury after blunt trauma include widening of the mediastinum, loss of the aortic knob, **loss of the aortopulmonary window (b),** left apical pleural cap/hemothorax, displaced nasogastric tube, widened paratracheal stripe, and rightward deviation of the trachea. **Pneumomediastinum (c)** may be seen but is a marker of aerodigestive injury; similarly, **Hamman sign (a)** (a crunching sound on auscultation of the chest) may be found on examination with aerodigestive injury but is not a radiographic sign nor is it directly suggestive of aortic disruption (although the two may coexist). **Westermark sign (d)** (loss of vascular markings with or without an associated radiodense pulmonary arterial shadow) is seen with pulmonary embolism.

11. Answer: a

Hypotension (c and d), hypercarbia (b) (resulting from hypoventilation), and acidemia cause cerebral vasodilatation in an attempt to increase cerebral perfusion in these suboptimal metabolic states. **Hypocarbia (a),** hypertension, and alkalosis cause *cerebral vasoconstriction.*

12. Answer: c

The classic finding with temporal lobe epidural hematomas causing increased ICP and **uncal herniation (c)** is an ipsilateral fixed/dilated pupil and contralateral paralysis. **Cerebellar tonsillar herniation (b)** and **transtentorial central herniation (a)** cause bilateral findings—both may feature pinpoint pupils. **Thiamine deficiency (d)** may cause altered sensorium and a sixth nerve palsy; not classically a third nerve palsy as seen in this case.

13. Answer: b

The patient appears to have **Class II hemorrhage,** as he is anxious, tachycardiac, tachypneic, and has a narrow pulse pressure. **Class I hemorrhage (a)** features normal HR, BP, and pulse pressure, although the HR could be slightly elevated for reasons other than shock (e.g., the anxiety produced by being the victim of a gunshot wound). **Class IV shock (d)** features a markedly elevated pulse and low blood pressure, narrow pulse pressure, and generally confusion, pallor, and obvious distress. **Class III shock (c)** is perhaps the most difficult to differentiate from Class II in this case; typically Class III features tachycardia as well (120 to 140 bpm), but also the BP is decreased (as well as pulse pressure narrowed). As the classes of hemorrhage escalate toward shock, the pulse becomes more rapid, and the pulse pressure is said to narrow in Classes II, III, and IV. By the time the BP begins to fall, it is either class III or IV. Note also that changes in BP and HR are relative and depend upon where the person rests natively—beware "normal" blood pressure (e.g., 110/70 mmHg) in a person with a history of hypertension.

14. Answer: b

Clinical signs of basilar skull fracture include periorbital (raccoon eyes) or mastoid (Battle sign) bruising, CSF oto/rhinorrhea, hemotympanum, and **post-traumatic vertigo or hearing loss (b). Cullen sign (c)** is periumbilical ecchymosis suggestive of hemorrhagic pancreatitis. **Papilledema (e)** is a sign of increased intracranial pressure, as is the **Cushing reflex (a)** triad (hypertension, bradycardia, respiratory depression). A **fixed and dilated pupil with decreased sensorium** and **contralateral hemiparesis (d)** is a sign of uncal herniation.

15. Answer: c

You suspect a *"blowout fracture" of the inferior orbital wall,* with traction injury to the infraorbital nerve causing the sensory disturbance, and must consider entrapment of the inferior rectus muscle—so **diplopia on upward gaze (c)** must be considered. **Nystagmus (b, d)** would not be a finding with globe or bony injury.

16. Answer: d

In penetrating neck trauma, Zone I runs from the sternal notch to the cricoid; Zone II from the cricoid to the mandibular angle, and Zone III from the mandibular angle to the base of the skull. Thus, this is a **Zone II injury,** making choices **a, c,** and **e** incorrect. Zone II injuries are managed by either mandatory operative neck exploration or selected surgical management complemented by diagnostic testing and serial examinations. It is **never sufficient to simply perform angiography in Zone II injuries (b),** since other injuries (laryngotracheal, esophageal) could be missed.

17. Answer: b

With traumatic hemothorax, urgent operative exploration is necessary when **1000 to 1500 mL of blood is seen from a newly placed chest tube;** other indications include 200 mL/hour for 3 hours.

18. Answer: d

A "positive" diagnostic peritoneal lavage in the setting of blunt trauma is generally considered to be (1) **≥10 mL of gross blood aspiration** on introduction of the needle, or (2) **after 1 L saline in followed by at least 250 mL return, an RBC count of >100,000 RBC/ mm^3 (d).**

19. Answer: d

The subtrochanteric fracture (d), seen in the elderly (osteoporosis) and in the younger patient with a high-energy injury, is associated with significant bleeding including shock, although other injuries (e.g., spine, abdominal, pelvic) should be sought as well if the mechanism of injury involves major trauma. All other hip fractures are not typically associated with major blood loss, with the exception of intertrochanteric fractures, which were not listed as a choice.

20. Answer: e

Isolated microscopic hematuria in the stable adult blunt trauma victim **does not mandate imaging (c, d), admission** and/or **serial urine microscopy (a),** or **urologic consultation in the ED (b)**—but is safely managed by **discharge with outpatient follow-up (e).** Caveats to this guideline include a lack of indication for CT to exclude associated injury (e.g., tenderness over the left upper quadrant), patients with rapid deceleration injury (to exclude renal pedicle injury), obvious signs of significant trauma (massive bruising and/or swelling over the flank—with or without hematuria), and transient but resolved hypotension.

Trauma II 20

Andrew D. Perron | Carl A. Germann

Spinal trauma

CERVICAL SPINE INJURIES

Flexion injuries

- **Atlanto-occipital dislocation**
    - Skull displaced from the cervical spine
    - Very unstable
    - Often seen in infants and young children given the relatively large head and poorly developed neck musculature

SIGNS AND SYMPTOMS

- Often associated with C1 spinal cord transection
- Typically fatal

DIAGNOSIS

- Lateral radiograph confirms diagnosis

TREATMENT

- Immediate neurosurgical consultation
    - Most patients do not survive to ED arrival

- **Bilateral facet dislocation**
    - Hyperflexion injury
    - Disruption of all ligamentous structures at the level of injury
    - Unstable

SIGNS AND SYMPTOMS

- Torticollis
- Neurological injury is common

DIAGNOSIS

- Widening of interspinous distance on AP radiograph
- Displacement and anterior subluxation on lateral view
- MRI is often performed to evaluate for disk herniation or associated fracture

TREATMENT

- Cervical spine immobilization
- Immediate spine surgeon consultation for reduction
- Disk herniation may be exacerbated by reduction
- Dislocations with fracture have higher incidence of redislocation and neurological injury. Therefore operative stabilization and fusion is often performed

- **Odontoid fracture** (Fig. 20-1)
    - Type 1: fracture through the tip of the dens

Type I

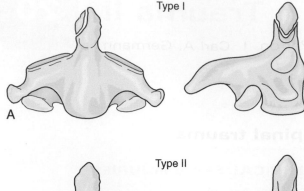

Type II

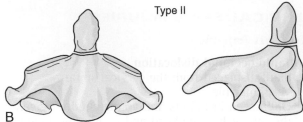

Type III

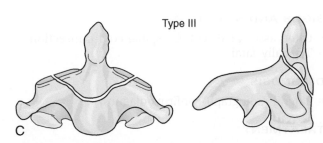

Figure 20-1. Three types of odontoid process fractures as seen in anteroposterior and lateral planes. *Type I* is oblique fracture through upper part of odontoid process. *Type II* is fracture at junction of odontoid process and body of second cervical vertebra. *Type III* is fracture through upper body of vertebra. (From Canale ST, Beaty JH: *Campbell's operative orthopaedics*, ed 11, Philadelphia, 2007, Mosby.)

- Type II: fracture traverses the dens at the junction of the body of C2
- Type III: fracture involves the body of C2

SIGNS AND SYMPTOMS

- Neck pain
- Neurological symptoms may be present with associated spinal cord or nerve root injury

DIAGNOSIS

- Radiographs show a lucency through the dens on AP view and/or an abnormal predental space on lateral view
- The normal predental space is 3 mm in an adult
- CT is often performed to better define the injury

TREATMENT

- Spinal immobilization
- Early consultation with a spine surgeon

- **Clay Shoveler's fracture**
  - Avulsion of the spinous process as a result of forced flexion or direct trauma

- Usually involves C6 through T3
- C7 is the most common site of injury
- Stable injury

SIGNS AND SYMPTOMS

- Posterior neck pain
- Usually not associated with neurologic injury

DIAGNOSIS

- Lateral radiograph will demonstrate an avulsion fragment of the spinous process

TREATMENT

- Analgesia
- Consultation with an a spine surgeon

Flexion rotation injuries

- **Unilateral facet dislocation**
  - Flexion and rotation injury
  - Mechanically stable unless associated with fracture

SIGNS AND SYMPTOMS

- Torticollis
- Axial rotation to contralateral side and lateral bend to injured side

DIAGNOSIS

- AP radiograph views show rotation
- Lateral radiograph shows forward displacement of the dislocated segment on the vertebra below

TREATMENT

- Immediate spine surgeon consultation
- Minimal subluxation is often treated with Philadelphia-type rigid cervical collar
- Dislocation is reduced and then immobilized with a halo device

Extension injuries

- **Hangman's fracture** (Fig. 20-2)
  - Fracture of the pedicle of C2 as a result of hyperextension
  - Rotatory instability may lead to spinal cord injury

SIGNS AND SYMPTOMS

- Neck pain
- Neurological symptoms may be present with associated spinal cord or nerve root injury

DIAGNOSIS

- Lateral radiograph views often show a fracture line through the posterior elements of C2 with anterior subluxation of C2 on C3
- CT is diagnostic

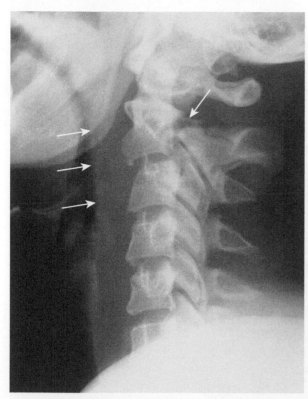

Figure 20-2. Hangman's fracture. The lateral view of the cervical spine demonstrates marked soft-tissue swelling anterior to C1, C2, and C3 *(small white arrows)*. A fracture line is seen just posterior to the body of C2 *(large arrow)*. (From Mettler FA, Jr: *Essentials of radiology*, ed 2, Philadelphia, 2005, Saunders.)

TREATMENT

- Spinal immobilization
- Early consultation with a spine surgeon

Flexion or extension injuries

- **Teardrop fracture** (Fig. 20-3)
- Hyperextension produces a triangular fragment displaced from the anterior-inferior corner of the vertebral body
- More commonly, hyperflexion produces a triangular fracture from the anterior-inferior aspect of the vertebral body
- Ligamentous injury and instability is more common with hyperflexion and is considered unstable

SIGNS AND SYMPTOMS

- Neck pain
- Neurological symptoms may be present with associated spinal cord or nerve root injury

DIAGNOSIS

- Lateral radiographs will often identify a displaced fragment

TREATMENT

- Spinal immobilization
- Early consultation with a spine surgeon

Vertical compression injuries

- **Jefferson fracture** (Fig. 20-4)
  - Burst fracture involving both the anterior and posterior arches of C1
  - Associated fractures of C2 are common

SIGNS AND SYMPTOMS

- Neck pain
- Neurological symptoms may be present with associated spinal cord or nerve root injury

DIAGNOSIS

- Lateral radiographs will demonstrate soft-tissue swelling anterior to the vertebral body and occasionally a fracture line through the cortex
- Widening of the predental space
- Best viewed by an open-mouth odontoid view with lateral displacement of both lateral masses

TREATMENT

- Spinal immobilization
- Early consultation with a spine surgeon

Cervical strains

- May involve injury to the muscles, ligaments, disks, or facet joints
- Often associated with neck hyperextension (i.e., rear-impact motor vehicle crash [MVC])
- Defining the exact tissues injured is extremely difficult

SIGNS AND SYMPTOMS

- Neck pain and often a decrease in range of motion
- Physical examination may show mild anterior, lateral, or posterior tenderness, although may be normal
- Radicular symptoms may be present
- Most symptoms resolve with conservative therapy within 6 weeks

DIAGNOSIS

- Clinical
- Using advanced imaging if examination suggests a deficit or to exclude other, more serious possibilities

TREATMENT

- Acetaminophen, nonsteroidal anti-inflammatory drugs (NSAIDs)
- Follow-up with primary care physician

Injury to nerve roots and peripheral nerves

- Neck trauma may cause injury to the brachial plexus, spinal roots, and peripheral nerves
- Neurological deficit may also result from vascular injury with associated ischemia

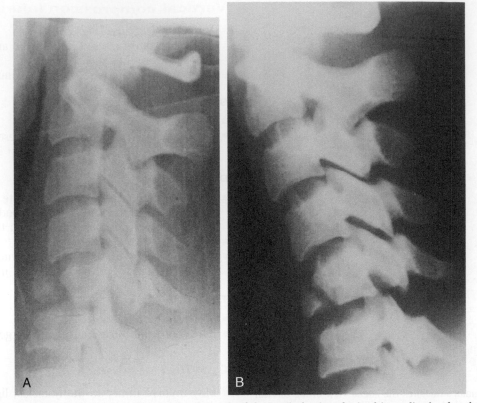

Figure 20-3. Flexion teardrop fracture **(A)** In the lateral radiograph of the cervical spine obtained immediately after the injury, the cervical spine is in the flexed attitude. A single large fragment consisting of the anteroinferior corner of the body of C5 is present. The fifth vertebral body is posteriorly displaced and, in addition, widening of the interfacetal and interspinous spaces between C5 and C6 indicates complete disruption of the posterior ligament complex and bilateral interfacetal dislocation. **B,** In the lateral examination carried out 2 weeks after the injury, the characteristic teardrop-shaped fragment is seen. In addition, the subjacent intervertebral disc space is abnormally widened, as are the interfacetal and interspinous spaces, indicating complete soft-tissue disruption at the involved level. (From Adam A, Dixon AK, Grainger RG, Allison DJ: *Grainger and Allison's diagnostic radiology,* ed 5, Philadelphia, 2008, Churchill Livingstone.)

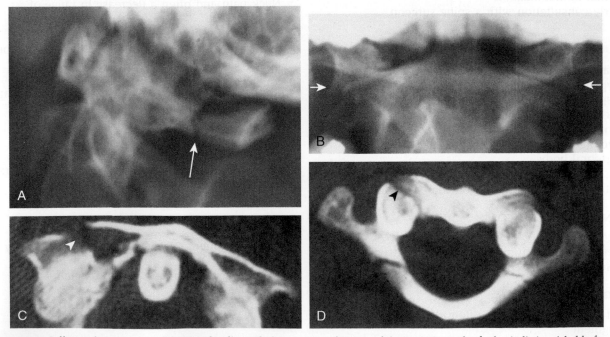

Figure 20-4. Jefferson fracture of C1 **(A)** Lateral radiograph demonstrates fracture of the posterior arch of atlas indistinguishable from the isolated fracture. **B,** The open-mouth view demonstrates bilateral displacement of the lateral masses relative to the lateral border of C1 and relative to the lateral margin of the vertebral body of C2 *(arrows).* Note also the widening of the space between the dens and medial border of the lateral masses of C1. These findings are characteristic of a Jefferson fracture. **C, D,** CT demonstrates a single fracture in the right portion of the anterior arch *(arrowhead)* and bilateral fractures of the posterior arch. (From Adam A, Dixon AK, Grainger RG, Allison DJ: *Grainger and Allison's diagnostic radiology,* ed 5, Philadelphia, 2008, Churchill Livingstone.)

SIGNS AND SYMPTOMS

- May result in both sensory and motor deficits
- Physical examination should identify corresponding cord level based upon specific motor and sensory deficit
- Neurapraxia results from stretching or contusion of the nerve and typically recovers within 6 weeks

DIAGNOSIS

- Clinical
- MRI if symptoms are severe or persistent

TREATMENT

- Acetaminophen, NSAIDs
- Most are treated conservatively
- Follow-up with primary care physician for reassessment and consideration for occupational and physical therapy
- Severe or persistent deficits may be referred to neurosurgery; however, variation exists in how these injuries are addressed surgically

SCIWORA

- **S**pinal **C**ord **I**njury **W**ithout **R**adiological **A**bnormality
- With advanced imaging techniques (e.g., MRI) this is rarely seen
- Children less than 8 years old are most susceptible given the elasticity of the spinal cord, larger head size, and less-developed neck muscles
- May result from direct trauma or a microvascular injury leading to ischemia

SIGNS AND SYMPTOMS

- Symptoms range from transient neurologic symptoms to complete paralysis
- Prognosis is based upon the severity of injury/deficit

DIAGNOSIS

- Neurological findings with a lack of bony abnormalities on plain radiograph or CT
- Most patients have positive MRI findings

TREATMENT

- Immobilize cervical spine
- Neurosurgical consultation and admission for observation

CAUDA EQUINA SYNDROME

- Injury to the lumbosacral nerve roots below the tip of the spinal cord
- Rarely caused by trauma

SIGNS AND SYMPTOMS

- Unilateral or bilateral sciatica and/or weakness
- Bowel or bladder incontinence
- Hypesthesia or analgesia in the saddle distribution

DIAGNOSIS

- Clinical
- MRI will confirm diagnosis

TREATMENT

- Immediate neurosurgical consultation
- Patients who undergo decompression within 24 hours of symptom onset have better outcome than those with late intervention

Penetrating extremity trauma

VASCULAR INJURIES

- Most result from penetrating trauma
- Major vessels of the upper extremity include the axillary, brachial, radial, and ulnar arteries
- Major vessels of the lower extremity include the femoral, popliteal, peroneal, and anterior and posterior tibial arteries

SIGNS AND SYMPTOMS

- **Hard signs of vascular injury**
  - Absent or diminished distal pulses
  - Active hemorrhage
  - Large, expanding, or pulsatile hematoma
  - Bruit or thrill
  - Signs of distal ischemia
- **The "5 P's" of vascular injury:** Pain, pallor, paresthesia, paralysis, poikilothermy
- **Soft signs of vascular injury**
  - Small, stable hematomas
  - Injury to an anatomically related nerve
  - Unexplained hypotension
  - History of hemorrhage no longer present
  - Proximity of injury to a major vessel

DIAGNOSIS

- If hard signs of vascular injury are present, the diagnosis is based on mechanism and clinical examination
- If only soft signs of vascular injury are present, start with arterial pressure index (API) testing and/or color-flow Doppler ultrasonography
  - API: Divide the Doppler pressure of the injured limb by the pressure of the uninjured limb. A value of <0.90 is considered abnormal
    - Angiography should be considered for those suffering gunshot wounds (without hard signs of vascular injury) as these injuries have a much higher degree of tissue destruction

TREATMENT

- Restore intravascular volume
- Evaluate for fracture, compartment syndrome, and other traumatic injuries
- Patients with hard signs of vascular injury or abnormal studies require immediate operative exploration and repair by a vascular surgeon
- Antibiotic therapy is not routinely recommended. However, it is suggested for wounds greater than

12 hours old, significantly contaminated wounds, and wounds involving joint spaces, tendons, or bones

Orthopedic extremity injuries

DISLOCATIONS

Shoulder dislocations

- Glenohumeral joint can dislocate anteriorly, posteriorly, inferiorly, or superiorly
- Anterior dislocation is the most common, accounting for 95% of cases
- Posterior dislocations are classically associated with seizures or electrical injury

SIGNS AND SYMPTOMS

- Severe pain and deformity of the shoulder
- In anterior dislocations, the arm is often held in abduction and external rotation
- In posterior dislocations, the arm is often held in adduction and internal rotation
- In inferior dislocations (aka luxatio erecta), the arm is locked overhead in 110 to 160 degrees of abduction
- A sensory deficit over the deltoid muscle or motor dysfunction of the deltoid represents an axillary nerve injury

DIAGNOSIS

- History and physical examination findings
- A focused neurological examination should be performed with particular attention to the axillary nerve, radial nerve, and axillary artery
- Radiographs will often confirm a displaced humeral head in anterior, inferior, and superior dislocations
- Standard AP radiographs of a posterior dislocation often appear normal while an axillary lateral or apical oblique view often confirm the diagnosis
- Associated fractures are common
  - *Hill–Sachs deformity:* compression fracture of the posterolateral aspect of the humeral head
  - *Bankart lesion:* fracture of the anteroinferior glenoid rim

TREATMENT

- Closed reduction of anterior dislocations
  - *Traction technique:* gentle downward traction with external rotation and abduction
  - *Traction–countertraction technique:* traction is applied along the abducted arm while an assistant uses a folded sheet wrapped around the chest for countertraction
  - *Stimson technique:* a prone patient hangs the dislocated arm over the edge of the bed while a 10- or 15-lb weight is attached to the wrist to provide traction
  - *Scapular manipulation:* application of downward traction to the arm of a prone patient while rotating the inferior tip of the scapula medially

- Posterior dislocations are reduced by applying axial traction and external rotation with gentle pressure on the displaced humeral head
- Inferior dislocations may be reduced by using traction–countertraction technique with gentle abduction followed by adduction
- Intravenous analgesia and sedatives may be required for muscle relaxation and successful reduction
- Reevaluate neurovascular status following relocation
- Sling and swathe bandage for immobilization of reduced shoulder
- Orthopedic referral

Elbow dislocation (Fig. 20-5)

- Majority are posterior and result from a fall on an outstretched arm

SIGNS AND SYMPTOMS

- Severe pain and deformity of the elbow
- Neurovascular injury may occur, particularly the brachial artery and median nerve

DIAGNOSIS

- History and physical examination findings
- A thorough neurological examination should be performed, with particular attention to the brachial artery and median nerve
- Radiographs will often confirm a displaced proximal ulna

TREATMENT

- Closed reduction using axial traction and flexion
- Intravenous analgesia and sedatives may be required for muscle relaxation and successful reduction

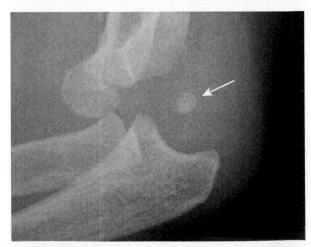

Figure 20-5. Radiograph of a posterior elbow dislocation. The medial epicondyle *(arrow)* is displaced and incarcerated in the joint. (From Green NE, Swiontkowski MF: *Skeletal trauma in children,* ed 4, Philadelphia, 2008, Elsevier.)

- Reevaluate neurovascular status following relocation
- Immobilize with a posterior arm splint with 90 degrees of flexion
- Orthopedic referral

Hip dislocation

- May occur in anterior or posterior direction
- **Posterior dislocations** are more common and usually result from MVCs, when the hip is adducted, flexed, and internally rotated
- **Anterior dislocation** results from a forceful extension, abduction, and external rotation of the femoral head

SIGNS AND SYMPTOMS

- Severe hip pain with shortening of the limb
- Posterior dislocations are typically held in hip flexion, adduction, and internal rotation
- Anterior dislocations are typically held in abduction, slight flexion, and external rotation
- Peroneal nerve injury may present with foot drop
- The likelihood of avascular necrosis of the femoral head is related to delay in reduction and severity of injury

DIAGNOSIS

- History and physical examination findings
- A focused neurological and vascular examination
- Radiographs

TREATMENT

- Early reduction using axial traction and slow flexion of the knee and hip
- Apply knee immobilizer to prevent movement of the joint
- Consultation with an orthopedic surgeon
- Irreducible dislocations or fracture dislocations should be reduced by an orthopedic surgeon under general anesthesia

Knee dislocation

- May occur in anterior or posterior direction and is described in relation of the tibia to the femur
- **Anterior dislocation** often occurs after a high-energy hyperextension injury
- **Posterior dislocations** are less common and are caused by a direct blow to the anterior tibia while the knee is flexed (dashboard injury)

SIGNS AND SYMPTOMS

- Massive swelling
- Spontaneous reduction may occur prior to presentation, so must check for instability
- Popliteal artery and nerve injuries are common
- Signs of arterial injury include a cool, cyanotic extremity with diminished distal pulses
- Irreversible muscle damage occurs 4 to 6 hours after injury to the popliteal artery

DIAGNOSIS

- History and physical examination findings
- A focused neurological examination should be performed with particular attention to the popliteal artery and nerve
- Radiographs will confirm displacement
- Ankle/brachial artery index (ABI) should be performed
- ABI less than 0.9 should necessitate a vascular surgery consultation ± arteriography

TREATMENT

- Early reduction using axial traction and anterior pressure on the distal femur
- Immobilize the knee with posterior splint in 15 degrees of flexion
- Strongly consider admitting the patient for observation
- Immediate vascular surgery consultation for signs of arterial injury or abnormal ABI

FRACTURES

Upper extremity

CLAVICULAR FRACTURE

- Most commonly involve the middle third of the clavicle
- Lateral trauma to the shoulder produces a shearing fracture to the midclavicle
- Fracture to the medial third result from a direct blow to the anterior chest
- Fracture to the lateral third are often due to a direct blow to the top of the shoulder

SIGNS AND SYMPTOMS

- Pain over the fracture site
- Extremity held close to the body
- Crepitus and palpable deformity on examination

DIAGNOSIS

- Radiography will confirm diagnosis

TREATMENT

- Pain control
- Immobilization with sling and swathe
- Arrange follow-up with orthopedic surgeon

SCAPULA FRACTURE

- Usually a high-force injury such as MVC or fall from height
- High potential for associated ipsilateral lung and chest wall injury
- Type I: body and spine
- Type II: involve acromion or coracoid processes
- Type III: involve scapular neck and glenoid fossa

SIGNS AND SYMPTOMS

- Pain over the fracture site
- Shoulder adducted and held close to the body

DIAGNOSIS

- History and physical examination
- AP and axillary lateral radiograph views
- CT is diagnostic if plain films are equivocal

TREATMENT

- Analgesia and immobilization with a sling
- Pendular shoulder exercises will reduce the risk of adhesive capsulitis

SUPRACONDYLAR FRACTURE (Fig. 20-6)

- Caused by forced hyperextension of the elbow joint often by falling on an outstretched hand
- 95% are displaced posteriorly
- The brachial artery and the median or radial nerves are at risk of associated injury

SIGNS AND SYMPTOMS

- Pain, swelling, and tenderness of the proximal elbow
- Often presents with obvious deformity and limited range of motion
- Risk of compartment syndrome and subsequent Volkmann ischemic contracture

DIAGNOSIS

- On lateral radiograph, a line drawn along the anterior border of the humeral shaft should transect the middle third of the capitellum
- A misplaced capitellum (usually posteriorly) suggests a supracondylar fracture
- An enlarged anterior fat pad and a posterior fat pad may be seen

TREATMENT

- Immediately assess neurovascular status
- Nondisplaced fractures may be splinted in 90 degrees of flexion with outpatient orthopedic follow-up
- Displaced fractures require orthopedic consultation for closed reduction and splinting (or casting) in the emergency department
- Reassess neurovascular status following reduction and splinting

OLECRANON FRACTURE

- Result from a flexion-type elbow injury or direct blow to the olecranon

SIGNS AND SYMPTOMS

- Pain and swelling of the olecranon
- Potential ulnar nerve injury

DIAGNOSIS

- Obtain full flexion and extension lateral radiographs as the olecranon fragment may not appear displaced at 90 degrees of flexion

TREATMENT

- Analgesia
- Assess distal neurovascular status

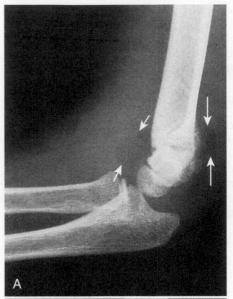

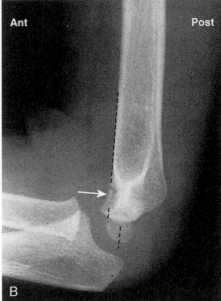

Figure 20-6. Supracondylar fractures. This is the most common elbow fracture in children. **A,** A lateral view of the elbow shows marked anterior displacement of the anterior fat and visualization of the posterior fat pad *(arrows)*, a sign that a fracture is almost certainly present. **B,** In a younger child, a fracture is seen because of the posterior displacement of the capitellum from the anterior humeral line. An incomplete cortical fracture also is seen *(arrow)*. (From Mettler FA, Jr: *Essentials of radiology,* ed 2, Philadelphia, 2005, Saunders.)

- Closed reduction (if needed) and immobilization with a sling
- Orthopedic referral

RADIAL HEAD FRACTURE

- Usually a result of a fall on an outstretched hand
- Associated with elbow dislocation

SIGNS AND SYMPTOMS

- Tenderness and swelling over the radial head

- Restricted range of motion especially with supination

DIAGNOSIS

- Nondisplaced fractures may not be apparent on radiograph
- An anterior or posterior fat pad sign is usually present
  - Anterior fat pad is normally visible as a thin stripe. An enlarged anterior fat pad is triangular resembling a sail and is pathologic
  - A visible posterior fat pad is always pathologic

TREATMENT

- Analgesia
- Nondisplaced fractures are treated with sling immobilization
- Closed reduction for displaced fractures with long arm posterior splint and sling
- Orthopedic referral

MONTEGGIA FRACTURE (Fig. 20-7)

- Fracture of the ulnar shaft with associated dislocation of the proximal radioulnar joint

SIGNS AND SYMPTOMS

- Pain and deformity at the fracture site
- Swelling of the elbow with restricted range of motion

DIAGNOSIS

- Lateral radiograph
- A normal lateral elbow radiograph should have a proximal radial line that bisects the capitellum

TREATMENT

- Analgesia
- Closed reduction and immobilization with a sling
- Orthopedic referral

GALEAZZI FRACTURE (Fig. 20-8)

- Fracture of the distal radius with associated distal ulnar dislocation
- Typically due to hyperpronation of an outstretched arm

SIGNS AND SYMPTOMS

- Prominent and tender ulnar styloid

DIAGNOSIS

- Lateral radiograph demonstrates a posteriorly displaced ulna with a fractured radius angulated anteriorly

TREATMENT

- Analgesia
- Closed reduction and splint
- Orthopedic referral

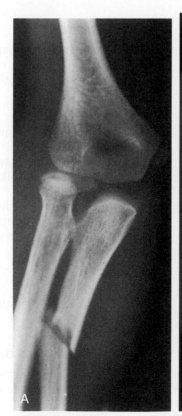 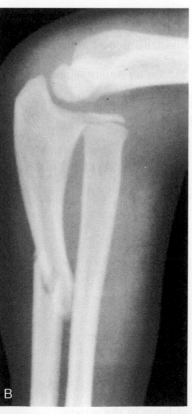

Figure 20-7. Monteggia fracture–dislocation of the proximal forearm. AP (A) and lateral (B) views demonstrate an anteriorly angulated fracture of the proximal ulna and anterior dislocation of the radius relative to the capitellum. (From Adam A, Dixon AK, Grainger RG, Allison DJ: *Grainger and Allison's diagnostic radiology,* ed 5, Philadelphia, 2008, Churchill Livingstone.)

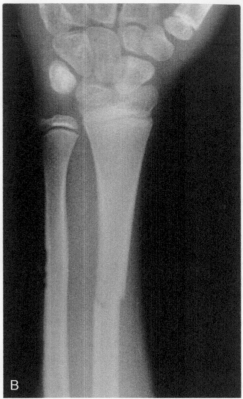

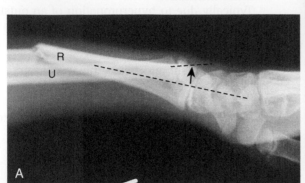

Figure 20-8. Galeazzi fracture. **A,** A lateral view of the distal aspect of the forearm shows a fracture of the distal radius and ulnar dislocation from the normal axis of the wrist. **B,** On the anteroposterior projection, only the radial fracture is seen. (From Mettler FA, Jr: *Essentials of radiology,* ed 2, Philadelphia, 2005, Saunders.)

COLLES FRACTURE

- Fracture of the distal radius with **dorsal** angulation of the distal fragment
- Most often a result of a fall on an outstretched hand
- A *Smith fracture* represents the converse fracture with **volar** angulation of the distal fragment

SIGNS AND SYMPTOMS

- Pain and deformity (dorsal displacement) of the distal radius
- Swelling of the proximal wrist

DIAGNOSIS

- Lateral radiograph
- Concomitant ulnar styloid fracture may be present

TREATMENT

- Analgesia
- Closed reduction and immobilization with a splint and sling
- Orthopedic referral

SCAPHOID FRACTURE

- Most commonly fractured bone in the wrist
- Often caused by falling on an outstretched hand
- Avascular necrosis is a common complication given the tenuous blood supply of the scaphoid

SIGNS AND SYMPTOMS

- Tenderness in the anatomic snuffbox
- Pain with axial loading of the thumb
- Pain with pronation against resistance

DIAGNOSIS

- Standard wrist radiographs may miss the fracture
- Scaphoid view films may provide a better view of the cortex and are taken in supination with ulnar deviation
- Physical examination findings suggestive of fracture necessitate treatment for an occult scaphoid injury; MRI is gold standard

TREATMENT

- Analgesia
- Immobilization with thumb spica splint
- Orthopedic referral

LUNATE FRACTURE AND DISLOCATION

- Often due to a fall on an outstretched hand
- May have associated lunate or perilunate dislocation
- *Kienböck disease:* avascular necrosis of the lunate that is often caused by repetitive trauma to the wrist
- Median nerve injury is common

SIGNS AND SYMPTOMS

- Central dorsal wrist pain and swelling
- Diminished range of motion of the wrist
- Tenderness at the dorsal aspect of the lunate
- Median nerve palsy and/or diminished grip strength

DIAGNOSIS

- Radiograph may miss subtle or nondisplaced fractures
- On lateral radiograph, a line drawn along the center of the radius should intersect the lunate and capitate
- **Lunate dislocation** (Fig. 20-9):
  - Radius and capitate remain partially aligned with displacement of the lunate anteriorly (spilled teacup sign)
  - PA film shows a triangular-shaped lunate "piece of pie" sign
- **Perilunate dislocation** (Fig. 20-10):
  - Radius and lunate align and the capitate and other carpal bones appear dorsally displaced
    - Lunate may appear triangular in shape on AP radiograph view with either type of dislocation

TREATMENT

- Analgesia
- Closed reduction and immobilization with volar splint or short arm cast
- Orthopedic referral

Lower extremity fractures

PATELLAR FRACTURE

- Majority are cause by MVCs when the knee strikes the dashboard
- May also be fractured after forceful contraction of the quadriceps

SIGNS AND SYMPTOMS

- Inability to maintain active extension of the knee
- Palpable defect and crepitus over the patella
- Knee effusion

DIAGNOSIS

- Imaged by AP, lateral, and tangential (sunrise) radiograph views

TREATMENT

- Analgesia
- Knee immobilizer
- Partial weight bearing with crutches
- Orthopedic referral

TIBIAL PLATEAU FRACTURE

- Usually occur after varus or valgus force with axial compression
- Associated with peroneal nerve and anterior tibial artery injury
- Ligamentous or meniscal injury may also be present

SIGNS AND SYMPTOMS

- Painful swelling of the knee
- Decreased range of motion
- Ligamentous instability may also be present

DIAGNOSIS

- AP radiographs may demonstrate fracture and/or effusion; oblique views may be helpful

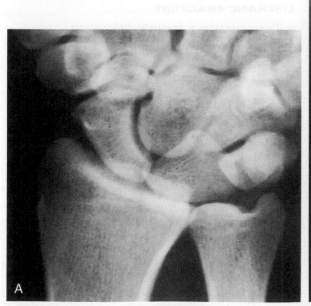
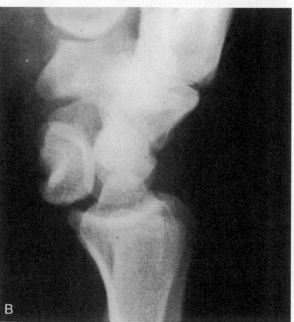

Figure 20-9. Lunate dislocation. PA view **(A)** can be indistinguishable from a perilunate dislocation. The lateral view **(B)** shows volar displacement, dislocation, and tilt of the lunate. The remainder of the carpus is normally aligned with the radius. (From Adam A, Dixon AK, Grainger RG, Allison DJ: *Grainger and Allison's diagnostic radiology*, ed 5, Philadelphia, 2008, Churchill Livingstone.)

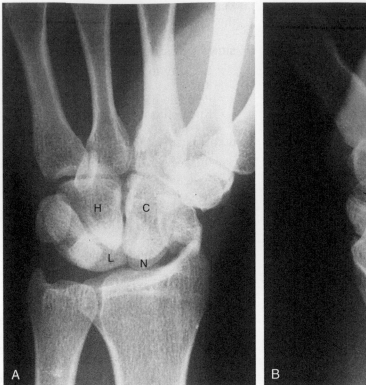
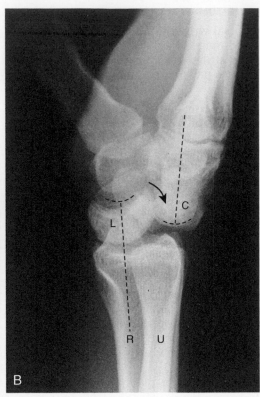

Figure 20-10. Perilunate dislocation. **A,** A posteroanterior view of the wrist does not show the normal two crescentic rows of carpal bones but rather shows a significant overlap of the hamate *(H)* and the lunate *(L)* as well as the capitate *(C)* with the navicular *(N)*. **B,** A lateral view shows that the lunate remains in alignment with the end of the radius, but the remainder of the carpal bones have been dislocated dorsally. (From Mettler FA, Jr: *Essentials of radiology,* ed 2, Philadelphia, 2005, Saunders.)

- Fractures can be radiographically subtle
- Joint aspiration may be positive for blood and fat

TREATMENT

- Immobilize the joint with knee immobilizer
- Orthopedic referral
- Often nonoperative treatment

CALCANEUS FRACTURE

- Most often due to significant axial force such as MVCs or fall from height
- 10% are bilateral and 10% are associated with compression fractures of the lumbar spine

SIGNS AND SYMPTOMS

- Pain and swelling at the heel
- Skin contusion or fracture blisters
- Lumbar spine pain

DIAGNOSIS

- AP, lateral, and oblique radiographs
- *Boehler angle* less than 20 degrees suggests calcaneus fracture
  - Intersection of a line drawn from the superior margin of the posterior tuberosity and superior tip of the posterior facet and a line drawn from the superior tip of the anterior process and the superior tip of the posterior facet (Fig. 20-11)
  - Normal: 20 to 40 degrees

TREATMENT

- Analgesia
- Nondisplaced fractures require immobilization with posterior splint, crutches, and orthopedic referral
- Displaced fractures require immediate orthopedic consultation

LISFRANC FRACTURE

- Tarso-metatarsal fracture dislocation
- May result from axial load, crush injury, or rotational forces

SIGNS AND SYMPTOMS

- Midfoot pain and swelling
- Decreased ability to bear weight

DIAGNOSIS

- Best seen on AP and oblique radiographs
- Loss of alignment of the second metatarsal and second cuneiform
- *Fleck sign:* fracture through the base of the second metatarsal suggestive of Lisfranc joint disruption

TREATMENT

- Immobilize with posterior splint and obtain orthopedic referral
- Displacement requires immediate consultation for closed or open reduction and fixation
- Non–weight bearing with crutches

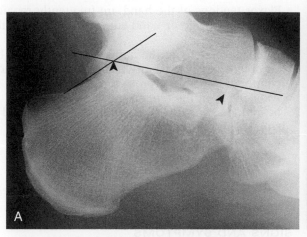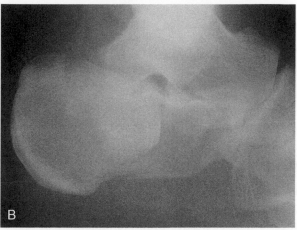

Figure 20-11. **A,** Lateral view of the calcaneus demonstrating the proper measurement of Boehler angle, which is normally 20 to 40 degrees. **B,** Fracture of the calcaneus causing flattening of Boehler angle. (From Adam A, Dixon AK, Grainger RG, Allison DJ: *Grainger and Allison's diagnostic radiology,* ed 5, Philadelphia, 2008, Churchill Livingstone.)

JONES FRACTURE

- Transverse fracture of the 5th metatarsal at the proximal diaphysis
- Generally caused by a forceful load to the ball of the foot
- Greater tendency for non-union than tuberosity avulsion fractures of the metatarsal

SIGNS AND SYMPTOMS

- Pain and swelling at the base of the 5th metatarsal

DIAGNOSIS

- AP and lateral radiograph

TREATMENT

- Short-leg cast or combination splint
- Non–weight bearing with crutches
- Orthopedic referral

Extremity soft-tissue injury

LACERATIONS

- Heal via inflammation, epithelialization, fibroplasia, and contraction

SIGNS AND SYMPTOMS

- May present with continued bleeding requiring direct pressure
- Extremity lacerations may present with signs of distal neurovascular compromise

DIAGNOSIS

- Physical examination primarily focuses on injury deep to the skin with attention to potential foreign bodies, tendon injury, or neurovascular insult
- Obtain radiographs for suspected bony injury or radiopaque foreign bodies

TREATMENT

- Simple lacerations require copious irrigation and closure
- Types of closure
  - **Primary:** immediate surgical or adhesive closure is recommended within 6 to 8 hours of injury
  - **Secondary intention:** contaminated wounds or puncture wounds are at high risk for infection and are cleansed and dressed to allow healing by granulation
  - **Tertiary** (delayed primary closure): Certain contaminated wounds and high-velocity missile wounds may be irrigated and dressed with delayed closure 4 to 5 days later if there is no evidence of infection
- High-risk wounds might benefit from prophylactic antibiotics that cover skin flora or suspected contaminants
  - Cephalexin 500 mg PO every 6 hours
  - Ampicillin/sulbactam 1.5 to 3.0 g IV every 6 hours
  - Tetanus toxoid as indicated

AVULSIONS

- Often more complex lacerations involving a tearing of soft tissue, resulting in a tissue bridge or tissue loss

SIGNS AND SYMPTOMS

- Tearing mechanism may cause underlying bony, tendon, or neurovascular injury
- Scalp avulsion may cause significant bleeding given the rich blood supply

DIAGNOSIS

- Represent a spectrum of injury, from superficial avulsion-style laceration to degloving with associated fracture and arterial tear

- Obtain radiographs for suspected bony injury or radiopaque foreign bodies

TREATMENT

- Irrigation and reattachment to surrounding tissue if possible
- Tetanus toxoid if indicated

PUNCTURE WOUNDS

- Generally depth exceeds the diameter of the visible surface injury

SIGNS AND SYMPTOMS

- Inoculation of organisms from the missile or skin surface to deeper tissues promote infection
- *Staphylococcus aureus* is the classic organism causing infection, followed by other staphylococcal and streptococcal species
- *Pseudomonas aeruginosa* is the classic pathogen in plantar foot infections
  - Typically results from puncture through a shoe sole
- Characteristics of the missile help predict the risk of foreign body and infection
- Physical examination should assess for depth, foreign bodies, tendon injury, and neurovascular integrity

DIAGNOSIS

- Radiographs may detect radiopaque foreign bodies
- Most organic substances such as wood are not identified by radiography

TREATMENT

- Debridement and aggressive irrigation
- Tetanus prophylaxis
- Use of prophylactic antibiotics is controversial
  - If used, oral fluoroquinolones offer antipseudomonal activity

TENDONS LACERATIONS

- Commonly involve the hand and foot given the proximity to the surface

SIGNS AND SYMPTOMS

- May be initially unsuspected and present as a simple and superficial laceration
- Up to 90% of the tendon may be lacerated, with preservation of range of motion without resistance

DIAGNOSIS

- Each flexor tendon of the injured extremity should be tested separately
- The laceration should be examined in full range of motion of the involved extremity in order to identify a proximal or distal tendon injury

TREATMENT

- Significant tendon lacerations of the lower extremity are usually repaired on an outpatient basis within a week after the initial injury

- Flexor tendons of the hand are frequently repaired by an orthopedic or hand surgeon in the operating room
- Extensor tendons of the hand may be repaired by an emergency physician who is experienced and comfortable with the procedure
- After repair of the tendon in the hand, the overlying skin should be repaired and the hand splinted in the position of function

COMPARTMENT SYNDROME

- Tissue pressures rise in a confined space to the point of compromising perfusion

SIGNS AND SYMPTOMS

- Common locations include forearm fractures, tibial fractures, hemorrhage, constrictive casts, crush injuries, and burns
- Pain is the earliest and most universal finding
- Other symptoms include paresthesia, pain with passive stretch, and paresis
- Prolonged ischemia may lead to necrosis and permanent muscle contracture, known as Volkmann ischemic contracture

DIAGNOSIS

- Commercial tissue pressure kits are most often used
- Normal tissue pressure is usually less than 10 mm Hg
- Capillary blood flow is compromised at around 20 mm Hg
- Muscle and nerves are at risk at pressures greater than 30 mm Hg

TREATMENT

- Remove constricting casts or dressings immediately
- Compartment pressures between 20 and 30 mm Hg need to be followed closely with repeat pressures
- Pressures greater than 30 mm Hg require emergent fasciotomy

AMPUTATIONS/REPLANTATION

- Often require immediate consultation and transfer to a reimplantation center

SIGNS AND SYMPTOMS

- Both the injured patient and the amputated part need immediate attention of this obvious injury

DIAGNOSIS

- Reimplantation may be appropriate for the following scenarios
  - Digits
  - Wrist and forearm
  - Sharp and clean amputations proximal to the elbow
  - All pediatric amputations

- Reimplantation may not be appropriate in the following scenarios
  - Unstable patients
  - Multiple levels of injury or amputation
  - Crush or avulsion injuries
  - Serious underlying disease
  - Extremes of age

TREATMENT

- Obtain IV access and keep the patient NPO
- Cleanse wound with normal saline irrigation
- IV antibiotics
- Wrap in sterile moist dressing
- Splint to protect from further injury
- Cold pack to prevent further ischemia
- Amputated digit(s) or extremity is similarly prepared but is wrapped in sterile moist dressing and placed in a watertight container that is then placed into a larger container of ice
- Address tetanus status

HIGH-PRESSURE INJECTION

- Potentially devastating consequences

SIGNS AND SYMPTOMS

- Often go unsuspected as they often initially present as a small, benign puncture wound
- Grease and oil-based compounds do not produce an immediate inflammatory response because of their high viscosity
- Severity of injury is based upon several factors
  - Properties of the injected material
  - Spread of the injectant
  - Time to diagnosis and treatment

DIAGNOSIS

- Radiographs often identify the foreign material, but may be normal

TREATMENT

- Immediate referral to a hand or plastic surgeon for operative debridement
- Amputation rate ranges from 16% to 55%

SPRAINS AND STRAINS

Sprains

- Ligamentous injuries from an abnormal motion of a joint

SIGNS AND SYMPTOMS

- May initially be indistinguishable from a fracture
- Physical examination may reveal swelling, tenderness, pain, or joint laxity in certain positions

DIAGNOSIS

- Clinical diagnosis although radiographs are sometimes indicated to evaluate for fracture

- First-degree sprain: minor tearing of ligamentous fibers
  - Minimal tenderness and swelling without any abnormal joint motion
- Second-degree sprain: partial tear of a ligament
  - Moderate swelling and tenderness with abnormal motion and/or loss of function
- Third-degree sprain: complete tearing of a ligament
  - Similar findings as a second-degree sprain with gross abnormal joint motion

TREATMENT

- NSAIDs
- Rest and immobilization for protection and comfort for the first 48 to 72 hours
- Orthopedic consultation or follow-up for third-degree sprains

Strains

- Musculotendinous injuries from an abnormal motion of a joint

SIGNS AND SYMPTOMS

- May initially be indistinguishable from a fracture
- Physical examination may reveal swelling, tenderness, pain, or joint laxity in certain positions
- Passive stretch of the involved muscle should be painful

DIAGNOSIS

- Clinical diagnosis although radiographs are sometimes indicated to evaluate for fracture
- First-degree strain: minor tearing of a musculotendinous unit
  - Minimal tenderness and swelling, with minor loss of function
- Second-degree strain: partial tear of a musculotendinous unit
  - Moderate swelling and tenderness with abnormal motion and/or loss of function
- Third-degree strain: complete tearing of a musculotendinous unit
  - Similar findings as a second-degree sprain with deformity and gross abnormal limb motion

TREATMENT

- NSAIDs
- Rest and immobilization for protection and comfort for the first 48 to 72 hours
- Urgent orthopedic consultation for third-degree strains

OTHER JOINT AND PERIARTICULAR INJURIES

Rotator cuff injuries

- Rotator cuff consists of **s**upraspinatus, **i**nfraspinatus, **t**eres minor, and **s**ubscapularis (SITS)

- Tendon tear may be full- or partial-thickness and related to acute or chronic injury
- Often caused by forced or repetitive hyperabduction or hyperextension
- Supraspinatus is the most commonly affected tendon of the rotator cuff

SIGNS AND SYMPTOMS

- More common in patients more than 40 years of age
- Chronic cuff tear may present with gradual pain in the lateral aspect of the upper arm that is worse at night
- Patients with acute cuff tears may report a "tearing" sensation with immediate pain and difficulty raising the arm
- Most patients will have weakness and pain on abduction, elevation, and external rotation
- *Drop arm test* is positive if the patient is unable to hold a fully extended arm at 90 degrees of shoulder abduction without dropping the extremity

DIAGNOSIS

- History and physical examination findings

TREATMENT

- Arm sling for support and comfort although prolonged immobilization should be avoided
- NSAIDs
- Ice for the acute injury
- Gentle range-of-motion exercises (walking fingertips up the wall, pendulum swings)
- Orthopedic referral for those with significant disability or suspected complete tears

Biceps tendon rupture

- Most injuries are proximal involving the long head of the biceps
- Result from overuse and/or a sudden or prolonged contraction against resistance

SIGNS AND SYMPTOMS

- A "snap" or "pop" may be described
- Pain in the anterior shoulder
- Swelling, tenderness, and crepitus over the bicipital groove
- Rarer distal biceps injuries present with pain, swelling, and tenderness in the antecubital fossa
- Flexion of the forearm will produce pain and may produce a midarm "ball" (retracted muscle)

DIAGNOSIS

- Clinical diagnosis based upon mechanism of injury and physical findings
- Radiographs should be obtained as avulsion fractures are common

TREATMENT

- Sling/immobilization
- Ice in the acute setting

- Analgesia
- Referral to an orthopedic surgeon

Adhesive capsulitis

- Frozen shoulder syndrome
- Painful inflammation of the glenohumeral joint followed by fibrosis of the joint capsule and restricted movement of the joint

SIGNS AND SYMPTOMS

- Pain may be diffuse and extend down the upper arm
- Often described as worse at night and present at rest
- Active and passive range of motion are limited, especially in abduction and external rotation

DIAGNOSIS

- Clinical

TREATMENT

- NSAIDs
- Progressive range of motion exercises
- Immobilization should be avoided
- Follow-up with primary care physician or orthopedic surgeon

Knee ligament injuries

- Include medial and lateral collateral ligaments and anterior and posterior cruciate ligaments
- Injuries may occur in isolation or involve other ligaments or menisci
- Medial collateral ligament (MCL) is the major restraint to valgus forces of the knee in all stages of flexion
- Lateral collateral ligament (LCL) is the major restraint to varus forces during flexion
- Anterior cruciate ligament (ACL) is the most commonly injured and usually caused by deceleration, hyperextension, or marked internal rotation or the tibia
- Posterior cruciate ligament (PCL) is usually injured by an anterior to posterior force applied to the tibia

SIGNS AND SYMPTOMS

- Injury may be associated with a "popping" sensation and swelling
- Approximately 75% of all knee hemarthroses are caused by disruption of the ACL

DIAGNOSIS

- MCL injury is noted by applying a valgus force to the knee at 30 degrees of flexion
- LCL injury is noted by applying a varus force to the knee at 30 degrees of flexion
- ACL injury is diagnosed clinically by noting laxity and/or pain by the Lachman test, the anterior drawer sign, and the pivot shift

- *Lachman test:* the knee is flexed to 15 to 30 degrees while an anterior force is applied to the proximal tibia
- *Anterior drawer sign:* with 45-degree flexion of the hip and 90-degree flexion of the knee, an anterior force is applied to the proximal tibia
- *Pivot shift:* With patient supine, the examiner lifts the heel to provide approximately 45 degrees of hip flexion with the knee fully extended. The opposite hand grasps the knee with the thumb behind the fibular head. The examiner then produces internal rotation of the ankle and knee with a valgus force and flexion to the knee.
- PCL injury may be determined by the *posterior drawer sign* where the hip is flexed at 45 degrees and the knee is flexed to 90 degrees, and a posterior force is applied to the proximal tibia
- MRI is often performed as an outpatient study

TREATMENT

- Knee immobilizer
- Ice packs in the acute setting
- NSAIDs
- Referral to orthopedic surgeon

Meniscal injuries

- Occur in isolation or with associated ligamentous injury
- Cutting, squatting, or twisting maneuvers
- Medial is twice as likely to be injured

SIGNS AND SYMPTOMS

- Locking of the knee joint on flexion or extension
- Effusion
- Sensation of "popping" or "clicking"
- Tenderness in the anterior joint space following excessive activity

DIAGNOSIS

- Clinical based upon suggestive history and physical examination
- The McMurray and Apley tests may aid in diagnosis
  - The *McMurray test* is preformed by placing the patient in a supine position and flexing and extending the knee while also internally and externally rotating the tibia on the femur
  - The *Apley test* is performed on a prone patient by flexing the knee to 90 degrees and internally and externally rotating the tibia with pressure applied to the heel
- MRI or arthroscopy is often performed as an outpatient

TREATMENT

- Partial weight bearing
- Ice packs in the acute setting
- NSAIDs
- Referral to orthopedic surgeon

Trauma in pregnancy

ABRUPTIO PLACENTAE

- Separation of the placenta from the uterine wall
- May occur following blunt abdominal trauma
- Atraumatic spontaneous abruption is more common
- May be complete, partial, or concealed

SIGNS AND SYMPTOMS

- Vaginal bleeding (unless concealed) and abdominal pain
- Coagulopathy is common

DIAGNOSIS

- Ultrasound is specific but not sensitive (50%)
- Cardiotocographic detection of fetal distress is sensitive but nonspecific
- History, physical examination, ultrasound, and cardiotocographic monitoring are often used in combination
- Laboratory test should include CBC, type and crossmatch, coagulation profile, and renal function studies

TREATMENT

- Intravenous fluid resuscitation to support maternal volume status
- Fresh frozen plasma should be given for coagulopathy
- Call for immediate obstetrical consultation

PERIMORTEM C-SECTION

- Should be performed with 5 minutes of maternal arrest
- Survival is unlikely if delivery occurs greater than 20 minutes after arrest
- May be attempted in gestational ages estimated beyond 23 weeks

SIGNS AND SYMPTOMS

- Fundal height is a quick way to estimate gestational age

DIAGNOSIS

- Doppler ultrasound can be used to confirm fetal life but should not delay intervention

TREATMENT

- Full maternal resuscitation should continue during the procedure
- Call for immediate pediatric, neonatal, and obstetrical consultation
- Should be performed quickly with one vertical incision to enter the peritoneum and another vertical incision to enter the uterus

PREMATURE CONTRACTIONS

- Most common finding after nonfatal maternal trauma
- May indicate uterus contusion or blood irritating the uterine musculature

SIGNS AND SYMPTOMS

- Intermittent lower abdominal pain or cramping

DIAGNOSIS

- Doppler ultrasound can be used to confirm fetal motion and heart rate

TREATMENT

- Call for immediate obstetrical consultation
- Monitoring should be continued until contractions cease

RUPTURE OF UTERUS

- Rare during the first trimester as the uterus is protected by the pelvis
- Prior uterine surgery is a risk factor

SIGNS AND SYMPTOMS

- Vary from minimal abdominal tenderness to peritonitis and shock
- Uterine fundus may be difficult to palpate

DIAGNOSIS

- Palpation of fetal extremities outside of the uterus
- Ultrasound may demonstrate extended fetal extremities or an oblique fetal lie

TREATMENT

- Intravenous fluid resuscitation to support maternal volume status
- Call for immediate obstetrical consultation

Trauma in pediatrics

GENERAL

- Trauma is the leading cause of death in children more than 1 year of age
- Head injury is the most frequent cause of death
- MVCs are the most common cause of injury

FRACTURES

Physis fractures (Fig. 20-12)

- Salter–Harris fracture classification is based upon the location of the fracture line in relation to the physis
- This system provides a prognosis for growth disturbance as bone growth may be interrupted because of injury to the epiphyseal circulation of the reproductive cells of the physis
- The risk of growth plate injury and premature growth arrest increases with each successive type of Salter–Harris fracture
- **Salter–Harris type I** fractures occur when the epiphysis separates from the metaphysis
- **Salter–Harris type II** fractures are the most common physeal fracture and extend along the physis and through the metaphyseal bone
- **Salter–Harris type III** fractures occur through the physis and epiphyseal bone
- **Salter–Harris type IV** fractures extend through the epiphysis, physis, and metaphysis
- **Salter–Harris type V** fractures occur as a result of a compressive force and produce a crush injury to the physis

SIGNS AND SYMPTOMS

- Injury and discomfort located at the end of a long bone (phalanges, tibia, radius, etc.)

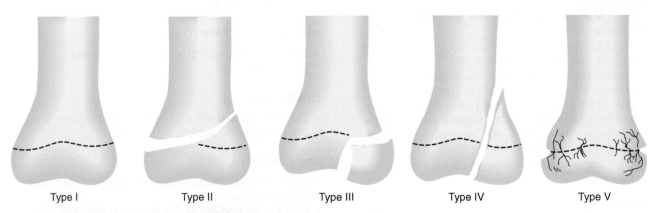

Type I   Type II   Type III   Type IV   Type V

Figure 20-12. Salter–Harris fracture classification of physeal fractures. In *type I* fractures, the fracture line traverses the physis, staying entirely within it. In *type II* fractures, the fracture line traverses the growth plate for a variable length, then exits obliquely through the metaphysis. *Type III* fractures also begin in the physis, but exit throughout the epiphysis toward the joint. *Type IV* fractures involve a vertical split of the epiphysis, physis, and metaphysis. *Type V* fractures are crush injuries to the physeal plate. (From Scott WN: *Insall and scott surgery of the knee*, ed 4, Philadelphia, 2005, Churchill Livingstone.)

DIAGNOSIS

- **Salter–Harris type I** fractures must be suspected clinically when point tenderness over the physis in present. Radiographic findings are typically subtle and include soft-tissue swelling or joint effusion
- Radiographically, **Salter–Harris type II** fractures have a triangular-shaped fragment of metaphysis
- **Salter–Harris type III** fractures will have a epiphyseal fragment without a metaphyseal fracture
- **Salter–Harris type IV** fractures have both metaphyseal and epiphyseal fragments
- **Salter–Harris type V** fractures may be radiographically normal or show narrowing of the physeal plate.

TREATMENT

- **Salter–Harris type I** fractures are treated with immobilization and referral to an orthopedic surgeon
- **Salter–Harris type II** fractures are treated with closed reduction of displaced fragments, immobilization and referral to an orthopedic surgeon
- **Salter–Harris type III** and **IV** fractures are often treated with open reduction and internal fixation of any displaced fragments, immobilization, and follow-up with orthopedic surgeon
- **Salter–Harris type V** fractures are treated with immobilization and referral to an orthopedic surgeon for close monitoring of bone growth arrest

Greenstick fractures

- Incomplete cortical fracture of compliant bone

SIGNS AND SYMPTOMS

- Often less painful than complete fractures

DIAGNOSIS

- Radiographic diagnosis showing periosteal tearing on convex side of the bone

TREATMENT

- Need for reduction is determined by the degree of angulation and location of the injury
- Orthopedic follow-up

Torus fractures (Fig. 20-13)

- Compressive forces result in buckling of periosteum rather than a true fracture line

SIGNS AND SYMPTOMS

- Visible deformity may not be present
- May present with soft-tissue swelling and pain over the metaphysis

DIAGNOSIS

- Deviation of the cortical margin and soft-tissue swelling is often present on radiograph

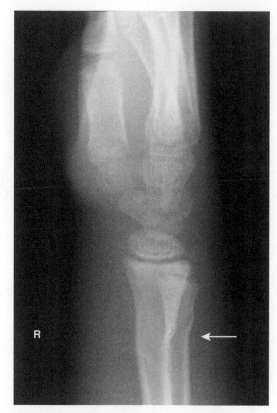

Figure 20-13. Torus fractures usually occur at the junction *(arrow)* of metaphyseal and diaphyseal bone. The more porous metaphyseal bone fails in compression. (From Green NE, Swiontkowski MF: *Skeletal trauma in children,* ed 4, Philadelphia, 2009, Elsevier.)

TREATMENT

- Splinting in position of function
- Orthopedic follow-up

Burns

THERMAL BURNS

- Risk highest in 18 to 35-year-old age group
- Mortality rate highest in 65-and-older age group

SIGNS AND SYMPTOMS

- Size of a burn is described by the percentage of body surface area (BSA) involved
  - Rule of Nines (Fig. 20-14)
  - Dorsum of patient's hand is approximately 1% BSA

DIAGNOSIS

- **First-degree** burns involve only the epidermis
- **Second-degree** or **partial-thickness** burns
  - Superficial partial-thickness burns involve the epidermis and superficial layers of the dermis
  - Deep partial-thickness burns extend to the deep (reticular) layer of the dermis
- **Third-degree** burns (full-thickness) destroy all epidermal and dermal structures
- **Fourth-degree** burns extend through subcutaneous fat, muscle, or bone

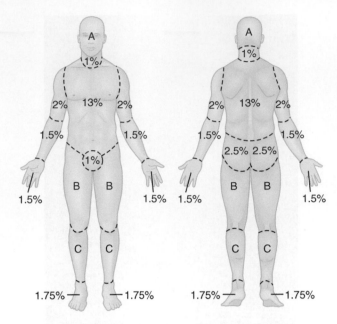

Relative percentages of areas affected by growth

Age	Half of head (A)	Half of one thigh (B)	Half of one leg (C)
Infant	9.5	2.75	2.5
1 yr	8.5	3.25	2.5
5 yr	6.5	4	2.75
10 yr	5.5	4.25	3
15 yr	4.5	4.25	3.25
Adult	3.5	4.75	3.5

Figure 20-14. Rule of Nines for determining the percentage of body surface area burned in adults. (Marx JA, Hockberger RS, Walls RM, Adams J, Rosen P: *Rosen's emergency medicine: concepts and clinical practice*, ed 6, Philadelphia, 2006, Mosby.)

- Possible laboratory studies may include carboxyhemoglobin level and urinalysis (for myoglobin) and creatine kinase levels

TREATMENT

- Assess airway, respiratory, and circulatory status with attention to inhalation or facial injury and potential airway compromise
  - Anticipate airway swelling and intubate early if there is concern for an airway burn
- Assess need for cervical spine stabilization
- Two peripheral large-bore IV lines should be placed
- Tetanus toxoid prophylaxis should be administered based on the patient's immunization history
- **Parkland formula**
  - 4 mL LR × weight (kg) × BSA (of second- and third-degree burns)
  - 1/2 over the first 8 hours from the time of burn
  - 1/2 over the subsequent 16 hours
- Pain control
- Wound care
  - Burns should be covered with a moist saline-soaked dressing while awaiting consultant assessment or transfer to a tertiary hospital or burn unit

- Circumferential burns of the limbs require escharotomy if there is circulatory compromise
- Circumferential burns of the chest or neck require escharotomy if there is mechanical restriction to ventilation
- 1% silver sulfadiazine, bacitracin, or triple antibiotic ointments may be used for minor burns
- American Burn Association Burn Unit Referral Criteria
  - Partial-thickness burns greater than 10% BSA
  - Burns that involve the face, hands, feet, genitalia, perineum, or major joints
  - Third-degree burns in any age group
  - Electrical burns, including lightning injury
  - Chemical burns
  - Inhalation injury
  - Burn injury in patients with medical problems that may complicate management or recovery
  - Patients with concomitant burn and trauma in which the burn injury may pose increased morbidity or mortality
  - Burned children in hospitals without qualified personnel or equipment for the care of children
  - Patients that may require special social or rehabilitative intervention

CHEMICAL BURNS

- Account for 5% to 10% of all U.S. burn center admissions
- Include lye, paint removers, phenols (disinfectants), sodium hypochlorite (disinfectants), methacrylic acid (artificial nail products), sulfuric acid (toilet bowel cleaners)

SIGNS AND SYMPTOMS

- Skin damage may appear with similar manifestations as thermal burns
- Tissue damage is determined by multiple factors
  - Concentration of agent
  - Quantity of agent
  - Duration of contact
  - Phase of agent (liquid or solid)
  - Extent of penetration

DIAGNOSIS

- **First-degree** burns involve only the epidermis and may present with erythema and/or blistering
- **Partial-thickness** burns involve the epidermis and some degree of the dermis, causing tissue edema and vesicle or bulla formation
- **Third-degree** burns (full-thickness) destroy all epidermal and dermal structures
- **Fourth-degree** burns extend through subcutaneous fat, muscle, or bone

TREATMENT

- Immediate removal of offending agent and contaminated garments
- Aggressive hydrotherapy

- pH indicator paper may help determine the continued presence of acid or alkali
- Pain control with systemic analgesics

Electrical Injuries (see Chapter 6, Environmental)

PEARLS

- Cauda equina syndrome may consist of sciatica, lower extremity weakness, analgesia in the saddle distribution, or bowel or bladder incontinence.

- Fractures associated with shoulder dislocation include Hill–Sachs deformity (compression fracture of the humeral head) and Bankart lesion (fracture of the anterior glenoid rim).

- Elbow dislocations are commonly associated with brachial artery and radial or median nerve injury.

- Monteggia fracture represents an ulnar shaft fracture with dislocation of the proximal radioulnar joint whereas a Galeazzi fracture corresponds to a distal radius fracture with associated distal ulnar dislocation.

- A Boehler angle of less than 20 degrees suggests a calcaneus fracture.

- Compartment syndrome is present with pressures measured at greater than 30 mmHg and requires emergent fasciotomy.

- The Parkland formula is calculated by using weight and the body surface area of second- and third-degree burns, with 1/2 of the total volume given over the first 8 hours and 1/2 given over the remanding 16 hours.

BIBLIOGRAPHY

Ferrera PC, Colucciello SA, Marx JA et al (eds): *Trauma management: an emergency medicine approach*, St. Louis, 2001, Mosby.

Germann CA, Perron AD, Brady WJ et al: Orthopedic pitfalls in the emergency department: calcaneal fractures, *Am J Emerg Med* 22:607–611, 2004.

Germann CA, Perron AD, Sweeney TW et al: Orthopedic pitfalls in the ED: tibial plafond fractures, *Am J Emerg Med* 23(3):357–362, 2005.

Marx JA, Hockberger RS, Walls RM (eds): *Rosen's emergency medicine: concepts and clinical practice*, ed 6, Philadelphia, 2006, Mosby.

Perron AD, Brady WJ, Keats TE: Orthopedic pitfalls in the emergency department: acute compartment syndrome, *Am J Emerg Med* 19(5):413–417, 2001.

Perron AD, Brady WJ, Keats TE: Orthopedic pitfalls in the emergency department: lisfranc fracture-dislocation, *Am J Emerg Med* 19(1):71–75, 2001.

Perron AD, Brady WJ, Keats TE, Hersch RE: Orthopedic pitfalls in the emergency department: lunate and perilunate injuries, *Am J Emerg Med* 19(2):157–162, 2001.

Perron AD, Brady WJ, Sing RF: Orthopedic pitfalls in the emergency department: vascular injury associated with knee dislocation, *Am J Emerg Med* 19(7):583–588, 2001.

Small SA, Perron AD, Brady WJ: Orthopedic pitfalls: cauda equina syndrome, *Am J Emerg Med* 23(2):159–163, 2005.

Tintinalli JE, Kelen GD, Stapczynski JS (eds): *Emergency medicine: a comprehensive study guide*, ed 6, New York, 2004, McGraw-Hill.

Wu MJ, Perron AD, Miller MD et al: Orthopedic pitfalls in the emergency department: pediatric supracondylar humerus fractures, *Am J Emerg Med* 20(6):544–550, 2002.

Questions and Answers

1. An 18-year-old man is brought into the emergency department after suffering a stab wound to the right arm. On physical examination, the patient has a 5-cm-deep linear laceration on the medial aspect of the arm just above the medial epicondyle. There is pallor and diminished distal pulses compared to the left upper extremity. The most appropriate management of this patient includes:
   a. angiography
   b. measure arterial pressure index (API)
   c. Doppler ultrasonography
   d. contact a vascular surgeon
   e. intravenous antibiotics

2. Which of the following Salter–Harris fractures contain a metaphyseal fracture fragment?
   a. Salter–Harris type I fracture
   b. Salter–Harris type II fracture
   c. Salter–Harris type III fracture
   d. Salter–Harris type IV fracture
   e. both **b** and **d**

3. All of the following cervical spine fractures are caused by flexion injuries EXCEPT:
   a. bilateral facet dislocation
   b. atlanto-occipital dislocation
   c. hangman's fracture
   d. odontoid fractures
   e. clay shoveler's fracture

4. A 55-year-old woman presents to the emergency department via ambulance after a high-speed MVC. She has severe left hip pain and the leg is noticeably shorter than the right lower extremity. The most likely injury and physical findings would be the following:
   a. anterior hip dislocation held in adduction, extension, and internal rotation
   b. anterior hip dislocation held in abduction, flexion, and external rotation
   c. posterior hip dislocation held in abduction, extension, and internal rotation
   d. posterior hip dislocation held in adduction, extension, and external rotation

e. posterior hip dislocation held in adduction, flexion, and internal rotation

5. Fracture of the anterior glenoid rim associated with shoulder dislocation is known as:

a. Hill–Sachs fracture
b. Milch fracture
c. Bennett fracture
d. Monteggia fracture
e. Bankart fracture

6. A 27-year-old man presents to the ED complaining of having stepped on a nail. The patient states that he is homeless and was walking along the railroad tracks when he stepped on a nail that went through his sneaker and into his foot. Physical examination is significant for a 0.5 cm puncture wound to the midportion of the sole of the foot with surrounding erythema. His tetanus status is unknown, but he has no other medical problems. Treatment of this injury should include consideration of antibiotic coverage for which specific organism?

a. *Staphylococcus aureus*
b. *Pseudomonas aeruginosa*
c. *Escherichia coli*
d. *Klebsiella pneumoniae*

7. An 18-year-old man presents complaining of pain in his left forearm. On examination, you notice a 1-cm soft-tissue defect on the volar aspect of the forearm and a 2-cm defect on the dorsal aspect. On further questioning, the patient states that he was shot in the arm the night before but did not seek medical attention for fear of the police. No other injuries are found on head-to-toe exam. The patient complains of intense pain in the whole forearm, particularly if you move or stretch his fingers or wrist. He states that his arm "feels asleep." The forearm is diffusely swollen and tense. A radial pulse is palpable. Definitive treatment of this condition requires:

a. surgical involvement for possible emergent fasciotomy
b. broad-spectrum antibiotics
c. angiography
d. CT imaging

8. Greater than what percentage disruption of a tendon results in loss of function when tested without resistance?

a. 20%
b. 40%
c. 60%
d. 80%
e. 90%

9. Correct packaging of an amputated part for transport is:

a. placing the part directly on ice
b. wrapping the part in dry gauze then placing it in a watertight container

c. wrapping the part in moist gauze, placing it in a watertight container, and placing the container on ice
d. keeping the part warm to promote patency of remaining vessels

10. A 27-year-old auto mechanic presents complaining of intense left hand pain. Examination reveals a small puncture wound on the palmar aspect of the hand and intense pain out of proportion to clinical findings. The hand is neurovascularly intact and x-rays show no fracture or dislocation. Further history reveals that the patient was working with a high-pressure grease gun when he sustained the injury. Immediate management includes:

a. ED fasciotomy
b. splint in position of function and follow-up with a hand specialist in 24 hours
c. antibiotics
d. immediate hand specialist consult in the ED
e. MRI imaging

11. 17-year-old male is brought to the ED by EMS after sustaining a high-voltage electrical injury. The patient stepped on a downed power line after a storm. Initially unconscious at the scene, he was resuscitated during transport and is now awake and complaining of pain in his left foot and his right arm. What type of dislocation is classically associated with electrical injuries?

a. anterior shoulder
b. posterior shoulder
c. posterior hip
d. anterior hip
e. elbow

12. A 48-year-old man arrives with EMS from the scene of a house fire. The man was trapped in an upstairs bedroom for 20 minutes before he was rescued. He arrives alert and oriented with approximately 40% body surface area second- and third-degree burns. He has burns to his entire face, his oropharynx is red, and there is soot in his mouth. His vital signs are heart rate (HR) = 110 beats per minute (bpm); blood pressure (BP) = 180/100 mmHg; respiratory rate (RR) = 20/minute; SaO_2 = 96% on room air. There is no stridor and his lungs are clear. He is asking for more pain medications. The first step in the management of this patient is:

a. fluid resuscitation via the Parkland formula
b. pain control
c. escharotomy
d. hyperbaric therapy
e. early RSI intubation

13. A 21-year-old woman who is 8 months pregnant arrives in the ED via EMS after a motor vehicle crash. She was the restrained driver of a car hit on the driver's side. Initially ambulatory at the

scene, she was placed in cervical spine immobilzation by EMS and now complains only of diffuse abdominal pain and vaginal bleeding that began after the accident. Her vital signs are HR = 115 bpm; BP = 100/50 mmHg; RR = 22/minute; SaO_2 = 99%. In addition to the history and physical examination, the most sensitive test for the patient's suspected condition is:

a. ultrasound
b. sterile speculum exam
c. cardiotocographic monitoring
d. digit vaginal exam
e. laparoscopy

14. Which of the following best describes the presentation of a patient with luxatio erecta?

a. the affected arm is locked in adduction and internal rotation
b. the affected arm is locked in adduction and external rotation
c. the arm is locked overhead in abduction
d. the leg is shortened and held in external rotation
e. the leg is shortened but remains in neutral position

15. Which of the following statements is **true** regarding knee dislocations?

a. knee dislocation always presents with a clinically obvious dislocation
b. anterior dislocation frequently occurs with a low-energy mechanism
c. posterior dislocation is far more common than anterior dislocation
d. popliteal artery and nerve injury are rare
e. irreversible muscle damage occurs within 4 to 6 hours of popliteal artery injury

16. Colles fracture is best described as:

a. a fracture of the distal radius with volar angulation
b. a fracture of the distal radius with dorsal angulation
c. a fracture of the proximal diaphysis of the 5th metatarsal
d. a fracture of the inferior glenoid rim
e. a fracture of the distal radius with associated distal ulnar dislocation

17. A 56-year-old man arrives in the ED with a complaint of foot pain. He states that he dropped a bowling ball on his right foot during a game. He is unable to bear weight on the foot. On exam, his midfoot is diffusely swollen and erythematous. There is no palpable crepitus and the foot is neurovascularly intact. You obtain plain films of the foot and you astutely note a positive Fleck sign. What is Fleck sign?

a. wedging of the calcaneus concerning for fracture

b. fracture of the cuboid
c. an avulsion fracture of the navicular bone that correlates with intra-articular injury
d. fracture through the base of the second metatarsal suggestive of a Lisfranc fracture
e. none of the above

18. Which of the following is **true** regarding a rotator cuff tear?

a. it occurs most commonly in the 2nd decade of life
b. it may be acute or chronic
c. patients are always able to hold a fully extended arm at 90 degrees of abduction without dropping the arm
d. the pain is generally greatest in adduction
e. the teres minor tendon is the most common tendon affected

19. Which of the following is true regarding perimortem caesarian section?

a. should be performed if maternal return of spontaneous circulation has not occurred within 20 minutes of loss of vitals
b. should be attempted at any gestational age
c. should be performed through a low-transverse incision
d. fetal survival is unlikely if delivery has not occurred within 20 minutes of maternal arrest
e. maternal resuscitation should be halted once the procedure has begun

20. A 27-year-old man presents to the ED after a 10-foot fall from a ladder. The patient landed on both feet and then fell to the ground. He complains of pain in both heels, and radiographs confirm bilateral calcaneus fractures. What other possible injuries should you be concerned about?

a. tibial plateau fracture
b. acetabular injury
c. lumbar spine fracture
d. aortic tear
e. all of the above

---

1. Answer: d

Vascular injuries are most often due to penetrating extremity trauma. Hard signs of vascular injury include absent or diminished pulses, active hemorrhage, expanding or pulsatile hematoma, bruit or thrill, or signs of distal ischemia. Signs of distal ischemia include pain, pallor, paresthesia, paralysis, and poikilothermia. All patients with hard signs of vascular injury require immediate operative exploration and repair by a **vascular surgeon** (thus **a**, **b**, and **c** are incorrect). **Antibiotic therapy** is not routinely recommended unless the wound is more than 12 hours old; the wound is significantly contaminated, or it involves a joint space, tendon, or bone (thus **e** is incorrect).

2. Answer: e

Salter–Harris fracture classification describes the location of the fracture line in relation to the physis and provides a prognosis for growth disturbance. **Salter–Harris type I** fractures are radiographically subtle without an obvious fracture through the metaphysis or epiphysis (**a**). **Salter-Harris type II** fractures (**b**) contain a metaphyseal fracture without an epiphyseal fragment, whereas **type IV** fractures (**d**) contain both metaphyseal and epiphyseal fragments. **Salter–Harris type III** fractures have an epiphyseal fragment without a metaphyseal fracture (**c**).

3. Answer: c

The mechanism of injury can often predict the expected pattern of injury in cervical spine fractures. **Bilateral facet dislocation (a), atlanto-occipital dislocation (b), odontoid fracture (d)**, and **clay shoveler's fracture** (avulsion of the spinous process) (**e**) are all due to *flexion injuries*. A **hangman's fracture,** which is a fracture of the C2 pedicle, is caused by extension forces.

4. Answer: e

This patient has a presentation that is typical of a *posterior hip dislocation.* As the knee strikes the dashboard during an MVC, the hip will be forced in a posterior direction. A significant amount of force is required to dislocate a hip and, therefore, hip dislocations are commonly associated with other injuries. *Anterior dislocations* are due to forceful extension, abduction, and external rotation and are typically held in **abduction, flexion,** and **external rotation** (thus, **a** and **b** are incorrect).

5. Answer: e

Bankart lesion (e) is a **fracture** of the anterior glenoid rim associated with shoulder dislocation. **Hill–Sachs deformity (a)** refers to a lesion caused by compression of the posterolateral humeral head. **Bennett fracture (c)** is a fracture of the base of the first metacarpal. **Monteggia fracture (d)** is fracture of the proximal ulna with associated radial head dislocation.

6. Answer: b

While **staph (a)** and **strep** species are the most common pathogens causing infection following puncture wounds to the foot, the history of a puncture wound through the sole of a shoe or sneaker should raise concern for possible **pseudomonal infection (b).**

7. Answer: a

The patient's presentation is most consistent with *compartment syndrome.* **Fasciotomy (a)** to relieve compartment pressure may be limb saving. The classic findings of compartment syndrome are pain, paresthesia, pain with passive stretch, and paresis. Swelling of the compartment impairs venous return, but arterial flow may not be affected until late in the course. Continued arterial flow and palpable pulses may give the examiner a false sense of security while actually worsening the condition. Diagnosis is based on clinical findings and measurement of compartment pressures. Normal pressure is ≤10 mmHg.

8. Answer: e

Complete range of motion of the affected digit may be preserved even if **90% of the tendon is disrupted (e).** However, functional testing against resistance will often reveal a deficit.

9. Answer: c

Correct packaging of an amputated part for transport is a critical aspect of care for these patients. Preservation of the part for possible reimplantation is essential. **Wrapping the part in moist gauze and placing it in a watertight container and then placing the container on ice** is the best option (**c**). Do not place the part directly on ice (**a**). This may lead to tissue freezing and death.

10. Answer: d

High pressure injection injuries may be limb threatening. They require **immediate specialty consultation in the ED (d)** for possible operative intervention. The external signs of injury may be deceptively minor. Amputation rates range from 15% to 55%.

11. Answer: b

Posterior shoulder dislocations (b) are relatively uncommon compared to anterior dislocations. Electrical injuries and seizures are classically described as causing posterior shoulder dislocation.

12. Answer: e

Early airway management (e) in the patient with a suspected airway burn is critical. Swelling of the airway may occur rapidly and complicate delayed attempts to definitively manage the airway. A high index of suspicion for airway burns must be maintained. Signs include burns to the face, burned facial or nasal hair, soot in the airway, erythema and edema in the mouth and oropharynx, and stridor.

13. Answer: c

This patient most likely has *abruptio placentae.* In this case, trauma has caused separation of the placenta from the uterine wall, leading to fetal distress. Painful vaginal bleeding in the third trimester is the classic presentation. Vaginal bleeding may be absent if the abruption is partial and bleeding is concealed. **Cardiotocographic evidence (c)** of fetal distress is considered the most sensitive modality. **Ultrasound (a)** is specific but lacks sensitivity. Immediate obstetrical consultation is required for emergent C-section.

14. Answer: c

Luxatio erecta refers to an *inferior shoulder dislocation* in which the patient presents with the

arm locked overhead in 110 to 160 degrees of abduction (c).

15. Answer: e

Knee dislocation is a potentially devastating injury, as associated **popliteal artery and nerve damage are common** (d is incorrect). **Irreversible muscle damage occurs within 4 to 6 hours** of popliteal artery injury (e is correct). Spontaneous reduction may occur prior to presentation, so the injury is **not always clinically obvious,** although massive swelling is generally present (a is incorrect). **Anterior dislocation is more common than posterior dislocation** and occurs due to **high-energy hyperextension injury** (b and c are incorrect). Posterior dislocation occurs as a result of a forceful blow to the anterior tibia with the knee flexed.

16. Answer: b

Colles fracture is often the result of a fall on an outstretched hand, and presents with a "dinner fork" deformity of the distal forearm. The injury is a fracture of the **distal radius with dorsal angulation (b).** A fracture of the **distal radius with volar angulation** is called a *Smith fracture* (a). A fracture of the **proximal diaphysis of the 5th metatarsal (c)** is called a *Jones fracture. Bankart lesion* is a fracture of the **anteroinferior glenoid rim (d)** associated with anterior shoulder dislocation. A fracture of the **distal radius with associated distal ulnar dislocation** is called a *Galeazzi fracture* (e).

17. Answer: d

A *Lisfranc fracture* is actually a tarso-metatarsal fracture dislocation. It is often the result of axial loading, crush, or rotational injuries. This injury is best seen on an AP projection as a loss of alignment of the second metatarsal on the second cuneiform. Fleck sign as described above **(d)** is a secondary finding that should raise suspicion of a Lisfranc fracture dislocation being present.

18. Answer: b

Rotator cuff tear is most frequent in patients **older than 40 years,** and most commonly affects the **supraspinatus tendon** (a and e are incorrect). Tears may be **acute or chronic** (b is correct). Patients frequently have a positive drop arm test, meaning that they are **unable to hold a fully extended arm at 90 degrees of abduction without dropping the arm** (c is incorrect). Pain related to rotator cuff tear is increased with **abduction, elevation,** and **external rotation** (d is incorrect).

19. Answer: d

Perimortem C-section should be performed if return of **maternal spontaneous circulation has not occurred within 5 minutes of the time of maternal arrest,** and should be considered only in **gestations of greater than 23 weeks** (a and b are incorrect). Perimortem C-section should be performed through a relatively **large vertical incision,** and **full maternal resuscitation should continue** (c and e are incorrect). Fetal survival is unlikely if **delivery has not occurred within 20 minutes of maternal arrest** (d is correct).

20. Answer: e

Falls that result in patients landing on their feet can generate any number of injuries such as those described above. The force of impact is conducted up the skeleton and a high index of suspicion must be maintained for associated injuries. Falls from a great enough height can cause deceleration type injuries to the aortic root.

21 Procedures

David A. Wald

General approach to procedures in the emergency department

- Explain the risks and benefits of the procedure
- Obtain written informed consent whenever possible
- Assemble necessary equipment or prepackaged kits
- Use appropriate monitoring equipment if performing procedural sedation
- Properly position patient
- Clean, prep, and drape the appropriate body part
- Adhere to aseptic or sterile technique, depending on procedure performed
- Anesthetize area as needed
- Provide post-procedure instructions

Additional procedural caveats

- Nonemergency/non–life-saving procedures may be contraindicated in the hemodynamically unstable patient
- *Coagulopathy* is often a relative contraindication in certain procedures and may be an absolute contraindication in others

Rapid sequence intubation (RSI)

- **Indications**
  - Patient requiring definitive airway management
    - Respiratory failure (oxygenation or ventilatory failure)
    - Loss of airway-protective reflexes
    - Worsening of expected clinical course leading to respiratory failure
- **Contraindications**
  - Able to manage airway with less-invasive means
  - Anticipated difficult intubation (relative)
- **Procedure preparating**
  - Prepare equipment and properly position patient
  - Preoxygenation
    - Nitrogen washout of the functional residual capacity
    - Passive administration of 100% oxygen for 3 to 5 minutes, or
    - Four vital capacity breaths within 30 seconds on 100% oxygen
  - **Pretreatment medications** *(LOAD)* (Optimal pretreatment medications and doses have not been determined)

- **Lidocaine**
  - Increased intracranial pressure scenarios
  - Reactive airway disease scenarios
  - 1.5 mg/kg intravenous push
- **Opioid** (fentanyl)
  - Vascular emergencies
  - 3 mcg/kg intravenous over 1 minute
- **Atropine**
  - Increased intracranial pressure scenarios
  - Pediatric intubations
  - Prevents bradycardia during RSI and intubation
  - 0.01 mg/kg intravenous push, minimum dose of 0.1 mg
- **Defasciculating agent**
  - One tenth the intubating dose of a competitive nondepolarizing neuromuscular blocking agent, intravenous push
- **Paralysis and induction**
  - Noncompetitive depolarizing neuromuscular blocker
    - **Succinylcholine**
      - Use with caution in patients at risk for hyperkalemia (includes myopathies, chronic immobilization, spinal cord injured, burn, crush injuries, extensive necrotic soft tissue infections—2 to 3 days before risk develops in burn and neurologically injured patients)
      - Contraindications if family or personal history of malignant hyperthermia;
      - 1.5 mg/kg (adults) intravenous push
      - 2 mg/kg (infants and small children)
  - Competitive nondepolarizing neuromuscular blocker
    - **Vecuronium**
      - 0.1 mg/kg intravenous push
    - **Rocuronium**
      - 1 mg/kg intravenous push
  - Induction agents
    - **Etomidate**
      - 0.3 mg/kg intravenous push
    - **Ketamine**
      - 1 to 2 mg/kg intravenous push
    - **Thiopental**
      - 3 to 5 mg/kg (adults) intravenous push
      - 5 to 6 mg/kg (children)
      - 6 to 8 mg/kg (infants)
- **Pass the tube**
- **Post intubation care**
  - Verification of tube placement—CO_2 detection/monitoring
  - Listen for equal breath sounds
  - Secure the endotracheal tube
  - Ventilator settings
    - Mode of ventilation
    - Tidal volume: 6 to 8 mL/kg
    - Respiratory rate: 12 to 14/minute on average
    - May be higher or lower depending on clinical scenario
  - FiO_2
    - Post-intubation arterial blood gas and chest radiograph
    - Continued sedation and paralysis if warranted

- **Complications**
  - Laryngeal, tracheal, or retropharyngeal trauma
  - Esophageal tube placement
  - Aspiration
  - Inability to intubate
  - Hypoxia
  - Hypotension

Nasotracheal intubation

- **Indications**
  - Spontaneously breathing patient requiring airway management
  - Considered an alternative method of intubation to RSI
- **Contraindications**
  - Apnea
  - Severe maxillofacial fractures
  - Basilar skull fracture
  - Head injury with elevated intracranial pressure
  - Nasopharyngeal obstruction
  - Coagulopathy
- **Procedure**
  - Preoxygenation
  - Application of vasoconstriction and topical anesthetic agent to nasal mucosa
  - Insert the endotracheal tube into the nostril with bevel facing the nasal septum
  - Advance the endotracheal tube through the nasopharynx into the laryngopharynx
  - While slowly advancing, listen for breath sounds through the proximal end of the endotracheal tube
  - Advance the tube through the vocal cords during inspiration
  - Inflate the endotracheal tube cuff, confirm placement, and secure the tube
  - Patients should not be able to phonate with cuff up if placed properly
  - Routine post-intubation care
- **Complications**
  - Epistaxis
  - Mucosal or nasal turbinate avulsion
  - Laryngeal, tracheal, or retropharyngeal trauma
  - Intracranial tube placement
  - Esophageal tube placement
  - Inability to intubate
  - Hypoxia

Retrograde intubation

- **Indications**
  - Patient requiring airway management when other less-invasive methods have failed or are contraindicated
- **Contraindications**
  - The ability to intubate or ventilate the patient by less-invasive methods
  - Trismus or an inability to open the mouth

- **Procedure**
    - Stabilize the patient's larynx and identify the cricothyroid membrane
    - Connect a 16- to 18-gauge catheter-over-the-needle to a 10-mL syringe containing 3 to 5 mL of sterile saline
    - Puncture the cricothyroid membrane at a 20- to 30-degree angle to the skin, pointed in the cephalad direction
    - Aspiration of air bubbles indicates proper placement
    - Advance the catheter-over-the-needle until the hub is against the skin of the neck and remove the needle and syringe
    - Feed the guidewire (retrograde airway kit or long J wire) through the catheter and out of the patient's mouth (preferred) or nose
    - Magill forceps may be used to retrieve the guidewire
    - Advance the guidewire out of the mouth or nose until 4 to 5 cm of wire is protruding from the neck, then remove the catheter
    - Place a hemostat on the guidewire where it enters the neck to secure it in place
    - If available, advance the introducer sheath (from commercially available retrograde kit) over the wire through the mouth or nose, until resistance is met at the cricothyroid membrane
    - Release the hemostat at the neck, secure the introducer sheath (at the mouth or nose), and remove the wire through the mouth or nose while advancing the introducer further into the trachea
    - Advance the endotracheal tube over the introducer into the trachea, remove the introducer
    - Confirm proper endotracheal tube placement
    - Secure the tube
    - Routine postintubation care
- **Complications**
    - Damage to tracheal cartilage or other airway structures
    - Inability to intubate
    - Hypoxia

Cricothyrotomy

- **Indications**
    - Inability to intubate or ventilate using a bag-valve mask
- **Contraindications**
    - The ability to intubate or ventilate the patient by less-invasive methods
    - Child younger than age 8 to 10 years
    - Significant trauma to the tracheal or cricoid cartilages
- **Procedure**
    - Stabilize the patient's larynx and identify the cricothyroid membrane
    - Midline vertical incision
    - Horizontal stab incision through the cricothyroid membrane

- Insert tracheal skin hook to elevate inferior border of tracheal cartilage
- Insert Trousseau dilator, remove skin hook, open the cricothyroid membrane vertically
- Insert the endotracheal (6.0 mm) or tracheostomy tube (4.0 Shiley)
- **Complications**
    - Esophageal perforation
    - Subcutaneous emphysema/subcutaneous placement of tube
    - Bleeding
    - Inability to intubate
    - Hypoxia
    - Subglottic stenosis
    - Damage to thyroid and cricoid cartilage

Tube thoracostomy

- **Indications**
    - Pneumothorax (24F or 28F tube)
    - Hemothorax (32F to 40F tube)
- **Contraindications**
    - Coagulopathy (relative)
- **Procedure**
    - Identify 4th–5th intercostal space, anterior axillary line (no lower than nipple level)
    - Abduct ipsilateral arm
    - Incision is made parallel to ribs at the above landmark
    - Blunt dissection upwards with Kelly clamp
    - Enter pleura above rib with clamp to avoid damaging neurovascular structures
    - Digitally explore tract
    - Insert chest tube, advance manually, and aim toward apex of lung for management of a pneumothorax and toward lung base for management of a hemothorax
    - Connect to pleural drainage system
    - Secure tube in place
    - Obtain confirmatory chest radiograph
- **Complications**
    - Bleeding and hemothorax
    - Perforation of visceral organs or major vascular structure
    - Subcutaneous tube placement/emphysema
    - Pneumonia
    - Empyema

Needle thoracostomy

- **Indications**
    - Tension pneumothorax
- **Contraindications**
    - None
- **Procedure**
    - Connect a 14- to 16-gauge catheter-over-the-needle to a 5- to 10-mL syringe without the plunger
    - Insert the needle into the 2nd intercostal space, midclavicular line on the side of the tension pneumothorax

- Advance the needle until a rush of air is heard, then advance the catheter until the hub is against the skin while withdrawing the needle and syringe
- Needle decompression of a tension pneumothorax is traditionally followed by the placement of a chest tube
- **Complications**
  - Local hematoma
  - Underlying lung injury
  - Intercostal vessels or nerve injury
  - Failure to decompress the tension pneumothorax

Paracentesis

- **Indications**
  - New onset ascites (diagnostic)
  - Suspected spontaneous bacterial peritonitis (diagnostic)
  - Tense, large-volume ascites requiring drainage (therapeutic)
- **Contraindications**
  - Overlying cellulitis
  - Pregnancy (perform with caution)
  - Organomegaly (perform with caution)
- **Procedure**
  - Identify site where paracentesis needle/catheter will be inserted
  - Recommended needle insertion sites include the midline, approximately 2 cm inferior to the umbilicus or in the right or left lower quadrant, 2 to 4 cm medial and cephalad to the anterior superior iliac spine
  - Ultrasound may be used to guide needle/catheter placement
  - Apply traction to the skin, cephalad, or caudad to the insertion site to pull the skin taut as the needle enters the peritoneum
  - Advance paracentesis needle/catheter
  - Aspirate peritoneal fluid
  - When complete, remove needle/catheter and cover site
  - Send fluid for analysis
    - Spontaneous bacterial peritonitis suggested by a polymorphonuclear cell count greater than 250 cells/mm^3 in the absence of an alternative infection
- **Complications**
  - Hypotension with large-volume paracentesis
  - Localized infection
  - Abdominal wall hematoma
  - Persistent fluid leak
  - Injury to abdominal organ

Thoracentesis

- **Indications**
  - Pleural effusion requiring fluid analysis or therapeutic drainage
- **Contraindications**
  - Overlying cellulitis

- Positive pressure ventilation (perform with caution)
- Coagulopathy (relative)
- **Procedure (diagnostic)**
  - Using an 18-gauge needle attached to a 50-mL syringe filled with 1 mL of heparin (100 U/mL), insert the needle 5 to 10 cm lateral to the spine, one or two intercostals spaces below the upper level of the pleural effusion, over the top of the rib to avoid the neurovascular bundle
  - Procedure is terminated when an adequate sample of pleural fluid is obtained
- **Procedure (therapeutic):** Catheter-over-the-needle technique
  - With a no. 11 blade, make a small skin incision at the needle insertion site
  - Using a 14- to 18-gauge catheter-over-the-needle attached to a 10-mL syringe, insert the needle 5 to 10 cm lateral to the spine, one or two intercostal spaces below the upper level of the pleural effusion
  - When fluid is aspirated, angle the needle caudally, advancing the catheter until the hub is against the skin
  - Withdraw the needle, leaving the catheter in place
  - Cover the catheter with a gloved finger to prevent air entry
  - Attach intravenous extension tubing to the catheter
  - A three-way stopcock attached to a 50-mL syringe can be connected to the extension tubing
  - Aspirate fluid into the 50-mL syringe then advance the fluid into a sterile container by adjusting the stopcock
  - Procedure is terminated upon the relief of the patient's dyspnea or when ~1000 mL of fluid has been withdrawn
  - Pleural fluid should be sent for analysis
  - A postprocedure chest radiograph is recommended to assess for a pneumothorax
- **Complications**
  - Pneumothorax
  - Hemothorax
  - Intra-abdominal organ injury
  - Intercostal vessels or nerve injury
  - Post-expansion pulmonary edema

Lumbar puncture

- **Indications**
  - Suspected meningitis
  - Suspected subarachnoid hemorrhage after negative CT scan of head
  - Condition requiring spinal fluid analysis
  - Delivery of anesthetic agents, antibiotics, or chemotherapy
- **Contraindications**
  - Coagulopathy
  - Cerebral herniation or increased intracranial pressure
  - Overlying cellulitis

- **Procedure**
  - Position patient in the lateral recumbent position with hips and knees flexed and identify landmarks (e.g., spinous processes; iliac crest)
  - Insert 20-gauge spinal needle between the L3-L4 or L4-L5 interspinous space
  - When inserting the spinal needle, orient the bevel facing upwards
  - This position aligns the bevel parallel to the dural fibers, more likely separating the fibers rather than cutting the fibers with the tip of the needle
  - If the patient is in the seated position, the bevel should be facing right or left to separate the dural fibers rather than cutting them with the tip of the needle
  - This positioning of the needle may decrease the incidence of post-dural puncture headaches
  - If bone is encountered when inserting the needle, withdraw the needle into the subcutaneous tissue and redirect in the midline
  - Obtain opening pressure when patient is in the lateral recumbent position
  - Collect 1 to 2 mL of spinal fluid in each collection tube
  - Reinsert stylet
  - Remove the spinal needle with stylet inserted
  - Cover skin puncture site with bandage
- **Complications**
  - Headache
    - Post-dural puncture headache occurs in up to 36% of patients within 48 hours after the procedure
  - Localized pain
  - Cerebral herniation
  - Subarachnoid epidermoid cyst

Intraosseous infusion

- **Indications**
  - Urgent need for vascular access when traditional methods have failed
- **Contraindications**
  - Diseased or osteoporotic bone
  - Overlying cellulitis or cutaneous burns (relative)
  - Failed placement in the same bone (relative)
- **Procedure**
  - Identify landmarks
  - Stabilize extremity with nondominant hand
  - Insert the intraosseous needle perpendicular to the long axis of the bone
  - Alternatively, the needle can be inserted at a 10- to 15-degree angle
  - Proximal tibial approach
  - Direct the needle caudad to avoid growth plate injury
  - Distal tibial or distal femoral approach
  - Direct the needle cephalad to avoid growth plate injury
- **Complications**
  - Subcutaneous and subperiosteal extravasation of fluid

- Compartment syndrome
- Localized infection
- Osteomyelitis
- Injury to the growth plate

Diagnostic peritoneal lavage

- **Indications**
  - Patients with abdominal trauma who do not have an indication for an exploratory laparotomy
- **Contraindications**
  - Abdominal trauma with an indication for an exploratory laparotomy
- **Procedure**
  - Using the closed technique, the introducer needle is inserted through the abdominal wall in the midline, 1 to 2 cm below the umbilicus at a 45-degree angle to the skin of the abdominal wall
  - Apply negative pressure to the syringe as it is slowly advanced caudally, aimed toward the pelvis
  - Three distinct pops should be felt as the needle penetrates skin, fascia, and peritoneum, respectively
  - After entering the peritoneum (third pop), advance the needle 2 to 3 mm
  - A return of blood at this step indicates hemoperitoneum (end of procedure)
  - If no blood is aspirated, remove the syringe and insert the guidewire
  - Withdraw the needle over the guidewire
  - Make a small incision in the skin adjacent to the guidewire
  - Place the lavage catheter over the guidewire and advance into the peritoneal cavity
  - Twisting the lavage catheter may aid in advancement
  - Remove the guidewire, leaving the lavage catheter in place
  - Infuse 1 L of normal saline or Ringer lactate solution through the lavage catheter (adult)
  - 10 to 20 mL/kg (maximum 1 L) in the pediatric patient
  - When complete, place the intravenous bag on the floor to allow the fluid to flow out of the peritoneum
  - At least 200 to 250 mL of lavage fluid should return from the peritoneal cavity to result in a reliable cell count
  - Remove the lavage catheter after obtaining as much return of fluid as possible from the peritoneal cavity
  - Cover puncture site with bandage
  - Send fluid for cell count
  - 100,000 RBCs/mm^3 is used as a threshold for laparotomy in patients with blunt abdominal trauma
- **Complications**
  - Localized infection
  - Bleeding or hematoma formation
  - Damage to intraabdominal organs

Lateral canthotomy

- **Indications**
  - Acute orbital compartment syndrome
- **Contraindications**
  - None
- **Procedure**
  - Insert a straight hemostat in the lateral canthal fold, clamp the tissue for 1 minute
  - Remove the hemostat, cut the tissue along the lateral canthal fold to the orbital rim
  - Grasp the lower eyelid retracting it outwards to identify the lateral canthal tendon (posterior and inferior to the lateral canthal fold)
  - The superior and inferior crus of the lateral canthal tendon are identified and released
  - Some operators prefer to release the inferior crus of the tendon and reassess the intraocular pressure before releasing the superior crus
  - Recheck intraocular pressure
- **Complications**
  - Bleeding
  - Localized infection
  - Globe perforation
  - Injury to the lacrimal gland
  - Injury of the lateral rectus muscle
  - Scleral laceration

Pericardiocentesis

- **Indications**
  - Pericardial tamponade
  - Pericardial effusion requiring analysis or therapeutic drainage
- **Contraindications**
  - Coagulopathy in the otherwise stable patient
  - Small, loculated or posteriorly located effusions in the stable patient
- **Procedure (subxiphoid approach)**
  - Insert an 18-gauge spinal needle between the xiphoid process and the left costal margin angled at 30 to 45 degrees to the skin
  - Aim the tip of the needle toward the patient's left shoulder
  - Aspirate fluid and send for analysis (diagnostic procedure)
  - Observe and evaluate for an improvement in clinical condition (therapeutic procedure)
  - Ultrasound guidance may assist placement of the needle
- **Complications**
  - Bleeding or hematoma formation
  - Pneumothorax
  - Damage to coronary vessels
  - Damage to intra-abdominal organs
  - Death

Peripheral venous cutdown

- **Indications**
  - Immediate need for vascular access in patients without peripheral access in whom central venous access is unobtainable or contraindicated
- **Contraindications**
  - Proximal extremity vascular injury or long bone fracture
  - Overlying skin infection (relative)
  - Coagulopathy (relative)
- **Procedure (greater saphenous vein [GSV] at the ankle)**
  - With lower leg externally rotated, identify medial malleolus
  - The GSV at the ankle is located 2.5 cm anterior and 2.5 cm superior to the medial malleolus
  - A transverse skin incision is made from the anterior tibial border to the posterior tibial border
  - Isolate the GSV
  - Insert curved hemostat, tip down and scrape along periosteum starting on the posterior border until the tip reaches the anterior border of the tibia
  - Rotate the hemostat 180 degrees, the tip will now be facing upward
  - Open the jaws of the hemostat and spread
  - The GSV should be visible between the jaws of the hemostat
  - Insert a straight hemostat between the jaws of the curved hemostat under the GSV, then remove the curved hemostat
  - The GSV at the ankle can be cannulated using an intravenous catheter technique
  - With the jaws of a straight hemostat opened under the GSV, insert a standard 16- to 18-gauge intravenous catheter-over-the-needle into the vein
  - Alternatively, the intravenous catheter can be inserted through the skin, into the vein
  - After a flash of blood is seen in the needle hub, advance the catheter over the needle into the vein and remove the needle
  - Attach intravenous tubing and begin fluid administration
- **Procedure (GSV at the groin)**
  - Identify where the scrotal or labial fold meets the thigh (approximately 2 cm below the site for placement of a femoral central venous line)
  - This is the area where the GSV is at its largest diameter
  - A transverse incision is made, medial to lateral, beginning where the scrotal or labial fold meets the thigh and extends until it meets a vertical line drawn from the lateral edge of the mons pubis
  - Dissect the subcutaneous tissue with a curved hemostat or sterile gauze to identify and isolate the GSV
  - The GSV at the groin can be cannulated using the Seldinger technique as if cannulating a central vein

- Required equipment is contained in a standard central line kit. Use a kit with an 8F or 9F introducer sheath
- Insert the catheter-over-the-needle into the vein
- After a flash of blood is seen in the needle hub, advance the catheter over the needle into the vein and remove the needle
- Insert the guidewire through the catheter and then remove the catheter
- Place the dilator and introducer sheath over the guidewire
- Secure the guidewire at the proximal end and advance the dilator and introducer sheath into the vein with a twisting motion
- Remove the guidewire and the dilator together
- Attach intravenous tubing and begin fluid administration
- Secure introducer in place and cover the incision site with saline moistened gauze
- **Complications**
  - Localized infection
  - Vascular injury
  - Nerve injury
  - Phlebitis
  - Thromboembolism
  - Wound dehiscence

Peritonsillar abscess incision and drainage

- **Indications**
  - Peritonsillar abscess
- **Contraindications**
  - Coagulopathy (perform with caution)
- **Procedure (aspiration)**
  - Identify the area of maximal fluctuance
  - Trim the needle cap so that the needle projects only 1 cm beyond the distal end of the cap
  - Limiting the depth of the needle insertion will prevent injury to the underlying carotid artery, which lies inferiorly and laterally
  - Depress the tongue with a tongue depressor
  - Insert the needle into the point of maximal fluctuance
  - Advance the needle posterior in a direction that is parallel to the floor
  - Aspirate while advancing the needle
  - Remove as much fluid as possible
  - Withdraw the needle
- **Complications**
  - Aspiration
  - Airway compromise
  - Bleeding
  - Vascular injury

Thrombosed external hemorrhoid excision

- **Indications**
  - Thrombosed external hemorrhoids with acute pain

- **Contraindications**
  - Grade IV internal hemorrhoids with thrombosed external hemorrhoids
  - Very large thrombosed external hemorrhoids
  - Thrombosed external hemorrhoids in patients with inflammatory bowel disease, anorectal fissures, perianal infections, portal hypertension, rectal prolapse, or anorectal tumors or those who are immunocompromised
  - Coagulopathy (perform with caution)
- **Procedure**
  - Identify the area to be incised
  - Excision can be achieved with two radial incisions starting near the center of the anus
  - The skin and underlying thrombosis are dissected free with scissors
  - Do not cut the anal sphincter at the base of the wound
  - Localized bleeding can often be controlled with the topical application of silver nitrate
  - Cover with dressing
- **Complications**
  - Localized infection
  - Bleeding or hematoma formation
  - Pain

Nail bed repair

- **Indications**
  - Nail bed injury
- **Contraindications**
  - None
- **Procedure**
  - Using fine scissors, insert the closed tip (angled up) between the nail plate and nail bed
  - Advance the tip, opening and closing to help separate the nail plate from the nail bed
  - Stop advancing the scissors when the tips of the blades are at the level of the eponychium
  - Grasp the nail plate with a hemostat, pull along the long axis of the finger and remove it from the finger
  - Repair nail bed laceration with absorbable suture
  - Replace the nail plate and suture in place for 7 days
  - Petroleum gauze can be substituted if nail plate is unavailable
- **Complications**
  - Localized infection
  - Complete nail loss
  - Nail growth abnormalities

Arthrocentesis

- **Indications**
  - To obtain synovial fluid for diagnostic analysis or therapeutic drainage
  - To inject local anesthetics or corticosteroids into nonseptic joints

- **Contraindications**
  - Overlying skin infection (relative)
  - Coagulopathy (relative)
  - Prosthetic joint (relative)
  - Septic or bacteremic patient (relative)
- **Procedure**
  - Palpate bony anatomy and identify proper anatomic landmarks
  - Insert the needle into the joint space
  - If bone is encountered, withdraw the needle slightly and redirect
  - Aspirate synovial fluid
  - Remove the needle from the skin when complete and bandage the skin
  - Send fluid for analysis
- **Complications**
  - Localized infection
  - Bleeding or hematoma formation

Incision and drainage of a felon

- **Indications**
  - A felon that is fluctuant
- **Contraindications**
  - Early infection that could be managed conservatively
  - Infection that can mimic a felon
    - Herpetic whitlow
- **Procedure**
  - Make a central longitudinal finger pad incision with a no. 11 scalpel if the area of greatest fluctuance is in the center of the pulp of the finger pad
  - An incision along the radial or ulnar surface of the finger pad can be made if the area of maximal tenderness is on the radial or ulnar aspect of the finger respectively
  - The incision should not cross the distal interphalangeal joint
  - Break up loculations
  - Irrigate the wound with sterile saline
  - Use iodoform gauze packing and dressing the wound
  - Prescribe antistaphylococcal antibiotics
  - Re-evaluate wound in 1 to 2 days
- **Complications**
  - Skin necrosis
  - Osteomyelitis
  - Extension of localized infection
  - Flexor tenosynovitis
  - Injury to neurovascular structures
  - Damage to finger pad

Escharotomy

- **Indications**
  - Circumferential deep partial thickness or full-thickness burns of the extremity which can lead to impaired perfusion

- Chest wall burn impairing chest wall movement and ventilation
- Neck burns leading to tracheal obstruction
- **Contraindications**
  - Overlying skin infection (relative)
  - Coagulopathy (relative)
  - Prosthetic joint (relative)
  - Septic or bacteremic patient (relative)
- **Procedure**
  - Sedation and local anesthesia may be warranted
  - Using a scalpel or electrocautery, make an incision along the medial and lateral aspect of the involved extremity
  - Incision should extend from 1 cm proximal to the burn to 1 cm distal to the involved area
  - The incision should extend through the full thickness of the skin only
  - When crossing a joint, care should be taken to avoid underlying neurovascular structures
  - Incisions on the chest should extend along the anterior axillary line from the clavicle to the costal margin (bilaterally) and can be joined by an inferior transverse incision
  - Incisions on the neck should be performed posterior and lateral to the vascular structures to avoid injury
- **Complications**
  - Bleeding
  - Localized infection
  - Damage to underlying neurovascular structures
  - Inadequate decompression
    - Muscle damage
    - Nerve injury
    - Renal failure
    - Hyperkalemia
    - Metabolic acidosis

Retrograde urethrogram and cystogram

- **Indications**
  - Suspected traumatic injury to the lower urinary tract (bladder and urethra)
    - Blood at the urethral meatus
    - High-riding prostate
    - Gross hematuria
    - Perianal or scrotal hematoma
- **Contraindications**
  - Hemodynamic instability
  - Acute urethritis in the patient with low clinical suspicion of lower urinary tract injury (relative)
  - Transurethral catheterization and retrograde cystogram are contraindicated if a urethral injury is identified on retrograde urethrogram
- **Procedure**
  - Urethral catheter method
    - Obtain a reference abdominal plain film (KUB) before injection of any contrast material
    - Cystographin, Renographin-60, or Hypaque (50%) can be used
    - Retract and secure the penile foreskin

- Prime the catheter tubing with contrast before inserting it into the urethra
- Insert the catheter until the retention balloon is within the distal urethra within the glans of the penis (fossa navicularis)
- Inflate the balloon with up to 3 mL of sterile saline to ensure a snug fit in the urethra
- Prior to the injection of contrast, straighten the penis across the patient's thigh to prevent urethral folding
- Inject 50 to 60 mL of contrast solution slowly over 5 to 10 seconds
- Alternatively, a 60-mL Toomey irrigating syringe can be used in place of a urethral catheter
  - Gently advance the syringe into the urethra until it fits snugly into the distal urethra
- An abdominal plain film is obtained during the injection of the last 10 mL of contrast
- If a urethral disruption is present, extravasation of contrast outside of the urethral contour should be seen
- If contrast is seen in the bladder with urethral extravasation, it is more likely that the injury is a partial rather than a complete tear of the urethra
- If a complete tear of the urethra is present, contrast should not be seen in the bladder
- If no extravasation is seen (normal study), proceed with retrograde cystogram
- Advance the urethral catheter into the bladder
- Inflate the balloon and gently pull back on the catheter to lodge the balloon at the neck of the bladder
- After removing the plunger, attach a 60 mL syringe to the catheter
- Fill the bladder with 300 to 350 mL of contrast (adult or older child), allowing it to drain into the bladder by gravity (holding the catheter and syringe above the patient's abdomen)
  - In younger children, estimate the amount of contrast to instill in milliliters by the formula (age in years + 2) × 30
    - After instilling contrast, clamp the catheter with a hemostat

- Obtain a plain supine abdominal radiograph with the bladder filled with contrast
  - Some recommend adding an oblique or lateral radiograph
- Evaluate the radiograph for adequate filling of the bladder and any extravasation
- Obtain a washout radiograph of the abdomen after releasing the hemostat and draining the bladder and review for extravasation
  - With an extraperitoneal bladder injury, extravasation of contrast appears as a flame-like projection within the pelvis. With an intraperitoneal bladder injury, extravasation of the contrast tends to outline the intraperitoneal organs
- As an alternative, a retrograde cystogram can be performed in conjunction with a contrast-enhanced CT scan of the abdomen and pelvis
- Consult a urologist for urethral or bladder injury
- All bladder injuries with intraperitoneal extravasation of contrast are managed surgically
- Some bladder injuries with extraperitoneal extravasation can be managed conservatively
- **Complications**
  - Complete urethral disruption if urethral catheter is inadvertently advanced into the bladder in a patient with a partial urethral disruption

BIBLIOGRAPHY

Dev SP, Nascimento B Jr, Simone C, Chien V: Chest tube insertion, *N Engl J Med* 357:e15, 2007.

Hsiao J, Pacheco-Fowler V: Cricothyroidotomy, *N Engl J Med* 358:e25, 2008.

Jankowski JT, Spirnak P: Current recommendations for imaging in the management of urologic trauma, *Urol Clin North Am* 33:365–376, 2006.

Reichman E, Simon RR: *Emergency medicine procedures*, New York, 2004, McGraw-Hill.

Roberts JR, Hedges J: *Clinical procedures in emergency medicine*, ed 4, Philadelphia, 2004, Saunders.

Thomsen TW, DeLaPena J, Setnik GS: Thoracentesis, *N Engl J Med* 355:e16, 2006.

Thomsen TW, Shaffer RW, White B, Setnik GS: Paracentesis, *N Engl J Med* 355:e21, 2006.

Thomsen TW, Shen S, Shaffer RW, Setnik GS: Arthrocentesis of the knee, *N Engl J Med* 354:e19, 2006.

Questions and Answers

1. Succinylcholine use during rapid sequence intubation should proceed with caution in patients at risk for developing:
   a. hypernatremia
   b. hyperglycemia
   c. hyperkalemia
   d. hypercalcemia

2. When performing nasotracheal intubation, the endotracheal tube should be inserted into the nostril with bevel facing:

   a. the nasal septum
   b. away from the nasal septum
   c. superiorly
   d. the floor of the nose

3. When performing a surgical cricothyrotomy, a tracheal skin hook is used to elevate the:

   a. superior border of tracheal cartilage
   b. inferior border of tracheal cartilage
   c. medial border of tracheal cartilage
   d. lateral border of tracheal cartilage

4. When inserting a chest tube for the management of a pneumothorax, in which direction should the tube be advanced and aimed?
   a. toward the posterior chest wall
   b. toward the mediastinum
   c. toward the base of the lung
   d. toward the apex

5. When placing a chest tube, the landmark for the skin incision is the:
   a. 5th–6th intercostal space, midaxillary line
   b. 5th–6th intercostal space, anterior axillary line
   c. 4th–5th intercostal space, midaxillary line
   d. 4th–5th intercostal space, anterior axillary line
   e. 4th–5th intercostal space, midclavicular line

6. When performing a needle decompression for a tension pneumothorax, the needle should be inserted into the:
   a. 1st intercostal space, midclavicular line
   b. 2nd intercostal space, midclavicular line
   c. 3rd intercostal space, midclavicular line
   d. 4th intercostal space, midclavicular line

7. Which of the following is an absolute contraindication to performing a paracentesis?
   a. pregnancy
   b. obesity
   c. prior abdominal surgery
   d. overlying cellulitis
   e. organomegaly

8. The threshold polymorphonuclear cell count suggestive of the diagnosis of spontaneous bacterial peritonitis in ascites fluid is:
   a. 50 cells/mm^3
   b. 150 cells/mm^3
   c. 250 cells/mm^3
   d. 350 cells/mm^3
   e. 450 cells/mm^3

9. When performing a thoracentesis, the insertion site for the needle should be in a position that is:
   a. 0 to 2 cm lateral to the spine
   b. 2 to 4 cm lateral to the spine
   c. 5 to 10 cm lateral to the spine
   d. 10 to 12 cm lateral to the spine

10. In which orientation should the bevel of the spinal needle be facing when performing a lumbar puncture?
    a. perpendicular to the long axis of the spinal cord
    b. parallel to ligamentum flavum
    c. perpendicular to the dural fibers
    d. parallel to the dural fibers
    e. specific orientation does not matter

11. When performing a lumbar puncture, an accurate opening pressure measurement can be obtained with the patient in the _____ position:
    a. supine
    b. prone
    c. lateral recumbent
    d. sitting

12. Post dural puncture headaches occur in up to what approximate percentage of patients within 48 hours after a lumbar puncture?
    a. 5%
    b. 15%
    c. 25%
    d. 35%
    e. 45%

13. After blunt abdominal trauma, when performing a diagnostic peritoneal lavage, how much lavage fluid should return from the peritoneal cavity, in the adult, for a reliable cell count?
    a. 100 to 150 mL
    b. 200 to 250 mL
    c. 300 to 350 mL
    d. 400 to 450 mL
    e. 500 to 550 mL

14. When performing a diagnostic peritoneal lavage on a child, how much normal saline or Ringer lactate solution is infused through the lavage catheter?
    a. 500 mL
    b. 5 to 10 mL/kg
    c. 10 to 20 mL/kg
    d. 20 to 30 mL/kg
    e. 30 to 40 mL/kg

15. What is the RBC threshold for laparotomy when performing a diagnostic peritoneal lavage in a patient with blunt abdominal trauma?
    a. 20,000 RBCs/mm^3
    b. 40,000 RBCs/mm^3
    c. 60,000 RBCs/mm^3
    d. 80,000 RBCs/mm^3
    e. 100,000 RBCs/mm^3

16. The greater saphenous vein at the ankle is located:
    a. anterior and superior to the medial malleolus
    b. anterior and inferior to the medial malleolus
    c. posterior and superior to the medial malleolus
    d. posterior and inferior to the medial malleolus

17. Excision of thrombosed external hemorrhoids is contraindicated in a patient with:
    a. rectal prolapse
    b. irritable bowel disease
    c. peptic ulcer disease
    d. gastroesophageal reflux
    e. pilonidal cyst

18. When performing an escharotomy for a full-thickness burn to the chest wall, the incision should extend along the:
    a. sternoclavicular line
    b. midclavicular line
    c. anterior axillary line
    d. midaxillary line
    e. posterior axillary line

19. When performing a retrograde urethrogram, a flame-like extravasation of contrast along with contrast seen in the bladder suggests which of the following injuries?
    a. complete urethral disruption
    b. normal urethral integrity
    c. partial urethral disruption
    d. urethral fistula
    e. penile fracture

20. A retrograde cystogram performed on a patient with a suspected bladder injury finds extravasation of contrast that outlines the intraperitoneal organs. The definitive management of this type of injury would include:
    a. insertion of a urethral catheter
    b. performing a suprapubic cystotomy
    c. placement of nephrostomy tubes
    d. placement of ureteral stents
    e. surgical repair

---

1. Answer: c

Succinylcholine administration should proceed with caution in any patient at risk for developing **hyperkalemia (c)**. It is safe to administer this medication to patients with acute burns, trauma, sepsis, spinal cord injury, and stroke.

2. Answer: a

When inserting the endotracheal tube, it is recommended to insert the tube with the **bevel facing the nasal septum (a)** to avoid injuring this structure.

3. Answer: b

The tracheal skin hook is inserted and used to elevate the **inferior border of the tracheal cartilage (b)**. This allows insertion of the Trousseau dilator to further open the cricothyroid membrane vertically.

4. Answer: d

When inserting a chest tube, advance manually and aim toward the **apex of the lung (d)** for management of a pneumothorax and **toward the lung base (c)** for management of a *hemothorax*.

5. Answer: d

The landmark for the skin insertion when inserting a chest tube is the **4th–5th intercostal space, anterior axillary line (d)**. The chest tube is inserted into the pleural cavity above the rib to avoid damaging neurovascular structures.

6. Answer: b

The landmark that is identified for the placement of the needle when decompressing a tension pneumothorax is the **2nd intercostal space, midclavicular line (b)** on the side of the tension pneumothorax.

7. Answer: d

The only absolute contraindication to performing a paracentesis is in the case of a patient with **overlying cellulitis (d)**. In patients who are **pregnant (a)** or with **organomegaly (e)**, the operator should be cautious, but the procedure is not contraindicated.

8. Answer: c

The cut-off value suggestive of bacterial peritonitis is in excess of **250 cells/mm^3 (c)**.

9. Answer: c

The recommended insertion site for the needle when performing a thoracentesis is **5 to 10 cm lateral to the spine (c)**, one to two intercostal spaces below the upper level of the pleural effusion.

10. Answer: d

When inserting the spinal needle, orient the bevel **parallel to the dural fibers (d)**, which run parallel to the long axis of the spinal cord. By doing so, you are more likely separating the fibers rather than cutting the fibers with the tip of the needle. Positioning the fibers in this orientation may also decrease the incidence of a post-dural puncture headache.

11. Answer: c

An accurate opening pressure can only be obtained from patients in the **lateral recumbent position (c)**. Lumbar punctures are at times performed in the **seated forward position (d)**; however, opening pressure measurements should not be obtained when performing the procedure in this position as they are unreliable.

12. Answer: d

Post-dural puncture headache occurs in up to **36.5% of patients (d)** within 48 hours after the procedure.

13. Answer: b

At least 200 to 250 mL of lavage fluid should return from the peritoneal cavity (b) to result in a reliable cell count.

14. Answer: c

When performing a diagnostic peritoneal lavage on a pediatric patient, infuse **10 to 20 mL/kg (c)** (maximum 1 L) of normal saline or Ringer lactate solution.

15. Answer: e

When performing a diagnostic peritoneal lavage, **100,000 RBCs/mm^3 (e)** is used as a threshold for laparotomy in patients with blunt abdominal trauma.

16. Answer: a

The location of the greater saphenous vein at the ankle is **2.5 cm *anterior* and 2.5 cm *superior* to the medial malleolus (a).**

17. Answer: a

Excision of thrombosed external hemorrhoids is contraindicated in patients with inflammatory bowel disease, anorectal fissures, perianal infections, portal hypertension, **rectal prolapse (a),** or anorectal tumors, and in those who are immunocompromised.

18. Answer: c

When performing an escharotomy, the incisions on the chest should extend along the **anterior axillary line (c)** from the clavicle to the costal margin (bilaterally) and can be joined by an inferior transverse incision.

19. Answer: c

If contrast is seen in the bladder with urethral extravasation, it is more likely that the injury is a **partial (c)** rather than a **complete (a) tear of the urethra.**

20. Answer: e

When a patient sustains a bladder injury with intraperitoneal extravasation, the contrast often outlines the intraperitoneal organs. All bladder injuries with intraperitoneal extravasation of contrast will require **surgical repair (e).**

Administration

CONTRACT PRINCIPLES

- From ACEP (American College of Emergency Physicians) Policy Statement "Emergency Physician Rights and Responsibilities"

Rights of emergency physicians

- Emergency physician autonomy in clinical decision making shall be respected and shall not be restricted other than through reasonable rules, regulations, and bylaws of his or her medical staff or practice group
- Emergency physicians have a right to expect adequate staffing and equipment to meet the needs of the patients seen at the facility and to have the institution provide support to improve patient safety. Emergency physicians shall be provided such support and resources as necessary to render high-quality emergency care in the ED setting and shall not be subject to adverse action for bringing to the attention of responsible parties deficiencies in such support or resources when done in a reasonable and appropriate manner
- Emergency physicians shall be reasonably compensated for clinical and administrative services and such compensation should be related to the physician qualifications, level of responsibility, experience, and quality and amount of work performed
- Emergency physicians shall not be required to purchase unnecessary, unneeded, or excessively priced administrative services from a hospital, contract group of any size, or other parties in return for privileges or patient referrals
- Emergency physicians shall be provided periodic reports of billings and collections in their name and have the right to audit such billings, without retribution
- Emergency physicians shall be accorded due process before any adverse final action with respect to employment or contract status, the effect of which would be the loss or limitation of medical staff privileges. Emergency physicians' medical and/or clinical staff privileges shall not be reduced, terminated, or otherwise restricted except for grounds related to their competency or professional conduct
- Emergency physicians who practice pursuant to an exclusive contract arrangement shall not be required to waive their individual medical staff due process rights as a condition of practice opportunity or privileges
- Emergency physicians shall not be required to render anything of value in return for referral of patients by a hospital (e.g., through the awarding of an exclusive contract) other than assurances of reliability and high-quality care, nor shall emergency physicians receive anything of value in return for referrals of patients to others
- Emergency physicians, both independent contractors and physician employees, shall be represented in the contract negotiation process between hospitals and those payers providing reimbursement for emergency services. Emergency physicians are entitled to fair rights and reimbursement pursuant to such contract agreements
- Emergency physicians shall not be required to agree to any restrictive covenant that limits the right to practice medicine after the termination of employment or contract to provide services as an emergency physician. Such restrictions are not in the public interest

Responsibilities of emergency physicians

- Emergency physicians bear a responsibility to practice emergency medicine in an ethical manner consistent with contemporary emergency medicine principles. Emergency physicians must maintain current emergency medicine knowledge and skills through independent study and continuing medical education (CME) activities
- Emergency physicians should exhibit attributes of professionalism in the ED, including altruism, accountability, duty, honor, integrity, and respect
- Emergency physicians should participate in medical staff and/or hospital affairs with the support of the ED medical director
- Emergency physicians should gain knowledge of the basic principles of documentation, coding and reimbursement, practice expense costs, and other applicable physician administration costs, to assist in accurate billing for their services and to properly interpret practice revenue and expense information that they receive
- Emergency physicians must maintain knowledge of and compliance with major federal and state regulations that affect the practice of emergency medicine, such as the Emergency Medical Treatment and Labor Act (EMTALA) and the Health Insurance Portability and Accountability Act (HIPAA)
- Emergency physicians who are employees, contractors, or principals of a practice group have certain duties and responsibilities to the group and are accountable to the best interests of the group. Efforts detrimental to the welfare of the group are inappropriate and may expose the individual to legal liability

FINANCIAL ISSUES

Budget and planning

- **Capital budget:** Comprises all major equipment expenditures or physical plant projects planned for the budget year
- **Revenue budget:** The projection of revenues by classification for the coming year
- **Expense budget:** Expenses based on the number of occasions of ED visits (e.g., medical and surgical billables, professional contracts, cleaning supplies, drugs, medical and office supplies, linens, food, repair and maintenance)
- **Salary budget:** Money for staffing expenses
  - One full-time equivalent (FTE) attending physician who works 36 hours a week for 48 weeks (3 weeks' vacation plus 1 week continuing medical education) will work 1728 hours per year
  - Will need FTEs for physicians, nurses, unit clerks, technicians and registration

Cost containment

- The emergency physician should make every effort to be cost conscious for the sake of the patient and health care system. Indiscriminate expenditures over the long run will negatively impact financial resources
  - Utilization of decision rules when applicable can reduce unnecessary costs, save time, and reduce patient exposures to potentially harmful tests (e.g., use of Ottawa ankles rules)
  - Ordering of "baseline labs" in the majority of cases may be wasteful and unnecessary
  - Cardiac monitoring or pulse oximetry may be expensive and unnecessary in some cases
  - Appropriate generic or low-cost medications will save the patient money
  - Use of oral, rather than parenteral, medications will reduce costs
  - The Joint Commission does not require documentation of cost-containment efforts

Reimbursement issues, billing, and coding

- The ED chart must be comprehensive enough to support billing and accurately documented to prevent fraud
- The majority of reimbursement comes from the five levels of evaluation and management Codes (Levels 1 to 5):
- **Level 1:** Problem focused; requires 1 to 3 elements of history of present illness plus 1 system of physical examination (e.g., insect bite)
- **Level 2:** Expanded problem focused, low-complexity; requires 1 to 3 elements of history of present illness; 1 review of systems; and 2 to 7 limited elements of physical examination (e.g., conjunctivitis)
- **Level 3:** Expanded problem focused, moderate-complexity; requires 1 to 3 elements of history of present illness; 1 review of systems; and 2 to 7 limited elements of physical examination (e.g., ankle sprain with radiographs indicated)
- **Level 4:** Detailed; requires 4 to 8 elements of history of present illness; 2 to 9 review of systems; 1 of 3 areas of past medical, family and social history; and 2 to 7 extensive elements of physical examination (e.g., a patient with abdominal pain who ultimately goes home)
- **Level 5:** Comprehensive; requires 4 to 8 elements of history of present illness; all review of systems; 2 of 3 areas of past medical, family, and social history; and 8+ extensive elements of physical examination (e.g., admitted chest pain)
- *Critical care billing* does not require evaluation and management level–specific requirements, but does require more than 30 minutes of a physician's constant cognitive attention to a patient who is unstable, critically ill, or injured. Critical care time reimbursement escalates in 30-minute increments and is supported by time:
  - Managing the patient's hemodynamics and vital signs
  - Ordering medications

- Interpreting or reviewing diagnostic studies or laboratory tests
- Obtaining history from outside sources (family, EMS, primary doctor)
- In management and discussion with consultants
- Reviewing the medical records
- And is NOT supported by time spent doing procedures
- *Observation billing* requires separate documentation from the ED chart and can increase billing on patients with an anticipated stay less than 24 hours
- The emergency physician is legally accountable for the claims on the ED chart, including criminal penalties in cases of up-coding. The emergency physician should document accurately without underrepresenting or overrepresenting the patient encounter, and physician groups or hospitals should systematically review charts to ensure the services match the documentation

OPERATIONS

Department administration

- Led by the ED clinical operations director who has the following qualifications:
  - EM board certified and currently practicing
  - Leader in the department
  - Excellent teacher, clinician, and administrator
  - Capable ambassador to the hospital for the ED
- Represents the ED within medical staff meetings
- Maintains daily clinical operations
- Maintains ED quality assurance and EM physician clinical competencies
- Organizes the clinical work schedule for the EM physicians

Documentation

- Serves to provide a detailed record of a patient's medical conditions and treatments; documentation must be legible
- Serves to minimize the medical liability risk of emergency physicians by documenting thought processes supporting treatment plans; patient instructions (discharge or against medical advice) must be specific
- Serves to support the charges billed to the patient by substantiating the services rendered; copies will go to the billing company, medical records, and the emergency department
- Joint Commission recommendations:
  - Record chief complaints in the patient's own exact words
  - Record history of present illness, past history, review of systems, physical examination (with vital signs), and pertinent laboratory and diagnostic testing
  - Record consent for all procedures
  - Record consultant input and timing
  - Record discharge instructions and follow-up plan

- Create an emergency department log including time/mode of arrival, patient demographics, chief complaint, laboratory/diagnostic testing, physician diagnosis, and admission location or time of discharge as appropriate

Facility design

- Parking and transportation
  - Patients and families need close access
  - Ambulances/helicopters need adjacent space and immediate access
- Emergency Department size
  - Related to the philosophy of hospital management since emergency services contribute substantially to hospital revenue
  - Must support anticipated patient load with capacity to increase in times of large patient flow or disaster
- Treatment spaces
  - Treatment spaces should have capacity for privacy and distant observation
  - Approximately requires one space for every 1500 to 2000 annual visits
  - Space should accommodate stretcher size and monitoring/acute care equipment
  - Specialty care spaces include medical/trauma resuscitation, decontamination, psychiatry, orthopedics, obstetrics and gynecology, wound care/procedures, otolaryngology, ophthalmology, oral surgery, and a family room
- Triage
  - Patients classified according to acuity
  - Major cases sent immediately to high-acuity emergency zone
  - Minor cases sent to a "fast track"
- Registration area must allow for patient privacy/confidentiality
- Waiting area
  - Must be completely visible to the staff to address sick patients
  - Must have enough space to accommodate patients and family members
  - Security must have immediate access to address disturbances
- Ancillary services space requirements
  - X-ray/CT—should be adjacent to the ED to prevent long distances for critically ill patients who need consistent monitoring
  - Laboratory—functions optimally with a separate ED lab with quick turnaround
  - Conference rooms/locker rooms/staff bathrooms/utility and equipment rooms
- Access to critical care and operating rooms must be immediate and under control of the ED staff

Human resource management

- Staffing for physicians, nurses, unit clerks, technicians, and registration is determined by number of patient visits, patient acuity, teaching program status, day and seasonal variation

- EM physicians can see 2 to 3 patients per hour of mixed acuity visits

Information management

- There is a movement to make all information electronic
- Patient health information is protected by the **Health Insurance Portability and Accountability Act (HIPAA):**
  - Requires institutions and providers to develop policies and procedures to protect patient health information
  - Allows use of this information for treatment, payment, and normal health care operations as long as there is patient consent
  - Requires written permission for use of protected information outside of normal health care operations
  - Allows patients the right to access, copy, and amend their records
  - Allows for certain health conditions (e.g., public health reporting) to be disclosed without the patient's consent
  - Carries significant penalties for violations including civil and criminal penalties with fines of up to $250,000 and/or imprisonment for up to 10 years

Overcrowding and patient throughput

- Overcrowding
  - 2006 Institute of Medicine (IOM) report *Hospital-Based Emergency Care: At the Breaking Point* brought overcrowding into the federal/national spotlight
  - ED visits have doubled in the last 15 years despite only a 10% to 15% population increase, whereas approximately 1000 hospitals have closed
  - Pressure exists to improve diagnostic accuracy in the emergency department while patient acuity becomes greater and more complex
    - Result is ED overcrowding, which is estimated by the IOM to have substantial cost and account for a considerable number of deaths due to system process failures
- Patient throughput: Divided into 3 phases (Input, Throughput, and Output)
  - Input refers to how many patients come into the emergency department:
    - Can reduce input burden by ambulance diversion (at large cost to the hospital) and by maintaining a "fast track" for minor acuity
    - Can reduce delays in input by bypassing triage and placing patients into empty beds during times of low ED census
  - Throughput refers to efficiency of patient management within the treatment area of the ED
    - Is maximized by early and appropriate decision making and resource utilization that is done in parallel and not in series/sequence

- Improved by use of nursing-initiated order sets, clinical decision rules, early consultations, and provider multitasking
- Slowed by overcrowding, physician distractions, poor laboratory and radiology turn-around times, and prolonged consultant decision making
- Output refers to getting patients out of the ED
  - The biggest hurdle to ED overall throughput is moving admitted/boarded patients out of the ED
  - Slowed down by transportation and social service issues related to discharging patients (e.g., waiting for an ambulance to a nursing home)

Policies and procedures

- Created and maintained by the ED director and ED leadership body; approved by hospital administration and the medical staff
- Should reflect the most current Joint Commission and institutional practice standards and be routinely reviewed

Safety and security

- Ensure safety and security through sound operational design and good practice patterns
  - Have departmental security clearly visible and able to respond quickly
  - Advise patients to preidentify toxic substances for decontamination
  - Detect weapons (using metal detectors and wands)
  - Have patients and coworkers in clear sight
  - Always have a clear path to exit a room
  - Observe universal precautions at all times
- Recognize risk factors and warning signs before violence occurs
- Use deescalation (communication) techniques to prevent violence
- Control the patient and situation with multiple coworkers to minimize further violence
- Protect the patient and others through appropriate restraint methods (physical and chemical)

PERFORMANCE IMPROVEMENT

Customer satisfaction and service

- Good service enhances patient attitudes regarding the ED
- Good customer satisfaction and service reduces the likelihood of potential lawsuit
- Patients most commonly are dissatisfied with long wait times and improper billing
- Studies show sitting down with the patient increases the perception of length of contact time

Patient safety

- The **Joint Commission**
  - Is the predominant health care accrediting body in the United States

- Has created multiple initiatives to promote patient safety and reduce errors
- Requires that any patient presenting to the ED must be evaluated and referred for follow-up
- Requires that all EDs be staffed by properly trained personnel
- Requires that a quality review/quality control program exist for the ED
- In 2002, announced its National Patient Safety Goals (NPSG) annual program
- 2009 Joint Commission NPSG goals:
  - Identify patients correctly
  - Improve staff communication
  - Use medicines safely
  - Prevent hospital-acquired infection
  - Check patient medicines
  - Prevent patients from falling
  - Help patients to be involved in their care
  - Identify patient safety risks (e.g., identify suicidal patients)
  - Watch patients closely for changes in their health, and respond quickly
  - Prevent errors in surgery
- Failure to comply results in automatic conditional accreditation
- The **Centers for Medicare and Medicaid Services (CMS)**
  - Promotes quality care agenda: "The right care for every person every time"
  - In 2005, released the CMS Quality Improvement Roadmap which implements major system strategies including public reporting, pay for performance, etc.
- The **Institute of Medicine**
  - Non-profit organization for science-based advice on medicine and health
  - In 2000, released *To Err Is Human*, placing error in the forefront of U.S. public health
  - Defines error as "a failure of a planned action to be completed as intended or the use of a wrong plan to achieve an aim"
  - Defines accident as "an event that damages a system and disrupts the ongoing or future output of the system"
  - Defines adverse event as "an injury caused by medical management rather than by the underlying disease or condition of the patient"
  - Requires that all EDs be staffed by properly trained personnel

Errors

- **Cognitive errors** are typically skill-based, rule-based, or knowledge-based
- **Violation-producing behaviors**
  - Premature closure: settling on a diagnosis before all the data are back
  - Availability bias: using recent encounters to influence future encounters disproportionately (e.g., CT scan on every chest pain to evaluate for pulmonary embolus after missing one)
  - Anchoring: committing too early to a diagnosis

- Triage queuing: location in the ED determines level of acuity
- Unpacking: incorrectly processing the diagnostic clues
- Representativeness heuristic: occurs when a clinician makes a subjective judgment of how similar an example is to a recognizable pattern
- **Error-producing conditions**
  - Diagnostic uncertainty: indecision about course of action
  - Low signal to noise: occurs when the incidence of a serious condition is low and is exceeded by the more common benign diagnosis
  - High cognitive load: the large amount of thinking in any given moment
  - Poor feedback: no reliable or timely feedback to ensure future accuracy
- **Error prevention**
  - Eliminate ambiguity and problem avoidance
  - Reduce cognitive load using clinical guidelines and pathways, mnemonics, computers (fact-finding and physician order entry), algorithms, and decision rules
  - Redesign jobs with correct work hours, workload, staffing, training, and resources
  - Incorporate technology
  - Conduct simulations
- **Mitigation:** enhancing the ability to recover from problems by preventing or minimizing their damage
  - Ensure a response to error reports, notify the patient and health system (e.g., risk management)
  - Make sure institutions and health care providers are accountable for safety
- **Disclosure**
  - In 2001, the Joint Commission required that hospitals document that "patients and their families be informed about the outcomes of care, including unanticipated outcomes"
  - Studies indicate that 88% of patients would wish to know everything about a mistake, whereas the remaining 12% would want to know about the mistake if it could or did affect their health
  - Strategies for disclosure of medical errors:
    - Make an explicit statement that an error occurred
    - Describe the error, explain why it happened, and discuss the steps to prevent similar errors in the future
    - Provide emotional support

Practice guidelines

- Be aware and follow national practice guidelines to meet the standard of care
- Current national and institutional guidelines should be available in the ED
- Follow quality measures specific to emergency medicine:
  - EKG performed for all nontraumatic chest pain and syncope

- Aspirin at arrival for acute myocardial infarction
- Vital signs, oxygen saturation, mental status assessment, and empiric antibiotics for community-acquired pneumonia

Ethics and professionalism

CONFLICT MANAGEMENT

- Conflict is the result of differing expectations, agendas, personal needs, backgrounds, and communication styles among individuals
- Principles of conflict resolution in emergency medicine:
  - Establish common goals and communicate effectively
  - Avoid accusations and public confrontations
  - Compromise and do not take conflict personally
  - Avoid rushing into premature solutions or positional bargaining
  - Move from positions to mutual interests
  - Invent options for mutual gain and accept differences of opinion
  - Establish shared expectations and use ongoing communication

Ethics

- Accepted social and bioethical values
  - Autonomy: a patient's ability to make personal decisions affecting care
  - Beneficence: a duty to do good
  - Confidentiality: an understanding that patient health information will not be revealed to another or other institution without the patient's consent
  - Justice: fairness in the allocation of resources and obligations
  - Nonmaleficence: doing no harm, prevention of harm and removal of harm
  - Personal integrity: adhering to one's own reasoned and defensible set of values and moral standards
- Bioethical dilemmas in emergency practice
  - Withholding and withdrawing treatment: higher standards exist to withhold care than to withdraw care later
  - **Advance directives**
    - **DNR order:** a physician's order in the hospital chart informing hospital personnel "do not resuscitate"
    - **Prehospital directives:** instructs prehospital personnel not to resuscitate in cases where EMS has been contacted
    - **Living will:** standardized form for resuscitative efforts once the patient loses decisional capacity; until then, the patient has free will
    - **Durable power of attorney:** allows for a surrogate decision maker to make health care decisions the patient would ordinarily make when the patient lacks decisional capacity

- **Nonstandard advance directive:** do not rely on these (e.g., a tattoo for "do not resuscitate") to determine care
- **Decision-making capacity**
  - Knowledge of the options (including no treatment if patient refuses care)
  - Awareness of the consequences of each option or refusal
  - Appreciation of personal costs, risks, consequences, and benefits of each option or refusal in relation to the patient's values and preferences
- **Consent**
  - **Implied consent:** presumed consent that any reasonable person would wish to have with or without decisional capacity
  - **Informed consent:** consent from a patient with decisional capacity who is given and understands all the options and voluntarily agrees to undergo the intervention
  - **Expressed consent:** a verbal or written willingness for treatment
- **Refusal of care**
  - Patient requires decisional capacity
  - Patients can refuse individual treatments and not the entire visit
  - Leaving against medical advice (AMA) forms should perhaps be signed by the patient using their own handwriting to document understanding of the risks and consequences ("I know I could die")
- **Surrogate decision makers:** when patients lack decisional capacity and have no advance directive
  - Surrogate list (in order of importance): spouse (not divorced or separated), adult children, parents (of an adult), domestic partner, sibling, close friend, and attending physician in consultation with a bioethics committee
- **Futile care:** Defined as <1% chance for a meaningfully positive outcome

Impairment

- According to an ACEP policy statement, "Physician impairment exists when a physician's professional performance is adversely affected because of illness, including mental or physical illness, aging, alcoholism, or chemical dependence." It is estimated there are 100 deaths annually among physicians attributable to chemical dependency

SIGNS AND SYMPTOMS

- Generally, a pattern of events rather than one single event
  - Family trouble (arguments, separation, extramarital affairs, or divorce)
  - Job changes and large intervals between employment
  - Substance abuse
  - Unkempt appearance

- Finally, professional duties degenerate such as tardiness, unprofessional behavior, poor clinical judgment, and neglect of patient care responsibilities

DIAGNOSIS
- Clinical

TREATMENT
- Prompt and careful intervention
  - Perform immediately after a precipitant crisis
  - Conduct a nonthreatening, nonjudgmental confrontation, working through expected physician denial
  - Document impaired behaviors
  - Plan intervention goals in advance, including choices of treatment facilities
- Prevent relapse
- Prognosis for recovery is excellent

Leadership (leading, directing, and mentoring)

- A leader can motivate others toward a common goal
- Leadership roles and skill sets
  - Visionary: the ability to see future options
  - Decision maker: the ability to choose among the options
  - Informant: the ability to communicate
  - Tone setter: creating the atmosphere that will allow for change to develop
  - Character: recognition by others that the leader is a person of strong ethical character
  - Fairness and justice: abiding by the highest standard without regard for personal gain
- People seek leadership and direction for mentorship

Personal well-being

- Wellness strategies
  - Promote wellness in the professional environment
    - Maintain a positive work environment
    - Work progressive shifts of reasonable length (<10 hours)
    - Management strategies for difficult and violent patients
    - Utilize professional organizations and support groups
  - Strengthen and maintain interpersonal relationships (family and social)
  - Be responsible with finances
  - Develop and continue physical fitness
  - Cultivate methods of relaxation, renewal, and personal growth

Professional development and lifelong learning

- The American Board of Emergency Medicine (ABEM) requires recertification every 10 years (ConCert exam); in addition, yearly lifelong learning and

self-assessment (LLSA) tests are required for 7 of the 10 years between recertification
- The American College of Emergency Physicians (ACEP) requires 150 hours of continuing medical education (CME) credit hours every 3 years

SYSTEMS-BASED MANAGEMENT

Managed care

- Insurance status of the patient influences patient treatment and follow up
  - Certain medications may not be covered by the patient's insurance
  - Patients may need to follow up with their primary care doctor for a specialist referral
  - Patients without insurance may need generic alternatives or get admitted to the hospital for specialty service intervention as they have poor access to outpatient follow-up

End-of-life issues

- Patients and families regard the end of life as one of the most important events in a person's life
- Importance: the desire to avoid dealing with the deaths of patients is one of the major causes of career disillusionment and change among ED staff
- **Barriers to end-of-life care**
  - Physician comfort: no preexisting relationship, stress of busy ED, fear of being blamed, survivor's guilt, and own mortality
  - Patient/family expectations: death viewed as preventable, physicians viewed as resistant to the emotional impact of death
- **Death telling**
  - Confirm identity of deceased and family
  - Identify yourself and sit down in a private location
  - Be organized with dialogue and with support staff (police, nurse, social work, religious advisor)
  - Use the patient's name and avoid euphemisms (e.g., do state that the patient "died," not that he "left us")
  - Let the family know in a way you would like to know
  - Address organ donation and referral to medical examiner/coroner
  - Allow the family to view the body and give opportunity to follow-up
- **Grief reaction**
  - Grief spike, denial, anger, bargaining, guilt/depression, and acceptance
- **Debriefing:** ensure systems are in place to allow for family and staff debriefing/grief

Medicolegal

ACCREDITATION

- Joint Commission approval for a hospital is for a maximum of 3 years

- The Resident Review Committee (RRC) of the Accreditation Council for Graduate Medical Education (ACGME) can approve a residency program in emergency medicine up to a maximum of 5 years

COMPLIANCE

- Physicians must comply with institutional requirements (e.g., TB testing, timely records)
- Physicians must comply with national requirements (e.g., Joint Commission and CMS) or face potential legal risk of not meeting the standard of care (see "Patient Safety")

CONFIDENTIALITY

- Patient records will be kept in the strictest of confidentiality (see HIPPA in Information Management)
- Confidential discussion with your own legal council is considered privileged and should not be discoverable except for a few exceptions

CONSENT AND REFUSAL OF CARE

- See "Ethics."

EMERGENCY MEDICAL TREATMENT AND ACTIVE LABOR ACT (EMTALA)

- Included in the COBRA legislation of 1986
- Created to prevent the discriminatory practice of hospitals transferring, discharging, or refusing to treat indigent patients coming to the emergency department because of the high cost of diagnosing and treating these patients with emergency medical conditions
- Protects anyone coming to the hospital seeking medical care
- EMTALA violations can lead to strict penalties including fines (not covered by the physician's malpractice policy) and exclusion from the Medicare program
- The EMTALA act has three primary requirements
  - The hospital must provide an appropriate medical screening examination to anyone coming to the Emergency Department seeking medical care
  - For anyone who comes to the hospital for whom the hospital determines that the individual has an emergency medical condition, the hospital must treat and stabilize the emergency medical condition
  - A hospital must not transfer an individual with an emergency medical condition that has not been stabilized unless several conditions are met, including that the transfer is not for financial reasons; the patient is being transferred to a higher level of care (benefits of transfer outweigh the risks); and the patient consents to transfer

LIABILITY, MALPRACTICE, AND RISK MANAGEMENT

- **Standard of care** (medically liable): defined as what an ordinary physician of like or similar training would reasonably do under like or similar circumstances
- **Medical malpractice/negligence lawsuit structure** has four components
  - **Duty:** the responsibility of caring for the patient
  - **Breach of duty:** the requirements for performance of that duty were not met
  - **Harm:** that damage actually happened
  - **Proximate cause:** the concept that the action or inaction of a physician was the exact cause that breached the duty and led to the patient's harm
- **Risk management**
  - Contact your institutional risk management for advice if you suspect a patient has been harmed or if an adverse event occurs
  - Mitigate risk with behavior and training
    - Communicate respectfully (e.g., be professional)
    - Value your patient's time (e.g., "Your time is valuable—I'm sorry for the wait")
    - Thank the patient and include his or her input into the health care
    - Document legibly and detail your thought processes and interactions ("If it's not documented, it didn't happen")
    - Manage patient expectations. (e.g., give the patient an anticipated timeline for reasonable recovery and explain how to navigate the health system)
    - Refrain from speaking in absolutes (e.g., "This could never be a heart attack")
    - Discharge patients with time and action specific instructions (e.g., "If abdominal pain does not get better in 6 hours, return to be examined")
    - Understand specific medical problems and their inherent future risks (e.g., never guarantee that there is not a foreign body when a patient has broken glass near a wound)

REPORTING (ASSAULT, COMMUNICABLE DISEASES, NATIONAL PRACTITIONER DATA BANK)

- Reportable assault
  - Gunshot and stab wounds
  - Physical assault (note that assault of a healthcare employee by a patient can be criminally elevated above simple assault)
  - Sexual assault
- Reportable communicable diseases
  - Venereal (gonorrhea, chlamydia, syphilis, AIDS)
  - Highly contagious (hepatitis, epidemic flu and gastroenteritis, whooping cough)

- Reportable abuse
  - Mandatory reporting for child and elder abuse
  - Spousal/intimate partner violence (formerly domestic violence)
- Reportable animal bites
  - Dog and cat (as pets)
  - Potentially rabid animals: dog, cat, fox, bat, skunk, raccoon (generally not rodents except beaver, woodchuck)
- Reportable deaths
  - Dead on arrival or dead in the emergency department
  - Abortions/miscarriages (may require separate fetal death certification based on gestational age)
- Reportable items on the National Practitioner Data Bank
  - Disciplinary action following formal peer review
  - Any amount paid in full or as partial settlement/ judgment of a written malpractice claim

PEARLS

- Reimbursement relies directly on the level of documentation; be aware of the rules of billing and coding to ensure that you are reimbursed for services provided.

- The Health Insurance Portability and Accountability Act (HIPAA) is designed to protect the confidentiality of the patient encounter and the patient's medical record; violations will be met with substantial fines and disciplinary action.

- The 2006 Institute of Medicine (IOM) report *Hospital-Based Emergency Care: At the Breaking Point* brought overcrowding into the federal/ national spotlight.

- Patient throughput is divided into 3 phases (input, throughput, and output). The greatest contributor to crowding is the inability to move admitted patients up to hospital beds.

- Be aware of the sources of cognitive errors, and strategies to minimize them.

- Signs of physician impairment include financial trouble, family problems, unkempt appearance, frequent job changes, frequent tardiness, unprofessional behavior, and poor clinical judgment.

- The Emergency Medical Treatment and Active Labor Act (EMTALA) was enacted as part of 1986 COBRA legislation in order to prevent the discriminatory practice of transferring, discharging, or refusing to treat indigent patients. It requires a medical screening examination for all patients presenting to the ED, treatment and stabilization of emergency medical conditions, and stabilization prior to patient discharge.

- Four components must exist in order to prove malpractice: duty, breach of duty, harm, and proximate cause.

BIBLIOGRAPHY

American College of Emergency Physicians: Emergency physician rights and responsibilities, *Ann Emerg Med* 52:187–188, 2008.

Biddinger P: Regulatory and legal issues in the emergency department. In Adams JG, Barton ED, Collings J et al (eds): *Emergency medicine*, ed 1, Philadelphia, 2008, Saunders, pp. 2193–2213.

DiGiacomo E: Optimal design features. In *Managing the emergency department*, vol 16, Texas, 1992, American College of Emergency Physicians, pp. 137–145.

EMTALA rules by AAEM. Available at http://www.aaem.org/ advocacy/emtala.php.

Garmel G: Conflict resolution in emergency medicine. In Adams JG, Barton ED, Collings J et al (eds): *Emergency medicine*, ed 1, Philadelphia, 2008, Saunders, pp. 2171–2185.

Goldberg R: Wellness, stress, and the impaired physician. In Marx JA, Hockberger RS, Walls RM et al (eds): *Rosen's emergency medicine: concepts and clinical practice*, ed 6, Philadelphia, 2006, Elsevier Mosby p. 3174.

Hamedani AG, Mort E: The quality movement in health care: a primer. In Adams JG, Barton ED, Collings J et al (eds): *Emergency medicine*, ed 1, Philadelphia, 2008, Saunders, pp. 2151–2159.

Henry GL: Medical-legal issues in emergency medicine. In Adams JG, Barton ED, Collings J et al (eds): *Emergency medicine*, ed 1, Philadelphia, 2008, Saunders, pp. 2199–2213.

Hobgood C: Patient safety in emergency medicine. In Adams JG, Barton ED, Collings J et al (eds): *Emergency medicine*, ed 1, Philadelphia, 2008, Saunders, pp. 2161–2170.

Honigman B: End of life. In Rosen P, Marx JA, Hockberger RS et al (eds): *Rosen's emergency medicine concepts and clinical practice*, ed 5, St. Louis, 2002, Mo, Mosby, pp. 2735–2747.

Iserson KV: Bioethics. In Marx JA, Hockberger RS, Walls RM et al (eds): *Rosen's emergency medicine: concepts and clinical practice*, ed 6, Philadelphia, 2006, Elsevier Mosby, pp. 3127–3138.

Issacs E: The violent patient. In Adams JG, Barton ED, Collings J et al (eds): *Emergency medicine*, ed 1, Philadelphia, 2008, Saunders, pp. 2047–2049.

Nicoll G: Financial management through budgeting. In *Managing the emergency department*, vol 2, Texas, 1992, American College of Emergency Physicians, pp. 5–7.

Takayesu JK: Coding and billing. In Adams JG, Barton ED, Collings J et al (eds): *Emergency medicine*, ed 1, Philadelphia, 2008, Saunders, pp. 2215–2220.

Twanmoh JR: Emergency department overcrowding, patient flow, and safety. In Croskerry P, Cosby KS, Schenkel SM, Wears RL (eds): *Patient safety in emergency medicine*, ed 1, Philadelphia, 2009, Lippincott Williams & Wilkins, pp. 149–157.

The Joint Commission. Available at www.jointcommision.org.

Questions and Answers

1. Which of the following is true about EMTALA?

   a. it is an EMTALA violation if tertiary care hospital A transfers a stable patient to tertiary care hospital B because hospital B has an electrophysiologist to take care of a patient's arrhythmia and hospital A does not

   b. EMTALA fines are covered by a physician's malpractice insurance

   c. it is an EMTALA violation if hospital A transfers an unstable patient to hospital B before making any attempts to stabilize the patient, even if hospital B is aware of the patient's condition and assumes responsibility

   d. it is an EMTALA violation to transfer stable patients from one emergency department to another emergency department

   e. it is an EMTALA violation to transfer a stable and medically low-risk psychiatric patient to a psychiatric crisis center after the patient has had an appropriate screening examination in the emergency department

2. Emergency physicians' rights and responsibilities include:

   a. being provided periodic reports of billings and collections in their name and having the right to audit such billings, without retribution

   b. agreeing to a restrictive covenant that limits the right to practice medicine after the termination of employment or contract to provide services as an emergency physician

   c. waiving the continuing medical education requirement if involved in a resident teaching program

   d. restricting clinical decision making when specialty services are required (e.g., neurologist prescribing systemic thrombolytic therapy for a stroke patient at 5 hours based on "cutting edge" research)

3. Which of the following statements is most correct regarding billing and coding?

   a. conjunctivitis can be coded a Level 4 if sufficient documentation exists

   b. observation billing does not require separate documentation from the ED chart

   c. emergency physicians are legally protected if a hospital billing service overcharges patients for Level 5 service when the physicians document at a Level 4

   d. with regard to these three areas, documenting two of three elements of past medical, family and social history will be sufficient to achieve a Level 5 coding

   e. critical care coding requires Level 5 evaluation and management documentation and coding plus supportive documentation; procedure time does not count

4. Which of the following statements is correct regarding HIPPA?

   a. violation fines can be covered by the provider's malpractice

   b. information on a positive case of syphilis can be reported to the appropriate authorities without the patient's consent

   c. patients have the right to access and copy their records, but not amend them

   d. institutions and providers require patient consent for treatment; payment does not require consent

   e. verbal consent is required for use of protected information outside of normal health care operations

5. Which of the following is most associated with the Joint Commission?

   a. customer satisfaction and service
   b. cost containment
   c. end-of-life issues
   d. the national patient safety goals
   e. the quality improvement roadmap

6. Which of the following increases patient perception of the amount of time they have had contact with the physician?

   a. shortening ED wait times
   b. offering food to patients
   c. ensure proper billing of the patient
   d. accurate diagnosis of the patient's problem
   e. sitting down while speaking with the patient

7. Which of the following describes the cognitive error related to committing too early to a diagnosis?

   a. anchoring
   b. availability bias
   c. premature stratification
   d. representativeness heuristic
   e. unpacking

8. Which of the following affects emergency department throughput the most?

   a. social service times prior to discharge
   b. distractions to the attending emergency physician
   c. laboratory and radiology turn-around times
   d. consultant decision making
   e. waiting time to go to a bed after an admission is placed in the ED

9. Cost-containment strategies include:

   a. ordering of baseline laboratory tests for future benefit
   b. ordering radiographs on all extremity injuries to ensure no missed fractures

c. prescribing a generic instead of a new antibiotic to treat an uncomplicated urinary tract infection despite a favorable *in vitro* study for the new antibiotic

d. cardiac monitoring of all patients to catch the unsuspected arrhythmia to prevent morbidity and a delayed diagnosis

e. administration of parenteral instead of oral medications which will work faster and obviate the need for multiple oral medications

10. Which of the following bioethical principles is most represented when a physician color-codes patients based on survivability during a mass causality?

a. autonomy
b. justice
c. nonmaleficence
d. confidentiality
e. personal integrity

11. Which of the following advance directives allows for a surrogate decision maker to make health care decisions?

a. prehospital directive
b. DNR order
c. nonstandard advanced directive
d. durable power of attorney
e. living will

12. Which concept is represented in a situation where a patient presents as a PEA code and it is determined that a needle thoracostomy procedure will be required to save a life?

a. expressed consent
b. decisional capacity
c. informed consent
d. refusal of care
e. implied consent

13. Which is typically the last outward sign or symptom of physician impairment?

a. neglect of professional duties
b. family troubles
c. substance abuse
d. job changes
e. unkempt appearance

14. Which of the following is NOT considered one of the four components of malpractice?

a. duty
b. breach of duty
c. harm
d. proximate cause
e. standard of care

15. Which of the following is reportable?

a. influenza
b. medical command call to your ED of a pronounced death at the scene

c. suspected elder abuse of a senior citizen who presents to the ED as failure to thrive
d. dismissed lawsuit
e. rat bite

---

1. Answer: c

EMTALA requires that a patient be stabilized prior to transfer. Although a patient may be unstable (even if the receiving hospital is aware), all appropriate measures to stabilize the patient must be performed prior to transfer. Transferring of stable patients to another hospital with **greater specialty resources (a), to another ED (d),** or to a specialty center **after an appropriate medical screening examination (e)** are appropriate transfers. EMTALA is **not covered by a physician's malpractice insurance (b).**

2. Answer: a

It is of paramount importance that an emergency physician be provided **periodic reports of billings and collections in their name and have the right to audit such billings, without retribution (a).** Certain physician groups have fired EM physicians after inquiries regarding collections, and this practice is completely unethical. EM physicians should not agree to **restrictive covenants** that limit the right to practice medicine after termination of employment or contract **(b).** The American Academy of Emergency Medicine (AAEM) has fought for EM physician rights in these 2 types of cases (closed collection books and restrictive covenants) and has won favorable judgments for the EM physicians. **CME is required for every EM physician (c),** and **EM autonomy in clinical decision making** shall be respected and shall not be restricted other than through reasonable rules, regulations, and bylaws of his or her medical staff or practice group **(d).**

3. Answer: d

Level 5 coding requires **2 of 3 areas of past medical, family and social history (d).** It also requires 4 to 8 elements of history of present illness, a complete review of systems, and 8 + extensive elements of physical examination. **Conjunctivitis cannot be up-coded to a Level 4 or 5** regardless of the documentation **(a). Observation billing** does require separate documentation from the ED chart **(b). EM physicians are responsible for overcharges to patients** and the level of documentation is required to reflect the level of service **(c). Critical care coding obviates the need for evaluation and management coding** but does require supportive documentation that cannot include time related to procedures **(e).**

4. Answer: b

Public health reporting can be disclosed without a patient's consent (b). Violations of HIPAA are **not**

covered by malpractice (a). Patients have the **right to access, copy, and amend their records (c)**. Institutions and providers **require patient consent for treatment and payment (d)**. **Written consent** is required for use of protected information outside of normal health care operations **(e)**.

5. Answer: d

The **national patient safety goals (d)** are a Joint Commission initiative. **Customer satisfaction and service (a), cost containment (b)**, and **end-of-life issues (c)** are not primarily associated with the Joint Commission. The **quality improvement roadmap (e)** is a Centers for Medicare and Medicaid Services (CMS) initiative.

6. Answer: e

While all of these choices are likely to result in greater patient satisfaction, **sitting down while interviewing the patient (e)** has been shown to increase the perceived amount of physician–patient interaction time.

7. Answer: a

Anchoring (a) is committing too early to a diagnosis. **Availability bias** is using recent encounters to influence future encounters **(b)**. **Premature closure** (not premature stratification) is settling on a diagnosis before all the data are back **(c)**. **Representativeness heuristic** is when a clinician makes a subjective judgment of how similar an example is to a recognizable pattern **(d)**. **Unpacking** is incorrectly processing the diagnostic clues **(e)**.

8. Answer: e

Waiting times for patients after an admission order has been placed (e) has the most effect on throughput. Long ED waiting times can have significant consequences on patient morbidity and mortality in the ED and in the waiting room (waiting for an ED bed). Choices **a**, **b**, **c**, and **d**, although important, have less effect on throughput.

9. Answer: c

Ordering and prescribing generic medications (c) (or writing for those covered by the patient's insurance company) **will help in cost containment**. **Ordering baseline laboratory tests (a)**, **indiscriminate cardiac monitoring (d)**, and **routine parenteral instead of oral medications (e)** will increase costs. Correct use of decision rules (e.g., the Ottawa ankle rule) will help in cost containment **(b)**.

10. Answer: b

Justice (b) is defined as fairness in the allocation of resources and obligations. **Autonomy** is a patient's ability to make personal decisions affecting care **(a)**. **Nonmaleficence** is doing no harm **(c)**. **Confidentiality** is an understanding that health care information will not be shared without patient permission **(d)**. **Personal integrity** is adhering to one's own set of values **(e)**.

11. Answer: d

A **durable power of attorney (d)** allows for a surrogate decision maker to make health care decisions the patient would ordinarily make when the patient lacks decisional capacity. A **prehospital directive** instructs prehospital people not to resuscitate **(a)**. A **DNR order** is a physician's order in the hospital chart informing the hospital not to resuscitate **(b)**. **Nonstandard advance directives** include medallions or tattoos that state not to resuscitate but are not legally binding **(c)**. A **living will** is a standardized form for resuscitative efforts once a patient loses decisional capacity **(e)**.

12. Answer: e

Implied consent (e) is presumed consent that any reasonable person would wish to have. **Expressed consent** is a verbal or written willingness for treatment **(a)**. **Decisional capacity** is knowledge, awareness, and appreciation of options prior to making choices **(b)**. **Informed consent** is consent from a patient who is given and understands all the options and voluntarily agrees to undergo the intervention **(c)**. **Refusal of care** requires an understanding of the risks and consequences and deciding against an intervention **(d)**.

13. Answer: a

The impaired physician will typically allow all aspects of his or her life to fall apart until ultimately there is **neglect of professional duties (a)**. It is for this reason it is so important to detect subtle changes in your colleagues before it becomes too late. The maladaptive patterns include, but are not limited to, tardiness, unprofessional behavior, poor clinical judgment, and neglect of patient care responsibilities. **Family troubles (b), substance abuse (c), job changes (d)** and **unkempt appearance (e)** usually come earlier in the spectrum of disease. An intervention is required for treatment and the prognosis for success is usually very good.

14. Answer: e

Duty is the responsibility of seeing a patient **(a)**. **Breach of duty** is the requirements of the care that were not met **(b)**. **Harm** is the actual damage that happens that will become quantified if a judgment is made against a physician **(c)**. **Proximate cause** is the concept that the action or inaction of a physician was the exact cause that breached the duty that led to the patient's harm **(d)**. **Standard of care** is defined as what an ordinary physician of like or similar training would reasonably do under like or similar circumstances **(e)**, and is not considered one of the four components of malpractice.

15. Answer: c

Elder abuse (c) requires mandatory reporting. **Epidemic flu** that is highly communicable requires reporting, **not the common flu (a).** Dead on arrival or dead in the emergency department requires reporting, **not dead at the scene (b).** Any amount paid in full or as partial settlement/judgment of a written malpractice claim will be reported to the national practitioner data bank, **dismissed lawsuits** are not **(d).** Animal bites (dogs or cats) and potentially rabid animals **(small rodents are not typically rabid)** require reporting **(e).**

Emergency Medical Services

Gerald C. Wydro | Ernest Yeh

EMS HISTORY

National Academy of Sciences-National Research Council Report (1966)

The Emergency Medical Services System Act (1973)

Prehospital providers: levels of care

EMS LEGAL ISSUES

MEDICAL OVERSIGHT AND MEDICAL COMMAND

EMS COMMUNICATION

EMS SYSTEM TYPES

Urban/suburban

Rural

Wilderness/frontier

Military

DISASTER PREPAREDNESS

Incident command system

Hazard vulnerability analysis (HVA)

Federal planning

SPECIFIC ISSUES RELATED TO DISASTER MANAGEMENT

Decontamination principles

Weapons of mass destruction (WMD)

Mass casualty incidents (MCIs)

EMS history

NATIONAL ACADEMY OF SCIENCES–NATIONAL RESEARCH COUNCIL REPORT (1966)

- "Modern Era of Prehospital Care" in the United States
- Report generated by NAS-NRC
- *Accidental Death and Disability: The Neglected Disease of Modern Society*
  - Failure of the U.S. healthcare system to provide for emergency patients
  - Identified key problems and issues
  - Summary report included a blueprint for EMS development
- Highway Safety Act of 1966
  - Established cabinet level Department of Transportation (DOT)
    - Legislative and financial authority to improve EMS
    - Specific emphasis on highway safety programs
    - Funded initial training and curriculum development of Emergency Medical Technician—Ambulance (EMT-A)
    - Late 1960s saw the arrival of new technologies for prehospital use
      - Drugs, defibrillation
      - Telemetry
      - Heartmobile Program, Columbus, Ohio (1969)
- National Registry of Emergency Medical Technicians
  - Founded in 1970
  - Developed standardized national certifying examination
  - Most states still required additional state specific certification

THE EMERGENCY MEDICAL SERVICES SYSTEM ACT (1973)

- Regionalization
- Funding from federal government to aid in development
- Identified 15 essential EMS components
  - Manpower
  - Training
  - Communications
  - Transportation
  - Facilities
  - Critical care units
  - Public safety agencies

- Consumer participation
- Access to care
- Patient transfer
- Coordinated record keeping
- Public information and education
- Review and evaluation
- Disaster plan
- Mutual aid

PREHOSPITAL PROVIDERS: LEVELS OF CARE

- EMT-A
  - Initially 70 hours of curriculum
  - Basic emergency care
  - CPR and basic first-aid skills
- EMT-B
  - Early 1990s
  - Evolution of EMT-A with new DOT national standard curriculum
- EMT-Paramedic (EMT-P)
  - Training times few hundred hours to 1200 hours of didactic and clinical time
  - Skills in addition to EMT-A
    - Defibrillation
    - Endotracheal intubation
    - Venipuncture
    - Medication administration
  - Initially required significant "on-line" medical oversight
    - Communication with a physician at a base hospital
- EMT–Intermediate (EMT-I)
  - Hybrid between EMT-A and EMT-P
  - Significant state-to-state variation

EMS legal issues

- Oversight and legislation of EMS will be variable dependent upon controlling entities
  - Federal, state, local level
- Immunity law "Good Samaritan" coverage varies by state
- Vicarious Liability: legal exposure for the acts of another even if not directly involved in caring for a patient
  - Physicians overseeing EMS providers may be responsible for:
    - Paramedic errors of omission/commission
    - Protocol violations
- Malpractice in EMS
  - Must establish key elements
    - A legal duty exists, the duty was breached, breach caused injury and damages
  - In EMS the malpractice may be through direct action (medical command order) or secondary to adherence to treatment protocol that is found to cause harm
- Legal exposures
  - Paramedic judgment errors leading to morbidity and mortality

- Failure to follow protocols
- Motor vehicle collisions (especially when emergency lights and sirens used)
- Patient nontransport/EMS initiated refusal
- Patient restraint
- EMTALA
- Nonclinical/administrative
- Legal protections
  - Separate liability coverage for EMS activities
  - Close involvement
    - Offline: protocols/quality assurance
    - Online: real-time communications with paramedics

Medical oversight and medical command

- Authority to provide medical oversight varies from state to state
  - State departments of health
  - Emergency medical services offices/divisions
- Establish guidelines
  - Medical protocol/policy development
  - Quality assurance and improvement
  - Education
  - Communication
  - System design
- Non–physician providers
  - "Borrowed servant" legal principle
    - Paramedic performs certain activities sanctioned by the responsible physician(s)
- Direct medical oversight
  - Physician and prehospital provider make contemporaneous medical decisions about patient care
    - Usually via telephone or radio communication
    - Online medical command/control
- Indirect medical oversight
  - Written protocols
    - Medical care guidelines
    - "Standing orders"
- Clinical protocols for typical cases
  - Minimize need for direct physician contact
  - Address other issues
    - Field pronouncement/termination of resuscitation
    - Transport vs. nontransport criteria
    - Refusal of care
    - Destination determination (decision to bypass the closest hospital in favor or specialty designated sites, e.g., trauma center, stroke center PCI facility)
    - Quality assurance
      - Evaluate effectiveness of protocols and modify as needed
- Training
  - Basic standards for initial education of providers
  - Continuing education for providers
- Monitor and establish standards for those providing medical command to EMS

- Medical Command Physician (also Medical Control Physician, Medical Control Authority)
- Nonlicensed medical providers require "supervision"
  - Acting as physician extenders
- Ensuring knowledge and skills proficiency of provider is adequate
- Authority varies from state to state
- Medical command assessment
  - Medical knowledge assessment
  - Protocol knowledge assessment
  - Skills verification
  - Retrospective review
- Restriction of medical command when deficiencies are identified
- Provide means for re-education
- Process to re-obtain medical command
- Mechanism for due process when medical command physician and provider disagree

EMS communications

- Consists of several intergrated steps that begins with a call for service
- Calls for service received in a single center
  - Calls for police assistance are majority of calls, therefore many 911 centers are run under the auspices of the police department
  - Initial information is gathered by a call taker, who then can transfer the necessary information to a dispatcher
  - Emergency Medical Dispatcher can then proceed to gather more details in order to
    - Prioritize the call in terms of type of response and resources needed
    - Provide Pre-Arrival Instructions (PAI) for the caller, such as: immediate medical care or interventions (i.e., starting CPR)
- Dispatch centers are responsible for sending the most needed resources, while preserving those not anticipated to be needed for the next call—Do the most good for the greatest number
  - Interagency communications, i.e., EMS to police, EMS to fire departments, EMS to EMS
  - Transport to the hospital
    - Priority of transport to the hospital is often left to the discretion of the on-scene crew
- **EMS traffic accidents are common and nonemergent transport is encouraged unless a true life or limb threat exists**
- Choice of receiving facility
  - Some EMS organizations mandate patients must go to closest appropriate facility
  - Some permit patients some latitude when a choice exists
  - EMS responsible for routing patients to specialty facilities when needed, i.e., trauma center, burn center, accredited stroke center, or facility with PCI capability

- Transfer of care
  - EMS personnel must give a report to hospital staff
  - Most systems require a written run report be left with hospital staff. Some permit a report to be generated up to 24 hours later
- Return to service
  - Restocking, filing run reports, and cleaning/disinfecting the unit
- Medical command
  - Many EMS systems will have standing orders, usually with some sort of indicator to inform the paramedic how far in a treatment algorithm they can proceed before contacting medical command
  - During disaster, or radio failure, medics can proceed with the protocol in its entirety, usually with subsequent documentation on communications failure in order to identify areas of system improvement
  - Communications may utilize any of the following modalities
    - Landline, radio, pager system, or advanced systems including mobile data terminals (MDTs), which are linked to the dispatch center. These may also permit responders to view data regarding the last few calls for service, and are often useful when incorporated into a GPS system to minimize response time to station to alert crew of emergency
    - Any system broadcasting over public airwaves can be monitored. Patient specific identifiers should be avoided

EMS system types

URBAN/SUBURBAN

- **Fire department–based**
  - Capitalizes on the existing fire suppression infrastructure
    - Community stations—referred to as the Fixed Deployment Model
    - Paramilitary chain of command
  - Utilizes a variety of staffing models across the spectrum of training (tiered response system) May include
    - A fire engine staffed by any combination of 1st Responders, EMT-Bs, EMT-Is, or EMT-Ps
    - BLS or ALS ambulance
    - ALS nontransport vehicle response to scene
    - Can result in understaffing/conflict of duties when all personnel are needed for fire suppression in dual-trained systems (FF/EMT, FF/Paramedic)
- **Separate third public safety agency/authority**
  - Separate public safety department dedicated to EMS
  - Also tiered system
- **Hospital-based EMS**
  - ALS, occasionally with some combination of EMT-Ps/Prehospital RNs
    - May function as interhospital transport or
    - Adjunct to primary 911-based system

- **Contracted private company(ies)**
  - May provide entire scope of prehospital response/transport
  - May share responsibilities with local government, i.e., local fire department
  - Urban units have minimal need for aircraft ambulances. Suburban services utilize aircraft more frequently, usually in the setting of trauma in order to speed arrival at a trauma center
  - Often have a higher percentage of nonemergent calls

RURAL

- Often volunteer services, sometimes augmented by paid crewpersons
- Some struggle to maintain continuing education and prevent skill erosion given paucity of funding and population, respectively
- Aircraft ambulances rise in importance, often being used to speed the critically ill and injured to hospitals that can be distant from the scene
- Often have higher percentage of higher acuity calls
- FARMEDIC program to train prehospital personnel about the injuries, and hazards, inherent in working farms and agricultural machinery

WILDERNESS/FRONTIER

- Newest of the recognized categories, often very different from more urbanized systems in their scope of practice (extensive)
- As a consequence of communication hurdles (caves, remote areas, mountainous terrain) and prolonged extrications/transport, often must support victim(s) for days
- Aircraft of marked importance, not only for transport, but also for Search & Rescue
- Some states delineate separate scopes of practice for prehospital wilderness responders

MILITARY

- Scope of practice of military personnel not necessarily congruent with civilian counterparts
- Aircraft, both rotary-wing and fixed-wing, are part of any modern military's evacuation plans
- EMS in peacetime, or on base
- Usually run out of the base hospital
- May or may not serve surrounding community in areas outside the United States
- Military may be used in times of disaster, or in areas of the country where civilian resources do not exist, to evacuate patients to either military or civilian hospitals

Disaster preparedness

- Disaster: An event that overwhelms the capacity of a local care system or community

- Organizing principles of disaster management are as follows.

INCIDENT COMMAND SYSTEM

- Complexity depends on the size of the event
- Establishes a common terminology
- Goal is to provide smooth flow of communication
- Incident Commander ultimately in charge
- Four section leaders
  - *Operations:* tasked with providing and directing all required duties to achieve required goals
  - *Finance:* track incident-related costs, maintain personnel records, and procurement of equipment and materials
  - *Logistics:* provide the resources, services, and support required by the incident
  - *Planning:* collection and display of incident information, as well as the status of involved personnel
- Other positions, divisions, or tasks may be added or removed as the incident requires

HAZARD VULNERABILITY ANALYSIS (HVA)

- Vulnerability assessment
- Review risks and potential exposures for planning

FEDERAL PLANNING

- Homeland Security Presidential Directive (HSPD)–5
  - Implemented in 2003 to enhance nation's ability to manage domestic incidents by establishing a single, comprehensive national incident management system
- **National Incident Management System (NIMS)**
  - Federal system of coordinating emergency response and incident management among federal, state, and local agencies
- **National Response Framework (NRF)**
  - Establishes a comprehensive, national, all-hazards approach to domestic incident response
  - Formerly known as the National Response Plan
  - Department of Homeland Security is lead agency
- **Disaster Medical Assistance Team (DMAT)**
  - Organized response team consisting of medical personnel with specialized equipment that is capable of response to local or national disaster to provide medical care when the local infrastructure has been disrupted
- **Urban Search and Rescue (USAR)**
  - Federal response unit under the Federal Emergency Management Agency that provides for disaster response in situations that require specially trained rescue (extrication) and medical care personnel to provide extrication and the initial medical stabilization of victims trapped in confined spaces

Specific issues related to disaster management

DECONTAMINATION PRINCIPLES

- The coordinated and organized application of removal of contaminated clothing and cleaning of contaminated subjects with water to remove potentially harmful agents
- **Zones of Decontamination**
  - **Hot Zone:** immediately dangerous to life or health. Accordingly, Level A personal protective equipment with self-contained breathing apparatus required
  - **Warm Zone:** uncontaminated environment into which contaminated victims, first responders, and equipment are brought. Often is located next to and upwind from the hot zone
  - **Cold Zone:** completely uncontaminated and a site at which definitive patient care, triage, and transport can occur
- **Personal protective equipment (PPE)**
  - **Level A:** a self-contained breathing apparatus and a totally encapsulating chemical-protective suit. Provides the highest level of respiratory, eye, mucous membrane, and skin protection
  - **Level B:** a positive-pressure respirator and nonencapsulated chemical-resistant garments, gloves, and boots
  - **Level C:** consists of an air-purifying respirator and nonencapsulated chemical-resistant clothing, gloves, and boots
  - **Level D:** consists of standard work clothes without a respirator

WEAPONS OF MASS DESTRUCTION (WMD)

- Weapons that are meant to kill a large number of people or destroy key infrastructure to disrupt normal activities for a large population. The end result of these acts is to cause panic, injury, or harm to a population and disrupt the society
- Chemical/biologic/radiological/nuclear/explosive (CBRNE)

Chemical

- Four main classes

BLISTER AGENTS (ALSO KNOWN AS VESICANTS)

- Agents that blister the skin, eyes, respiratory system
- Main vesicant is **sulfur mustard,** used mainly in World War I
- Lewisite—a more potent vesicant, but no known use has occurred to date
- Vesicants are liquids that aerosolize when weaponized
- Most commonly, symptoms are related to skin exposure

- Initially, erythema and itching
- Progress quickly to large blisters similar to second-degree burns
- Management involves decontamination and wound care similar to that of patients with equivalent burns
- Eye exposures should be treated as corneal chemical burns
- Inhalational injury
  - May present with cough, dysphonia, dyspnea
  - Treated supportively, intubation if severe dyspnea
- GI—abdominal pain, nausea, vomiting, diarrhea
- Systemic absorption may occur through mucous membranes
  - Hematologic, CNS, immunologic effects are possible
  - Monitor WBCs and platelets after large exposures

BLOOD AGENTS: AFFECT RESPIRATION, CARRYING OF OXYGEN

- **Cyanide**—easily manufactured (hydrogen cyanide has "bitter-almond" odor)
  - Inhalation of vapor, or transcutaneous absorption
  - Cyanide salts may be used to contaminate food or water supply
  - Inhibition of electron transport chain, leading to anaerobic metabolism and lactic acidosis
  - Decontamination is necessary, as ongoing absorption may occur
  - Supportive care of cardiovascular and respiratory effects
  - Antidotes available- hydroxocobalamin or nitrite plus sodium thiosulfate
  - **See Chapter 18, Toxicologic II, for further information on cyanide**

CHOKING/PULMONARY AGENTS: DIRECTLY DAMAGE RESPIRATORY SYSTEM

- **Phosgene** (smell of fresh-mowed hay) and **chlorine gases**
- Phosgene used in manufacturing pesticides and plastics
- Direct toxicity to the alveolar-capillary membrane
  - Pulmonary edema, hypoxemia, respiratory failure
- Irritation to skin or eyes
- Symptoms within 30 minutes
  - Cough, shortness of breath, nausea, vomiting
  - Pulmonary edema occurs later
- Some cases of very delayed symptoms (2 days), so those exposed must be observed for that time period
- Decontamination is necessary to avoid provider exposure
- No antidote exists
- Supportive care

NERVE AGENTS: AGENTS THAT EFFECT NERVE-MUSCLE FUNCTION

- Organophosphates developed as chemical weapons
- Five known agents—**sarin, tabun, soman, GF, VX**

- Liquid at room temperature, vaporized to weaponize
- Inhibit acetylcholinesterase, leading to increased acetylcholine in the CNS, neuromuscular junction, and autonomic nervous system
- Onset of symptoms depends on dose and route of exposure
- Symptoms include:
  - CNS: anxiety, restlessness, emotional lability, tremor, headache, dizziness, mental confusion, delirium, hallucinations, seizures, coma
  - Parasympathetic: salivation, lacrimation, urination, defecation, GI pain, emesis, bronchorrhea, bronchospasm, bradycardia (SLUDGE and the killer Bs)
  - Neuromuscular: fasciculations, weakness, paralysis
- Decontamination is necessary
- Supportive care (avoid succinylcholine if intubating)
- Antidotes
  - Atropine titrated to drying of secretions
  - Pralidoxime (2-PAM) to prevent irreversible binding (aging) of enzyme
- **See Chapter 18, Toxicologic II, for more detail on organophosphates**

Biologic

- Bioterrorism agents classified into three categories based on impact on public health; ability to be produced, distributed, and delivered; potential for interpersonal transmission; need for a specialized public response; and potential for civil disruption
- **Category A:** Highest Priority Agents can be easily disseminated or transmitted from person to person, result in high mortality rates, and have the potential for major public health impact
  - Anthrax, smallpox, plague, botulism, tularemia, viral hemorrhagic fever
- **Category B:** High Priority Agents that are moderately easy to disseminate, result in moderate morbidity rates and low mortality rates, and require specific enhancements of diagnostic capacity and enhanced disease surveillance
  - Brucellosis, food borne (e.g., Salmonella, Escherichia coli 0157:H7), Q fever, ricin toxin, staphylococcal enterotoxin B, typhus, viral encephalitis, waterborne illness
- **Category C:** Third priority agents representing emerging pathogen production and use. Carries a high risk for morbidity and mortality
  - Nipah virus, Hantavirus
- Category A agents are considered the most dangerous and likely possibilities (Table 23-1)

ANTHRAX

- Causative agent is *B. anthracis*
- Inhaled form is greatest concern, with high mortality rates
- Cutaneous form may naturally occur or occur due to terrorism
- Disease is caused by exposure to spores, not bacteria

- Usual incubation period is 4 to 5 days
- **Inhalational anthrax**
  - Initial flulike illness
  - Within days, dyspnea, chest pain, pleural effusions, mediastinitis, overwhelming sepsis, multiple organ failure, and death may occur
- **Cutaneous anthrax**
  - Initial papule or vesicle enlarges, then ruptures, leaving a painless eschar with surrounding edema
  - May progress to systemic infection

DIAGNOSIS

- Generally clinical, usually in the face of suspicion for this agent
- Chest radiograph may show hilar adenopathy, pleural effusions, wide mediastinum, with or without infiltrate (Fig. 23-1)
- Recovery of causative agent from blood or skin site
- Distinct appearance of cutaneous form (Fig. 23-2)

TREATMENT

- Inhalational or cutaneous with systemic toxicity
  - Ciprofloxacin OR doxycycline two times a day for adults and children
  - 60 days of treatment—start IV and transition to PO when toxicity resolves
  - IV penicillin G and amoxicillin can be substituted if the strain proves susceptible
- Cutaneous without systemic toxicity
  - PO ciprofloxacin OR doxycycline two times a day
  - 7 to 10 days of treatment typically, but prolonged course (60 days) suggested if related to bioterrorism

PREVENTION

- FDA-approved vaccine—18 months for full course
- Postexposure prophylaxis—same as for nontoxic cutaneous anthrax patients (prolonged course)

SMALLPOX

- Causative agent is Variola major or Variola minor virus
- Considered ideal agent because of virulence and ease with which it is aerosolized and cultured
- Approximately 2-week incubation period
- Person-to-person spread through aerosolized droplets, with patients becoming contagious when the rash appears
- First 2 to 3 days, high fever, severe malaise, and headache
- Rash then begins as maculopapular, progressing to vesicular, then pustular (Fig. 23-3)
- First on face and arms, then spreads to trunk and legs
- All lesions at same stage (different from chicken pox)

TABLE 23-1 Clinical Features of Category A Agents

A	Anthrax (Inhalation)	Smallpox	Plague (Pneumonia)	Tularemia	Botulism	Viral Hemorrhagic Fever
Cases in U.S. per year	0	0	8-10	100-200	100-200	0
Clinical features	Flulike, then shock	Fever, then characteristic rash	Pneumonia, hemoptysis	Pneumonia	Descending paralysis and involvement of cranial nerves	Hemorrhage and fever
Diagnosis	Blood culture, CT of the chest	BSL-4 laboratory for virus	Blood and sputum culture	Sputum culture and radiograph	Toxin assay of blood, GI specimens; EMG	BSL-4 laboratory for virus
Mortality	40%-50%	30%	10%-20%	1%-2%	60%	Variable
Treatment*	Cipro, Doxy, or Levo + 2nd agent,† 60-100 days	None	Gent/Strep (Cipro/Doxy), 10 days	Gent/Strep (Cipro/Doxy), 10 days	Antitoxin, ventilator	Ribavirin (some), 7 days
Prevention*	Cipro/Doxy	Vaccine	Cipro/Doxy	Cipro/Doxy	None	None
Infection control	Not transmitted	Contact and airborne precautions	Masks	Not transmitted	Not transmitted	Contact precautions

From Barlett JG: Bioterrorism. Goldman L, Ausiello D (eds): *Cecil medicine*, ed 23, Philadelphia, 2007, Saunders.

BSL, Biologic Safety Level; *Cipro*, ciprofloxacin; *CT*, computed tomography; *EMG*, electromyography; *GI*, gastrointestinal; *Levo*, levofloxacin; *Doxy*, doxycycline; *Gent*, gentamicin; *Strep*, streptomycin; (), alternative to preferred.

*Doses: ciprofloxacin, 400 mg IV q8-12h or 500-750 mg PO bid; levofloxacin, 500-750 mg IV qd or 500 mg PO qd; doxycycline, 100 mg PO or IV bid; gentamicin, 5 mg/kg/day IM or IV; streptomycin, 1 g IM bid; ribavirin, 16 mg/kg/day IV × 4 days, then 8 mg/kg/day × 3 days or 1000-1200 mg/day PO × 7.

†Imipenem (500 mg IV q6h), rifampin (600 mg IV or PO qd), chloramphenicol (1 g IV q6h), clarithromycin (500 mg PO bid), vancomycin (1 g IV bid), or clindamycin (600 mg IV q8h).

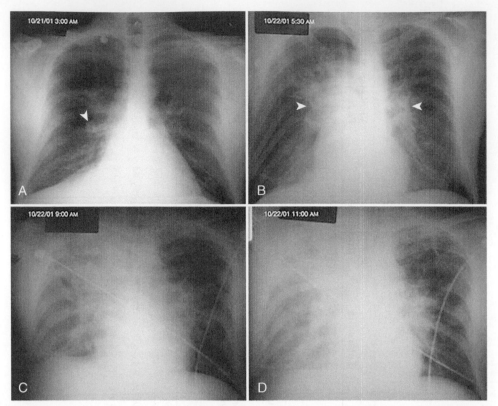

Figure 23-1. Chest radiograph of a patient with inhalational anthrax in 2001. The arrows emphasize the widened mediastinum due to the characteristic mediastinal adenopathy. (From Borio L, Frank D, Mani V et al: Death due to bioterrorism-related inhalational anthrax: report of 2 patients, *JAMA* 286:2554-2559, 2001.)

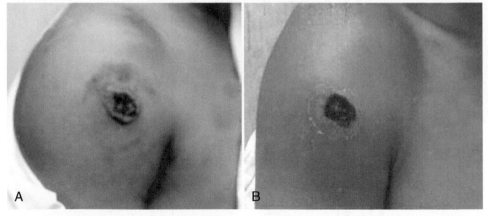

Figure 23-2. Sequential lesion of cutaneous anthrax, progressing from a painless ulcerative vesicle with surrounding erythema **(A)** to black eschar with persisting erythema **(B).** (From Centers for Disease Control and Prevention; Long SS, Pickering LK, Prober CG: *Principles and practice of pediatric infectious disease,* ed 3, Philadelphia, 2008, Churchill Livingstone.)

DIAGNOSIS

- Primarily clinical based on severity of illness and all lesions being at the same stage
- Fluid can be taken from vesicles for testing

TREATMENT

- Supportive—there is no known beneficial therapy

PREVENTION

- Respiratory isolation of affected patients

- Vaccination—not completely without risks
- Useful within several days after exposure

PNEUMONIC PLAGUE

- Causative agent is *Yersinia pestis*
- Three forms of plague—pneumonic, bubonic, and septicemic
- **Pneumonic** is the major bioterrorism concern, as aerosolization is the most likely form of terrorist delivery
- Incubation is 1 to 6 days

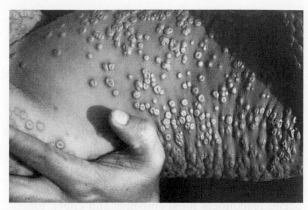

Figure 23-3. Smallpox lesions on skin of trunk. (From the U.S. Centers for Disease Control and Prevention (CDC) Public Health Information Library (PHIL). Available at http:phil.cdc.gov/phil/default.asp. Image ID 5 284. Photograph taken in 1973 by James Hicks, CDC)

- Initial flulike syndrome, followed by pneumonia, hemoptysis, sepsis, and death
- 100% mortality if not treated
- Coagulation abnormality, DIC, or gangrene in fingers, toes, or nose may occur
- Person-to-person spread may occur

DIAGNOSIS

- Lobar consolidation most common, but may have differing x-ray findings
- Hemoptysis is a key finding
- Sputum Gram stain or culture may identify organism

TREATMENT

- Respiratory isolation of affected patients
- Streptomycin, gentamicin, doxycycline, ciprofloxacin, chloramphenicol all effective— start with IV and transition to PO when stable
- Treatment duration is 10 days

BOTULISM

- Causative agent is *Clostridium botulinum* toxin
- Lethal in minute amounts
- Inhibits release of acetylcholine at the neuromuscular junction
- Descending flaccid paralysis, with early symptoms most prominent at the bulbar muscles
- Clinically indistinguishable from food-borne botulism

DIAGNOSIS

- Primarily clinical based on symmetric descending paralysis

TREATMENT

- Primarily supportive, and may require mechanical ventilation
- Lack of ventilators could be a problem in wide-scale event

- Antitoxin is available, must be given early
- **See Chapter 10, Infectious Disorders, for more information on botulism**

TULAREMIA

- Causative agent is *Francisella tularensis*
- Naturally occurring in the United States.
- Incubation period is 3 to 5 days
- Presents with fever and nonspecific flulike illness
- Progresses to bronchitis, pneumonitis, pharyngitis, pleurisy
- Hilar adenopathy is common

DIAGNOSIS

- Hilar adenopathy, along with pleurisy and typical symptoms
- Gram stain may be helpful, but specialized testing is necessary to isolate organism

TREATMENT

- Streptomycin, gentamicin are first-line
- Doxycycline and ciprofloxacin are second-line
- Treatment is for 10 days

PREVENTION

- Presumptively treat exposed persons who develop fever

VIRAL HEMORRHAGIC FEVERS

- Four families of RNA viruses
- Include Ebola hemorrhagic fever, Lassa fever, Marburg disease, Rift Valley fever, Crimean-Congo hemorrhagic fever, Yellow fever, among others
- High mortality rates, highly infectious when aerosolized, transmissible from person-to-person (mostly through bodily fluids)
- Duration of incubation period and time of symptom progression varies among causative agents
- Early symptoms include fever, headache, myalgias, malaise, vomiting, diarrhea
- Later develop increased vascular permeability, with mucosal hemorrhage, petechiae, hematuria, bloody vomit or diarrhea, and eventually DIC and shock

DIAGNOSIS

- Based on the presence of acute fever and unexplained hemorrhagic complications
- Suspected case must be reported, and testing must be done by designated secure facilities

TREATMENT

- Aggressive supportive care, including fluids, pressors, and blood products as needed
- Ribavirin is useful against some forms of viral hemorrhagic fever, and should be started empirically when the diagnosis is ascertained

- Once testing is complete, ribavirin can be continued if the agent is susceptible

Radiologic/Nuclear

- Terrorist detonation of military nuclear weapons or sabotage of a nuclear power plant are considered unlikely, as they are very hard to obtain, move, and detonate
- More likely candidates for terrorist use include:
  - Simple devices—many available (such as those used in radiation therapy), could be placed in high foot-traffic areas
  - Dispersal devices ("dirty bombs") —conventional explosive used to disperse commonly available radioactive materials
- Tissues with the highest cell turnover rates are affected the most
  - GI, hematopoetic, and CNS effects predominate
- Generally, the greater the radiation dose, the earlier the onset of symptoms
  - Doses greater than 10 Gray are generally fatal
- Patients will have either been irradiated (exposed, but pose no threat to providers) or contaminated (need to be decontaminated). If the nature of the event is unclear, all patients exposed should be decontaminated
- Emergency Departments need protocols in place to deal with the exposed patient before an incident occurs
- The hospital radiation safety officer needs to be contacted immediately to institute these protocols
- **Decontamination** should be done outside of the hospital or in a dedicated decontamination area
  - Removal of clothing
  - Showering with soap and water
  - Monitoring of radiation levels by the radiation safety officer
  - Staff needs appropriate personal protective equipment, and should wear dosimeters
- **Treatment** is generally supportive, but blockage of absorption or end-organ uptake may be based on the radioactive isotope used in the attack
  - Potassium iodide may be used to prevent thyroid uptake of radioactive iodine isotopes
  - Chelating agents or Prussian blue may be used for certain isotopes
- **See Chapter 6, Environmental, for further information on radiation-induced illness**

Explosive

- Terrorist weapon of choice, accounts for more than 70% of incidents
- **Ammonium nitrate (fertilizer)** and **diesel oil** has been one common method
- **Four categories of blast injury**
  - **Primary**—tissue damage from the blast wave passing through the body
    - Affects air containing organs—lungs, GI tract, ears

- **Secondary**—trauma caused by objects/debris thrown by the explosion
- **Tertiary**—trauma from persons being thrown onto other objects
- **Quaternary**—miscellaneous other injuries caused by explosions, such as inhalational injury, thermal burns, or crush injury
- Remain aware of the possibility of dual explosions, with a second delayed explosion meant to injure bystanders and first responders ("second hit")
- **Triage** is key in these settings, and mass casualty protocols must be enacted
- Scene responders must consider and check for chemical and nuclear threats
- **Decontamination** should occur in the field if nuclear or chemical contamination is suspected, and hospitals should be notified
- Markers of severity of injury that have correlated with requiring more urgent care and a higher level of triage include:
  - TM rupture (may be a marker for blast lung injury), penetrating torso trauma, shrapnel wounds, signs of blast lung injury, amputation, burns >30% BSA, open skull fracture
- Lungs, abdomen, and TMs should be examined for all those exposed to the blast
- GI injuries may be initially occult, so serial examinations may be necessary
- Pulmonary contusion evolves slowly, so initial chest radiography followed by observation (and potentially repeat radiography) is prudent
- Acute Gas Embolism (AGE) is a concern, and neurologic findings should be evaluated for whether they are the result of trauma or AGE

MASS CASUALTY INCIDENTS (MCIs)

- Incident that overwhelms the local or regional resources in which it occurs
- Natural or man-made
- Produces large number of casualties
- Requires a rapid response by multiple agencies to prevent further casualties
- **Types**
  - Natural (earthquakes, floods, hurricanes)
  - Technological (fires, hazardous materials, collapses)
  - Intentional (terrorism, bombings)
- **Phases**
  - **Planning/preparedness**
    - Command/Incident command system (ICS) structure
    - Communications plan
    - Mutual aid agreements
    - Resource cataloging
    - Tiered response levels
    - Regular drills
  - **Activation**
    - Notification and response
    - Establishment of ICS

- **Implementation**
  - Search and rescue
  - Triage/treatment/transport
  - Scene management, safety, and security
- **Recovery**
  - Postdisaster analysis/planning changes
  - Critical incident stress debriefing
  - Patient care
- **Triage**—based on French term "trier" (to sort)
  - The categorization of patients by severity of illness or injury to allow for the organized treatment and transport from an MCI incident location
  - Multiple systems available
  - Generally accepted color coding
    - Red (immediate/unstable)
    - Yellow (delayed/stable)
    - Green (minor)
    - Black (dead/ not salvageable)
  - Tag patient and move on
- **Treatment**
  - ALS and BLS
  - Periodic reassessment and retriage
- **Transport**
  - Track hospital availabilities/capacities
  - Determine needed transport resources
  - Determine patient destination hospital
  - Track patient by name/number, unit, hospital

PEARLS

- **National Academy of Sciences–National Research Council Report (1966)** *Accidental Death and Disability: The Neglected Disease of Modern Society*—ushered in the "modern era of prehospital care" in the United States, and included a blueprint for EMS development.

- **Highway Safety Act of 1966** established cabinet level Department of Transportation (DOT) and established authority to improve EMS.

- **The Emergency Medical Services System Act of 1973** identified the 15 key EMS components.

- In EMS, the malpractice may be through direct action (medical command order) or secondary to adherence to treatment protocol that is found to cause harm.

- EMS oversight may be direct (contemporaneous decision making) or indirect (using established "standing" orders.

- The four section leaders for incident command are operations, finance, logistics, and planning.

- The four main classes of chemical agents include vesicants (blistering agents), blood agents, nerve agents, and pulmonary/choking agents.

- The antidotes for nerve agent toxicity are atropine and pralidoxime (2-PAM).

- Pulmonary anthrax patients typically have hilar adenopathy and a widened mediastinum on chest radiograph.

- The severity of radiation exposure typically correlates with the onset of symptoms, with very early symptoms predicting poor prognosis.

- The air-filled structures (GI tract, lungs, ears) are most susceptible to the effects of an explosion.

- Consider pulmonary blast injury in patients with a TM rupture after an explosion.

BIBLIOGRAPHY

Centers for Disease Control and Prevention Emergency Preparedness and Response (website). Available at http://emergency/cdc.gov.
Fry DE: Chemical threats, *Surg Clin North Am* 86:637–647, 2006.
Goldman L, Ausiello D (eds): *Cecil medicine*, ed 23, Philadelphia, 2007, Saunders Elsevier.
Kuehl AE (ed): *Prehospital systems and medical oversight*, ed 3, Dubuque, IA, 2002, Kendall Hunt.
Marx JA (ed): *Rosen's emergency medicine concepts and clinical practice*, ed 6, Philadelphia, 2006, Mosby.
Tintinalli JE (ed): *Emergency medicine: a comprehensive study guide*, ed 6, New York, 2003, McGraw-Hill.
Townsend CM (ed): *Sabiston textbook of surgery*, ed 18, Philadelphia, 2008, Saunders Elsevier.

Questions and Answers

1. Which federal legislation identified 15 essential components of an EMS System?
   - a. Highway Safety Act of 1966
   - b. Emergency Medical Services System Act of 1973
   - c. National Standard Curriculum
   - d. Consolidated Omnibus Budget Reconciliation Act of 1985

2. *Vicarious liability* is defined as:
   - a. failure to legally maintain controlled substances on ambulance units
   - b. exposure for the acts of a subordinate even if not directly involved in care
   - c. restraint of a patient against their will
   - d. the proximate cause in a medical malpractice case

3. Common areas for risk exposure in EMS include:

   a. paramedic errors in judgment
   b. EMS initiated refusal
   c. motor vehicle collisions
   d. workplace harassment issues
   e. all of the above

4. Oversight in which paramedics and physicians make real-time decisions about patient care is best described as:

   a. direct medical oversight
   b. special operations
   c. indirect medical oversight
   d. standing orders

5. Verbal guidance from dispatchers to callers to provide aid until rescuers arrive is:

   a. computer-aided dispatch
   b. mobile data terminals
   c. prearrival instructions
   d. public service answering point

6. An event that overwhelms the capacity of the local care system of a community is considered what?

   a. incident command
   b. hazard vulnerability analysis
   c. disaster
   d. triage systems

7. The four (4) section leaders in the Incident Command System are?

   a. Finance, Security, Operations, Planning
   b. Public Information, Incident Commander, Planning, Operations
   c. Finance, Logistics, Operations, Planning
   d. Transportation, Finance, Logistics, Planning

8. A federal response team that provides specialized rescue and medical teams for victims of collapse and confined-space disasters?

   a. Disaster Medical Assistance Team
   b. Urban Search and Rescue Team
   c. National Response Framework
   d. Metropolitan Medical Strike Team

9. The level of personal protective equipment (PPE) that includes an air-purifying respirator and nonencapsulated chemical-resistant clothing, gloves, and boots:

   a. Level A
   b. Level B
   c. Level C
   d. Level D

10. The group of biologic agents that are all considered Category A?

   a. smallpox, botulism, and tularemia
   b. smallpox, ricin, and Hantavirus

   c. Nipah virus, botulism, and ricin
   d. ricin, typhus, and botulism

11. Nerve agents are chemical weapons that increase the amount of what neurotransmitter at the neuromuscular junction?

   a. dopamine
   b. norepinephrine
   c. epinephrine
   d. acetylcholine
   e. serotonin

12. Vesicants cause skin findings that appear much like, and should be treated similarly to, which of the following?

   a. third-degree burns
   b. urticaria
   c. second-degree burns
   d. lightning injury
   e. scombroid

13. Pralidoxime (2-PAM) acts to prevent which of the following?

   a. copious secretions in the airway
   b. irreversible binding of the nerve agent to acetylcholinesterase
   c. CNS irritability
   d. inhibition of the electron transport chain
   e. the need for decontamination

14. The classic chest radiographic finding in a patient with inhalational anthrax would show which of the following?

   a. no acute findings
   b. an air-fluid level in the upper lobe
   c. widened mediastinum with hilar adenopathy
   d. diffuse increased vascular markings
   e. pneumothorax

15. One way of differentiating smallpox from chicken pox is based on what skin finding?

   a. chicken pox lesions are all in the same stage of development
   b. smallpox lesions are in various stages of development
   c. smallpox lesions are all in the same stage of development
   d. chicken pox lesions are located only on the scalp and torso
   e. smallpox lesions slough and leave a black eschar

---

1. Answer: b

The **Emergency Medical Services System Act of 1973** provided funding for the development of EMS systems and identified the 15 essential components of an EMS system.

2. Answer: b

The medical command physician is vicariously liable for the acts of a **prehospital provider practicing under that physician's license.**

3. Answer: e

These are all common areas for risk exposure in EMS.

4. Answer: a

Direct oversight involves real-time physician involvement in EMS operations. **Indirect oversight** involves standing orders and protocol-based EMS care.

5. Answer: c

Verbal guidance given to callers by the dispatcher on the phone is called **prearrival instructions.** They are meant to help institute such necessary care as CPR before the arrival of the rescue personnel.

6. Answer: c

This is the definition of a **disaster.** A **hazard vulnerability analysis,** the establishment of **incident command** and **triage systems** are part of the early response to a disaster.

7. Answer: c

Operations: tasked with providing and directing all required duties to achieve required goals. **Finance:** track incident-related costs, maintain personnel records, and procurement of equipment and materials. **Logistics:** provide the resources, services, and support required by the incident. **Planning:** collection and display of incident information as well as the status of involved personnel.

8. Answer: b

This describes an **Urban Search and Rescue Team.** A **Disaster Medical Assistance Team** is an organized response team consisting of medical personnel with specialized equipment that is capable of response to local or national disaster to provide medical care when the local infrastructure has been disrupted.

9. Answer: c

Level A: a self-contained breathing apparatus and a totally encapsulating chemical-protective suit. It provides the highest level of respiratory, eye, mucous membrane, and skin protection. **Level B:** a positive-pressure respirator and nonencapsulated chemical-resistant garments, gloves, and boots. **Level C:** consists of an air-purifying respirator and nonencapsulated chemical-resistant clothing, gloves, and boots. **Level D:** consists of standard work clothes without a respirator.

10. Answer: a

Category A: Highest Priority Agents can be easily disseminated or transmitted from person to person; result in high mortality rates and have the potential for major public health impact. These include anthrax, **botulism,** plague, **smallpox, tularemia,** viral hemorrhagic fevers.
Category B: High Priority Agents that are moderately easy to disseminate; result in moderate morbidity rates and low mortality rates; and require specific enhancements of diagnostic capacity and enhanced disease surveillance. These include brucellosis, foodborne illness (e.g. *Salmonella, Escherichia coli* 0157:H7), Q fever, ricin, staphylococcal enterotoxin B, typhus, viral encephalitis, waterborne illness
Category C: Third priority agents representing emerging pathogen production and use. Carries a high risk for morbidity and mortality. These include Nipah virus and Hantavirus.

11. Answer: d

Nerve agents are *organophosphates* that act by inhibiting acetylcholinesterase, thus increasing the amount of **acetylcholine** at the neuromuscular junction. This action leads to fasciculations, muscle weakness, and ultimately paralysis.

12. Answer: c

Vesicants, also known as blistering agents, initially cause erythema and itching. They quickly progress to blisters that appear similar to those of **second-degree burns.** Patients who have been exposed to blistering agents should be decontaminated, and then treated as if they have sustained second-degree burns.

13. Answer: b

Pralidoxime, when given early, may **prevent the irreversible binding of the nerve agent to the acetylcholinesterase enzyme** (known as aging). Atropine is used to **dry airway secretions. CNS irritability** is treated with benzodiazepines. Cyanide (a blood agent) works through **inhibition of the electron transport chain,** leading to anaerobic metabolism. All patients exposed to nerve agents **need to be decontaminated.**

14. Answer: c

A **widened mediastinum with hilar lymphadenopathy** is classic for inhalational anthrax. Other findings may include pleural effusions, and possibly an infiltrate.

15. Answer: c

Smallpox lesions appear to be **all in the same stage of development,** while chicken pox lesions are typically in **various stages of development.** A **black eschar** is typical of cutaneous anthrax.

24 Pediatrics*

Ghazala Q. Sharieff | Kenneth T. Kwon

CARDIOPULMONARY RESUSCITATION
Supraventricular tachycardia (SVT)
Tachycardia with poor perfusion
Bradycardia
PEA/asystole
Pulseless V-tach/V-fib
Neonatal resuscitation

CARDIOVASCULAR
Congenital heart defects

EARS, NOSE, AND THROAT
Acute otitis media
Epiglottitis
Retropharyngeal abscess
Croup (laryngotracheobronchitis)
Bacterial tracheitis
Tonsillitis/peritonsillar abscess
Gingivostomatitis

ENDOCRINE/METABOLIC
Congenital adrenal hyperplasia
Hyponatremia, hyperkalemia,
   hypoglycemia

GASTROINTESTINAL
Pyloric stenosis
Intussusception
Malrotation with midgut volvulus
Appendicitis
Gastroenteritis/enterocolitis
Gastrointestinal bleeding
Meckel diverticulum
Hirschsprung disease/aganglionic
   megacolon
Colic/formula intolerance

GENITOURINARY/RENAL
Testicular torsion
Paraphimosis
Balanoposthitis
Hemolytic uremic syndrome (HUS)

NEUROLOGIC
Seizures
Status epilepticus
Febrile seizures
Infant botulism

ORTHOPEDICS
Physeal injuries
Elbow fractures
Slipped capital femoral epiphysis
Legg–Calve–Perthes disease
Osgood–Schlatter disease
Transient synovitis of the hip

RESPIRATORY
Airway foreign bodies
Bronchiolitis
Pneumonia
Pertussis
Asthma

BACTEREMIA AND SEPSIS

RHEUMATOLOGIC
Kawasaki disease
Henoch–Schönlein purpura

SKIN AND SOFT-TISSUE INFECTIONS
Orbital cellulitis
Periorbital cellulitis
Impetigo
Erythema infectiosum (fifth disease)
Roseola (exanthem subitum)
Varicella (chicken pox)
Scarlet fever
Staphylococcal scalded skin syndrome
Candida
Herpangina
Hand–foot–mouth disease
Tinea capitis

PSYCHIATRIC
Physical Abuse
Shaken baby syndrome
Sexual abuse

SUDDEN INFANT DEATH SYNDROME/ APPARENT LIFE-THREATENING EVENT

Cardiopulmonary resuscitation

- Two-person CPR 30:2 compressions to ventilations
- Health care provider or trained individual 15:2
- Once an advanced airway is placed, do not give more than 8-10 rescue breaths per minute
- Avoid cessation of compressions

*This chapter has been adapted from the Pediatrics chapter as printed in Emergency Medicine: A Focused Review of the Core Curriculum, Copyright © 2008 American Academy of Emergency Medicine Resident and Student Association.

FLUIDS

- Newborns 10 mL/kg NS
- Older children: 20 mL/kg NS
- 10 mL/kg PRBCs

DRUGS (Fig. 24-1)

- If IV access attempts are delayed or unsuccessful, proceed immediately to intraosseous access (IO)
- All administration routes are IV or IO unless otherwise indicated
  - Avoid giving medications via the endotracheal tube (ETT) if at all possible
- Medications that can be given down the ETT
  - Epinephrine, atropine, lidocaine, naloxone
    - **Epinephrine**
      - 0.1 mL/kg of 1:10,000 (or 0.01 mg/kg)
      - Use the 1:1000 form for ETT drug dosing (except neonates)
      - PALS has "deemphasized" high-dose epinephrine IV
    - **Atropine**
      - 0.02 mg/kg, minimum dose is 0.1 mg
      - Only PALS indication is symptomatic bradycardia
      - Not used for neonatal resuscitation
    - **Lidocaine**
      - 1 mg/kg
    - **Adenosine** for supraventricular tachycardia (SVT)
      - 0.1 mg/kg (maximum 6 mg), repeat dose 0.2 mg/kg (maximum 12 mg)

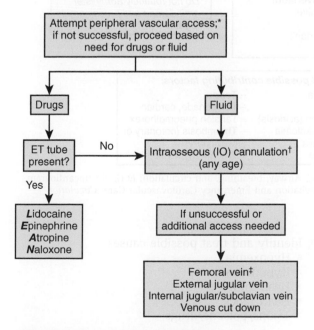

* Attempt site you are most successful with.
† Pursue IO cannulation immediately if CPR/severe shock.
‡ Femoral vein is safest central venous site during CPR.

Figure 24-1. Vascular access and drug delivery algorithm in pediatric advanced life support. *CPR*, Cardiopulmonary resuscitation; *ET*, endotracheal. (From Marx JA, Hockberger RS, Walls RM: *Rosen's emergency medicine: concepts and clinical practice*, ed 6, Philadelphia, 2006, Mosby.)

- Must be given as centrally as possible, as adenosine has a very short half-life
  - **Amiodarone**
    - 5-mg/kg bolus for pulseless VT and VF
    - 5 mg/kg over 20 to 60 minutes for VT with pulse or SVT
- Cardioversion
  - Start with 0.5 to 1 J/kg for unstable SVT or VT with a pulse; 2 J/kg for subsequent shocks
- Defibrillation
  - 2 J/kg followed by 2 minutes or 5 cycles of CPR; if no response, the subsequent voltage is 4 J/kg for VF and pulseless VT
  - Stacked shocks are no longer recommended
- If no change in rhythm after first shock then proceed to appropriate PALS medication regimens

SUPRAVENTRICULAR TACHYCARDIA (SVT) (Fig. 24-2)

- **Stable**
  - Vagal maneuvers
    - Ice to face in infants
    - Blowing through occluded straw in children
  - Adenosine: 0.1 mg/kg rapid IV push (maximum 6 mg)
    - Double dose if first not effective (maximum 12 mg)
  - Consider alternative medications
    - Amiodarone 5 mg/kg over 20 to 60 minutes or
    - Procainamide 15 mg/kg over 30 to 60 minutes
  - Verapamil not used in infants
- **Unstable**
  - Cardioversion 0.5 to 1 J/kg first dose, 2 J/kg subsequent doses

TACHYCARDIA WITH POOR PERFUSION

- **Narrow complex** (≤0.08 seconds)
- If HR >220 in infants or 180 in children, probable SVT
  - Consider vagal maneuvers
  - If IV/IO access
    - Adenosine 0.1 mg/kg (maximum 6 mg first dose)
    - Adenosine 0.2 mg/kg (maximum 12 mg), can repeat one time
      - Use rapid IVP *or*
  - Consider cardioversion
    - 0.5 to 1 J/kg 1st dose
    - 2 J/kg subsequent doses
    - Sedate prior to cardioversion if possible
- **Wide complex** (>0.08 seconds); probable ventricular tachycardia
  - Immediate cardioversion
    - 0.5 to 1 J/kg first dose
    - 2 J/kg subsequent doses
  - Consider alternative medications
    - Amiodarone 5 mg/kg over 20 to 60 minutes *or*
    - Procainamide 15 mg/kg over 30 to 60 minutes *or*
    - Lidocaine 1 mg/kg bolus

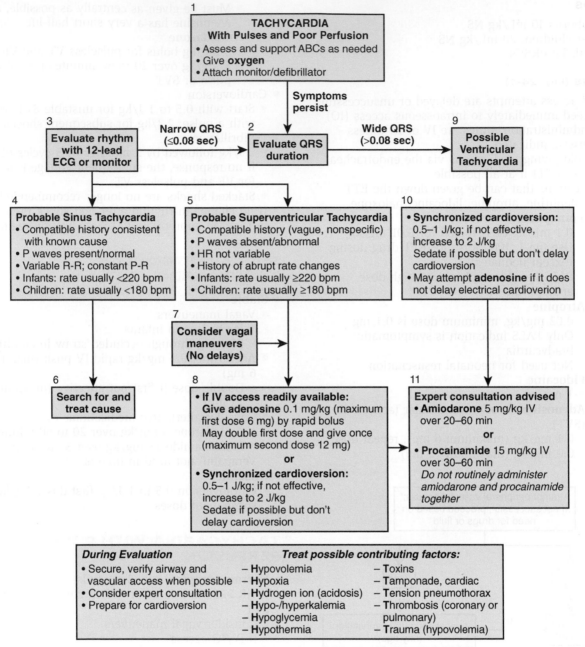

Figure 24-2. Pediatric advanced life support tachycardia algorithm. *ABC,* Airway, breathing, and circulation; *ECG,* electrocardiogram. (From American Heart Association Guidelines for Cardiopulmonary Resuscitation and Emergency Cardiovascular Care: *Circulation* 112:IV-167-IV-187, 2005.)

BRADYCARDIA

- If cardiorespiratory compromise and HR <60 despite oxygenation/ventilation
  - Chest compressions 100/minute
  - Epinephrine 0.01 mg/kg (1:10,000; 0.1 mL/kg), repeat q3-5 minutes
    - If ETT, 0.1 mg/kg (1:1000; 0.1 mL/kg)
  - Atropine 0.02 mg/kg (minimum dose 0.1 mg)
    - Can repeat one time
  - Consider dopamine or epinephrine drip
    - Dopamine 5 to 20 mcg/kg/minute
    - Epinephrine 0.1 to 1 mcg/kg/minute
  - Consider cardiac pacing

- Identify and treat possible causes
  - Hypoxemia
  - Hypothermia
  - Head injury
  - Heart block
  - Toxins/poisons/drugs

PEA/ASYSTOLE

- Verify electrode placement
- CPR/chest compressions
- Intubation
- IV/IO access

- Medications
  - Epinephrine 0.01 mg/kg (1:10,000; 0.1 mL/kg)
    - If ETT, 0.1 mg/kg (1:1000; 0.1 mL/kg)
- Identify and treat causes
  - Hypoxemia
  - Hypovolemia
  - Hypothermia
  - Hyper-/hypokalemia and metabolic disorders
  - Tamponade
  - Tension pneumothorax
  - Toxins/poisons/drugs
  - Thromboembolism

PULSELESS V-TACH/V-FIB

- CPR
- Defibrillation 2 J/kg, 2 minutes of CPR, epinephrine, defibrillate 4 J/kg
- Medications
  - Epinephrine 0.01 mg/kg (1:10,000; 0.1 mL/kg) every 3-5 minutes
    - If ETT, 0.1 mg/kg (1:1000; 0.1 mL/kg)
  - Antiarrhythmics
    - Amiodarone 5 mg/kg bolus *or*
    - Lidocaine 1 mg/kg bolus *or*
    - Magnesium 25 to 50 mg/kg for torsades de pointes or hypomagnesemia (maximum 2 g)
- Defibrillate 4 J/kg every 3 to 5 minutes

NEONATAL RESUSCITATION

- Position, suction
- Tactile stimulation
- Keep baby warm, dry
- Heart rate most important factor
  - If >100/minute, okay
  - If <100, give PPV
  - If <60 despite stimulation, PPV, and O₂, start CPR, and give epinephrine
- Bradycardia reflects hypoperfusion/hypoxia
- Atropine not used for neonatal resuscitation
- Epinephrine: always use 1:10,000
  - 0.01 mg/kg IV/IO/UVC (umbilical vein catheter)
  - 0.02 to 0.03 mg/kg ETT
- Umbilical vein can be used for fluids and medications
- Give glucose as 2-4 mL/kg of 10% dextrose
- No need to suction meconium at perineum
- May resuscitate initially with room air; however, move quickly to 100% oxygen if there is no response
- CPR ratio of compressions to ventilations is 3:1

Cardiovascular

CONGENITAL HEART DEFECTS

- 8 to 10 cases per 1000 live births
- **Neonatal circulation**
  - First breath: pulmonary vascular resistance decreases with resultant increase in pulmonary blood flow; peripheral vascular resistance continues to decrease, and the right ventricle reaches adult pressures by day 10 of life; when the umbilical cord is clamped, systemic vascular resistance increases, resulting in an increase in left ventricular afterload and an increase in left atrial pressure; this normally leads to physiologic closure of the foramen ovale, ductus arteriosus, umbilical arteries, and umbilical vein
- **PDA-dependent lesions:**
  - Usually sudden onset and present in the first week of life with cyanosis and shock when the ductus closes
- **Categories**
  - *Blue baby:* cyanotic heart disease with right to left shunt
  - *Mottled baby:* outflow tract obstruction with shock
  - *Pink baby:* congestive heart failure with left to right shunt
- **Cyanotic Congenital Heart Disease** (The "Terrible T's)
  - Tetralogy of Fallot (6% to 10%)
  - Transposition of the great arteries (3 to 5%)
  - Tricuspid atresia (1 to 2%)
  - Truncus arteriosus (1%)
  - Total anomalous pulmonary venous return (1%)
  - Pulmonary atresia (<1%)
  - Hypoplastic left heart (<1%)

SIGNS AND SYMPTOMS

- Difficulty feeding, sweating with feeds, failure to thrive, tachypnea
- Cardiac cyanosis worsens with crying, whereas pulmonary cyanosis usually improves
- Sudden onset of lethargy, pallor, or central cyanosis
  - Central cyanosis: tongue, conjunctiva, and body are cyanotic
  - Peripheral cyanosis: tongue and conjunctiva are pink
- Tachypnea, retractions, grunting
- Poor perfusion
- Murmur is present in most cyanotic CHD; single S2 also common
- Hepatomegaly
- Weakened/absent femoral pulses
  - Seen in coarctation; check four extremity blood pressures and simultaneous pre- and post-ductal saturations (right hand and either foot)
- Hyperoxia test: 100% supplemental oxygen for 10 minutes, then ABG; PaO₂ <150 mmHg or O₂ saturations <75% suggest cyanotic CHD

TREATMENT

- ABCs
  - Adequate perfusion and oxygenation is the goal NOT an oxygen saturation of 100%
  - Intubation may not be necessary

- If ductal-dependent lesion is suspected, start PGE1 infusion (prostaglandin E1):
  - 0.05 to 0.1 mcg/kg/minute IV; usually see improvement in 15 minutes; side effects are apnea, tachycardia, fevers, and hypotension
  - Intubation may be required because of risk of apnea
- If the patient presents with congestive heart failure
  - Furosemide 1 mg/kg
  - Consider morphine, dobutamine, and dopamine
- Search for underlying cause of decompensation
  - Maintain a high suspicion for sepsis
  - Start empiric antibiotics and send appropriate cultures
- Admit to NICU or PICU

Ears, nose, and throat

ACUTE OTITIS MEDIA

- Peak incidence in the preschool years, declines with increasing age
- *Streptococcus pneumoniae, Haemophilus influenzae, Moraxella catarrhalis*

SIGNS AND SYMPTOMS

- Acute onset of symptoms
- Signs/symptoms of middle ear **effusion**:
  - Bulging TM
  - Limited/absent TM mobility
  - Air/fluid level behind TM
  - Otorrhea
- Signs/symptoms of middle ear **inflammation**:
  - Distinct TM erythema
  - Distinct otalgia

TREATMENT

- Management per *American Academy of Pediatrics* (2004)
- Observation without antibiotics is an option if:
  - Age >2 years
  - Age 6 months to 2 years with uncertain diagnosis and nonsevere symptoms (T <39.0° C, mild otalgia)
  - Observation for 48 to 72 hours an option only if assurance of follow-up
  - If none of the above criteria are met, then treat with antibiotics
- Initial antibiotics
  - Amoxicillin 80 to 90 mg/kg/day in most cases
  - Alternatives:
    - Cefdinir, cefuroxime, cefpodoxime, macrolides
    - Ceftriaxone 50 mg/kg IM × 1 dose
- Treatment failures
  - Amoxicillin/clavulanate
  - Clindamycin, ceftriaxone × 3 doses are alternatives

EPIGLOTTITIS

- *H. influenzae* type B—decreasing secondary to vaccine
- Reported cases of *S. pneumoniae, Staphylococcus aureus,* and group A beta-hemolytic streptococci

- Wide age range: newborns to adults
  - Average pediatric age 3 to 7 years

SIGNS AND SYMPTOMS

- Several hours of fever, sore throat with rapid progression
- Irritability, lethargy, drooling
- Viral prodrome usually absent
- Dysphagia
- Severe stridor usually absent
- Tripod/sniffing position

DIAGNOSIS

- Clinical
- Lateral neck radiograph
  - Classic "thumb" sign
  - Do not send patient out of department for films
- Confirmed by direct visualization in the operating room
- 70% to 90% of blood cultures yield the offending organism
- WBC count will be elevated with bandemia

TREATMENT

- Keep patient in position of comfort
- Mobilize OR team
- Start IV in OR
- If emergent intubation required, use 0.5 to 1.0 mm smaller endotracheal tube than predicted
- Third-generation cephalosporins are antibiotics of choice
- Steroids are not indicated

RETROPHARYNGEAL ABSCESS

- Group A beta-hemolytic streptococci, *S. aureus,* and anaerobes are most common causes
- Age: 50% of cases occur in patients between 6 months and 12 months of age; 96% of cases occur in patients less than 6 years of age
- Abscess may rupture into esophagus or mediastinum

SIGNS AND SYMPTOMS

- Prodromal nasopharyngitis with abrupt onset of high fever, dysphagia, respiratory distress
- Drooling
- Meningismus
- Neck held in hyperextension

DIAGNOSIS

- Lateral neck radiograph (Fig. 24-3)
  - Widening of the retropharyngeal space
  - Normal measurements:
    - Anterior to C1-C4 <7 mm in children and adults
    - Anterior to C4-C7 <14 mm in children less than 15 years and <22 mm in adults
  - Alternative is to consider abnormal if width of retropharyngeal space is greater than the width of corresponding vertebral body above C4 or >2 times the width below C4

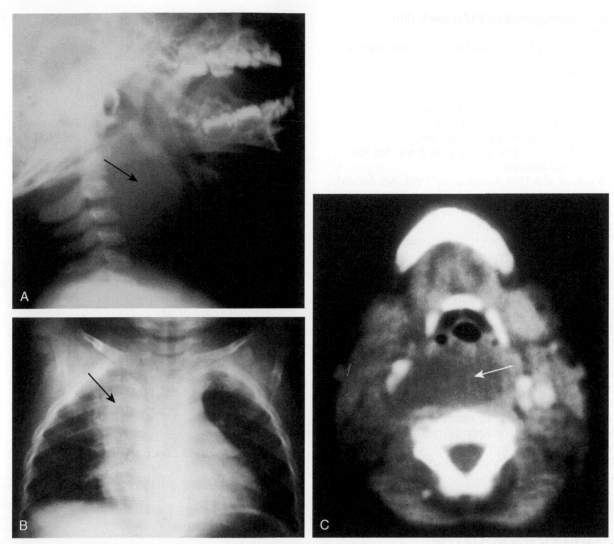

Figure 24-3. Lateral neck radiograph **(A)** of an 18-month-old toddler with retropharyngeal abscess from *Staphylococcus aureus* infection. Note marked retropharyngeal soft-tissue density *(arrow)* with anterior displacement of the hypopharynx and laryngotracheal airway. Note the normal sharp appearance of the epiglottis, glottis, and subglottic airway. **B,** Chest radiograph. Note extension of infection into the mediastinum *(arrow)*. **C,** Computed tomographic scan of upper cervical region without injection of contrast material. Note abscess in the retropharyngeal space *(arrow)* with anterior displacement and compression of the airway and lateral displacement of the great vessels. Bony structures are the mandible *(top)*, hyoid bone, and the cervical vertebrae. (From Long SS, Pickering LK, Prober CG: *Principles and practice of pediatric infectious diseases,* ed 3, Philadelphia, 2008, Churchill Livingstone.)

- Mild neck extension and end-inspiration is ideal, otherwise can get false-positive findings
- CT scan: can differentiate between true abscess and cellulitis

TREATMENT

- IV antibiotics
  - Nafcillin ± ceftriaxone or cefotaxime; consider clindamycin for anaerobes
- Emergent surgical drainage and admission

CROUP (LARYNGOTRACHEOBRONCHITIS)

- Parainfluenza type 1 is most common cause; also respiratory syncytial virus (RSV), adenovirus, influenza A
- Typically from 6 months to 6 years of age; peak incidence at 2 years

SIGNS AND SYMPTOMS

- 1- to 3-day history of URI
- Barking cough and hoarse voice
- Fever
- Stridor: in severe cases can be inspiratory and expiratory

DIAGNOSIS

- Radiographic confirmation (rarely needed, consider to exclude other causes)
- Lateral neck film findings
  - Hypopharyngeal overdistension
  - Subglottic narrowing
  - Normal epiglottis

- Frontal (anteroposterior [AP]) neck film findings
  - Classic "steeple sign" in the subglottic region

TREATMENT

- Cool mist humidification
  - Not proven but has little downside
- Racemic epinephrine via nebulizer
  - Indicated in moderate/severe croup
  - 0.25 mL of a 2.25% solution in 2 mL NS for patients <6 months
  - 0.5 mL of a 2.25% solution in 2 mL NS for older patients
  - Observation for rebound of symptoms 2 to 4 hours after administration
  - Steroids should be given to all patients who are given racemic epinephrine
- Dexamethasone
  - Should be administered to all patients with croup, including those with mild disease
  - 25 times more potent than hydrocortisone
  - Dose: 0.15 to 0.6 mg/kg IM, PO, IV (maximum 16 mg)
  - Long biological half-life (up to 54 hours), so single dose usually sufficient
- **Admission criteria**
  - Stridor at rest, despite above interventions
  - Incomplete response to racemic epinephrine
  - Multiple doses of racemic epinephrine required
  - Persistent respiratory distress or poor oxygen saturation
  - Dehydration
  - Poor social situation

BACTERIAL TRACHEITIS

- *S. aureus* most common
- Also *S. pneumoniae*, group A beta-hemolytic streptococci, *H. influenzae*, *M. catarrhalis*, and mixed flora with anaerobes

SIGNS AND SYMPTOMS

- Presents in two ways
  - Initial mild/moderate croup-like symptoms for days followed by sudden worsening
  - Previously well with acute onset of symptoms and airway obstruction
- Preceding upper respiratory tract infection (URI)
- High fever
- Stridor
- Retractions, wheezing may be present
- Dysphagia
- No improvement or deterioration with standard croup interventions

DIAGNOSIS

- Clinical suspicion: child appears toxic
- Radiographs: subglottic narrowing similar to croup

- Blood cultures usually not positive, but culture of tracheal aspirate may be

TREATMENT

- Emergent intubation is usually necessary; management similar to epiglottitis
- IV antibiotics
  - Nafcillin 100 to 150 mg/kg/day divided every 6 hours + ceftriaxone 50 mg/kg/day pending culture data

TONSILLITIS/PERITONSILLAR ABSCESS

- Polymicrobial with Group A streptococci, anaerobes, *Peptostreptococcus*, *Fusobacterium*
  - Uncommon: *S. pneumoniae*, *S. aureus*, *H. influenzae*
  - Can occur simultaneously with Epstein–Barr virus (EBV)
  - Age: >8 years of age

SIGNS AND SYMPTOMS

- Gradually increasing sore throat
- Ipsilateral ear pain
- Trismus, dysphagia, "hot potato" voice
- Fever

DIAGNOSIS

- Peritonsillar mass effect: uvula deviates away from involved side
- Ipsilateral cervical adenopathy
- Fluctuance
- WBC elevated
- Throat culture often positive

TREATMENT

- Surgical drainage or tonsillar aspiration if abscess present
- Antibiotics
  - IV antibiotics occasionally needed

GINGIVOSTOMATITIS

- Herpes simplex virus (HSV), Coxsackie virus, *Candida albicans*
- Vesicles and ulcerations are more common in viral causes
- HSV: anterior portion of the mouth and lip involvement is more common
- Coxsackie virus: Only soft palate/tonsillar pillar involvement
- Inspect the palms and soles for Hand–Foot–Mouth disease
- *C. albicans*: white plaques

SIGNS AND SYMPTOMS

- Fever usually present before the oral lesions
  - May present as "fever without a source"
- Pain
- Decreased oral intake

TREATMENT

- Supportive with appropriate pain control
  - "Magic mouthwash" (diphenhydramine, aluminum hydroxide/magnesium hydroxide, lidocaine) or equivalent
  - Be careful sending parents home with too much solution to avoid possible lidocaine toxicity
- Nystatin suspension or fluconazole if treating *Candida*
- Dehydrated patients may require in-house therapy with IV fluids

Endocrine/Metabolic

CONGENITAL ADRENAL HYPERPLASIA

- 1/10,000 to 1/15,000 live births; higher in Eskimos (up to 1/300)
- Deficiency in one of 5 enzymes involved in the production of cortisol
- Most common is 21-hydroxylase deficiency, seen in 90% to 95%
- Simple virilizing (1/3) vs. salt wasting (2/3)

SIGNS AND SYMPTOMS

- Vomiting
- Dehydration
- Fever
- Circulatory collapse during the first 2 weeks of life unresponsive to IV fluids
- Females may have enlarged clitoris, and fusion of the labial folds
- Males more prone to missed diagnosis; may have a small phallus
- Some children have hyperpigmentation because of the increased melanin production that is concurrent with an increased ACTH level

HYPONATREMIA, HYPERKALEMIA, HYPOGLYCEMIA

- May see arrhythmias because of hyperkalemia and acidosis
- Patient may have seizures because of hypoglycemia

TREATMENT

- Volume repletion with NS, then switch to maintenance fluid of D5 0.9% NS at 100 to 125 mL/kg/day
- Replace cortisol with hydrocortisone
  - 25 mg IV, then 25 to 50 mg/m^2/day divided every 6 to 8 hours
- Prior to administering hydrocortisone, draw blood for 17-hydroxyprogesterone, dehydroepiandrosterone, androstenedione, and testosterone levels
- Usually hyperkalemia responds to fluid replacement
- Severe hyperkalemia should be treated
  - 10% calcium gluconate (100 mg/kg)
  - Sodium bicarbonate 1 mEq/kg

- Insulin 0.1 unit/kg with 10% dextrose 2 to 4 mL/kg
- Sodium-potassium exchange resin
- Monitor glucose
- Hypoglycemia is common
- Hypoglycemia and glucose replacement
  - Normal blood glucose: >30 mg/dL in infants, >40 mg/dL in children
  - Treatment of hypoglycemia: glucose 0.25 to 1 g/kg
  - Neonates: D10, 2 to 10 mL/kg (4 mL/kg = 0.5 g/kg)
  - Infants and young children: D25, 2 to 4 mL/kg (2 mL/kg = 0.5 g/kg)
  - Glucagon: 0.1 to 0.2 mg/kg IM if known insulin excess
  - D10 in newborns and small infants to avoid vein damage and intracranial hemorrhage

Gastrointestinal

- Differential diagnosis of pediatric abdominal pain (Table 24-1)

PYLORIC STENOSIS

- Narrowing of the pyloric canal due to muscle hypertrophy
- 1/250 live births; more common in Caucasians, rare in Asians
- Usual onset of symptoms is during the third to fifth week of life
- Male-to-female ratio is 4:1

SIGNS AND SYMPTOMS

- Initially presents with occasional vomiting after meals and then progresses to vomiting after each meal and can result in the classic "projectile" vomiting
- The baby is hungry and will refeed immediately after vomiting
- Weight loss may be seen
- Constipation can occur due to the fluid loss and resultant dehydration
- Palpable "olive" in right upper quadrant (RUQ); passing an nasogastric (NG) tube before trying to palpate will decompress the stomach to improve accuracy
- Visible peristaltic waves from left to right after feeding

DIAGNOSIS

- Labs
  - Metabolic alkalosis: hypochloremic, hypokalemic early in the course
  - Acidosis develops in the setting of dehydration
- Ultrasound
  - Normal pyloric wall thickness is <2 mm
  - Pyloric stenosis: wall thickness is ≥4 mm and the canal length is also elongated ≥14 mm

TABLE 24-1 **Differential Diagnosis of Pediatric Abdominal Pain**

Infancy	Adolescence
Incarcerated hernia	Ectopic pregnancy
Intussusception	Appendicitis
Pyloric stenosis	Pelvic inflammatory disease
Hirschsprung disease	Inflammatory bowel disease
Colic	Biliary disease
Malrotation with volvulus	Gastroenteritis
Perforation	Torsion
Necrotizing enterocolitis	Henoch–Schönlein purpura
Gastroenteritis	Epididymitis
	Renal stone
	Pancreatitis
	Mittelschmerz
	Pregnancy
	Ovarian torsion/cyst
	Peptic ulcer disease
Childhood	
Appendicitis	
Constipation	
Gastroenteritis	
Pancreatitis	
Gallbladder disease	
Ulcers	
Urinary tract infection	
Hemolytic uremic syndrome	
Henoch–Schönlein purpura	
Inflammatory bowel disease	
Renal stone	
Mesenteric adenitis	
Extra-abdominal causes of GI distress	
Pneumonia	
Sepsis	
Pharyngitis—especially streptococcal	
Abdominal migraine	
Abdominal epilepsy	
Ingestions—think of iron	
Black widow spider bite	

- Upper GI
  - Shows the "string sign"—contrast going through the stenotic and elongated channel; false positives can result from pyloric spasm
- NG aspirate
  - >5 mL of gastric volume after 3 to 4 hours of NPO status; specificity is 94% with an accuracy of 96%

TREATMENT

- IV hydration with correction of electrolyte abnormalities
- Surgical treatment—incision of the pylorus (pyloromyotomy)

INTUSSUSCEPTION

- Prolapse of one part of the intestine into the lumen of an immediately adjacent distal part; most common location is ileo-colic
- Age: most common between 3 months and 5 years of age

- 60% of all cases occur in the first year of life, with peak incidence in children 6 months to 11 months of age

SIGNS AND SYMPTOMS

- Classic triad: only seen in 20% to 40% of patients
  - Intermittent colicky abdominal pain: 50% to 90% of cases
  - Vomiting: 60% to 90%
  - "Currant jelly" stools (diarrhea containing mucus and blood): 21% to 60%
- RUQ mass (may also be in RLQ)
- Colicky pain
  - Child will draw the knees up in pain, cry for 4 to 5 minutes and then look better between episodes; gradually the child becomes more irritable with vomiting, which may be bilious
- Mental status changes:
  - Irritability progressing to lethargy
  - Lethargy is frequently the presenting complaint
  - Thought to be from endogenous opioid production
- Stools highly variable
  - "Currant jelly" stool is late finding
  - Occult blood seen in 75% of intussusception with nonbloody stools; therefore, a rectal examination is imperative
- Low-grade fever may be present
- Vomiting without diarrhea or fever is suspicious for intussusception

DIAGNOSIS

- Abdominal films
  - May be normal early in the course
  - Later show evidence of obstruction such as air-fluid levels, paucity of air, and dilated loops of small bowel, particularly in the right lower quadrant
- Ultrasound
  - Classic finding is "target" or "doughnut" sign, which is a single hypoechoic ring with a hyperechoic center (Fig. 24-4)
  - "Pseudokidney" sign is superimposed hypoechoic and hyperechoic rings consisting of edematous walls of intestine and compressed mucosal layers

ENEMA

- Barium: has been the gold standard and is still performed at many institutions
  - Rule of 3's: no more than 3 attempts, barium column no higher than 3 feet, 3 minutes per attempt
- Air: advantages of air versus barium
  - Less radiation exposure
  - Less expensive
  - Higher success rate
  - Easier administration
  - If perforation does occur, air is safer for peritoneum
- Contraindications: perforation, hypovolemic shock, peritonitis

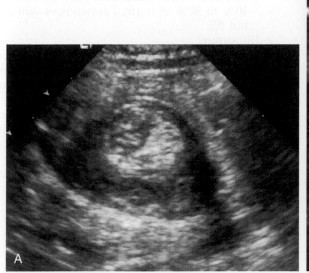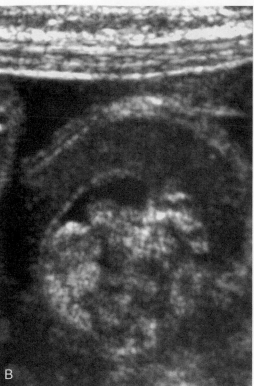

Figure 24-4. Intussusception. Ultrasound showing **(A)** crescent in doughnut appearance and **(B)** fluid trapped between the intussusceptum and intussuscipiens, and some free intraperitoneal fluid. (From Adam A, Dixon AK, Grainger RG, Allison DJ: *Grainger and Allison's diagnostic radiology*, ed 5, Philadelphia, 2008, Churchill Livingstone.)

- Recurrence
  - 80% to 90% are reduced successfully, remainder need to go to the OR
  - After successful reduction, 5% to 10% can recur usually within 24 hours

TREATMENT

- Call pediatric surgeon before performing definitive treatment

MALROTATION WITH MIDGUT VOLVULUS

- Abnormal fixation of bowel mesentery (Ladd bands), which can lead to twisting of loop of bowel around mesenteric attachments
- Age: usually occurs in the first months of life, but can occur anytime
- Gender: male-to-female ratio is 2:1
- 75% of malrotations will develop volvulus, most within the 1st month of life
  - Mortality rate with volvulus up to 15%

SIGNS AND SYMPTOMS

- Sudden onset of bilious vomiting
- Abdominal distension
- Constant pain
- Hematochezia is a late sign
- Jaundice
- Shock

DIAGNOSIS

- Abdominal films: classic "double bubble sign" (Fig. 24-5)
  - Overall there is a paucity of gas with two air bubbles, one in the duodenum and one in the stomach
- Upper GI: the gold standard
  - Imaging decisions should be made with specialist input
  - The small intestine is rotated to the right side of the abdomen with narrowing of the contrast at the site of obstruction; "cork-screw" or "apple core" sign is seen, which is the spiraling of the small intestine around the superior mesenteric artery
- Ultrasound: may show a distended, fluid-filled duodenum, dilated loops of small bowel to the right of the spinal column

TREATMENT

- Rehydrate aggressively
- Place NG tube
- Start antibiotics: ampicillin, gentamicin, and metronidazole (or clindamycin)
- Contact pediatric surgeon immediately upon suspicion of midgut volvulus

APPENDICITIS

- Most common surgical cause of abdominal pain in children

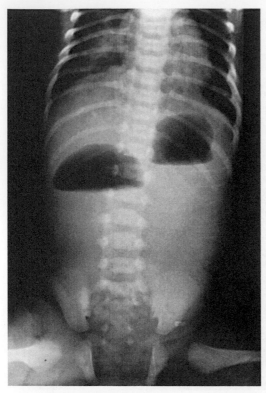

Figure 24-5. The classic finding of malrotation with midgut volvulus on abdominal plain films is the "double bubble sign," which shows a paucity of gas (airless abdomen) with two air bubbles, one in the stomach and one in the duodenum. (From McCollough M, Sharieef G: Abdominal pain in children, *Pediatr Clin N Am* 53(1), 2006.)

- 4/1000 children; peak incidence is 9 to 12 years of age
- Approximately 6% of the population will develop appendicitis
- Male to female ratio is 2:1

SIGNS AND SYMPTOMS

- Anorexia and vomiting
- Fever
- Diarrhea: may be present in 10% of patients
- Pain is initially periumbilical and progresses to RLQ pain
- Tenderness over McBurney point; Rovsing sign, psoas sign, obturator sign
- Peritonitis due to higher perforation rates (15% to 40%; 90% rate under 2 years)

DIFFERENTIAL DIAGNOSIS

- Gastroenteritis: most common misdiagnosis
- *Yersinia* is known as the great imitator and can cause RLQ pain
- Also consider mesenteric adenitis, lymphoma, UTI, constipation

DIAGNOSIS

- Laboratory data: >96% of patients have an elevated WBC count >10,000/mm³ or a left-shifted differential with >75% neutrophils

- Abdominal films
  - Fecalith is only seen in 10% of patients; other findings—loss of psoas shadow, lumbar spine scoliosis, localized ileus in right lower quadrant
- Barium enema
  - Nonfilling of the appendix with contrast and resultant nonvisualization; false positives as 10% to 30% of normal appendices will also not fill
- Ultrasound
  - The inflamed appendix is not compressible, and measures >6 mm in diameter; fecalith may be present; periappendiceal fluid collection may be evidence of early perforation
  - Sensitivity and specificity is operator dependent
  - Sensitivity, specificity, and overall accuracy up to 95% in experienced hands
- Helical CT
  - Inflamed appendix, fecalith, abscess, stranding of peri-appendiceal fat which indicates an inflammatory process

TREATMENT

- Surgical consultation
- IV rehydration
- Initiate antibiotics
  - Consider triple antibiotics (ampicillin, gentamicin, and metronidazole or clindamycin) or cefoxitin; consider meropenem if perforation

GASTROENTERITIS/ENTEROCOLITIS

- Viral 60%, bacterial 20%, parasitic 5%
- Rotavirus accounts for 30% to 60% of all cases of severe diarrhea in children between the ages of 3 and 15 months
- Bloody diarrhea is uncommon; fever and vomiting precede the onset of diarrhea
- Norwalk virus is responsible for 40% of cases of diarrhea in older children or adults in schools and camps

SIGNS AND SYMPTOMS

- Signs of dehydration (Table 24-2)
- Stool can vary from watery to grossly bloody
- Fever: more likely to be bacterial if temperature is >40° C
- Seizures may be seen with *Shigella*
- *Escherichia coli* 0157:H7 (enterohemorrhagic)
  - Hallmark is visibly bloody stool, abdominal pain, and absence of fevers

DIAGNOSIS

- CBC: *Shigella* gives a normal or low WBC but a marked left shift
- Electrolytes help to determine degree and type of dehydration
  - Bicarbonate less than 17 mEq/L present in up to 94% of patients with greater than 10% loss of body weight

TABLE 24-2 Signs and Symptoms of Dehydration

Clinical Findings	Mild, ≤5%	Moderate, 10%	Severe, ≥15%
Mental status	Alert	Irritable	Lethargic
Tears	Present	Decreased	Absent
Mucous membranes	Moist	Dry	Very dry
Urine output	Normal	Oliguric	Anuric
Systolic BP	Normal	Normal	Decreased
Heart rate	Normal	Normal-rapid	Rapid
Fontanelle	Normal	Flat	Sunken
Eyes	Normal	Sunken	Glassy
Capillary refill	<2 s	2-3 s	>3 s

TABLE 24-3 Antimicrobial Therapy Recommendations for Specific Causes of Diarrhea

Organism	Antibiotic
Shigella	Trimethoprim/sulfamethoxazole or azithromycin
Campylobacter	Erythromycin or azithromycin
Clostridium difficile	Oral vancomycin or metronidazole
Salmonella	Antibiotics generally not needed in mild disease (also thought to prolong carrier state), but may need IV antibiotics (ceftriaxone) in severe disease, immunocompromised patients, sickle cell, or patients less than 4 months of age
E. coli 0157:H7	If suspected, avoid treatment with antibiotics until cultures return, as antibiotics may enhance toxin release and increase rate of hemolytic uremic syndrome

- Stool studies: fecal leukocytes, culture, Rotazyme, ova and parasites

TREATMENT

- Oral rehydration therapy, with quick return to formula or breast milk
  - BRAT (bananas, rice, applesauce, toast) diet not recommended
  - Consider NG tube placement if needed for oral rehydration
  - Oral ondansetron (0.15 mg/kg) has been shown to help prevent vomiting and facilitate oral rehydration
  - Phenergan: FDA black-box warning against use in children under 2 years of age due to fatal respiratory depression
- IV hydration, if attempts at oral rehydration fail
- Admit for dehydration >5%, poor social situation
- Selected antimicrobial therapy (Table 24-3)
- AAP does not recommend antidiarrheals

TABLE 24-4 Causes of Gastrointestinal Bleeding

AGE	Upper GI	Lower GI
0-1 month	Idiopathic	Anal fissure (most common)
	Esophagitis	Upper GI bleed
	Maternal blood	Volvulus
	Blood dyscrasias	Necrotizing enterocolitis
	Arteriovenous malformation	Swallowed maternal blood
	Stress ulcer	Infectious colitis
		Milk allergy
1 month-1 year	Esophagitis	Anal fissure
	Mallory–Weiss	Intussusception
	Stress ulcer	Volvulus
	Arteriovenous malformation	Meckel diverticulum
	Stress ulcer	Infectious colitis
		Milk allergy
		Pseudomembranous colitis
1-12 years	Esophagitis	Anal fissure
	Mallory–Weiss	Intussusception
	Stress ulcer	Volvulus
	Foreign body	Meckel
	Esophageal varices	Infectious colitis
	Peptic ulcer disease	Henoch–Schönlein purpura
		Hemolytic uremic syndrome
		Polyps
		Pseudomembranous colitis

GASTROINTESTINAL BLEEDING
(Table 24-4)

MECKEL DIVERTICULUM

- Most common congenital abnormality of the small intestine, and is the remnant of the omphalomesenteric duct that connected the embryo's gut to the yolk sac
- Rule of "2s": found in 2% of the population, 45% of symptomatic patients are less than 2 years of age, 2 cm wide, 2 cm long, and 2 feet from the ileocecal valve
- Symptomatic patients are more likely to be male

SIGNS AND SYMPTOMS

- Isolated rectal bleeding is common in pts less than 5 yrs of age
  - Classic presentation is painless GI bleeding
- Abdominal pain, distension, vomiting if obstruction has occurred
- May mimic appendicitis
- May be the cause of intussusception
- Heterotopic gastric tissue may be present and result in bleeding from a peptic ulcer within the diverticulum or in adjacent ileum

DIFFERENTIAL DIAGNOSIS

- Peptic ulcer disease, polyps, tumors, intussusception, volvulus, appendicitis

DIAGNOSIS

- Abdominal film: may show signs of obstruction
- Meckel scan: injection of technetium-pertechnetate IV
  - Test relies on the presence of gastric mucosa, which has an affinity for the radionucleotide
  - 95% accuracy rate for detecting the presence of gastric mucosa within the diverticulum
- Arteriography: can detect the site of active bleeding

TREATMENT

- Large-bore IV line
- NPO/NG tube
- Transfusion may be necessary
- Start antibiotics if there are peritoneal signs
- Diverticulotomy versus more extensive resection if there is irreversible ischemia

HIRSCHSPRUNG DISEASE/ AGANGLIONIC MEGACOLON

- The absence of intramural ganglion cells in the rectum
- Extends to the sigmoid colon in 77% of patients
- Involves the entire colon in 15% of patients
- 1/5000 births; no ethnic predilection; male-to-female ratio 4:1

SIGNS AND SYMPTOMS

- Suspect the diagnosis if there is no passage of meconium stool in the newborn within the first 24 to 48 hours
- Vomiting
- Abdominal distension
- Chronic constipation
- Toxic megacolon
- Do not do rectal examination: it interferes with the barium enema by giving a false negative

DIAGNOSIS

- Abdominal films: may show signs of obstruction
- Barium enema: cone-shaped transition zone with dilated segment of proximal colon
- Rectal manometry: shows paradoxical contraction of the internal anal sphincter
- Rectal biopsy: definitive diagnosis; reveals the lack of ganglion cells in the rectal submucosa

TREATMENT

- Surgical repair: decompressing colostomy followed by closure at 1 year of age vs. a one-step repair
- Complications of surgery
  - Perineal abscess formation
  - Enterocolitis in up to 9% of patients; symptoms are bloody stools, fever, abdominal distension, elevated WBC count

COLIC/FORMULA INTOLERANCE

- Classically defined as unexplained paroxysmal crying for greater than 3 hours for greater than 3 days in greater than 3 weeks, in an otherwise healthy child
- Affects 10% to 30% of infants; typically occurs in the late afternoon and evening; usually starts in the third week of life and resolves by 3 months of age

DIFFERENTIAL DIAGNOSIS

- Do not assume the patient has colic
- Must consider other causes such as infection, obstruction, hernia, hair tourniquet syndrome, corneal abrasion, testicular torsion, fracture, child abuse

DIAGNOSIS

- History is usually classic; physical examination is directed at finding other possible causes
- Colic is a diagnosis of exclusion

TREATMENT

- Reassure the parents that the infant is not medically ill
- The parent can try rocking the baby, going for a drive, swaddling the baby, or pacifier use; make sure that the parents take a break from the crying; at times, formula changes can be tried as well as simethicone; patient usually self-improves by 3 months of age

Genitourinary/renal

TESTICULAR TORSION

- Most involve "bell clapper" deformity, where testis lacks normal attachment to tunica vaginalis
- Peak incidence 13 years, with a smaller peak in the first year of life
- Salvage rate: 80% to 100% within 6 hours, <10% after 24 hours

SIGNS AND SYMPTOMS

- Abrupt onset scrotal pain, can be inguinal/abdominal pain
- Nausea and vomiting
- Absent cremasteric reflex; horizontal lie of testicle

DIAGNOSIS

- Usually clinical
- Urinalysis: pyuria does not rule out torsion
- Ultrasound with color-flow Doppler

MANAGEMENT

- Surgical exploration
- Manual detorsion as temporizing measure may be attempted (opening book technique)

PARAPHIMOSIS (Fig. 24-6)

- Inability to reduce foreskin over glans penis

TREATMENT

- Circumferential compression of the glans and penis

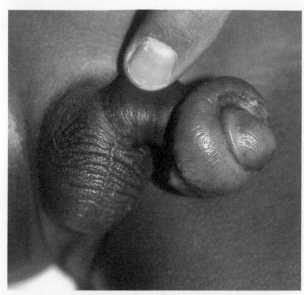

Figure 24-6. Paraphimosis. The foreskin has been retracted proximal to the glans penis and has become markedly swollen secondary to venous congestion. (From Kliegman RM, Behrman RE, Jenson HB, Stanton BMD: *Nelson textbook of pediatrics*, ed 18, Philadelphia, 2007, Saunders.)

- Needle fluid aspiration of foreskin
- Urologic consultation

BALANOPOSTHITIS

- Inflammation of glans penis (balanitis) and/or foreskin (posthitis), usually from infection

TREATMENT

- Hygiene/sitz baths; 0.5% hydrocortisone cream sparingly; oral antibiotics if cellulitis; topical antifungal if candidal, urologic referral
  - Consider diabetes in patients with recurrent candidal balanoposthitis

HEMOLYTIC UREMIC SYNDROME (HUS)

- Most common in infants and children less than 5 years of age. Most commonly associated with verotoxin-producing *E. coli* 0157:H7 (up to 10%)

SIGNS AND SYMPTOMS

- Severe abdominal cramping
- Watery diarrhea followed by grossly bloody stools
- Emesis and URI symptoms may be also be present
- Enteritis is followed by acute renal failure, petechiae, GI bleeding, and CNS symptoms such as irritability, seizures, hemiparesis, or coma
- HTN is seen in 40% to 50 % of patients

DIAGNOSIS

- CBC shows a microangiopathic hemolytic anemia, thrombocytopenia (platelet count less than 50,000 mm³)

TREATMENT

- Early peritoneal dialysis for severely affected patients
- Rehydration, treatment of hyperkalemia
- RBC transfusion, platelet transfusion for active bleeding or counts below 20,000 mm³
- HTN can be treated with nifedipine, labetalol, captopril or hydralazine
- Treat seizures with benzodiazepines and phenytoin

Neurologic

SEIZURES

- **Definitions**
- **Seizure:** paroxysmal electrical discharge of neurons resulting in either behavioral or motor change
- **Epilepsy:** Two or more unprovoked seizures not immediately preceded by fever, trauma, head injury, or chemical imbalance
- **Status epilepticus:** any single seizure lasting longer than 5 minutes or any two seizures between which normal cognitive function is not regained

INCIDENCE

- 3.5% of all children will experience a seizure by age 15
- 2% to 5% of children between the age of 6 months and 5 years have febrile seizures
- 1% of children develop epilepsy

ETIOLOGY (Table 24-5)

DIFFERENTIAL DIAGNOSIS

- Syncope
- Breath-holding spells
- Migraines
- Night terrors
- Psychiatric disturbances/pseudoseizures

HISTORY

- Known epileptic versus first time seizure
- Change in seizure type, pattern, frequency or duration
- Medication history
- Fever/stiff neck/rash
- Drugs/alcohol
- Head trauma
- Sleep cycle history
- Medical history: coagulopathy, diabetes, cardiac, immunosuppression
- Last menstrual cycle

STATUS EPILEPTICUS

TREATMENT

- ABCs
- Obtain glucose, electrolyte panel, calcium, magnesium
- Treat hyponatremia <120 mEq/L
  - 5 mL/kg of 3% saline over 10 to 15 minutes
  - Should raise sodium by 5 mEq/L

TABLE 24-5 **Etiologies of Seizures**

Infections						**Trauma**	
Meningitis/encephalitis						Epidural/subdural	
Brain abscess						Intracerebral	
Shigella gastroenteritis						Post-traumatic	
Cysticercosis						**Tumors**	
Inborn errors of metabolism						**Metabolic**	
Psychological						Hypoglycemia	
Breath holding spell						Hypomagnesemia	
Hyperventilation						Hypophosphatemia	
Hypoxic/ischemic						Hypocalcemia/hypercalcemia	
Ingestions (*PLASTIC* – mnemonic for substances that can cause seizures)							

P	L	A	S	T	I	C
Propoxyphene	Lead	Antihistamine	Salicylates	TCAs	Insulin	Cocaine
PCP	Lithium	Anticholinergic	Strychnine	Tegretol	Inderal	Caffeine
Pesticides	Lidocaine	Antidepressant	Serotonin-agonists	Theophylline	INH	Camphor
Phenothiazine	Lindane		Sympathomimetics		Industrial acids	CO

Adapted from Roberts JR: Pocket guide, *EM-News*, 1996.

- Obtain drug levels, toxicology screen in suspected ingestion
- **Medications**
- Lorazepam: onset 1 to 2 minutes, duration of action up to 13 to 15 hours
  - Dose: 0.05 to 0.1 mg/kg IV/IO, rectal dose 0.5 mg/kg
  - Considered a first-line agent
- Diazepam: onset <1 minute, duration of action 15 to 20 minutes
  - Dose: 0.1 to 0.3 mg/kg IV/IO, rectal dose 0.5 mg/kg
- Midazolam: onset 1 to 2 minutes , duration of action: 15 to 30 minutes
  - Dose: 0.1 mg/kg IV/IO, 0.2 mg/kg IM
  - Drip: loading dose of 0.15 mg/kg then maintenance of 0.75 to 10 mg/kg/minute
- Phenytoin
  - Load 15 to 20 mg/kg IV/IO, no faster than 1 mg/kg/minute
  - Peak CNS levels in 10 to 30 minutes
- Fosphenytoin
  - Load 15 to 20 mg/kg, can give 3 mg/kg/minute
  - Peak IV level: 7 minutes, IM: 30 minutes
- Phenobarbital
  - Load 15 to 20 mg/kg IV, no faster than 1 mg/kg/minute
  - Peak CNS levels reached in 20 to 60 minutes
- Pentobarbital
  - Load 10 to 20 mg/kg over 1 hour, then infusion 0.5 to 2 mg/kg/hour
- Valproic acid
  - 10 to 30 mg/kg IV bolus over 15 minutes has been successful for both generalized tonic–clonic status and nonconvulsive status epilepticus
- **Newborn seizures: Special considerations**
- Acyclovir (20 mg/kg per dose every 8 hours) if there are increased WBCs and elevated protein without organisms on CSF examination, xanthochromia, focal neurologic findings, or maternal history of herpes, vesicular rash, pneumonitis, or hepatitis
- Consider calcium gluconate 10%, 100 to 300 mg/kg IV, if seizures are refractory

- Consider pyridoxine 100 mg IV if refractory seizures
- Intubation and ventilatory support as needed

FEBRILE SEIZURES

- Incidence 2% to 5%
- Risk increases to 10% to 30% with parent or sibling with history of febrile seizures
- Recurrence rate of 25% to 30%
  - 75% of recurrences occur within first year and 50% within 6 months
- **Simple febrile seizures**
  - Brief duration of less than 15 minutes
  - Occurs only once in a 24-hour period
  - Generalized seizure without focal findings
  - No evidence of CNS infection
  - Age range: 6 months to 5 years
- **Complex febrile seizures**
  - Seizure duration greater than 15 minutes
  - Focal seizure
  - More than 1 seizure in a 24-hour period
- **Risk factors for recurrence**
  - Age <12 months with initial seizure
  - Lower temperature with initial seizure (<39° C)
  - Complex seizure
  - Parent or sibling with history of febrile seizures

DIAGNOSIS

- No need for routine CT or MRI in cases of simple febrile seizures
- Fever evaluation based on patient age: consider UA and culture, CBC and blood culture, chest x-ray, LP as per standard evaluation for febrile illness
- No need for routine electrolyte or calcium and magnesium levels
- Lumbar puncture after first febrile seizure? ACEP recommendations:
  - LP should be strongly consider in <18 months with febrile seizure if any following exists:
    - History of irritability, decreased feeding, lethargy
    - Abnormal appearance or mental status in initial assessment of child after postictal state

- Any signs of meningitis (bulging fontanelle, Kernig/Brudzinski signs, photophobia, severe HA)
- Any complex features of seizure
- Any slow postictal clearing of mentation
- Prior treatment of child with antibiotics
- If these factors are absent, then LP can be safely deferred

INFANT BOTULISM

SIGNS AND SYMPTOMS

- Ptosis
- Constipation
- Loss of developmental milestones
- "Floppy child"

TREATMENT

- Supportive
- Trial of antitoxin, but usually not effective because of minimal amounts of circulating toxin
- Antibiotics also not effective, but if used avoid aminoglycosides

Orthopedics

PHYSEAL INJURIES

- Occur at growth plate (physis)
- Up to one third of all pediatric fractures involve physis; usually upper extremities

- Peak incidence 11 to 13 years of age
- **Salter–Harris classification** (Fig. 24-7)
  - **Type I** (6%): involves separation of metaphysis from the epiphysis through zone of provisional calcification
    - May be suspected on clinical grounds alone
    - May not be radiographically evident if the epiphysis is not displaced
    - Only visible radiographically if the physis is widened, distorted, or the epiphysis is displaced
  - **Type II** (75%): most common; involves metaphysis, good prognosis
  - **Type III** (10%): epiphysis, intra-articular
    - anatomic position must be reestablished to restore normal joint mechanics and prevent growth arrest or chronic disability
  - **Type IV** (10%): contiguous fracture through epiphysis, physis and metaphysis, intra-articular
  - **Type V** (1%): crush injury due to axial compression of germinal growth plate
    - Difficult to see on x-ray, may be confused with Salter-Harris type 1
    - Base diagnosis on x-ray and if mechanism of injury suggests an axial compression along the long axis of the bone
    - Use comparison views if needed
- Distal radius most common site of injury (30% to 60%)
- Ligaments tend to be stronger than physis: physeal separation/fracture more common than sprain

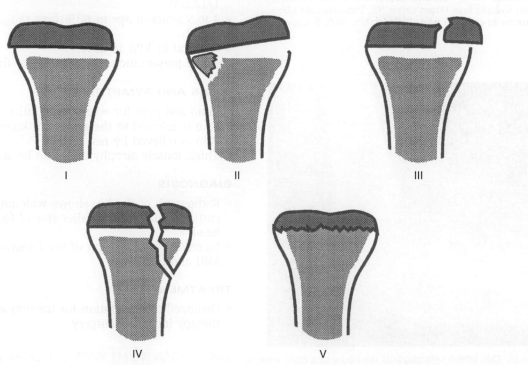

I   II   III

IV   V

Figure 24-7. **Salter–Harris classification** of epiphyseal fractures in children. A **type I fracture** is straight across the epiphyseal plate and a **type II fracture** is a corner fracture through the metaphysis. This occurs 75% of the time. A **type III fracture** involving part of the epiphysis occurs only about 10% of the time. A **type IV fracture** involving part of the epiphysis and part of the metaphysis occurs about 10% of the time. A **type V fracture** is direct impaction and has the most serious consequences for further growth. (From Mettler FA, Jr: *Essentials of radiology*, ed 2, Philadelphia, 2005, Saunders.)

ELBOW FRACTURES

- Supracondylar most common (60%)
- Posterior fat pad/large anterior fat pad alone highly predictive of elbow fracture (Figs. 24-8 and 24-9)
  - Assume nondisplaced (Type 1) supracondylar fracture in children; occult radial head fracture in adult

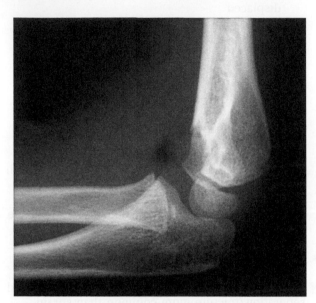

Figure 24-8. A lateral elbow radiograph shows no obvious fracture, but both an anterior and a posterior elevated fat pad can be noted. The child was treated for a supracondylar fracture that became evident 3 weeks later after observation of the periosteal reaction and fracture line. (From Green NE, Swiontkowski MF: *Skeletal trauma in children,* ed 4, Philadelphia, 2008, Saunders.)

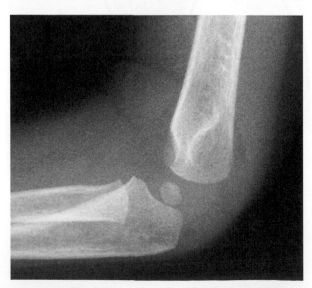

Figure 24-9. This lateral radiograph of the elbow in a child who sustained a nondisplaced supracondylar fracture shows a markedly displaced anterior fat pad. (From Green NE, Swiontkowski MF: *Skeletal trauma in children,* ed 4, Philadelphia, 2008, Saunders.)

SLIPPED CAPITAL FEMORAL EPIPHYSIS

- Medial slip of the femoral epiphysis; associated with obesity and puberty
- May present acutely as a result of trauma or may be chronic
- Peak incidence is 12 to 16 years of age in boys and 10 to 14 years in girls
- Bilateral in 10% to 25%

SIGNS AND SYMPTOMS

- Pain in the groin, thigh, and knee, usually gradual onset, but may be acute
- Lower limb is held in external rotation; restricted full flexion
- Limb shortening and proximal thigh muscle atrophy

DIAGNOSIS

- Obtain AP and frog leg views of the hip
  - *Klein's line:* in the AP view, a line across the lateral (superior) aspect of the femoral neck should transect the lateral portion of the femoral epiphysis

TREATMENT

- Orthopedic consultation and admission; operative reduction and fixation to avoid avascular necrosis

LEGG–CALVE–PERTHES DISEASE

- Avascular necrosis of the femoral head; 1/1200 to 1/12,500
- 4 to 9 years of age in 80% (age range 3 to 12 years)
- Bilateral in 10% to 20%
  - Age presentation of LCP younger than SCFE

SIGNS AND SYMPTOMS

- Limp and pain for weeks to months
- Pain is referred to the groin and knee
- Pain is relieved by rest
- Thigh muscle atrophy may also be seen

DIAGNOSIS

- Radiograph of the hip shows widening of the cartilage space and smaller size of femoral head
- Increased opacification of the femoral head
- MRI and bone scan

TREATMENT

- Orthopedic consultation for traction and future therapy including surgery

OSGOOD–SCHLATTER DISEASE

- Seen in early adolescence, boys more commonly affected

- Repetitive injury from inflammation of the tibial tubercle apophysis; partial or complete avulsion of the tibial tubercle may occur

SIGNS AND SYMPTOMS

- Swelling, pain, and tenderness over the tibial tubercle

TREATMENT

- Rest, NSAIDs, knee immobilization for 2 to 4 weeks for severe symptoms
- Avulsion may require surgery

TRANSIENT SYNOVITIS OF THE HIP

- Peak age: 3 to 6 years of age; right hip is more common than the left

SIGNS AND SYMPTOMS

- Gradual or acute
- Preceding viral syndrome (URI)
- Low-grade fever
- Pain on palpation of the anterior hip
- Decreased range of hip motion

DIAGNOSIS

- Diagnosis of exclusion
- WBC and ESR/CRP are usually normal, if elevated then consider joint aspiration to rule out septic arthritis
- Hip radiographs or ultrasound may show a mild hip effusion

TREATMENT

- NSAIDs and close follow-up

Respiratory

AIRWAY FOREIGN BODIES

ETIOLOGY

- Organic debris most frequently found on bronchoscopy
  - Nuts, seeds, hot dogs, vegetable/fruits
- Airway foreign bodies are rarely radiopaque
- Age: 75% of all cases occur in patients less than 3 years of age
- Most FB lodge in mainstem bronchus
  - 3% to 11% involve trachea or larynx
- 50% to 90% of patients have suggestive history of acute paroxysmal cough
- Only 50% are diagnosed in the first 24 hours after aspiration

SIGNS AND SYMPTOMS

- Paroxysmal cough, wheezing, and decreased breath sounds in 40%
- 25% may be asymptomatic

- 39% may have no helpful physical examination findings
- Recurrent pneumonia

DIAGNOSIS

- Inspiratory/expiratory films or lateral decubitus films
  - Persistent hyperinflation is suspicious for foreign body
  - Mediastinal shift toward unaffected side
  - Pulmonary infiltrates

TREATMENT

- Position of comfort with supplemental oxygen
- Complete obstruction: BLS maneuvers if age <1 year: 5 back blows and 5 chest thrusts; age >1 year: Heimlich maneuver
- Direct laryngoscopy with McGill forceps removal of visualized foreign body
- Avoid blind finger sweep
- Bronchoscopy
- Intubation with dislodgment of the object into a mainstem bronchus
- Needle cricothyrotomy

BRONCHIOLITIS

ETIOLOGY

- Respiratory syncytial virus (RSV) most common cause (75% of brochiolitis admissions)
- Also parainfluenza, influenza, adenovirus, rhinovirus, enterovirus, herpes simplex, *Mycoplasma pneumoniae*
- Age: highest incidence in patients <1 year of age
- Winter and early spring predominance

SIGNS AND SYMPTOMS

- Usually preceded by URI symptoms, fever
- Cough may be paroxysmal
- Irritability, poor feeding
- Tachypnea, tachycardia
- Intercostal retractions, wheezing
- Rales may be present
- Apnea: especially in infants <2 months or <6 months with history of prematurity
- Acute otitis media associated in 53%

DIAGNOSIS

- Clinical, but RSV probe can be sent
- Chest x-ray may reveal flattened diaphragms with hyperinflation

TREATMENT

- Nasal saline drops and bulb suction
- Humidified oxygen
- Beta-agonist nebulization may be helpful
- Steroids of no known benefit
- Racemic epinephrine of questionable benefit
- IV hydration may be needed
- Heliox therapy

TABLE 24-6 **Causes of Pneumonia**

	Bacterial	**Viral**	**Other**
Neonates	Group B streptococci *E. coli* Listeria Pseudomonas Klebsiella	RSV Varicella	Chlamydia
3 weeks to 3 months	*Streptococcus pneumoniae* *Staphylococcus aureus* Pertussis Group A/B streptococci *Haemophilus influenzae* (type/non-type)	RSV Parainfluenza Adenovirus Influenza	Chlamydia
4 months to 4 years	*S. pneumoniae* *S. aureus* *H. influenzae* (type/non-type) Group A streptococci Pertussis	RSV Parainfluenza Adenovirus Influenza Enterovirus Rhinovirus	Mycoplasma
Older children ≥5 years	*S. pneumoniae* *H. influenzae* Group A streptococci	Parainfluenza Influenza Adenovirus Rhinovirus	Mycoplasma *Chlamydia pneumoniae*

- Admission criteria
  - Persistent oxygen requirement
  - Tachypnea with respiratory distress
  - Inability to tolerate liquids
  - Poor social situation
  - History suggestive of apnea
  - Age <2 months
  - Underlying cardiopulmonary disease

PNEUMONIA

- Causes by age (Table 24-6)
- 60% to 90% viral overall

SIGNS AND SYMPTOMS

- Tachypnea
  - Most reliable sign in children
- Cough
- Grunting, flaring, retractions
- Fevers
- Vomiting, poor feeding, irritability, lethargy in infant/toddlers

TREATMENT

- Age less than 3 months
  - Admission with IV ampicillin and cefotaxime (also consider erythromycin for afebrile pneumonias due to chlamydia or suspected pertussis
- 3 months to 4 years
  - Amoxicillin 80 to 100 mg/kg/day PO or cefuroxime, amoxicillin/clavulanate, macrolide, trimethoprim–sulfamethoxazole (TMP/SMX)
  - IV medications include cefuroxime, cefotaxime, and ceftriaxone
- Children ≥5 years of age
  - Macrolide (azithromycin, erythromycin, clarithromycin) to cover for *M. pneumoniae*
  - Consider doxycycline if >8 years

TABLE 24-7 **Stages of Pertussis Infection**

Stage	Duration	Features
Catarrhal	1-2 weeks	Lacrimation, rhinorrhea, mild cough, low-grade fever to 101°F
Paroxysmal	2-4 weeks	Paroxysmal cough, apnea, cyanosis, emesis, neurologic, and respiratory symptoms
Convalescent	1-4 months	Cough may persist up to 6 months

- Admit all patients with suspected *Staph. aureus* pneumonia
- *Chlamydia pneumoniae*
  - Young infants
  - Usually afebrile
  - Classic cough is staccato-like that may be associated with post-tussive emesis
  - May be a history of concurrent or previous chlamydial conjunctivitis
  - Hyperinflation or increased interstitial markings on CXR
  - Treatment is with oral erythromycin or sulfonamide

PERTUSSIS

- *Bordetella pertussis*: gram-negative organism
- Transmitted by respiratory droplets
- Incubation period: 6 to 20 days
- Stages (Table 24-7)

DIAGNOSIS

- WBC greater than 15,000 with lymphocytosis
- Characteristic coughing paroxysm
- Fluorescent antibody staining
- Nasopharyngeal culture

TREATMENT

- IV hydration may be necessary
- Supplemental oxygen
- Erythromycin 50 mg/kg/day eliminates organisms from nasopharynx in 3 to 4 days
- May use trimethoprim–sulfamethoxazole 8 mg/kg/day if erythromycin is not tolerated
- Antibiotic therapy does not shorten the paroxysmal stage
- Treat household contacts with 14-day course of erythromycin
- Admission criteria
  - History of apnea
  - Inability to tolerate fluids
  - Poor social situation or unreliable parents
  - Age <6 months, history of prematurity
  - Persistent O_2 requirement

ASTHMA

- Mucosal edema, bronchospasm, increased secretions
- Cough, wheezing, dyspnea
- Three categories
  - Symptoms in presence of URI
  - Continued wheezing after 3 years of age
  - Those associated with atopic disease

DIFFERENTIAL DIAGNOSIS OF WHEEZING

- Asthma, bronchiolitis, pneumonia, CHF, PE, anaphylaxis/allergic reaction, cystic fibrosis, laryngotracheomalacia, tracheoesophageal fistula, bronchopulmonary dysplasia, mediastinal masses, vascular anomalies, foreign body aspiration

TREATMENT

- ABCs
- Beta agonists are the cornerstone of management
  - Albuterol
  - Levalbuterol gives no significant advantage over standard albuterol
- Epinephrine: subcutaneous dose
  - 0.01 mL/kg of 1:1000 concentration (maximum 0.5 mL)
  - May use IV if in extremis 0.1 mL/kg of 1:10,000, use 1/10th to 1/3rd of code dose
- Steroids: 2 mg/kg/day of prednisolone, prednisone, methylprednisolone
  - Decadron (0.6 mg/kg) single-dose or two-dose therapy has also been effective
- Anticholinergics: ipratropium bromide
- Magnesium sulfate
  - 50 to 75 mg/kg up to 2 g over 20 to 30 minutes
- Intubation
  - Use ketamine for sedation 2 mg/kg (reduces bronchospasm)
  - Anticipate difficulty with ventilator management
  - Avoid unless absolutely necessary
- Admission criteria
  - Persistent respiratory distress
  - Hypoxia
  - Poor response to treatment

- Concurrent pneumonia
- Multiple visits for same episode
- Poor parental compliance or poor social situation
- Inability to tolerate fluids
- Hypercapnia or normal CO_2 on blood gas indicates distress
- Low threshold for patients with history of intubation

Bacteremia and sepsis

- **Common pathogens by age**
- **Neonates**
  - Group B Streptococcus, *E. coli*, *Listeria monocytogenes*, *Enterococcus* species
- **30 to 90 days**
  - As above, also *S. pneumoniae*, *Neisseria meningitides*, *H. influenzae* B, Group A Streptococcus, *Salmonella* species, *Staph. aureus*
- **3 to 36 months**
  - *S. pneumoniae*, *N. meningitides*, *H. influenzae* B, Group A Streptococcus, *Escherichia coli*, *Salmonella* species, *Staph. aureus*
- **Fever without source**
- Fever definition
  - ≥38.0° C (100.4° F) rectal if <3 months
  - ≥39.0° C (102.2° F) rectal if ≥3 months
- **Serious bacterial infection** (SBI)
  - Bacteremia
  - Bacterial meningitis, pneumonia, gastroenteritis
  - Urinary tract infection
  - 7.5% rate in febrile infants <2 months
  - Cellulitis
  - Osteomyelitis
  - Septic arthritis
- **Under 3 months of age**
  - SBI up to 7%
  - Bacteremia or bacterial meningitis 2% to 3%
  - Up to 13% under 29 days old
  - Otitis media not considered source at this age
- **3 to 36 months of age**
  - Pre-HIB SBI prevalence up to 5%
  - Post-HIB <2%
  - Post-Pneumovax <1%
- **Occult pneumococcal bacteremia**
  - 10% to 25% complication rate, of which 3% to 6% develop meningitis
  - Evaluation based on age (Table 24-8)
- Lab screening and empiric antibiotics may not be necessary in the highly febrile, well-appearing 6- to 36-month-old child who has received the primary pneumococcal conjugate vaccine series
  - CBC and blood cultures being deemphasized

Rheumatologic

KAWASAKI DISEASE (Fig. 24-10)

- Also called mucocutaneous lymph node syndrome

TABLE 24-8 **Evaluation of Children with Fever**

Age	Temp (C)	Workup	ED treatment	Disposition
0-28 days	≥ 38.0 R or	Full septic	Ampicillin & cefotaxime ± acyclovir*	Admit
28 days-2 months	≥ 38.0 R	Full septic	Ceftriaxone	Admit or discharge if low-risk Next day follow up
2-3 months	≥ 38.0 R	Complete blood count (CBC), blood culture (Cx), urinalysis (UA), urine Cx ± lumbar puncture (LP) and chest x-ray (CXR) and stool Cx	± Ceftriaxone no antibiotics if no LP	Discharge if workup negative Next day follow-up
3 months-3 years	>39.0 R and without source	UA and Ur Cx in girls <2 years UA and Ur Cx in boys <6 months or <12 months if uncircumcised Consider CBC/blood Cx ± LP, CXR, and stool Cx	± Ceftriaxone Treat if WBC > 15,000 or <5000 or other studies abnormal	Discharge if workup negative and child nontoxic, or if workup positive, child nontoxic, and the infection is commonly treated as an outpatient, the patient can be discharged with next day follow-up Admit if ill-appearing

*Consider Acyclovir 20 mg/kg per dose q 8 hours if CSF pleocytosis or elevated protein, vesicular lesions, focal neurologic findings/seizures, hepatitis, pneumonia, or positive maternal history of herpes.

- A generalized vasculitis of unclear etiology which involves the coronary arteries and the small-to-medium sized arteries
- Toxins from *Staph. aureus* and *Strep. pyogenes* may produce superantigen toxins
- Common childhood vasculitis
  - Up to 5000 children are affected annually in the United States
  - Male-to-female ratio is 1.5:1
  - Peak age is 1 to 2 years of age and 80% of patients present before 4 years
  - Most common cause of acquired heart disease in the United States

SIGNS AND SYMPTOMS

- Fever of at least 5 days' duration plus at least four of the following:
  - Bilateral nonexudative conjunctivitis
  - Changes of the lips and oral mucosa (fissured lips, strawberry tongue)
  - Changes in the extremities (erythema of the palms and soles, edema, periungal desquamation)
  - Polymorphous rash
  - Cervical adenopathy (1.5 cm in diameter or greater)
- Incomplete KD with only two or three of above features requires close follow-up and possible treatment
- Acute phase lasts 7 to 14 days and is followed by the subacute phase (2 to 4 weeks)

COMPLICATIONS

- Coronary artery aneurysms
  - 15% to 25% without treatment
  - Up to 4% despite treatment
  - More common in infants, as they can present with fever only and none of the classic features

- MI, CHF, peripheral artery occlusion, hydrops of the gallbladder, arthritis, aseptic meningitis

DIAGNOSIS

- Criteria above
- ESR/CRP and WBC usually elevated
- Sterile pyuria due to urethritis
- Elevated liver enzymes, thrombocytosis after 1 week
- Check ECG and echocardiogram

TREATMENT

- Aspirin 80 to 100 mg/kg/day until day 14, then 3 to 5 mg/kg/day until platelet count returns to normal
- Single infusion of intravenous immunoglobulin (IVIG) 2 g/kg over 10 hours is effective

HENOCH–SCHÖNLEIN PURPURA

- IgA-mediated vasculitis involving the small vessels of the skin, GI and renal tracts, and musculoskeletal
- Most common acute vasculitis in children

SIGNS AND SYMPTOMS

- Presentation: "ARENA"
  - A = Abdominal pain (bloody stools, intussusception)
  - R = Rash, purpuric, classically "palpable purpura" (Fig. 24-11)
    - Rash of some form occurs in all
    - Rash is presenting symptom in >50%
    - Starts in lower extremities—ankles/feet and buttocks

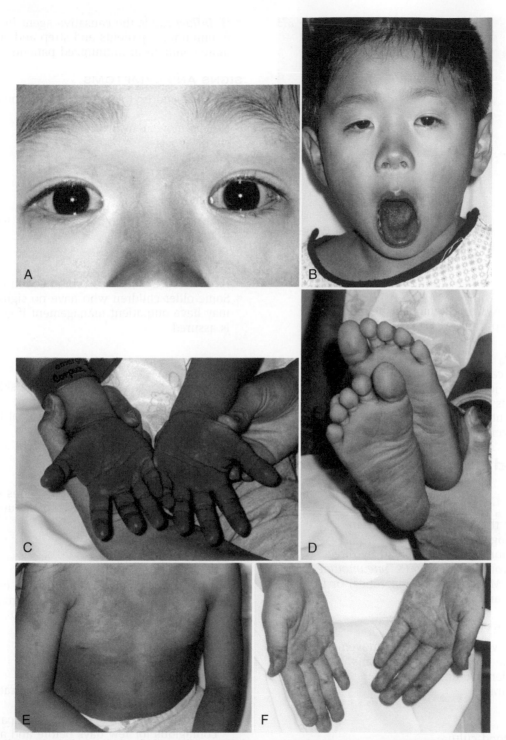

Figure 24-10. Classic physical examination findings of Kawasaki disease. Note the bilateral nonexudative scleral injections **(A)** with perilimbic sparing (the thin margin of white sclera around the cornea), red-cracked lips with a strawberry tongue **(B)**, diffuse palmar erythema **(C)**, red soles **(D)**, and the polymorphous exanthema **(E)**. The diffuse palmar erythema of Kawasaki disease **(C)** is distinct from the palmar findings seen in other viral illnesses such as the discrete macular lesions on the palms in this child with measles **(F)**. (From Marx JA, Hockberger RS, Walls RM: *Rosen's emergency medicine: concepts and clinical practice*, ed 6, Philadelphia, 2006, Mosby.)

- Face, trunk, palms/soles usually spared
- Typically no itching
- E = Edema
- N = Nephritis
- A = Arthralgias

DIAGNOSIS

- Hemoglobin, platelets usually normal
- ESR normal or mild elevation
- WBC frequently elevated
- Positive ASO titer or GABHS throat culture common

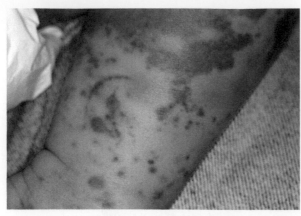

Figure 24-11. Purpura of the lower leg in HenochSchönleinn purpura (HSP). (From Kliegman RM, Behrman RE, Jenson MP, Stanton BMD: *Nelson textbook of pediatrics,* ed 18, Philadelphia, 2007, Saunders.)

- Elevated BUN/Cr or significant hematuria → glomerulonephritis

TREATMENT

- Arthralgias can be treated with NSAIDs
- Renal/GI or joint involvement sometimes treated with steroids and IVIG
- Admit patients with severe symptoms, HTN, or renal involvement

Skin and soft-tissue infections

ORBITAL CELLULITIS

- Infection of the orbit is considered an ophthalmologic emergency
- Most common is bacteria spread by direct extension from the sinuses (*S. pneumoniae, H. influenzae, M. catarrhalis,* anaerobes) or from the skin (staph and strep)

SIGNS AND SYMPTOMS

- Decrease in visual acuity, globe movement, and proptosis are the hallmark symptoms
- Fever, swollen eye lid, red eye
- Toxic appearance

DIAGNOSIS

- CBC and blood culture
- Orbital CT

TREATMENT

- Admit for IV antibiotics
  - Third-generation cephalosporin ± vancomycin or nafcillin ± clindamycin

PERIORBITAL CELLULITIS

- May develop after a break in the skin from trauma, insect bites, or chicken pox

- *H. Influenzae* is the causative agent in unimmunized patients and strep and staph are more common in immunized patients

SIGNS AND SYMPTOMS

- Swelling and erythema of the periorbital region
- No eye movement involvement
- No proptosis
- Warmth
- Not toxic appearing

DIAGNOSIS

- With marked swelling, may need CT to differentiate from orbital cellulitis

TREATMENT

- IV antibiotics similar to orbital cellulitis
- Some older children who have no signs of toxicity may have outpatient management if good follow-up is assured

IMPETIGO

- Superficial bacterial infection of the skin
- Due to *S. aureus* and Group A Strep;
- Usually no systemic symptoms except local lymphadenopathy
- Erythematous papules with transient small vesicles

SIGNS AND SYMPTOMS

- The hallmark is honey-crusted lesions with the characteristic site lying between the upper lip and nose
- Glomerulonephritis is rare

TREATMENT

- Topical antibiotics (mupirocin) or an oral course of either cephalexin, penicillin or erythromycin; combination therapy is not necessary

ERYTHEMA INFECTIOSUM (FIFTH DISEASE)

- Due to Parvovirus B19, usually respiratory transmission, also maternal–fetal
  - Incubation period is 4 to 20 days; patients are contagious for few days before and after rash

SIGNS AND SYMPTOMS

- Low-grade fever in 15% to 30% of patients
- Classic rash (Fig. 24-12)
  - Slapped cheeks on face
  - Lacy rash on arms, trunk
  - Rash recurs with heat, sunlight
  - Teens and adults can develop arthralgia, arthritis

COMPLICATIONS

- Aplastic crisis in hemolytic disease (sickle cell)
- Fetal hydrops in pregnancy

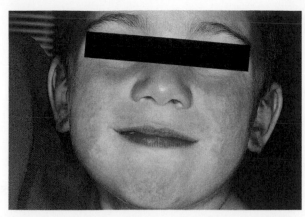

Figure 24-12. Erythema infectiosum. Erythema of the bilateral cheeks, which as been likened to a "slapped cheeks" appearance. (From Paller AS, Macini AJ: *Hurwitz clinical pediatric dermatology,* ed 3, Philadelphia, 2006, Saunders, p. 431.)

TREATMENT

- Supportive, isolate pregnant women

ROSEOLA (EXANTHEM SUBITUM)

- Caused by human herpes virus 6
- Incubation 5 to 15 days
- Common infection in children 6 months to 2 years

SIGNS AND SYMPTOMS

- High fever 3 to 5 days
- Febrile seizures possible
- Maculopapular rash develops immediately after defervescence

TREATMENT

- Antipyretics

VARICELLA (CHICKEN POX)

SIGNS AND SYMPTOMS

- Macules, papules, and vesicles that develop and spread over 24 hours
- Lesions described as dew drops on rose petals
- Rash starts on trunk, then spreads to face and extremities
- Highly contagious until all lesions have crusted

COMPLICATIONS

- Cellulitis
- Pneumonia
- Encephalitis: seizures, coma (early)
  - Cerebellitis: benign ataxia (late)
  - Reye syndrome (especially in association with aspirin use)

TREATMENT

- Antipruritics
- Antipyretics: use acetaminophen

- Consider acyclovir
  - 20 mg/kg/dose maximum 800 mg/dose QID for 5 days
  - Must be started within 24 hours of symptoms
  - Should be given to children at risk if exact exposure has been documented
- VZIG for children at high risk for development of severe disease
  - Must be given within 96 hours of exposure (48 hours preferred)
  - 125 U/10 kg IM, maximum 625 U
- Prevention with the varicella vaccine, given between 12 and 18 months of age
  - After 13 years, two doses are needed to be effective

SCARLET FEVER

- Commonly associated with Group A beta-hemolytic streptococci

SIGNS AND SYMPTOMS

- **Sand paper rash** first noted in skin folds such as the axillae, groin, and antecubital areas (Pastia lines)
- Circumoral pallor
- Rash usually develops 12 to 48 hours after the onset of sore throat, fever, and chills; may be accentuated by heat, and can last 4 to 5 days
- Desquamation may occur over the next 2 weeks, especially on the hands and feet

TREATMENT

- Penicillin VK (25 to 50 mg/kg/day four times a day) or erythromycin (20 to 50 mg/kg/day three or four times a day)
- No school until 24 hours after starting the antibiotics

STAPHYLOCOCCAL SCALDED SKIN SYNDROME

- Usually seen in children less than 5 years of age

SIGNS AND SYMPTOMS

- Irritability when skin is touched
- Fever
- Generalized skin erythema followed by bullae formation and skin desquamation (Fig. 24-13)
- **Nikolsky sign:** Pressure applied to bullae causes separation of the dermal layers
- Mucous membranes are not involved

TREATMENT

- Aggressive IV hydration
- All but the most mildly affected children should be admitted for IV cefazolin or nafcillin
- All newborns should be admitted regardless of degree of symptoms

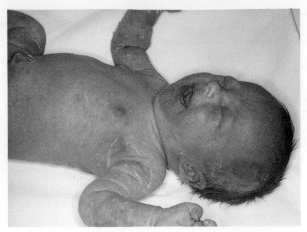

Figure 24-13. Staphylococcal scalded skin syndrome. Exfoliative phase, during which the upper epidermis is shed. (From Habif TP: *Clinical dermatology: a color guide to diagnosis and therapy,* ed 4, Philadelphia, 2004, Mosby.)

CANDIDA

- **Oral candidiasis**
  - Causes inflammation of the tongue, palate, and buccal mucosa
  - White plaques cannot be wiped off the mucous membranes
  - Rare in newborns, more common in children over 2 months of age
  - Treat with oral nystatin suspension (100,000 units/mL) 1 mL in each side of the mouth four times a day
- **Cutaneous candidiasis**
  - Erupts in the moist, warm areas of the body; axillae, neck folds, and diaper area
  - Satellite lesions are common along the edge of the eruption
  - Treatment is with topical antifungal agents (nystatin, clotrimazole)

HERPANGINA

- Vesicular stomatitis in the posterior pharynx
- High fever and sore throat, with drooling
- Recovery in 4 to 6 days
- Symptomatic therapy

HAND-FOOT-MOUTH DISEASE

- Coxsackie virus
- Typically in children less than 10 years of age
- Fever
- Vesicular rash in mouth, hands and feet (palms and soles are included)
- Treatment is symptomatic

TINEA CAPITIS

- *Trichophyton tonsurans* (most common, 90%) transmitted from person to person via fomites (e.g., barber's razor)

SIGNS AND SYMPTOMS

- Alopecia
- "Black dot" appearance on scalp
- Kerion (swollen boggy abscess of scalp)

DIFFERENTIAL DIAGNOSIS

- Alopecia areata
- Trichotillomania
- Traction alopecia

DIAGNOSIS

- Clinical, or if unclear, may send culture of scraping from hair roots

TREATMENT

- Must be oral
- Griseofulvin 20 mg/kg/day for 6 weeks
  - Routine LFTs do not need to be done
- Selenium sulfide shampoo should be used 2 times a week for first 2 weeks of oral treatment to prevent spread of spores
- Prednisone may be added at 1 mg/kg/day for 5 days in the treatment of a severe kerion
- Discharge home with follow-up with primary care physician (PCP) at end of treatment

Psychiatric

- ***Child abuse*** is broadly defined as maltreatment of a child by parents, guardians, or other caregivers, and may take the form of physical, sexual, or emotional abuse; denial of nutrition, medical care, or a safe environment can also be considered abuse

PHYSICAL ABUSE

RED FLAGS

- Child claims to have been injured
- No history at all is offered
- History of inflicted injury
- History changes over time or different caretakers give different histories
- Serious injury blamed on another child
- Child is developmentally incapable of acting as described
- History provided is inconsistent with injuries suffered
- Delay in seeking medical care

CLINICAL INDICATORS

- A lack of physical findings does not exclude abuse
- Lethargy, poor feeding, colic, bulging fontanelle, apnea, seizures
- Retinal hemorrhages outside the neonatal period
- Multiple injuries of various types and ages
- Pathognomonic injuries: loop marks, cigarette burns, immersion burns, fractures of posterior ribs, metaphyseal or "bucket handle" fractures, spiral femur fractures in non–weight-bearing infants, retinal hemorrhages

CHARACTERISTIC FRACTURES OF ABUSE

- High specificity
  - Fractures of metaphyseal corner "bucket-handle" fracture (Fig. 24-14), posterior rib, sternum, long bone shaft in non–weight-bearing age
- Medium specificity
  - Complex skull fractures, vertebral body fractures, multiple fractures of different ages
- Low specificity
  - Long bone shaft fracture in weight-bearing age, linear skull fracture

MANAGEMENT OF SUSPECTED PHYSICAL ABUSE

- Radiographic studies
  - Complete skeletal survey indicated for children <2 years of age with evidence of abuse
  - Other x-rays as clinically indicated
- Call the Child Protection Team (CPT)

SHAKEN BABY SYNDROME

- Subdural hematoma
- Retinal hemorrhage
- Long bone fracture
- Minimal signs of external trauma

SEXUAL ABUSE

- More commonly committed by family or household members than by strangers
- Historical components suggestive of sexual abuse
  - Inappropriate knowledge of adult sexual behavior
  - Compulsive masturbation
  - Excessive sexual curiosity
  - Sleep disturbances
  - Aggressive behavior
  - Running away
  - Suicide attempt
  - Abrupt behavioral change
  - Diminished school performance
  - Abdominal pain
  - Sexually provocative behavior and promiscuity

PHYSICAL EXAMINATION

- Genital injury
- Rectal injury
- Vaginal/urethral discharge
- Vaginal/rectal pain or bleeding
- Pregnancy
- Evidence of physical abuse
- Sexually transmitted diseases (gonorrhea, syphilis, chlamydia) are definitive of sexual abuse in children and infants

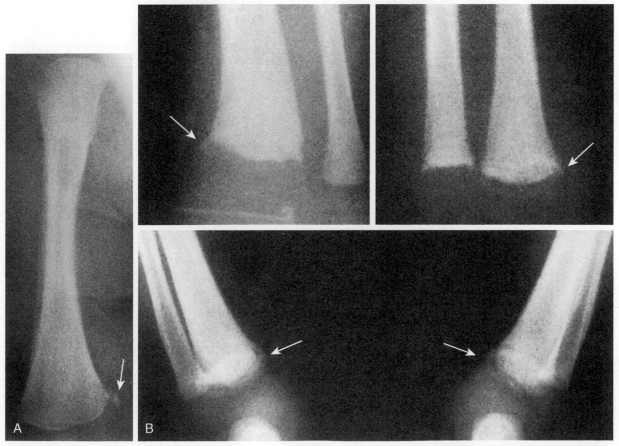

Figure 24-14. Metaphyseal fractures. **(A, B)** Radiographs of the right femur **(A)** and both ankles **(B)** of a 2-month-old abused infant demonstrating metaphyseal corner fractures of the distal femur and both distal tibia *(arrows)*. The angled tangential view reveals the "bucket handle" appearance of the fracture.

Continued

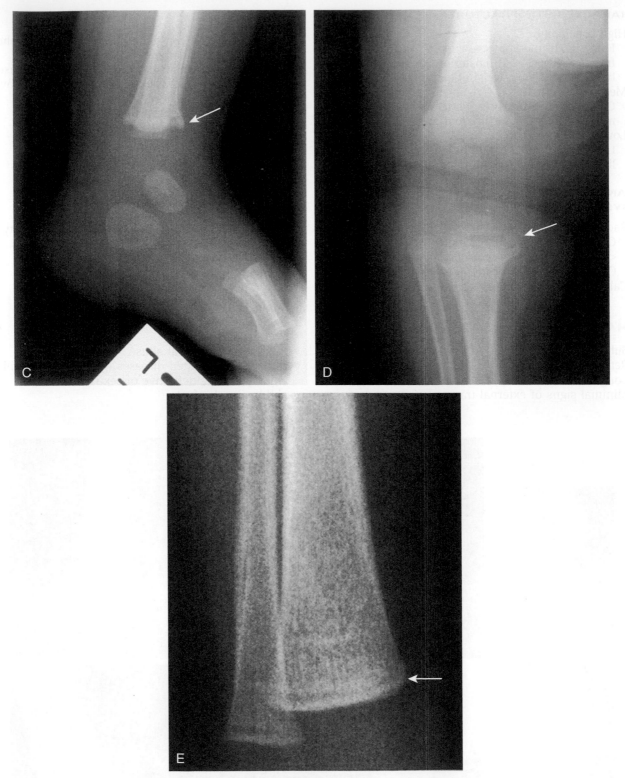

Figure 24-14, cont'd. **(C)** Radiograph of the left ankle of an infant demonstrates a metaphyseal corner fracture of the distal tibia *(arrow)*. (From Adam A, Dixon AK, Grainger RG, Allison DJ: *Grainger and Allison's diagnostic radiology,* ed 5, Philadelphia, 2008, Churchill Livingstone.)

MANAGEMENT

- Laboratory studies
  - Cultures for *Neisseria gonorrhea* from the oropharynx, rectum, vagina/cervix should be obtained for girls, and from the oropharynx, rectum, and urethra for boys as indicated
  - *Chlamydia trachomatis* cultures should be obtained from the vagina/cervix or urethra
  - DNA probes are not acceptable
  - Urinalysis and pregnancy tests should be obtained as indicated
  - A vaginal wet mount for *Trichomonas* is indicated for vaginal discharge
- Consider postexposure prophylaxis for pregnancy and HIV as indicated
- Unless medically indicated, the physician should not perform a pelvic examination—instead, the genital examination and cultures can be deferred to the examiner from the Child Protection Team
- Call the Child Protection Team

Sudden infant death syndrome/apparent life-threatening event

- SIDS
  - Sudden death of an infant less than 1 year of age, which remains unexplained after a thorough case investigation
- Apnea
  - Absence of respirations for 20 seconds or any length of time if associated with a decrease in heart rate, hypotonia, or change in color (pallor or cyanosis)
- Apparent life-threatening event (ALTE)
  - Characterized by apnea, color change (cyanosis or pallor), marked change in muscle tone, choking or gagging
  - Usual age is 2 to 3 months, but can occur at any time
  - Unknown association with SIDS
  - Differential
    - Seizure, gastroesophageal reflux, bronchiolitis, pertussis, choking, URI, head injury, breath holding

EVALUATION

- CBC
- Electrolytes
- Pan-cultures, including respiratory syncytial virus in infants who were premature and patients with congenital heart disease
- Consider a lumbar puncture if <2 months of age
- Pertussis and chlamydia cultures should be obtained if clinically suspected
- Chest radiograph and, if upper-airway obstruction is suspected, anteroposterior and lateral soft-tissue radiographs of the neck
- ECG
- Toxicologic screen
- Head CT should be obtained in patients with an altered level of consciousness, abnormal muscle tone, focal neurologic findings or retinal hemorrhages

DISPOSITION

- Admit all children who meet the criteria for an ALTE, despite a normal workup and physical examination

PEARLS

- 6 months to 6 years—peak ages for both croup and retropharyngeal abscess.

- Virtually all patients with croup should receive dexamethasone.

- Lethargy with a history of colicky abdominal pain mandates a rectal examination for blood in the stool (peak ages 3 months to 5 years).

- In gastroenteritis with leucopenia/bandemia and/or associated seizures, think shigellosis.

- "Rule of 2s" for Meckel diverticulum.

- Fracture more common than a sprain to pediatric population.

- Fractures highly suggestive of abuse include: "bucket-handle"; posterior rib, sternum, and long-bone (if the child is not yet weight-bearing).

Questions and Answers

1. A 7-year-old boy weighing 20 kg presents with bradycardia unresponsive to epinephrine. What is the recommended initial IV dose of atropine?
   a. 0.10 mg
   b. 0.20 mg
   c. 0.30 mg
   d. 0.40 mg
   e. 0.50 mg

2. A 1-year-old toddler has been vomiting for 6 days. In the ED she is somnolent but responsive, with a pulse of 195 and capillary refill time >4 seconds. Her weight is 10 kg. The serum sodium is 110. What is the most appropriate initial therapy?
   a. infusion of 3% hypertonic saline at 1 mL/kg/hour and concomitant administration of furosemide

b. infusion of 3% hypertonic saline at 5 mL/kg over 15 minutes

c. normal saline at 40 mL/hour

d. rapid infusion bolus of normal saline at 20 mL/kg

e. D5 ½ normal saline at 80 mL/hour

3. Which of the following symptoms is NOT consistent with Henoch–Schönlein Purpura?

   a. abdominal pain
   b. weight loss
   c. joint pain
   d. rash
   e. hematuria

4. You are managing a nontoxic infant with stridor and suspected viral croup. Despite cool mist therapy and intramuscular dexamethasone at a dose of 0.6 mg/kg, the patient continues with stridor at rest. Racemic epinephrine nebulization is administered with complete resolution of stridor. What is the most appropriate management immediately after initial racemic epinephrine administration?

   a. admit to hospital
   b. repeat another dose of dexamethasone
   c. obtain lateral soft-tissue neck radiograph
   d. observe in ED for stridor recurrence
   e. discharge home

5. What is the most common type of Salter–Harris physeal fracture seen in children?

   a. Type I
   b. Type II
   c. Type III
   d. Type IV
   e. Type V

6. A 18-month-old toddler presents with a 1-day history of fever to 39.8° C rectal and clutching his left ear in pain. He has never had an ear infection before. Physical examination reveals a bulging and erythematous tympanic membrane with limited mobility with insufflation. What is the most appropriate treatment?

   a. amoxicillin 40 mg/kg/day
   b. amoxicillin 80 mg/kg/day
   c. amoxicillin/clavulanate 40 mg/kg/day
   d. observation only with follow up in 2 days
   e. observation with a wait and see prescription (WASP) for oral antibiotics with instructions to fill and take antibiotics if symptoms do not improve in 1 day

7. Which of the following is NOT considered a form of cyanotic congenital heart disease?

   a. transposition of the great arteries
   b. Tetralogy of Fallot
   c. tricuspid atresia
   d. patent ductus arteriosus
   e. truncus arteriosus

8. A 14-year-old male presents with pain in the left hip and knee for 3 weeks. There has been no associated trauma, fevers, or chills. Physical examination reveals normal vital signs and a left hip held in mild external rotation. Which of the following is the most likely diagnosis?

   a. transient synovitis of the hip
   b. slipped capital femoral epiphysis (SCFE)
   c. Legg–Calve–Perthes (LCP) disease
   d. septic arthritis
   e. hip avulsion fracture

9. Which of the following concerning pyloric stenosis is true?

   a. occurs more frequently in first-born females
   b. vomiting is projectile and bilious
   c. usual onset of symptoms is during the third to fifth week of life
   d. electrolyte abnormalities include hyperchloremic hypokalemia
   e. plain radiographs are the study of choice

10. A 1-week-old male neonate presents with vomiting and poor feeding. He had an unremarkable birth and prenatal history. Vital signs reveal a temperature of 37.2° C rectal, heart rate (HR) = 200 beats per minute (bpm), blood pressure (BP) = 60/35 mmHg, RR = 70/minute, and oxygen saturation of 97%. Physical examination is notable for a listless neonate with dry mucous membranes, clear lungs, no cardiac murmur, and palpable femoral pulses. Blood tests are notable for a normal CBC but with electrolytes showing a sodium of 122 mEq/L, potassium of 6.4 mEq/L, and glucose of 30 mg/dL. He receives an intravenous glucose bolus and normal saline bolus of 40 mL/kg, and resultant blood pressure is 65/40 mmHg. Empiric antibiotics are started after cultures are obtained. What is the most appropriate next step in management?

    a. start IV epinephrine infusion
    b. start IV prostaglandin E infusion
    c. administer phenobarbital 20 mg/kg IV over 15 minutes
    d. obtain stat bedside echocardiogram
    e. administer hydrocortisone 25 mg IV

11. Which of the following is NOT a diagnostic criterion for Kawasaki disease (mucocutaneous lymph node syndrome)?

    a. leukocytosis
    b. rash
    c. conjunctivitis
    d. strawberry tongue
    e. cervical adenopathy

12. A 6-year-old boy falls on an outstretched hand and is complaining of elbow pain. Where is the most likely fracture site?

    a. radial head
    b. olecranon

c. supracondylar
d. lateral condyle
e. medial condyle

13. A 6-week-old infant boy is brought into the ED with a 2-day history of tactile fevers without cough, vomiting, or diarrhea. He is otherwise feeding well and vigorous. Physical examination reveals a nontoxic infant with a temperature of 38.8° C rectal. What is the most appropriate diagnostic workup?

    a. urinalysis, urine culture, CBC, blood culture, and cerebrospinal fluid (CSF) studies
    b. urinalysis, urine culture, CBC and blood culture only
    c. CBC and blood culture only
    d. urinalysis and urine culture only
    e. no diagnostic laboratories needed

14. What medication is considered first-line therapy in an actively seizing child in the ED?

    a. phenobarbital
    b. phenytoin
    c. pyridoxine
    d. valproic acid
    e. lorazepam

15. A 14-month-old infant is brought into the ED by her father with the chief complaint of lethargy and nonbilious vomiting. There is no history of fevers or diarrhea, although her father states that she appears to have episodes of crying and drawing her knees up to her chest. Physical examination reveals an afebrile, well-hydrated infant with no nuchal rigidity. The abdomen is nontender, and rectal examination shows brown stool that is occult blood positive. What is the most likely diagnosis?

    a. meningitis
    b. bacterial gastroenteritis
    c. intussusception
    d. appendicitis
    e. malrotation with midgut volvulus

16. A 2-week-old neonate is found to have a blood glucose level of 20 mg/dL. What is the correct glucose replacement fluid?

    a. dextrose 5% 2 mL/kg
    b. dextrose 10% 4 mL/kg
    c. dextrose 25% 2 mL/kg
    d. dextrose 50% 1 mL/kg
    e. lactated Ringer 20 mL/kg

17. A 9-month-old infant female infant presents with a fever to 39.6° C rectal but is vigorous and feeding well without vomiting per parents. She was born full-term without complications and has no other medical problems. Laboratories reveal a catheterized urinalysis with 35 WBCs/hpf but negative leukocyte esterase. What is the most appropriate management?

    a. hospitalize and administer IV antibiotics
    b. hospitalize but do not administer antibiotics pending urine culture results
    c. hospitalize, perform full septic workup including lumbar puncture, and administer IV antibiotics
    d. administer parenteral antibiotics in ED and discharge on oral antibiotics pending urine culture results
    e. discharge home and do not administer antibiotics pending urine culture results

18. An 11-year-old boy weighing 30 kg presents to the emergency department (ED) in cardiopulmonary arrest. What is the initial dose of IV epinephrine?

    a. 0.03 mg
    b. 0.10 mg
    c. 0.30 mg
    d. 1 mg
    e. 3 mg

19. A 5-year-old boy who was previously healthy presents with a 2-day history of grossly bloody diarrhea and diffuse crampy abdominal pain with no fever or vomiting. Physical examination reveals normal vital signs and a nontoxic and well-hydrated boy with minimal diffuse abdominal tenderness. Blood tests are normal and stool specimen is collected and sent for culture. What is the most appropriate management?

    a. start trimethoprim/sulfamethoxazole
    b. start azithromycin
    c. start metronidazole
    d. discharge home on no antibiotics and close follow-up of stool culture
    e. admit to hospital for IV antibiotics

20. What is the most appropriate initial antibiotic to treat a 7-year-old child with suspected pneumonia?

    a. amoxicillin
    b. azithromycin
    c. cefuroxime
    d. doxycycline
    e. trimethoprim-sulfamethoxazole

---

1. Answer: d

The weight-based dosing of atropine is 0.02 mg/kg with a maximum single dose of 0.5 mg in children and 1 mg in adolescents. Minimal single dose is 0.1 mg because lower dosing can cause paradoxical bradycardia.

2. Answer: d

Initial fluid resuscitation therapy in pediatrics consists of **20-mL/kg boluses** of **isotonic crystalline solution** (normal saline or lactated Ringer solution). **Hypertonic saline** is only indicated in severe hyponatremia with significant symptoms, such as seizures or coma.

3. Answer: b

Peripheral edema, **not weight loss,** is associated with Henoch–Schönlein purpura. All the other symptoms are commonly seen in this disease.

4. Answer: d

If racemic epinephrine is given, the patient should be **observed in the ED for 2 to 4 hours** after administration. If the stridor does not recur, patient can be discharged home; if the stridor does recur, additional racemic epinephrine can be given and **hospital admission** should be considered. **Dexamethasone** dosing is up to 0.6 mg/kg and generally will not need to be repeated during a croup illness due to its limited course and dexamethasone's long duration of action. **Radiographs** are not needed in viral croup unless another diagnosis is being entertained, such as retropharyngeal abscess or foreign body.

5. Answer: b

Approximately one third of all pediatric fractures involve the physis. **Salter–Harris classification Type II** (metaphyseal) fractures comprise 75% of all physeal fractures.

6. Answer: b

This patient has acute otitis media. **Observation with or without a wait-and-see prescription** is only an option under 2 years of age if nonsevere symptoms (temperature <39.0° C and/or mild otalgia) and assurance of follow-up. Otherwise, treatment is with **high-dose amoxicillin** because of the high rate of penicillin-resistant *Streptococcus pneumoniae*. Amoxicillin/clavulanate is usually reserved for amoxicillin treatment failures or recurrent infections.

7. Answer: d

Remember the "Terrible T's" of cyanotic congenital heart disease, which includes total anomalous pulmonary venous return in addition to the above 4 entities. **Patent ductus arteriosus** in isolation does not cause cyanosis.

8. Answer: b

Both SCFE and LCP have similar presenting symptoms. However, the age of usual presentation is different. **SCFE** usually presents between 10 and 15 years of age, whereas **LCP** usually presents in children less than 10 years of age. **Transient synovitis** usually presents before 5 years of age. This presentation is not consistent with **septic arthritis** or **hip avulsion fracture.**

9. Answer: c

Pyloric stenosis is more common in **first-born males. Vomiting is nonbilious** as emesis material is proximal to the pylorus. Symptoms are usually not seen immediately at birth, but rather a **few weeks into life** as the pylorus begins to hypertrophy. **Hypochloremic hypokalemia** is seen due to vomiting. **Ultrasound** or **upper GI** is the diagnostic study of choice.

10. Answer: e

This patient most likely has *adrenal crisis* from *congenital adrenal hyperplasia* as evidenced by his presentation, laboratory abnormalities, and unresponsiveness to IV fluid administration. Sepsis can mimic adrenal crisis, so **empiric antibiotics** are appropriate for a patient with this presentation. Congenital heart disease such as coarctation of the aorta is unlikely given the lack of murmur and normal femoral pulses.

11. Answer: a

The diagnostic criteria for Kawasaki disease is fever of at least 5 days' duration with the presence of at least four of the following: **bilateral conjunctivitis, changes of the lips** and **oral mucosa** such as **strawberry tongue,** changes of the extremities such as **erythema** or **edema, polymorphous rash,** and **cervical lymphadenopathy. Leukocytosis,** in addition to thrombocytosis and elevation of other acute phase reactants, are frequently seen but are not part of the diagnostic criteria for Kawasaki disease.

12. Answer: c

Supracondylar fractures comprise up to 60% of elbow fractures in children and are typically the result of a hyperextension mechanism. **Radial head** fractures are uncommon in children and more common in adults. **Olecranon fractures** are usually the result of direct elbow trauma after falls. **Lateral** and **medial condylar fractures** comprise a smaller percentage of pediatric elbow fractures.

13. Answer: a

In any infant under 2 months of age with a rectal temperature ≥38.0° C, a **full septic workup** should be performed including **urine, blood** and **CSF studies.** Chest radiograph or stool studies should also be obtained if any respiratory symptoms or diarrhea.

14. Answer: e

Benzodiazepines, particularly **lorazepam,** are considered the first-line antiepileptic drug of choice in active seizures and status epilepticus in the pediatric population. **Pyridoxine** can be considered in refractory seizures in newborns.

15. Answer: c

This presentation is most characteristic of **intussusception.** This disease frequently presents with lethargy as the chief complaint, thought to be related to endogenous endorphin release associated with intussuscepting bowel. Currant jelly stools are typically a late finding, whereas occult blood is frequently seen with non–bloody-appearing stools.

16. Answer: b

Treatment of hypoglycemia is with glucose 0.25 to 1 gm/kg. Using a midlevel dose of 0.5 gm/kg equates to **dextrose 10% 4 mL/kg, dextrose 25% 2 mL/kg, or dextrose 50% 1 mL/kg. Dextrose 10% solution is used in neonates** and small infants to avoid vein damage and risk of intracranial hemorrhage. Dextrose 25% is used in older infants and children, while dextrose 50% is used in adolescents and adults.

17. Answer: d

This patient has pyuria and *presumed acute pyelonephritis* and thus should be treated with antibiotics pending culture results. In neonates and infants with pyelonephritis, leukocyte esterase or even pyuria may be falsely negative because of their limited leukocytic response. Urine cultures are mandatory in suspected cases of urinary tract infection in this age group regardless of urinalysis results. In patients that are older than 3 months of age who appear well without comorbidities and with good follow-up, **outpatient management with oral antibiotics after parenteral antibiotic administration** in the ED is recommended. Cerebrospinal fluid studies are generally not needed in nontoxic infants older than 3 months.

18. Answer: c

The weight-based dose of epinephrine for cardiopulmonary arrest is **0.01 mg/kg** (0.1 mL of 1:10,000 solution). High-dose epinephrine (0.1 mg/kg) has been deemphasized and is no longer recommended in standard pediatric arrest algorithms.

19. Answer: d

This patient may have **enterohemorrhagic *E. coli* (0157:H7),** which is characterized by grossly bloody stools and abdominal pain with the absence of fevers. **Empiric antibiotics should be avoided in nontoxic children with bloody diarrhea without fevers until cultures return,** as antibiotics may enhance toxin release and increase rate of hemolytic uremic syndrome with *E. coli* 0157:H7.

20. Answer: b

After 4-5 years of age, a macrolide such as **azithromycin** should be used for pneumonia to cover for *Mycoplasma* pneumonia. Under 4 years of age, *Mycoplasma* is uncommon, and high dose **amoxicillin** is the antibiotic of choice. Amoxicillin, **cefuroxime** and **trimethoprim-sulfamethoxazole** do not cover *Mycoplasma* pneumonia. **Doxycycline** can cause staining of primary teeth and is generally not recommended under 8 years of age.

Note: Page numbers followed by f indicate figures; those followed by t indicate tables; those followed by b indicate boxes.